3608040782

KU-705-258

WITHDRAWN

# FOUNDATIONS OF
# ADULT
# NURSING

9781529713664
Found Adult Nur 2E

**How to access your e-book via Kortext**

-Go to www.kortext.com .
-Click on the 'Login' button.
-Enter your Access Code in the relevant box.
-Enter your personal details to set up an account.
-Access your book online!
-Download the App for offline access.

Access Code

MUHZADEPE8

WITHDRAWN

Sara Miller McCune founded SAGE Publishing in 1965 to support the dissemination of usable knowledge and educate a global community. SAGE publishes more than 1000 journals and over 800 new books each year, spanning a wide range of subject areas. Our growing selection of library products includes archives, data, case studies and video. SAGE remains majority owned by our founder and after her lifetime will become owned by a charitable trust that secures the company's continued independence.

Los Angeles | London | New Delhi | Singapore | Washington DC | Melbourne

# FOUNDATIONS OF ADULT NURSING

EDITED BY

*Dianne Burns*

2ND EDITION

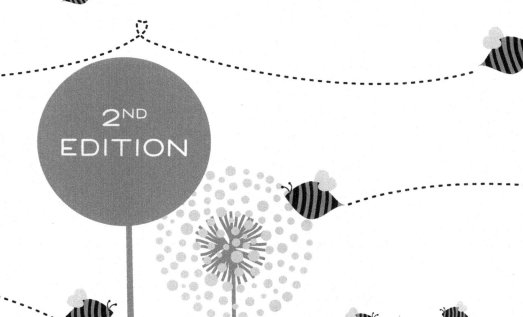

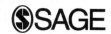

Los Angeles | London | New Delhi
Singapore | Washington DC | Melbourne

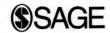

Los Angeles | London | New Delhi
Singapore | Washington DC | Melbourne

SAGE Publications Ltd
1 Oliver's Yard
55 City Road
London EC1Y 1SP

SAGE Publications Inc.
2455 Teller Road
Thousand Oaks, California 91320

SAGE Publications India Pvt Ltd
B 1/I 1 Mohan Cooperative Industrial Area
Mathura Road
New Delhi 110 044

SAGE Publications Asia-Pacific Pte Ltd
3 Church Street
#10-04 Samsung Hub
Singapore 049483

Editor: Alex Clabburn
Editorial assistant: Jade Grogan
Assistant editor, digital: Chloe Statham
Project manager: Swales & Willis Ltd, Exeter, Devon
Marketing manager: Tamara Navaratnam
Cover design: Wendy Scott
Typeset by: C&M Digitals (P) Ltd, Chennai, India
Printed in the UK

Editorial arrangement and Introduction
© Dianne Burns 2019
Chapter 1 © Joanne Timpson,
Elizabeth Lee-Woolf and Jane
Brooks 2019
Chapter 2 © Caroline Jagger, Heather
Iles-Smith and Dianne Burns 2019
Chapter 3 © Dianne Burns, Mark Cole
and Penelope Stamford 2019
Chapter 4 © Jean Rogers and Sarah
Booth 2019
Chapter 5 © Julie Gregory and
Charlotte Middleton 2019
Chapter 6 © Ann Wakefield and Nicola
Olleveant 2019
Chapter 7 © Mary Cooke 2019

Chapter 8 © Dianne Burns 2019
Chapter 9 © Dianne Burns 2019
Chapter 10 © Helen Davidson, Karen
Iley and Susan Ramsdale 2019
Chapter 11 © Emma Stanmore and
Christine Brown Wilson 2019
Chapter 12 © Judith Ormrod and
Dianne Burns 2019
Chapter 13 © Paul Tierney and Julie
Gregory © 2019
Chapter 14 © Samantha Freeman,
Colin Steen and Greg Bleakley
2019
Chapter 15 © John Costello 2019
Chapter 16 © Karen Heggs and
Samantha Freeman 2019

This second edition first published 2019
First edition published 2015. Reprinted 2015, 2017 (twice)

Apart from any fair dealing for the purposes of research or private study, or criticism or review, as permitted under the Copyright, Designs and Patents Act, 1988, this publication may be reproduced, stored or transmitted in any form, or by any means, only with the prior permission in writing of the publishers, or in the case of reprographic reproduction, in accordance with the terms of licences issued by the Copyright Licensing Agency. Enquiries concerning reproduction outside those terms should be sent to the publishers.

**Library of Congress Control Number: 2018948377**

**British Library Cataloguing in Publication data**

A catalogue record for this book is available from the British Library

ISBN 978-1-4739-9792-9
ISBN 978-1-4739-9793-6 (pbk)

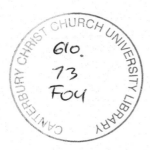

610.
73
FOU

3608040782

At SAGE we take sustainability seriously. Most of our products are printed in the UK using responsibly sourced papers and boards. When we print overseas we ensure sustainable papers are used as measured by the PREPS grading system. We undertake an annual audit to monitor our sustainability.

# CONTENTS

## 13  Caring for the Acutely Ill Adult                                           365
*Paul Tierney and Julie Gregory*

## 14  Caring for the Critically Ill Adult                                        404
*Samantha Freeman, Colin Steen and Greg Bleakley*

## 15  The Provision of Effective Palliative Care for Adults                      433
*John Costello*

# ABOUT THE EDITOR
# AND CONTRIBUTORS

## Editor

**Dianne Burns**, BSc(Hons), MSc (Clinical Leadership), PGCE, RGN, RNT, SFHEA, is a Senior Lecturer in Adult Nursing at the University of Manchester where she teaches across a variety of programmes within the Faculty of Biology, Medicine and Health. She is Co-Director of the Faculty PG Cert in Teaching and Learning, and Faculty Lead for the Higher Education Academy/AdvanceHE LEAP Fellowship and Staff Development Programmes. She also leads the postgraduate Leadership and Managing Change modules within the Division of Nursing, Midwifery and Social Work. A Registered General Nurse since 1984, Dianne worked in a variety of acute clinical settings (Acute Medical/Surgical, Orthopaedics, Accident and Emergency) before moving into a community setting to work as a practice nurse then Nurse Practitioner/Nursing Team Co-ordinator within a large semi-rural GP practice. She is also the Lead University Link Lecturer for Tameside & Glossop Integrated Care NHS Foundation Trust. Each of these roles provides a perfect opportunity for her to draw upon her enthusiasm and passion for engaging with students, colleagues and healthcare practitioners in order to enhance teaching and learning within the university and the wider community.

## Contributors

**Greg Bleakley**, BSc(Hons), PG Cert(Critical Care), DProf, DipN, RN, RNT, AFHEA, is a Lecturer in Adult Nursing at the University of Manchester. He teaches on a variety of undergraduate units on the BNURS(Hons) programme. Qualifying as a Registered Nurse in 1999, he has worked largely in critical care and more recently as a Specialist Nurse (Organ Donation) for almost a decade. Initially, this was a dual focus role and Greg provided care for patients awaiting kidney/pancreas transplantation. His research interests include critical illness management, organ donation and transplantation, critical care and end of life care.

**Sarah Booth**, RN, BSc(Hons), Community Health (with District Nurse Qualification), PGCE, PG Cert in Business and Executive Coaching (Distinction), qualified as a Registered Nurse in 1994. She has always been very keen to support learners in practice and to enthuse students about the reality of working within the NHS. Sarah has always had a passion for community nursing. She is currently working as Practice Education Facilitator at Stockport NHS Foundation Trust and leads on the Inter-professional Learning (IPL) developments at the Trust, for which she has won two national awards. Sarah is a trustee for a local charity working with vulnerable and homeless people.

**Jane Brooks**, PhD, RN, SFHEA, is a Senior Lecturer at the University of Manchester, Communications Officer for the UK Association for the History of Nursing and Chair of Publications for the American Association for the History of Nursing. Her first monograph, *Negotiating Nursing:*

*British Army Sisters and Soldiers in the Second World War*, has been published by Manchester University Press (2018) and she is also co-editor of *One Hundred Years of Wartime Nursing Practices, 1854–1953* (Manchester University Press, 2015). Her work on nursing in the Second World War has been supported by the Queen Alexandra's Royal Army Nursing Corps Association and the Monica Baly Bursary from the Royal College of Nursing, History of Nursing Society. She has previously published on the history of nursing work with older adults in the UK.

**Christine Brown Wilson** is a Registered Nurse with an international research and practice profile in ageing and dementia. She has established links with industry and service user organisations in the UK, enabling older people, family caregivers and staff to be active participants in the research process. Christine has also supported organisations and teams in changing practice through quality improvement workshops and developing relationship-centred services in dementia care. Through this process, Christine has developed relationship-based strategies that can be embedded at all levels of an organisation, including a facilitated model of practice development that supports staff in identifying practical strategies to implement person-centred care. Christine is a Senior Fellow of Advanced HE with extensive experience of teaching undergraduate nursing students in the UK, Singapore and Australia.

**Mark Cole**, BA(Hons), MSc, PhD, RNT, RGN, RMN, is a Senior Lecturer in Adult Nursing at the University of Manchester. He teaches on a variety of undergraduate and postgraduate units. He worked as an Infection Prevention and Control Nurse for 10 years before transferring to higher education. His research interests include hand hygiene and policy compliance.

**Mary Cooke**, BSc(Hons), RN, CM, MSc (Econ), PGDipEd, is a Lecturer in Emergency and Urgent Care Nursing at the University of Manchester. Her most recent publications report research into modelling the cost comparisons of diabetic wound dressings, research waste, service user and carer involvement in research, and carers' needs for looking after people with cancer at their end of life in the home, among others. This interest in outcomes when involving patients, service users and carers in changing health services, policy, and relationships with professionals has developed over 20 years. Her clinical specialism in emergency and trauma nursing is the basis for the decision-making chapter, where theory in decision making is explored.

**John Costello**, PhD, RN, is an Honorary Senior Lecturer in palliative care nursing. He has extensive experience of palliative care research, education and practice, having published 5 books and over 100 papers. He has presented his work at conferences internationally, and is committed to education and palliative care. His latest book is based on service user needs and the experiences of patients with non-cancer conditions who require palliative care.

**Helen Davidson**, BNurs(Hons), MSc, PGCE, HV Cert, is a Lecturer at the University of Manchester. After graduating from the University of Manchester in 1998, Helen worked for a number of years as a health visitor in south Manchester, while also developing an interest in practice education and mentorship. Helen recognises the increased emphasis on health promotion and public health across the field of adult nursing, within a range of settings.

**Samantha Freeman**, MSc, BSc(Hons), PGCE, RN, is a Senior Lecturer at the University of Manchester. She teaches across both undergraduate and postgraduate provision, focusing on acute and critical care as well as leadership. She is currently the Programme Director of the MSc in Leadership for

Professional Practice. Before this she was a Senior Sister on the Critical Care unit Manchester Foundation Trust, where she had a 15-year clinical post. She is currently undertaking a PhD to explore the ways in which patient agitation is best managed in the critical care environment.

**Julie Gregory**, BA(Hons), MSc (Pain Management), PhD, RN, INP (V300), is a Nurse Lecturer at the University of Manchester. She strongly believes educated nurses with knowledge and skills are essential to provide high-quality compassionate care for the increasingly complex individual patient requirements. Julie has extensive clinical experience, initially in orthopaedics and trauma, caring for a wide range of age groups and conditions. She was a clinical nurse specialist for acute pain until 2011 and has been an independent nurse prescriber since 2005. Teaching has been an important aspect of her roles in clinical practice, providing education about pain management and as a member of the team delivering the Acute Illness Management (AIM) course for all the members of the healthcare team.

**Karen Heggs**, BSc(Hons), MA, PG Dip, PG Cert in Teaching and Learning, DPSN, RN, RSCPHN – HV, FHEA, is a Lecturer in Adult Nursing and Academic Lead for Practice Development at the University of Manchester. Qualifying as a Registered Nurse in 1997, she has extensive clinical experience, predominantly as a nurse specialist in palliative care. Most recently, she worked as a health visitor before joining the University of Manchester in 2015, where she teaches on undergraduate provision and also the Supportive and Palliative Care Continuing Professional Development (CPD) unit. Karen has a keen interest in role transition from student to Registered Nurse, supportive and palliative care, and innovations in the use of information technology to enhance teaching and learning.

**Heather Iles-Smith**, MSc, PhD, RGN, is Head of Nursing Research and Innovation, Leeds Teaching Hospitals Trust (LTHT) and Honorary Clinical Associate Professor, Faculty of Health, University of Leeds. Her role includes senior leadership of Research and Innovation at LTHT, the development of clinical academic careers for nurses, midwives and allied healthcare professionals and other non-medical professions, and leadership and development of the clinical research delivery workforce. Having completed her PhD in 2012, Heather continues to be an active applied health researcher.

**Karen Iley**, BSc(Hons), MSc, RN, RNT, is a Lecturer in Adult Nursing at the University of Manchester and has worked in higher education for over 19 years at several universities, teaching nursing and social sciences including public health to both pre-registration nursing students and postgraduate healthcare professionals. Karen has an interest in the role transition from student to registrant. She is the Lead University Link Lecturer for Manchester University NHS Foundation Hospitals Trust. Her research interests include social inequalities concerning ethnicity and she is currently investigating undergraduate black, Asian and minority ethnic (BAME) healthcare students' experiences of studying at university, and the impact on their degree classification, with colleagues from the School of Health Sciences at the University of Manchester. Karen previously spent 16 years working in London as a staff nurse in trauma, burns and plastic surgery, and as a senior nurse in acute medicine.

**Caroline Jagger**, BSc(Hons), MSc, Dip HE, RN, NMP, qualified as a nurse in 2001. For the past 11 years she has been a specialist osteoporosis nurse and more recently a teaching fellow at the University of Manchester. She currently teaches students on the BNurs undergraduate programme, leading the medicines management unit. She is also deputy programme director for the independent prescribing short course for nurses and pharmacists.

**Elizabeth Lee-Woolf**, BSc, MSc (BOE), DipN, RN, RM, RNT, was, until her recent retirement, a Lecturer at the University of Manchester. Her experience in nurse education spans the last 30 years and she has been involved in the development and delivery of several curricula, with particular emphasis on the biosciences applied to nursing and the development of e-learning strategies. Understanding the changing needs of students as they make their transition from new students to registrants has been a major influence in facilitating a caring, yet thorough, student experience to ensure that they are ready for the challenge of their first post. Liz has significant experience in the development of processes through which challenges to a student's fitness to practise are managed, including how a student is supported before, during and after a fitness-to-practise hearing.

**Charlotte Middleton**, BSc, MClinRes, RN, SCPHN/HV, spent the first years of her career in perioperative practice, before later qualifying as a Specialist Community Public Health Nurse (health visiting) in 2013 and practising as a health visitor. Following a MClinRes at the University of Manchester (2015), Charlie was appointed as a Lecturer in Adult Nursing at the School of Nursing, Midwifery and Social Work at the University of Manchester in 2015. She joined the School of Nursing in Dundee in 2018.

**Nicola Olleveant**, BSc(Hons), PhD, PGCE, RGN, is a Lecturer in Nursing at the University of Manchester. She has extensive experience of teaching students in acute and critical care and in evidence-based practice. She trained in London and spent most of her nursing experience working as a sister on a busy intensive care unit, where she undertook her PhD part-time while working clinically. She currently leads the undergraduate complex care unit, and has a wealth of research experience in many clinical environments and using many research methodologies. She is particularly interested in working with students to ensure that they have a positive undergraduate experience in higher education.

**Judith Ormrod**, BEd, BSc, MA, MSc, PhD, RGN, spent most of her clinical nursing experience working as a staff nurse and senior ward sister in intensive care units and acute admission wards in central London Hospitals. Since moving to Manchester she has taught undergraduate and postgraduate nursing students at the University of Manchester. Her clinical and research interests include psychosocial factors affecting women across the lifespan, interpersonal violence and female genital mutilation/cutting (FGM/C), family estrangement, clinical supervision and the ethics of research. Her PhD considered the psychosocial factors affecting pregnant women who were living with type 1 diabetes mellitus. She is also a Chartered Psychologist and works part-time in a local NHS trust.

**Susan Ramsdale**, BSc(Hons), MA, EdD, PGCE, DipHE, RN(MH), RNT, FHEA, is employed as a Senior Lecturer and Mental Health Field Lead at the University of Manchester. She qualified as a mental health nurse in 1996 and worked across the north-west in a range of acute and crisis care settings, responsible for developing the first mental health crisis response service in Lancashire in 1999. She began her career in nurse education in 2003 and has managed a range of programmes including BSc Nursing Programmes in both Mental Health and Adult Nursing, and held external examiner roles relating to these programmes. She was awarded a Doctorate in Education in 2017.

**Jean Rogers**, BSc(Hons), MSc, CertEd (FE), RGN, is a Practice Educator Facilitator at Stockport NHS Foundation Trust. She has a passion for encouraging, supporting and educating the educators and supervisors in practice, so they can develop the nurse force for the future. Jean has been qualified since 1988 and worked in numerous areas of practice before embarking on her current role. Her area of expertise is orthopaedics and trauma, having undertaken the orthopaedic course at the Robert Jones and Agnes Hunt Hospital, at the same time completing a certificate in education. She is the co-author of the Oxford University Press book *Handbook in Orthopaedic and Trauma Nursing*.

**Penelope Stamford,** BSc(Hons), MSc, PhD, PGDE, RN, OND, RNT, SFHEA, is a Senior Lecturer in Adult Nursing at the University of Manchester. Penelope's clinical background is in ophthalmic nursing. She trained at the Manchester Royal Eye Hospital and worked there as Senior Sister. Penelope is the Academic Lead for Quality and Enhancement in the Division of Nursing, Midwifery and Social Work and Chair of the RCN Ophthalmic Forum. She teaches on undergraduate and postgraduate education programmes and leads the degree and master's level ophthalmic course at the University of Manchester.

**Emma Stanmore,** BNurs(Hons), MRes, PhD, DN, RN, is a Senior Lecturer in the Division of Nursing, Midwifery and Social Work at the University of Manchester and the Deputy Lead for the Healthy Ageing Research Group for the Institute of Population Health. Emma has, over 25 years, combined experience in healthcare, research and teaching, with a particular focus on the promotion of healthy ageing and health innovation. Emma is committed to improving the care of older people in practice, research, and through the education of undergraduate and postgraduate nurses. She has held numerous grants as principal investigator from funders such as Arthritis Research UK, Innovate UK, ESRC and the Wellcome Trust on projects investigating falls prevention, evaluation of new roles and services, telemedicine and health technologies in rehabilitation.

**Colin Steen,** MSc, PGCE, RN, FHEA, is a Lecturer in the Division of Nursing, Midwifery and Social Work at the University of Manchester. He teaches acute and critical care nursing to undergraduate and post-registration nurses. Before his current post he worked clinically for 20 years as a senior nurse in critical care nursing, with a particular emphasis on general, cardiac surgery, thoracic medicine and surgery, heart transplant, lung transplant, and heart and lung transplant, as well as the use of ventricular assist devices as a bridge to transplantation. He has a number of interests related to the discipline but is an award winner in medical innovation and the development of new devices to assist in healthcare. As an educator he has an interest in students from BAME backgrounds and their engagement in higher education and is about to commence a research project in this area as part of an EdD.

**Paul Tierney,** RGN, BSc, MSc, PGCHET, is a Lecturer (Education) in the School of Nursing and Midwifery, Queen's University Belfast. He teaches on the undergraduate nursing programme and is Pathway Coordinator for the postgraduate Specialist Practice Cardiology programme. Paul's clinical background began in the Coronary Care Unit in the Royal Victoria Hospital, Belfast. He subsequently worked in a variety of cardiology posts progressing to Deputy Ward manager in a medical cardiology ward. Later, Paul worked as a clinical trials research nurse before moving into nurse education.

**Joanne Timpson,** BA(Hons) Nurs Ed, MSc Nursing, Nurse Tutor, Dip, Oncology, Cert Counselling, is a Senior Lecturer who currently enacts the dual roles of Directorate Lead for Adult Nursing and Chair of Workload Planning within the Division of Nursing, Midwifery and Social Work at the University of Manchester, having previously held the Academic Lead for the Student Experience and Senior Academic Advisor roles. Joanne currently leads the undergraduate Core Values for Professional Nursing and postgraduate Supportive and Palliative Care units. She instils both her teaching and leadership roles with the enduring belief of nursing as privilege, empowering colleagues and nursing students to enact informed, holistic, therapeutic frames by which to enhance nursing practice and secure positive patient outcomes, underpinned by a shared ethos of partnership and reciprocity.

**Ann Wakefield**, MSc, PhD, Cert Ed, RGN, RMN, RCNT, RNT, Dip Nursing Part A (London), PFHEA, is a Professor of Nursing Education at the University of Manchester. She has extensive experience of teaching both undergraduate and postgraduate students about evidence-based practice. She is particularly interested in qualitative research methods and teaches students across a range of programmes about how to undertake research as well as supervising masters' and PhD students. Ann has undertaken research using ethnomethodological approaches to investigating the organisation of surgical nursing work, as well as using more general qualitative and mixed method approaches to educationally based research.

# ACKNOWLEDGEMENTS

We are particularly grateful to all of the practitioners, educators, students and others we have met over the years who have helped and guided us in our own nursing and teaching practice. We would like to thank families, friends and colleagues for their support.

On behalf of the authors, SAGE would like to thank all of the academics who provided original material for the previous edition or reviewed the content of the book, helping to shape and influence it for the better:

Lesley Andrews

Darren Brand

Beryl Cooledge

Kevin Crimmons

Yvonne Dexter

Catherine Hill

Angela Hudson

Jan Hunter

Julia Jones

Mhairi Kidd

Erin King

Scott Macpherson

Georgia Taylor

Suzan Thompson

Deborah Ward

# PUBLISHER'S ACKNOWLEDGEMENTS

On behalf of the Editor and the Contributors, the publisher would like to extend their thanks to all third parties who granted us permission to reproduce the following material:

Figure 6.3 Hierarchies of evidence, adapted from Porzsolt, F., Ohletz, A., Thim, A., Gardner, D., Ruatti, H., Meier, H., Schlotz-Gorton, N. & Schrott, L. (2003). 'Evidence-based decision making – the six step approach', *BMJ Evidence-Based Medicine*, 8(6): 165–6. © 2001–2017, The Board of Regents of the University of Wisconsin System.

Table 6.8 Examples of database information related to nursing and healthcare, reproduced with permission from Wakefield, A. (2014). 'Searching and critiquing the research literature', *Nursing Standard*, 28(39): 49.

Figure 7.1 A hypothetico-deductive approach to clinical decision making, Tanner, C., Padrick, K., Westfall, U. and Putzier, D. (1987) 'Diagnostic reasoning: strategies for nurses and nursing students', *Nursing Research*, 36: 358–63. Wolters Kluwer.

Figure 7.2 From novice to expert, 1982 Benner, P. (1982) 'From novice to expert', *American Journal of Nursing*, 82: 402–7. Wolters Kluwer.

Figure 7.4 Carper's interconnected 'patterns of knowing', Carper (1978) 'Fundamental patterns of knowing in nursing', *Advanced Nursing Science*, 1(1): 1113–23. Wolters Kluwer.

Figure 7.6 Schematic representation of the Situated Clinical Decision Making Framework, Gillespie, M. and Paterson, B.L. (2009) 'Helping novice nurses make effective clinical decisions: the situated clinical decision-making framework', *Nursing Education Perspectives*, May/June, 9(3): 165–70. Wolters Kluwer.

Figure 8.4 Grol's (1997) 5-stage implementation process, Grol, R. (1997), Beliefs and evidence in changing clinical practice, *BMJ*, 315: 418–25.

Figure 8.5 Illustrative tools and methods in improvement, Batalden, P.B. and Davidoff, F. (2007) 'What is "quality improvement" and how can it transform healthcare?', *Quality and Safety in Healthcare*, 16: 2–3. BMJ Publishing Group Ltd and the Health Foundation.

Table 8.2 Stakeholder engagement approaches, reproduced with permission of stakeholdermap.com.

Figure 8.8 Plan, Do, Study, Act Cycle, Langley, G.L., Nolan, K.M., Nolan, T.W., Norman, C.L. and Provost, L.P. (2009) *The Improvement Guide: A Practical Approach to Enhancing Organizational Performance*, 2nd edition. San Francisco, CA: Jossey-Bass.

Figure 9.2 Valuing older workers (RCN, 2012), 'Valuing older workers', Royal College of Nursing: London.

Figure 11.2 The overlap between long-term conditions and mental health problems, Naylor, C., Parsonage, M., McDaid, D., Knapp, M., Fossey, M. and Galea, A. (2012) *Longterm Conditions and Mental Health: The Cost of Co-morbidities*. London: The King's Fund.

Figure 11.3 The NHS and Social Care Long Term Conditions Model (2007). Department of Health: London. © Crown copyright.

Figure 11.5 The House of Care Model, Coulter, A., Roberts, S. and Dixson, A. (2013) Delivering Better Services for People With Long-Term Conditions: Building the House of Care. London: The King's Fund.

Figure 11.7 Continuum strategies to support self-management, de Longh, A., Fagan, P., Fenner, J. and Kidd, L. (2015) A practical guide to self-management support. Available from: www.health.org.uk/publication/practical-guide-self-management-support. London: The Health Foundation.

Table 12.4 NEWS score and Table 12.5 Outline clinical response to NEWS triggers, Royal College of Physicians, 2012.

Figure 16.1 The Eatwell Guide, Public Health England in association with the Welsh government, Food Standards Scotland and the Food Standards Agency in Northern Ireland.

Figure 16.2 Influences on health, Dahlgren, G. and Whitehead, M. (1991) *Policies and Strategies to Promote Social Equity in Health*. Stockholm: Institute for Future Studies. World Health Organization: Denmark.

Figure 16.3 Herd immunity, National Institute of Allergy and Infectious Diseases.

# ONLINE RESOURCES

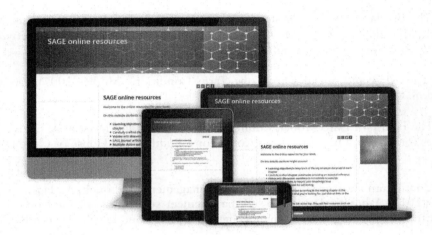

The 2nd edition of *Foundations of Adult Nursing* is supported by a variety of online resources for students and lecturers. These resources will aid your learning and teaching respectively, covering core nursing theory and the important transition to practice for nurses at the pre-registration level.

All resources are available at: https://study.sagepub.com/Burns2e

## Resources for lecturers

**Seminar slides** for use in teaching and as discussion points cover a range of central topics from the book. Including but not limited to Clinical Decision Making, Evidence Based Practice, Health Promotion, Medicines Management and Clinical Leadership.

## Resources for students

**Read more widely!** A selection of *free* **SAGE journal articles** that support each chapter to help deepen your knowledge and reinforce your learning of key topics. An ideal place to start for literature reviews/dissertations/assignments. Preceding each article is an annotation from the chapter author and the editor, Dianne Burns, introducing its relevance for practice and or revision.

**Weblinks** direct you to relevant resources to broaden your understanding of chapter topics and expand your knowledge by linking to real world organisations and/or conversations on being a professional nurse today. Preceding each article is an annotation from the chapter author and the editor, Dianne Burns, introducing its relevance for practice and or revision.

**MCQs – Multiple Choice Questions** per chapter, written by the chapter authors, test your core knowledge of the topic covered, making sure you understand the material covered, highlighting areas for further revision and reading.

# INTRODUCTION

This book aims to provide a concise, easy-to-read introductory text for those individuals who are undertaking their studies focusing on *adult nursing at undergraduate level* (i.e. students on the Nursing and Midwifery Council [NMC] approved undergraduate programmes) leading to Registered Nurse status. However, we recognise that it will be of interest to students undertaking *nursing associate* programmes and *nursing apprenticeships* along with students from other fields of nursing. Practice supervisors, assessors, mentors, coaches and those involved in supporting nursing students (e.g. lecturers, nurse teachers and academic assessors) will also find the book and accompanying resources useful.

As a core text for 'beginners', the book is written in an easy-to-access, user-friendly style and examines in detail the essential knowledge and skills needed to provide therapeutic care to adults with a range of health needs. Taking a broad rather than a deep approach, we will be encouraging you as the reader to explore the core principles and key aspects of an adult nurse's role, reflecting upon current nursing theory and the factors that underpin high-quality, evidence-based care delivery in practice. By incorporating a variety of activities and case scenarios we intend to bring to life many of the contemporary issues faced by adult nurses today. By also guiding you to other resources as appropriate, our primary aim is to assist you in the development of an understanding of the importance of *person-centred care* using an *evidence-based approach* to inform adult nursing. In doing so, we hope not only that this will help you demonstrate your knowledge in written assignments and examinations, but also more importantly that you will use your knowledge and understanding of each of these fundamental aspects to underpin the care you provide for your patients.

The *Modernising Nursing Careers Framework* (Department of Health, Social Services and Public Safety or DHSSPS, 2006) identifies the changing context for healthcare and a need for the current nursing workforce to reflect those changes and become more adaptable. This approach will be illustrated throughout this book in terms of its relevance to current UK healthcare provision and policy, namely with regard to:

- An expanding older population;
- The increasing incidence of long-term conditions;
- The growing impact of preventable conditions due to lifestyle choices (i.e. smoking, obesity, alcohol intake, etc.); and
- The need for nurses to demonstrate skills in caring for people in a variety of settings.

The content of the book is underpinned throughout by the Nursing and Midwifery Council's *Future Nurse: Standards of Proficiency for Registered Nurses* (NMC, 2018a), which clearly defines what nursing students must achieve before entering the professional register (and what registered nurses must continue to meet throughout their professional career), and *The Code* (NMC, 2018b), which presents the professional standards that nurses and midwives must uphold in order to be registered to practise in the UK. It will also reflect current UK policy, taking into account the fact that contemporary adult nursing is delivered to a diverse client group in a number of settings.

Focusing primarily on the top morbidity and mortality indicators across the UK (i.e. circulatory disease, cardiovascular disease, respiratory disease, diabetes, cancers, infectious disease and dementia), it includes specific content to support the development of knowledge and skills related to the EU Directive 2005/36EC (European Commission, 2011) which demands that adult nurses gain exposure to the following:

- General and specialist medicine;
- General and specialist surgery;
- Child care and paediatrics;
- Maternity care;
- Mental health and psychiatry;
- Care of the older person (geriatrics);
- Home nursing (community nursing).

The book is composed of two parts.

# Part 1: Theory and Context in Relation to Adult Nursing

Made up of Chapters 1–9, this part of the book provides an introduction to the overarching theoretical and contemporary practice issues faced by adult nurses today.

## Chapter 1: Essentials of Nursing: Values, Knowledge, Skills and Practice

This chapter introduces you to the key principles, core values, and legal and professional issues that inform contemporary nursing practice, recognising the importance of self-awareness and professional regulation in developing your own practice. The significance of core values is explored (e.g. empathy, compassion, dignity, respect, cultural competence, communication) to help you develop an appreciation of how such values must underpin your nursing practice. We also briefly introduce the importance of evidence-based care and nursing research.

## Chapter 2: Nursing Therapeutics

In this chapter we encourage you to consider appropriate philosophies, models and frameworks for the delivery of *safe* and *competent* care. We identify the factors that contribute to the development of therapeutic partnerships, exploring the concept of safe and effective *person-centred care*. The overall focus of the chapter is on challenging routine and tradition in nursing practice and the importance of effective communication, which assists in the development of a therapeutic relationship with all patients, clients and their families, including those individuals who are vulnerable and therefore most at risk.

## Chapter 3: Fundamental Aspects of Adult Nursing

This chapter introduces you to the application of systematic approaches to nursing care, the nature of nursing interventions and the mechanisms by which interventions can be selected and evaluated.

Focusing on the activities of daily living (Roper et al., 2000), we explore ways in which nurses can undertake a holistic nursing assessment, considering requirements for making 'reasonable adjustments' and identifying some of the clinical nursing skills needed in order to be able to provide high-quality nursing care. In doing so we also consider the key concepts of 'confidentiality', 'informed consent', 'mental capacity' and 'infection control'.

## Chapter 4: Interprofessional and Multidisciplinary Team Working

This chapter explores how multi-agency working has the potential to positively impact on health, highlighting the importance of accurate record keeping, effective communication, accountability and delegation. You will begin to understand the significance and the benefits of team working in the provision of effective healthcare. We also identify useful strategies for overcoming common barriers to interprofessional and multidisciplinary working in practice settings.

## Chapter 5: Medicines Management

This chapter outlines the theoretical underpinning knowledge related to the management and review of medicines, exploring the role and responsibilities of adult nurses to promote patient safety in the context of medicines management. We review current policies, legal and ethical requirements, and the practical application of medicines. We also consider various procedures intended to improve the safe management and administration of medicines. Concentrating on the mechanisms and actions of medicines administered for commonly encountered adult medical and mental health conditions, we encourage you to identify and evaluate the likely side effects and interactions of commonly used medications.

## Chapter 6: Evidence-based Practice and the Importance of Research

This chapter aims to nurture your ability to critically appraise evidence in order to help you to make informed decisions about the care you administer. It begins by exploring the origins of evidence-based practice and examines why evidence-based medicine (EBM) and research are important in today's healthcare systems. It goes on to examine how you can implement evidence-based principles into your own clinical practice, by supporting the development of critical appraisal skills, and outlining strategies that can also be employed to encourage others to use evidence as part of their everyday work.

## Chapter 7: Clinical Decision Making

This chapter explores the underpinning theories related to clinical judgement and decision-making processes within a healthcare setting, examining the key issues in managing complexity and critically reviewing determinants that can impact on your own clinical decision-making processes. It also includes a critical consideration of the higher-order intellectual skills associated with clinical (diagnostic) reasoning, empirical (diagnostic) judgements and discerning clinical decision making.

## Chapter 8: Leadership and Management

This chapter reviews current leadership approaches within contemporary healthcare settings and encourages you to reflect upon the importance of key leadership and management skills, recognising potential areas for personal improvement in order to enhance your own leadership skills. It also seeks to explain the difference between 'risk aversion' and 'risk management', and explores effective strategies for risk assessment and management in order to provide a safe and healthy environment for patients, staff and visitors.

## Chapter 9: Developing Practice and Managing Change

In this chapter we appraise the concept of quality, focusing on quality assurance frameworks and methods of monitoring and improving the quality of care and service provision. We outline current legal, ethical and professional drivers for change/service improvement and critically discuss the role of a change agent(s) in developing and leading teams to effective change. We also discuss barriers to service improvement implementation, appraising effective strategies for change management and sustaining service improvements.

# Part 2: Caring for Adults in a Variety of Settings

This section of the book highlights specific areas of care that are commonly encountered within adult nursing practice.

## Chapter 10: Supporting and Promoting Health

This chapter begins by introducing you to the principles and practice of epidemiology, public health, health promotion/health education and preventative healthcare, thereby enabling you to gain a basic understanding of how demographic health information and epidemiological data inform national and global priorities for health and health promotion/public health initiatives. We explore the role of the adult nurse in contemporary public health practice and the interrelationship of the health of the public, the social determinants influencing health, and the tools and structures that underpin the assessment of health and healthcare needs. In particular we look at the impact of 'risky behaviours' (unhealthy eating, physical inactivity, alcohol and substance misuse, and sexual health), focusing on national health promotion initiatives and services to provide a clear overview of both the government agenda and legislative practice. We also consider the range of opportunities available to promote health within any contemporary healthcare setting, emphasising the requirements of adult nurses to be able to recognise and respond appropriately to the various health needs of individuals, for example: babies, children and young people; pregnant and postnatal women; people with mental health problems; people with physical disabilities; people with learning disabilities; older people; and those with long-term problems such as cognitive impairment.

## Chapter 11: Specialist Care of the Older Person: A Person-centred, Biographical Approach

This chapter considers the knowledge, skills and attitudes required by nurses for the optimum care of the older person, and explores how we might promote individualised, person-centred care in our everyday practice. You will develop an understanding of the principles of health promotion, quality of life, dignity in care, independence, empowerment and choice in relation to older people. We explore the needs of older people and their carers in a variety of care settings, taking into account the nature of care that older people may require. A key focus of the chapter is promoting an understanding of the principles of anti-discriminatory practice with reference to age and considering how this is applied in practice with an emphasis on the 'frail' older person. In particular, we look at the challenges faced by those with dementia with reference to physical activity and falls prevention.

## Chapter 12: Caring for Adults with Long-term Conditions

This chapter examines the bio-psychosocial impact of living with and caring for individuals experiencing long-term ill health, exploring ways in which you can work effectively to support individuals and their families/carers by promoting self-care and empowerment within a variety of settings. It identifies the common problems encountered by individuals living with a long-term condition and the relevant government policies that aim to support self-management, personalised care planning, and partnership working with patients and carers. It seeks to help you to develop a greater understanding of how the concepts of *patient empowerment, shared decision making* and *concordance* can be used to inform the adult nurse's role.

## Chapter 13: Caring for the Acutely Ill Adult

This chapter considers the impact of acute illness on normal daily functioning and explores the principles of working towards recovery from acute illness, utilising contemporary surgical and medical approaches with a particular focus on acute assessment. Highlighting the significance of risk assessment, prioritising care and the prevention of deterioration, the importance of the application of critical thinking and evaluation to provide safe, knowledgeable and competent individualised client care competently is explored.

## Chapter 14: Caring for the Critically Ill Adult

This chapter focuses on the comprehensive assessment of a critically ill adult who requires specialist care within a critical care environment. We provide an outline of the nurse's role in recognising and responding to critically ill adults using appropriate evidence-based strategies and an ABCDE approach (Resuscitation Council UK, 2015). We also explore some of the legal and ethical issues relating to the individual in critical care settings, including consent, confidentiality, best interest principles, after-care rehabilitation and organ donation.

## Chapter 15: The Provision of Effective Palliative Care for Adults

This chapter focuses on the role of the nurse in supporting patients with a life-limiting illness within a palliative care context. It centres around the provision of care within a multidisciplinary framework that involves the holistic assessment of physical and bio-psychological needs in relation to patients with malignant and non-malignant conditions. We provide a summary of the way in which palliative care for adults has been developed in the UK. Explaining the principles of palliative care and identifying key policies, standards, and legal and ethical issues that underpin an evidence-based approach, we discuss the importance of effective communication and therapeutic relationships in exploring patient choice and preferences in the provision of culturally competent and sensitive end of life care. We also include an exploration of contemporary palliative care services, including hospice care and care at home, highlighting the provision of care to family members and significant others who are associated with grief and bereavement after care.

## Chapter 16: Managing the Transition to Registered Nursing Practice

This final chapter explores the challenge of managing role transition to help you to prepare for the start of a professional registered nursing career. We consider how best to approach your final placement, describe the process of application for employment and explain how best to promote yourself to prospective employers. We also explain how preceptorship can support you in your transition from student nurse to registrant, outline the process of revalidation and consider the role of a registered nurse when responding to a major incident.

# References

Department of Health, Social Services and Public Safety (2006) *Modernising Nursing Careers: Setting the Direction*. Belfast: DHSSPS.

European Commission (2011) *European Union Directive 2005/36/EC* (consolidated version). Available at: https://eur-lex.europa.eu/legal-content/EN/TXT/?uri=celex%3A32005L0036 (last accessed 21 July 2018).

Nursing and Midwifery Council (2018a) *Future Nurse: Standards of Proficiency for Registered Nurses*. London: NMC.

Nursing and Midwifery Council (2018b) *The Code: Professional Standards of Practice and Behaviour for Nurses and Midwives*. London: NMC.

Resuscitation Council UK (2015) *Resuscitation Guidelines*. Available at: www.resus.org.uk/resuscitation-guidelines (last accessed 21 July 2018).

Roper, N., Logan, W.W. and Tierney, A.J. (2000) *The Roper–Logan–Tierney Model of Nursing: Based on Activities of Living*. London: Churchill-Livingstone.

# NMC PROFICIENCIES MAP FOR REGISTERED NURSES

**Platform 1: Being an accountable professional** Registered nurses act in the best interests of people, putting them first and providing nursing care that is person-centred, safe and compassionate. They act professionally at all times and use their knowledge and experience to make evidence-based decisions about care. They communicate effectively, are role models for others and are accountable for their actions. Registered nurses continually reflect on their practice and keep abreast of new and emerging developments in nursing, health and care. The outcomes set out below reflect the proficiencies for accountable professional practice that must be applied across the standards of proficiency for registered nurses, as described in platforms 2–7, in all care settings and areas of practice. At the point of registration, the registered nurse will be able to:

| NMC Proficiencies for Registered Nurses | Main Chapter/s *(but also referred to in other chapters as appropriate)* |
|---|---|
| 1.1 Understand and act in accordance with The Code: Professional standards of practice and behaviour for nurses and midwives and fulfil all registration requirements | Chapter 1 |
| 1.2 Understand and apply relevant legal, regulatory and governance requirements, policies and ethical frameworks to all areas of practice, differentiating where appropriate between the devolved legislatures of the United Kingdom | Chapter 1 |
| 1.3 Understand and apply the principles of courage, transparency and the duty of candour, recognising and reporting any situations, behaviours or errors that could result in poor care outcomes | Chapters 1 & 8 |
| 1.4 Demonstrate an understanding of and the ability to challenge discriminatory behaviour | Chapter 1 |
| 1.5 Understand the demands of professional practice and demonstrate how to recognise signs of vulnerability in themselves or their colleagues and the action required to minimise risks to health | Chapters 1 & 8 |
| 1.6 Understand and maintain the level of health, fitness and wellbeing required to meet people's needs for mental and physical care | Chapters 1 & 16 |
| 1.7 Demonstrate an understanding of research methods, ethics and governance in order to critically analyse, safely use, share and apply research findings to promote and inform best nursing practice | Chapters 6 & 7 |
| 1.8 Demonstrate the knowledge, skills and ability to think critically when applying evidence and drawing on experience to make evidence-informed decisions in all situations | Chapters 7 & 10–15 |
| 1.9 Understand the need to base all decisions regarding care and interventions on people's needs and preferences, recognising and addressing any personal and external factors that may unduly influence decisions | All Chapters |
| 1.10 Demonstrate resilience and emotional intelligence and be capable of explaining the rationale that influences judgements and decisions in routine, complex and challenging situations | Chapters 1, 7 & 8 |
| 1.11 Communicate effectively using a range of skills and strategies with colleagues and people at all stages of life and with a range of mental, physical, cognitive and behavioural health challenges | Chapters 3 & 10–15 |
| 1.12 Demonstrate the skills and abilities required to support people at all stages of life who are emotionally or physically vulnerable | Chapters 2 & 10–15 |
| 1.13 Demonstrate the skills and abilities required to develop, manage and maintain appropriate relationships with people, their families, carers and colleagues | All Chapters |

*(Continued)*

(Continued)

| | |
|---|---|
| 1.14 Provide and promote non-discriminatory, person-centred and sensitive care at all times, reflecting on people's values and beliefs, diverse backgrounds, cultural characteristics, language requirements, needs and preferences, taking account of any need for adjustments | Chapters 3 & 10–15 |
| 1.15 Demonstrate the numeracy, literacy, digital and technological skills required to meet the needs of people in their care to ensure safe and effective nursing practice | Chapters 3 & 5, 10–15 and web resources |
| 1.16 Demonstrate the ability to keep complete, clear, accurate and timely records | Chapters 4 & 10–15 |
| 1.17 Take responsibility for continuous self-reflection, seeking and responding to support and feedback to develop their professional knowledge and skills | Chapters 1 & 16 |
| 1.18 Demonstrate the knowledge and confidence to contribute effectively and proactively in an interdisciplinary team | Chapters 4 & 8, 10–15 |
| 1.19 Act as an ambassador, upholding the reputation of the profession and promoting public confidence in nursing, health and care services | Chapters 1 & 16 |
| 1.20 Safely demonstrate evidence-based practice in all skills and procedures stated in Annexes A and B | Chapters 2, 3, 5 and 10–15 |
| **Platform 2: Promoting health and preventing ill health** Registered nurses play a key role in improving and maintaining the mental, physical and behavioural health and wellbeing of people, families, communities and populations. They support and enable people at all stages of life and in all care settings to make informed choices about how to manage health challenges in order to maximise their quality of life and improve health outcomes. They are actively involved in the prevention of and protection against disease and ill health and engage in public health, community development and global health agendas and in the reduction of health inequalities. The proficiencies identified below will equip the newly registered nurse with the underpinning knowledge and skills required for their role in health promotion and protection and prevention of ill health. At the point of registration, the registered nurse will be able to: | |
| 2.1 Understand and apply the aims and principles of health promotion, protection and improvement and the prevention of ill health when engaging with people | Chapter 10 |
| 2.2 Demonstrate knowledge of epidemiology, demography, genomics and the wider determinants of health, illness and wellbeing and apply this to an understanding of global patterns of health and wellbeing outcomes | Chapter 10 |
| 2.3 Understand the factors that may lead to inequalities in health outcomes | Chapter 10 |
| 2.4 Identify and use all appropriate opportunities, making reasonable adjustments when required, to discuss the impact of smoking, substance and alcohol use, sexual behaviours, diet and exercise on mental, physical and behavioural health and wellbeing, in the context of people's individual circumstances | Chapter 10 |
| 2.5 Promote and improve mental, physical, behavioural and other health-related outcomes by understanding and explaining the principles, practice and evidence base for health screening programmes | Chapter 10 |

| | |
|---|---|
| 2.6 Understand the importance of early years and childhood experiences and the possible impact on life choices, mental, physical and behavioural health and wellbeing | Chapter 10 |
| 2.7 Understand and explain the contribution of social influences, health literacy, individual circumstances, behaviours and lifestyle choices to mental, physical and behavioural health outcomes | Chapter 10 |
| 2.8 Explain and demonstrate the use of up to date approaches to behaviour change to enable people to use their strengths and expertise and make informed choices when managing their own health and making lifestyle adjustments | Chapters 10 & 12 |
| 2.9 Use appropriate communication skills and strength-based approaches to support and enable people to make informed choices about their care to manage health challenges in order to have satisfying and fulfilling lives within the limitations caused by reduced capability, ill health and disability | Chapters 2 & 10–15 |
| 2.10 Provide information in accessible ways to help people understand and make decisions about their health, life choices, illness and care | Chapters 2 & 10–15 |
| 2.11 Promote health and prevent ill health by understanding and explaining to people the principles of pathogenesis, immunology and the evidence base for immunisation, vaccination and herd immunity | Chapter 10 |
| 2.12 Protect health through understanding and applying the principles of infection prevention and control, including communicable disease surveillance and antimicrobial stewardship and resistance | Chapter 3 |
| **Platform 3: Assessing needs and planning care** Registered nurses prioritise the needs of people when assessing and reviewing their mental, physical, cognitive, behavioural, social and spiritual needs. They use information obtained during assessments to identify the priorities and requirements for person-centred and evidence-based nursing interventions and support. They work in partnership with people to develop person-centred care plans that take into account their circumstances, characteristics and preferences. The proficiencies identified below will equip the newly registered nurse with the underpinning knowledge and skills required for their role in assessing and initiating person-centred plans of care. At the point of registration, the registered nurse will be able to: | |
| 3.1 Demonstrate and apply knowledge of human development from conception to death when undertaking full and accurate person-centred nursing assessments and developing appropriate care plans | Chapters 3 & 10–15 |
| 3.2 Demonstrate and apply knowledge of body systems and homeostasis, human anatomy and physiology, biology, genomics, pharmacology, social and behavioural sciences when undertaking full and accurate person-centred nursing assessments and developing appropriate care plans | Chapters 3 & 10–15 |

(Continued)

(Continued)

| | |
|---|---|
| 3.3 Demonstrate and apply knowledge of all commonly encountered mental, physical, behavioural and cognitive health conditions, medication usage and treatments when undertaking full and accurate assessments of nursing care needs and when developing, prioritising and reviewing person-centred care plans | Chapters 3, 5 & 10–15 |
| 3.4 Understand and apply a person-centred approach to nursing care, demonstrating shared assessment, planning, decision making and goal setting when working with people, their families, communities and populations of all ages | Chapters 2, 3 & 10–15 |
| 3.5 Demonstrate the ability to accurately process all information gathered during the assessment process to identify needs for individualised nursing care and develop person-centred evidence-based plans for nursing interventions with agreed goals | Chapters 3 & 10–15 |
| 3.6 Effectively assess a person's capacity to make decisions about their own care and to give or withhold consent | Chapters 3 & 10–15 |
| 3.7 Understand and apply the principles and processes for making reasonable adjustments and best interest decisions where people do not have capacity | Chapters 3 & 10–15 |
| 3.8 Recognise and assess people at risk of harm and the situations that may put them at risk, ensuring prompt action is taken to safeguard those who are vulnerable | Chapters 3, 8 & 10–15 |
| 3.9 Undertake routine investigations, interpreting and sharing findings as appropriate | Chapters 3 & 10–15 |
| 3.10 Interpret results from routine investigations, taking prompt action when required by implementing appropriate interventions, requesting additional investigations or escalating to others | Chapters 3 &10–15 |
| 3.11 Demonstrate an understanding of co-morbidities and the demands of meeting people's complex nursing and social care needs when prioritising care plans | Chapters 3 & 10–15 |
| 3.12 Identify and assess the needs of people and families for care at the end of life, including requirements for palliative care and decision making related to their treatment and care preferences | Chapter 15 |
| 3.13 Demonstrate the ability to work in partnership with people, families and carers to continuously monitor, evaluate and reassess the effectiveness of all agreed nursing care plans and care, sharing decision making and readjusting agreed goals, documenting progress and decisions made | Chapters 3 & 10–15 |
| 3.14 Demonstrate knowledge of when and how to refer people safely to other professionals or services for clinical intervention or support | Chapters 4, 8 & 10–15 |

**Platform 4: Providing and evaluating care** Registered nurses take the lead in providing evidence-based, compassionate and safe nursing interventions. They ensure that care they provide and delegate is person-centred and of a consistently high standard. They support people of all ages in a range of care settings. They work in partnership with people, families and carers to evaluate whether care is effective and the goals of care have been met in line with their wishes, preferences and desired outcomes. The proficiencies identified below will equip the newly registered nurse with the underpinning knowledge and skills required for their role in providing and evaluating person-centred care. At the point of registration, the registered nurse will be able to:

| | |
|---|---|
| 4.1 Demonstrate and apply an understanding of what is important to people and how to use this knowledge to ensure their needs for safety, dignity, privacy, comfort and sleep can be met, acting as a role model for others in providing evidence-based person-centred care | Chapters 2, 3 & 10–15 |
| 4.2 Work in partnership with people to encourage shared decision making, in order to support individuals, their families and carers to manage their own care when appropriate | Chapters 2, 3, 4, 5, 7 & 10–15 |
| 4.3 Demonstrate the knowledge, communication and relationship management skills required to provide people, families and carers with accurate information that meets their needs before, during and after a range of interventions | Chapters 2, 3 & 10–15 |
| 4.4 Demonstrate the knowledge and skills required to support people with commonly encountered mental health, behavioural, cognitive and learning challenges and act as role model for others in providing high-quality nursing interventions to meet people's needs | Chapters 3, 8 & 10–15 |
| 4.5 Demonstrate the knowledge and skills required to support people with commonly encountered physical health conditions, their medication usage and treatments and act as role model for others in providing high-quality nursing interventions when meeting people's needs | Chapter 3, 5 & 10–15 |
| 4.6 Demonstrate the knowledge, skills and ability to act as a role model for others in providing evidence-based nursing care to meet people's needs related to nutrition, hydration and elimination | Chapters 3 & 10–15 |
| 4.7 Demonstrate the knowledge, skills and ability to act as a role model for others in providing evidence-based, person-centred nursing care to meet people's needs related to mobility, hygiene, oral care, wound care and skin integrity | Chapters 3 & 10–15 |
| 4.8 Demonstrate the knowledge and skills required to identify and initiate appropriate interventions to support people with commonly encountered symptoms including anxiety, confusion, discomfort and pain | Chapters 3 & 10–15 |
| 4.9 Demonstrate the knowledge and skills required to prioritise what is important to people and their families when providing evidence-based person-centred nursing care at end of life including the care of people who are dying, families, the deceased and bereaved | Chapter 15 |

*(Continued)*

(Continued)

| | |
|---|---|
| 4.10 Demonstrate the knowledge and ability to respond proactively and promptly to signs of deterioration or distress in mental, physical, cognitive and behavioural health and use this knowledge to make sound clinical decisions | Chapters 7 & 10–15 |
| 4.11 Demonstrate the ability to manage commonly encountered devices and confidently carry out related nursing procedures to meet people's needs for evidence-based, person-centred care | Chapters 3 & 10–15 |
| 4.12 Demonstrate the knowledge, skills and confidence to provide first aid procedures and basic life support | Chapter 16 & web resources |
| 4.13 Understand the principles of safe and effective administration and optimisation of medicines in accordance with local and national policies and demonstrate proficiency and accuracy when calculating dosages of prescribed medicines | Chapter 5 & web resources |
| 4.14 Demonstrate knowledge of pharmacology and the ability to recognise the effects of medicines, allergies, drug sensitivities, side effects, contraindications, incompatibilities, adverse reactions, prescribing errors and the impact of poly-pharmacy and over the counter medication usage | Chapter 5 |
| 4.15 Demonstrate knowledge of how prescriptions can be generated, the role of generic, unlicensed, and off-label prescribing and an understanding of the potential risks associated with these approaches to prescribing | Chapter 5 |
| 4.16 Apply knowledge of pharmacology to the care of people, demonstrating the ability to progress to a prescribing qualification following registration | Chapter 5 |
| 4.17 Demonstrate the ability to coordinate and undertake the processes and procedures involved in routine planning and management of safe discharge home or transfer of people between care settings | Chapters 11–15 |
| **Platform 5: Leading and managing nursing care and working in teams**<br>Registered nurses provide leadership by acting as a role model for best practice in the delivery of nursing care. They are responsible for managing nursing care and are accountable for the appropriate delegation and supervision of care provided by others in the team including lay carers. They play an active and equal role in the interdisciplinary team, collaborating and communicating effectively with a range of colleagues. The proficiencies identified below will equip the newly registered nurse with the underpinning knowledge and skills required for their role in leading and managing nursing care and working effectively as part of an interdisciplinary team. At the point of registration, the registered nurse will be able to: | |
| 5.1 Understand the principles of effective leadership, management, group and organisational dynamics and culture and apply these to team working and decision making | Chapters 8 & 9 |
| 5.2 Understand and apply the principles of human factors, environmental factors and strength-based approaches when working in teams | Chapters 4, 8 & 9 |

| | |
|---|---|
| 5.3 Understand the principles and application of processes for performance management and how these apply to the nursing team | Chapters 8 & 9 |
| 5.4 Demonstrate an understanding of the roles, responsibilities and scope of practice of all members of the nursing and interdisciplinary team and how to make best use of the contributions of others involved in providing care | Chapters 4, 8 & 9 |
| 5.5 Safely and effectively lead and manage the nursing care of a group of people demonstrating appropriate prioritisation, delegation and assignment of care responsibilities to others involved in providing care | Chapter 8 |
| 5.6 Exhibit leadership potential by demonstrating an ability to guide, support and motivate individuals and interact confidently with other members of the care team | Chapter 8 |
| 5.7 Demonstrate the ability to monitor and evaluate the quality of care delivered by others in the team and lay carers | Chapters 8 & 9 |
| 5.8 Support and supervise students in the delivery of nursing care, promoting reflection and providing constructive feedback and evaluating and documenting their performance | Chapter 8 |
| 5.9 Demonstrate the ability to challenge and provide constructive feedback about care delivered by others in the team, and support them to identify and agree individual learning needs | Chapter 8 |
| 5.10 Contribute to supervision and team reflection activities to promote improvements in practice and services | Chapters 8 & 9 |
| 5.11 Effectively and responsibly use a range of digital technologies to access, input, share and apply information and data within teams and between agencies | Chapters 4, 8, 9 & 10–15 & web resources |
| 5.12 Understand the mechanisms that can be used to influence organisational change and public policy, demonstrating the development of political awareness and skills | Chapter 8 |

## Platform 6: Improving safety and quality of care

Registered nurses make a key contribution to the continuous monitoring and quality improvement of care and treatment in order to enhance health outcomes and people's experience of nursing and related care. They assess risks to safety or experience and take appropriate action to manage those, putting the best interests, needs and preferences of people first. The proficiencies identified below will equip the newly registered nurse with the underpinning knowledge and skills required for their role in contributing to risk monitoring and quality of care improvement agendas. At the point of registration the registered nurse will be able to:

| | |
|---|---|
| 6.1 Understand and apply the principles of health and safety legislation and regulations and maintain safe work and care environments | Chapters 3, 8 & 10–16 |

*(Continued)*

(Continued)

| | |
|---|---|
| 6.2 Understand the relationship between safe staffing levels, appropriate skills mix, safety and quality of care, recognising risks to public protection and quality of care, escalating concerns appropriately | Chapters 8 & 9 |
| 6.3 Comply with local and national frameworks, legislation and regulations for assessing, managing and reporting risks, ensuring the appropriate action is taken | Chapters 5, 8 & 10–16 |
| 6.4 Demonstrate an understanding of the principles of improvement methodologies, participate in all stages of audit activity and identify appropriate quality improvement strategies | Chapter 9 |
| 6.5 Demonstrate the ability to accurately undertake risk assessments in a range of care settings using a range of contemporary assessment and improvement tools | Chapters 3, 8 & 10–15 |
| 6.6 Identify the need to make improvements and proactively respond to potential hazards that may affect the safety of people | Chapters 8, 9 & 10–15 |
| 6.7 Understand how the quality and effectiveness of nursing care can be evaluated in practice and demonstrate how to use service delivery evaluation and audit findings to bring about continuous improvement | Chapter 9 |
| 6.8 Demonstrate an understanding of how to identify, report and critically reflect on near misses, critical incidents, major incidents and serious adverse events in order to learn from them and influence their future practice | Chapters 5, 8 & 9 |
| 6.9 Work with people, their families, carers and colleagues, to develop effective improvement strategies for quality and safety, sharing feedback and learning from positive outcomes and experiences, mistakes and adverse outcomes and experiences | Chapters 4 & 9 |
| 6.10 Apply an understanding of the differences between risk aversion and risk management and how to avoid compromising quality of care and health outcomes | Chapter 8 |
| 6.11 Acknowledge the need to accept and manage uncertainty, and demonstrate an understanding of strategies that develop resilience in self and others | Chapters 1, 7 & 16 |
| 6.12 Understand the role of registered nurses and other health and care professionals at different levels of experience and seniority when managing and prioritising actions and care in the event of a major incident | Chapter 16 & web resources |

## Platform 7: Coordinating care

Registered nurses play a leadership role in coordinating and managing the complex nursing and integrated care needs of people at any stage of their lives, across a range of organisations and settings. They contribute to processes of organisational change through an awareness of local and national policies. The proficiencies identified below will equip the newly registered nurse with the underpinning knowledge and skills required for their role in coordinating and leading and managing the complex needs of people across organisations and settings. At the point of registration, the registered nurse will be able to:

| | |
|---|---|
| 7.1 Understand and apply the principles of partnership, collaboration and interagency working across all relevant sectors | Chapters 4 & 10–15 |
| 7.2 Understand health legislation and current health and social care policies, and the mechanisms involved in influencing policy development and change, differentiating where appropriate between the devolved legislatures of the United Kingdom | Chapters 1 & 9 |
| 7.3 Understand the principles of health economics and their relevance to resource allocation in health and social care organisations and other agencies | Chapter 9 |
| 7.4 Identify the implications of current health policy and future policy changes for nursing and other professions and understand the impact of policy changes on the delivery and coordination of care | Chapters 8, 9 & 10–15 |
| 7.5 Understand and recognise the need to respond to the challenges of providing safe, effective and person-centred nursing care for people who have co-morbidities and complex care needs | Chapters 10–15 |
| 7.6 Demonstrate an understanding of the complexities of providing mental, cognitive, behavioural and physical care services across a wide range of integrated care settings | Chapters 10–15 |
| 7.7 Understand how to monitor and evaluate the quality of people's experience of complex care | Chapters 8, 9 & 14 |
| 7.8 Understand the principles and processes involved in supporting people and families with a range of care needs to maintain optimal independence and avoid unnecessary interventions and disruptions to their lives | Chapters 3 & 10–15 |
| 7.9 Facilitate equitable access to healthcare for people who are vulnerable or have a disability and demonstrate the ability to advocate on their behalf when required and make necessary reasonable adjustments to the assessment, planning and delivery of their care | Chapters 3 & 10–15 |
| 7.10 Understand the principles and processes involved in planning and facilitating the safe discharge and transition of people between caseloads, settings and services | Chapters 3 & 10–15 |
| 7.11 Demonstrate the ability to identify and manage risks and take proactive measures to improve the quality of care and services when needed | Chapters 2, 9 & 10–15 |

(Continued)

(Continued)

| | |
|---|---|
| 7.12 Demonstrate an understanding of the processes involved in developing a basic business case for additional care funding, by applying knowledge of finance, resources and safe staffing levels | Chapter 9 |
| 7.13 Demonstrate an understanding of the importance of exercising political awareness throughout their career, to maximise the influence and effect of registered nursing on quality of care, patient safety and cost effectiveness | Chapter 9 |

## Annexe A: Communication and relationship management skills

The communication and relationship management skills that a newly registered nurse must be able to demonstrate in order to meet the proficiency outcomes outlined previously are set out in this annexe. Effective communication is central to the provision of safe and compassionate person-centred care. Registered nurses in all fields of nursing practice must be able to demonstrate the ability to communicate and manage relationships with people of all ages with a range of mental, physical, cognitive and behavioural health challenges. This is because a diverse range of communication and relationship management skills is required to ensure that individuals, their families and carers are actively involved in and understand care decisions. These skills are vital when making accurate, culturally aware assessments of care needs and ensuring that the needs, priorities, expertise and preferences of people are always valued and taken into account. Where people have special communication needs or a disability, it is essential that reasonable adjustments are made in order to communicate, provide and share information in a manner that promotes optimum understanding and engagement and facilitates equal access to high-quality care. The communication and relationship management skills within this annexe are set out in four sections. For the reasons above, these requirements are relevant to all fields of nursing practice and apply to all care settings. It is expected that these skills would be assessed in a student's chosen field of practice. Those skills outlined in Annexe A, Section 3: Evidence-based, best practice communication skills and approaches for providing therapeutic interventions also apply to all registered nurses, but the level of expertise and knowledge required will vary depending on the chosen field of practice.

Registered nurses must be able to demonstrate these skills to an appropriate level for their intended field(s) of practice. At the point of registration, the registered nurse will be able to safely demonstrate the following skills:

## 1 Underpinning communication skills for assessing, planning, providing and managing best practice, evidence-based nursing care

| | |
|---|---|
| 1.1 Actively listen, recognise and respond to verbal and non-verbal cues | Chapter 3 |
| 1.2 Use prompts and positive verbal and non-verbal reinforcement | Chapter 3 |
| 1.3 Use appropriate non-verbal communication including touch, eye contact and personal space | Chapter 3 |
| 1.4 Make appropriate use of open and closed questioning | Chapter 3 |
| 1.5 Use caring conversation techniques | Chapter 3 |
| 1.6 Check understanding and use clarification techniques | Chapter 3 |

| | |
|---|---|
| 1.7 Be aware of own unconscious bias in communication encounters | Chapter 3 |
| 1.8 Write accurate, clear, legible records and documentation | Chapter 4 |
| 1.9 Confidently and clearly share and present verbal and written reports with individuals and groups | Chapter 4 |
| 1.10 Analyse and clearly record and share digital information and data | Chapter 4 |
| 1.11 Provide clear verbal, digital or written information and instructions when delegating or handing over responsibility for care | Chapter 4<br>Chapter 8 |
| 1.12 Recognise the need for and facilitate access to translator services and material | Chapters 2 & 3 |
| **2 Evidence-based, best practice approaches to communication for supporting people of all ages, their families and carers in preventing ill health and in managing their care** | |
| 2.1 Share information and check understanding about the causes and implications and treatment of a range of common health conditions including anxiety, depression, memory loss, diabetes, dementia, respiratory disease, cardiac disease, neurological disease, cancer, skin problems, immune deficiencies, psychosis, stroke and arthritis | Chapters 10–15 |
| 2.2 Use clear language and appropriate written materials, making reasonable adjustments where appropriate in order to optimise people's understanding of what has caused their health condition and the implications of their care and treatment | Chapters 2 & 10–15 |
| 2.3 Recognise and accommodate sensory impairments during all communications | Chapters 2, 3 & 10–15 |
| 2.4 Support and manage the use of personal communication aids | Chapters 2 & 10–15 |
| 2.5 Identify the need for and manage a range of alternative communication techniques | Chapters 2 & 10–15 |
| 2.6 Use repetition and positive reinforcement strategies | Chapters 3 & 10–15 |
| 2.7 Assess motivation and capacity for behaviour change and clearly explain cause and effect relationships related to common health risk behaviours including smoking, obesity, sexual practice, alcohol and substance use | Chapter 10 |
| 2.8 Provide information and explanation to people, families and carers and respond to questions about their treatment and care and possible ways of preventing ill health to enhance understanding | Chapters 10–15 |
| 2.9 Engage in difficult conversations, including breaking bad news and support people who are feeling emotionally or physically vulnerable or in distress, conveying compassion and sensitivity | Chapters 2 & 11–16 |

*(Continued)*

(Continued)

**3 Evidence-based, best practice communication skills and approaches for providing therapeutic interventions**

| | |
|---|---|
| 3.1 Motivational interview techniques | Chapter 3 |
| 3.2 Solution focused therapies | Chapter 3 web resources |
| 3.3 Reminiscence therapies | Chapter 3 web resources |
| 3.4 Talking therapies | Chapter 3 web resources |
| 3.5 De-escalation strategies and techniques | Chapter 3 web resources |
| 3.6 Cognitive behavioural therapy techniques | Chapter 3 web resources |
| 3.7 Play therapy | Chapter 10 |
| 3.8 Distraction and diversion strategies | Chapter 13 |
| 3.9 Positive behaviour support approaches | Chapter 10 |

**4 Evidence-based, best practice communication skills and approaches for working with people in professional teams**

**4.1 Demonstrate effective supervision, teaching and performance appraisal through the use of:**

| | |
|---|---|
| 4.1.1 clear instructions and explanations when supervising, teaching or appraising others | Chapters 8, 9 & 16 |
| 4.1.2 clear instructions and check understanding when delegating care responsibilities to others | Chapter 8 |
| 4.1.3 unambiguous, constructive feedback about strengths and weaknesses and potential for improvement | Chapters 8, 9 & 16 |
| 4.1.4 encouragement to colleagues that helps them to reflect on their practice | Chapters 8, 9 & 16 |
| 4.1.5 unambiguous records of performance | Chapters 8 & 9 |

**4.2 Demonstrate effective person and team management through the use of:**

| | |
|---|---|
| 4.2.1 strengths-based approaches to developing teams and managing change | Chapter 9 |
| 4.2.2 active listening when dealing with team members' concerns and anxieties | Chapters 8 & 9 |
| 4.2.3 a calm presence when dealing with conflict | Chapter 8 |
| 4.2.4 appropriate and effective confrontation strategies | Chapter 8 |
| 4.2.5 de-escalation strategies and techniques when dealing with conflict | Chapter 8 |
| 4.2.6 effective coordination and navigation skills through | Chapter 8 |
| 4.2.6.1 appropriate negotiation strategies | Chapter 8 |
| 4.2.6.3 appropriate approaches to advocacy | Chapters 8 & 10–15 |

## Annexe B: Nursing procedures

The nursing procedures that a newly registered nurse must be able to demonstrate in order to meet the proficiency outcomes, outlined previously above are set out in this annexe. The registered nurse must be able to undertake these procedures effectively in order to provide, compassionate, evidence-based person-centred nursing care. A holistic approach to the care of people is essential and all nursing procedures should be carried out in a way which reflects cultural awareness and ensures that the needs, priorities, expertise and preferences of people are always valued and taken into account. Registered nurses in all fields of practice must demonstrate the ability to provide nursing intervention and support for people of all ages who require nursing procedures during the processes of assessment, diagnosis, care and treatment for mental, physical, cognitive and behavioural health challenges. Where people are disabled or have specific cognitive needs it is essential that reasonable adjustments are made to ensure that all procedures are undertaken safely. The nursing procedures within this annexe are set out in two sections. These requirements are relevant to all fields of nursing practice although it is recognised that different care settings may require different approaches to the provision of care. It is expected that these procedures would be assessed in a student's chosen field of practice where practicable. Those procedures outlined in Annexe B, Part I: Procedures for assessing needs for person-centred care, sections 1 and 2 also apply to all registered nurses, but the level of expertise and knowledge required will vary depending on the chosen field(s) of practice. Registered nurses must therefore be able to demonstrate the ability to undertake these procedures at an appropriate level for their intended field(s) of practice.

At the point of registration, the registered nurse will be able to safely demonstrate the following procedures:

## Part I: Procedures for assessing people's needs for person-centred care

| | |
|---|---|
| 1 Use evidence-based, best practice approaches to take a history, observe, recognise and accurately assess people of all ages | Chapter 3 |
| 1.1 Mental health and wellbeing status | Chapter 3 |
| 1.1.1 signs of mental and emotional distress or vulnerability | Chapter 3 |
| 1.1.2 cognitive health status and wellbeing | Chapter 3 |
| 1.1.3 signs of cognitive distress and impairment | Chapter 3 |
| 1.1.4 behavioural distress-based needs | Chapter 3 |
| 1.1.5 signs of mental and emotional distress including agitation, aggression and challenging behaviour | Chapter 3 |
| 1.2 Physical health and wellbeing | Chapters 3 & 10–15 |
| 1.2.1 symptoms and signs of physical ill health | Chapters 3 & 10–15 |
| 1.2.2 symptoms and signs of physical distress | Chapters 3 & 10–15 |
| 1.2.3 symptoms and signs of deterioration and sepsis | Chapters 13 & 14 |

*(Continued)*

(Continued)

| 2 Use evidence-based, best practice approaches to undertake the following procedures | |
|---|---|
| 2.1 Take, record and interpret vital signs manually and via technological devices | Chapters 3 & 10–15 & web resources |
| 2.2 Undertake venepuncture and cannulation and blood sampling, interpreting normal and common abnormal blood profiles and venous blood gases | Chapters 3, 13 & 14 & web resources |
| 2.3 Set up and manage routine electrocardiogram (ECG) investigations and interpret normal and commonly encountered abnormal traces | Chapters 13–14 & web resources |
| 2.4 Manage and monitor blood component transfusions | Chapters 13–14 & web resources |
| 2.5 Manage and interpret cardiac monitors, infusion pumps, blood glucose monitors and other monitoring devices | Chapters 3 & 13 and web resources |
| 2.6 Accurately measure weight and height, calculate body mass index and recognise healthy ranges and clinically significant low/high readings | Chapter 3 |
| 2.7 Undertake a whole body systems assessment including respiratory, circulatory, neurological, musculoskeletal, cardiovascular and skin status | Chapter 3 |
| 2.8 Undertake chest auscultation and interpret findings | Chapter 3 |
| 2.9 Collect and observe sputum, urine, stool and vomit specimens, undertaking routine analysis and interpreting findings | Chapter 3 |
| 2.10 Measure and interpret blood glucose levels | Chapter 3 |
| 2.11 Recognise and respond to signs of all forms of abuse | Chapters 3 & 10–15 |
| 2.12 Undertake, respond to and interpret neurological observations and assessments | Chapter 3 |
| 2.13 Identify and respond to signs of deterioration and sepsis | Chapters 13–14 |
| 2.14 Administer basic mental health first aid | Chapter 10 |
| 2.15 Administer basic physical first aid | Chapter 16 (web resources) |
| 2.16 Recognise and manage seizures | Chapter 16 (web resources) |
| 3 Use evidence-based, best practice approaches for meeting needs for care and support with rest, sleep, comfort and the maintenance of dignity, accurately assessing the person's capacity for independence and self-care and initiating appropriate interventions | |
| 3.1 Observe and assess comfort and pain levels and rest and sleep patterns | Chapters 3 & 10–15 |
| 3.2 Use appropriate bed-making techniques including those required for people who are unconscious or who have limited mobility | Web resources |

| | |
|---|---|
| 3.3 Use appropriate positioning and pressure relieving techniques | Chapters 3 & 10–15 |
| 3.4 Take appropriate action to ensure privacy and dignity at all times | Chapters 3 & 10–15 |
| 3.5 Take appropriate action to reduce or minimise pain or discomfort | Chapters 3 & 10–15 |
| 3.6 Take appropriate action to reduce fatigue, minimise insomnia and support improved rest and sleep hygiene | Chapters 3 & 10–15 |
| **4 Use evidence-based, best practice approaches for meeting the needs for care and support with hygiene and the maintenance of skin integrity, accurately assessing the person's capacity for independence and self-care and initiating appropriate interventions** | |
| 4.1 Observe, assess and optimise skin and hygiene status and determine the need for support and intervention | Chapter 3 |
| 4.2 Use contemporary approaches to the assessment of skin integrity and use appropriate products to prevent or manage skin breakdown | Chapter 3 |
| 4.3 Assess need for and provide appropriate assistance with washing, bathing, shaving and dressing | Chapter 3 |
| 4.4 Identify and manage skin irritations and rashes | Chapter 3 |
| 4.5 Assess need for and provide appropriate oral, dental, eye and nail care and decide when an onward referral is needed | Chapter 3 |
| 4.6 Use aseptic techniques when undertaking wound care including dressings, pressure bandaging, suture removal and vacuum closures | Chapter 3 |
| 4.7 Use aseptic techniques when managing wound and drainage processes | Chapter 3 |
| 4.8 Assess, respond and effectively manage pyrexia and hypothermia | Chapters 3 & 10–15 |
| **5 Use evidence-based, best practice approaches for meeting needs for care and support with nutrition and hydration, accurately assessing the person's capacity for independence and self-care and initiating appropriate interventions** | |
| 5.1 Observe, assess and optimise nutrition and hydration status and determine the need for intervention and support | Chapters 3 & 10–15 |
| 5.2 Use contemporary nutritional assessment tools | Chapters 3 & 10–15 |
| 5.3 Assist with feeding and drinking and use appropriate feeding and drinking aids | Chapters 3 & 11–15 |
| 5.4 Record fluid intake and output and identify, respond to and manage dehydration or fluid retention | Chapters 3 & 11–15 |
| 5.5 Identify, respond to and manage nausea and vomiting | Chapters 3 & 11–15 |

*(Continued)*

(Continued)

| | |
|---|---|
| 5.6 Insert, manage and remove oral/nasal/gastric tubes | Chapters 3 & 11–15 & web resources |
| 5.7 Manage artificial nutrition and hydration using oral, enteral and parenteral routes | Chapters 13 & 14 & web resources |
| 5.8 Manage the administration of IV fluids | Chapters 13 & 14 |
| 5.9 Manage fluid and nutritional infusion pumps and devices | Chapters 13 & 14 & web resources |
| 6 Use evidence-based, best practice approaches for meeting needs for care and support with bladder and bowel health, accurately assessing the person's capacity for independence and self-care and initiating appropriate interventions | |
| 6.1 Observe and assess level of urinary and bowel continence to determine the need for support and intervention assisting with toileting, maintaining dignity and privacy and managing the use of appropriate aids | Chapter 3 |
| 6.2 Select and use appropriate continence products; insert, manage and remove catheters for all genders; and assist with self-catheterisation when required | Chapters 3 & 11–15 |
| 6.3 Manage bladder drainage | Chapters 11–15 |
| 6.4 Assess elimination patterns to identify and respond to constipation, diarrhoea and urinary and faecal retention | Chapter 3 |
| 6.5 Administer enemas and suppositories and undertake rectal examination and manual evacuation when appropriate | Chapters 3 & 11–15 |
| 6.6 Undertake stoma care identifying and using appropriate products and approaches | Chapter 3 |
| 7 Use evidence-based, best practice approaches for meeting needs for care and support with mobility and safety, accurately assessing the person's capacity for independence and self-care and initiating appropriate interventions | |
| 7.1 Observe and use evidence-based risk assessment tools to determine need for support and intervention to optimise mobility and safety, and to identify and manage risk of falls using best practice risk assessment approaches | Chapters 3 & 11–15 |
| 7.2 Use a range of contemporary moving and handling techniques and mobility aids | Chapters 3 & 11–15 |
| 7.3 Use appropriate moving and handling equipment to support people with impaired mobility | Chapters 3 & 11–15 |
| 7.4 Use appropriate safety techniques and devices | Chapters 3 & 10–15 |

| | |
|---|---|
| 8 Use evidence-based, best practice approaches for meeting needs for respiratory care and support, accurately assessing the person's capacity for independence and self-care and initiating appropriate interventions | |
| 8.1 Observe and assess the need for intervention and respond to restlessness, agitation and breathlessness using appropriate interventions | Chapters 3 & 11–15 |
| 8.2 Manage the administration of oxygen using a range of routes and best practice approaches | Chapters 12, 13–14 and web resources |
| 8.3 Take and interpret peak flow and oximetry measurements | Chapter 3 & web resources |
| 8.4 Use appropriate nasal and oral suctioning techniques | Chapters 3, 13–14 & web resources |
| 8.5 Manage inhalation, humidifier and nebuliser devices | Chapter 3 (web resources) |
| 8.6 Manage airway and respiratory processes and equipment | Chapters 13–14 |
| 9 Use evidence-based, best practice approaches for meeting needs for care and support with the prevention and management of infection, accurately assessing the person's capacity for independence and self-care and initiating appropriate interventions | |
| 9.1 Observe, assess and respond rapidly to potential infection risks using best practice guidelines | Chapter 3 |
| 9.2 Use standard precautions protocols | Chapter 3 |
| 9.3 Use effective aseptic, non-touch techniques | Chapter 3 |
| 9.4 Use appropriate personal protection equipment | Chapter 3 |
| 9.5 Implement isolation procedures | Chapter 3 |
| 9.6 Use evidence-based hand hygiene techniques | Chapter 3 |
| 9.7 Safely decontaminate equipment and environment | Chapter 3 |
| 9.8 Safely use and dispose of waste, laundry and sharps | Chapter 3 |
| 9.9 Safely assess and manage invasive medical devices and lines | Chapters 3, 13 & 14 |
| 10 Use evidence-based, best practice approaches for meeting needs for care and support at the end of life, accurately assessing the person's capacity for independence and self-care and initiating appropriate interventions | |
| 10.1 Observe and assess the need for intervention for people, families and carers, identify, assess and respond appropriately to uncontrolled symptoms and signs of distress including pain, nausea, thirst, constipation, restlessness, agitation, anxiety and depression | Chapters 11–15 |

*(Continued)*

(Continued)

| | |
|---|---|
| 10.2 Manage and monitor effectiveness of symptom relief medication, infusion pumps and other devices | Chapters 11–15 |
| 10.3 Assess and review preferences and care priorities of the dying person and their family and carers | Chapter 15 |
| 10.4 Understand and apply organ and tissue donation protocols, advanced planning decisions, living wills and health and lasting powers of attorney for health | Chapters 14 & 15 |
| 10.5 Understand and apply DNACPR (do not attempt cardiopulmonary resuscitation) decisions and verification of expected death | Chapters 14 & 15 |
| 10.6 Provide care for the deceased person and the bereaved respecting cultural requirements and protocols | Chapter 15 |
| 11 Procedural competencies required for best practice, evidence-based medicines administration and optimisation | |
| 11.1 Carry out initial and continued assessments of people receiving care and their ability to self-administer their own medications | Chapter 5 |
| 11.2 Recognise the various procedural routes under which medicines can be prescribed, supplied, dispensed and administered; and the laws, policies, regulations and guidance that underpin them | Chapter 5 |
| 11.3 Use the principles of safe remote prescribing and directions to administer medicines | Chapter 5 |
| 11.4 Undertake accurate drug calculations for a range of medications | Chapter 5 |
| 11.5 Undertake accurate checks, including transcription and titration, of any direction to supply or administer a medicinal product | Chapter 5 |
| 11.6 Exercise professional accountability in ensuring the safe administration of medicines to those receiving care | Chapter 5 |
| 11.7 Administer injections using intramuscular, subcutaneous, intradermal and intravenous routes and manage injection equipment | Chapter 5 |
| 11.8 Administer medications using a range of routes | Chapter 5 |
| 11.9 Administer and monitor medications using vascular access devices and enteral equipment | Chapter 5 |
| 11.10 Recognise and respond to adverse or abnormal reactions to medications | Chapter 5 |
| 11.11 Undertake safe storage, transportation and disposal of medicinal products | Chapter 5 |

# THEORY AND CONTEXT IN RELATION TO ADULT NURSING

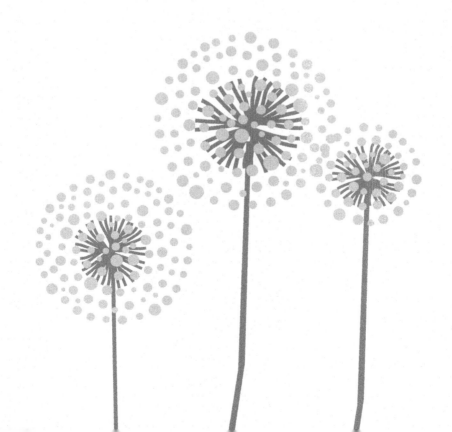

# ESSENTIALS OF NURSING: VALUES, KNOWLEDGE, SKILLS AND PRACTICE

## JOANNE TIMPSON, ELIZABETH LEE-WOOLF AND JANE BROOKS

---

### CHAPTER OBJECTIVES

- Outline the landmarks of nursing history and highlight how these have influenced nursing practice across the UK;
- Explain how legal and ethical principles provide a core framework for our professional practice;
- Define the core values that underpin nursing and recognise their application to practice;
- Understand the principles of *The Code* (Nursing and Midwifery Council or NMC, 2018a) by which we practise and how these define our fitness to practise;
- Highlight the challenges to modern nursing and relate these to our professional values in regard to cultural competence, emotional IQ and resilience.

---

As you begin your studies in nursing we hope that you will be as full of questions, as you are enthusiasm, for your chosen profession and trust that you are prepared for the challenge ahead. Our aim is to engage you with our passion for nursing and instil an ethos of nursing as a privilege. Together, we will review the essentials of nursing knowledge and values, exploring how these will underpin your practice in a way that we hope will excite your professional imagination, intelligence and curiosity.

# Related NMC proficiencies for registered nurses

The overarching Nursing and Midwifery Council (NMC) requirement is that all nurses act in the best interests of people, putting them first and providing nursing care that is person centred, safe and compassionate. They should act professionally at all times and use their knowledge and experience to make evidence-based decisions about care. They communicate effectively, are role models for others and are accountable for their actions. Registered nurses continually reflect on their practice and keep abreast of new and emerging developments in nursing, health and care (NMC, 2018b).

## To achieve entry to the nursing register you must be able to

- Understand and act in accordance with *The Code: Professional Standards of Practice and Behaviour for Nurses and Midwives* and fulfil all registration requirements (NMC, 2018a);
- Act as an ambassador, upholding the reputation of your profession and promoting public confidence in nursing, health and care services;
- Understand and apply relevant legal, regulatory and governance requirements, policies and ethical frameworks to all areas of practice, differentiating where appropriate between the devolved legislatures of the United Kingdom;
- Demonstrate resilience and emotional intelligence and be capable of explaining the rationale that influences your judgements and decisions in routine, complex and challenging situations;
- Understand and maintain the level of health, fitness and wellbeing required to meet people's needs for mental and physical care;
- Understand the demands of professional practice and demonstrate how to recognise signs of vulnerability in yourself or your colleagues and the action required to minimise risks to health;
- Understand and apply the principles of courage, transparency and the duty of candour, recognising and reporting any situations, behaviours or errors that could result in poor care outcomes;
- Demonstrate an understanding of and the ability to challenge discriminatory behaviour;
- Take responsibility for continuous self-reflection, seeking and responding to support and feedback to develop your professional knowledge and skills.

(Adapted from NMC, 2018b)

# Background

To understand the role of the contemporary adult nurse in the UK, it is useful to know a little of nursing's history and to recognise key landmarks over the last 150 years that signal the development towards the professional nursing practice we have today. However, it is not our intention to provide a detailed history of nursing here and you are advised to explore the Further Reading section at the end of this chapter, which illustrates in more detail the historical threads that bring us to this point.

Although caring, and the role of carer, has existed throughout history, nursing in its modern sense is a relatively recent concept. It is recognised that the words 'nurse' and 'nursing' are derived from the Old French *nourice* and the Late Latin *nutrire*, meaning to nourish and care (*Oxford English*

*Dictionary*, 2014a), but their use in today's sense has occurred only from the seventeenth century onwards. It is often suggested that nursing can be traced back through history to its earliest times. If you accept that this reflects the act of carer and caring then this is undoubtedly true. The themes that run through the earliest annals of history involve those who provided succour (i.e. assistance and support in times of hardship or distress) for families, communities or for those injured in battle, for example. What is perhaps more important here for modern notions of nursing are those involved with what Reverby, O'Brian D'Antonio, and Mann Wall have called 'professed-nursing', namely the care of sick strangers (Reverby, 1987; O'Brien D'Antonio, 1993; Mann Wall, 1998). This distinction is crucial because, if we understand modern professional nursing as caring for those people who are not our friends or family, this means that it is a very different undertaking from caring for those who are. Nevertheless, often the carers who nursed 'sick strangers' were influenced by religious values and altruism, believing that it would be wrong to gain monetarily from their work. There was, however, a more insidious ideology at work: once a lady worked for money, she was no longer considered a lady. To cite historian Hawkins, 'they forfeited their respectability' (Hawkins, 2010: 29). Given that nursing reformers in the nineteenth century wished to increase the number of educated middle-class women in the occupation this was clearly a problem. Hence the vocation or calling to nurse has been the province of those who had a desire to care with little thought of reward or perhaps, more pertinently, were felt not to want such financial reward because they were respectable. Either way, whilst philanthropy may indeed be admirable, such notions influenced the status of the nurse and, perhaps, some might argue, limited the evolution of nursing as a highly skilled profession (Helmstadter, 1993, 1996).

Throughout the eighteenth century we can see the appearance of what might be termed the 'modern hospital' in Britain. This was also the Age of Enlightenment – a movement made up of intellectuals who wished to see development in many areas of life through reasoned argument and science rather than adhering to traditions without thought. This influence can be seen in the funding of modern 'voluntary hospitals' by wealthy benefactors such as Thomas Guy who funded Guy's Hospital in London (1719), followed by the Edinburgh Royal Infirmary (founded in 1729), St Bartholomew's Hospital (opened in 1730, funded by public subscription), the Middlesex Hospital (opened in 1745, funded by public subscription) and the Manchester Royal Infirmary (in 1752). These hospitals had a charitable remit to provide treatment for the poor which was recognised by an Act of Parliament in 1836. However, they needed to provide care only for the 'deserving poor', and all voluntary hospitals tended to focus on acute illnesses that could be treated and would therefore provide excellent advertisements for future possible benefactors. This system excluded the chronically sick, the elderly and infirm, the mentally ill and those with learning disabilities. The last two types of patients were cared for in separate 'asylums for the insane' whereas the elderly and chronically sick were cared for in Poor Law Hospitals. The Poor Law Hospitals were described as 'murderous pesthouses' into which 'the dense mass of living creatures were crammed' (cited in White, 1978: 18).

- How do people today consider the work carried out by nurses in intensive care units in acute hospitals?
- How do people view the nursing of older people with dementia?
- What sort of facilities do we offer to each of these groups of patients?
- The thing about history is that there are often reasons in our past that go some way to explaining the ways in which services develop over time.
- Are you able to identify any links with history for the care of older people that exist today?

Modern nursing has its roots in the nineteenth century (please note, we do not wish to ignore the notion that there were significant examples of nursing-type activities in earlier times, but it would be difficult to present their importance here without sounding superficial). As the Industrial Revolution changed the face of our national landscape the need to care and manage the sick faced equal challenges. The choices surrounding who did what were primarily influenced by industry and the developing urban communities employed therein, but also by gender role. As a result, those individuals who nursed tended to be women. Living conditions were often crowded, unsanitary and polluted. Disease flourished and work-based accidents were common.

## ———— SOME EARLY NURSING PIONEERS IN BRITAIN ————

**Florence Nightingale** was born in 1820 to a wealthy family. She was encouraged and taught to think and question in a way that was unusual for a girl of those times. Her parents did not approve of her wish to nurse which they deemed unconventional. However, in 1851 she travelled to Kaiserswerth for three months to learn to be a nurse and two years later Nightingale became superintendent of a hospital for gentlewomen in Harley Street. The outbreak of the Crimean War, and the plight of wounded soldiers in terrible conditions, saw her initiate a campaign to take a team of nurses to military hospitals in Turkey where, despite relentless opposition, she improved the care and conditions for patients. Even before her return to Britain in 1856 the Nightingale Fund – which the grateful public of Britain had established in her name following her work in the Crimea – had accrued significant monies. Although initially not enthused by the project, in 1860 the Nightingale Training School for nurses at St Thomas's Hospital in London was established in her name (Baly, 1997; Bostridge, 2008). The purpose of the school was to train nurses who would then establish similar schools based on her principles. By 1867 probationer nurses were able to pay to attend and this facilitated a two-tier system of nurses where, by the turn of the twentieth century, only those who had paid for their training would be offered a post as Sister.

**Mary Seacole** was another Crimean pioneer (Alexander and Dewjee, 1984; Griffon, 1998). Born in Jamaica in 1805 (her father was a Scot and her mother Jamaican), Seacole was well travelled and had gained perspectives on medicines and care wherever she went. Like Florence Nightingale, in 1854 Seacole asked the British government to send her to the Crimea to assist in the army hospital. In her autobiography, Seacole recalled being turned down. However, she did then fund her own travel to the Crimea, where she cared for soldiers. On returning to the UK her health was poor and she had little money and no family to support her. She achieved a great deal but died in 1881 and thus did not live to see the achievement of nurse registration.

**Ethel Gordon Manson** (who later became known as Mrs Bedford Fenwick) was passionate about the improvements to nursing and nurse training. She trained as a nurse at the Nottingham Children's Hospital and then at Manchester's Royal Infirmary between 1878 and 1879. She became the matron of St Bartholomew's Hospital in London at the age of only 24 years. In 1888 she married Dr Bedford Fenwick, retired from nursing, and devoted her life to national and international nursing matters. As the founder of the Royal British Nurses' Association (1887) and the International Council of Nurses (1899), and editor of the first professional nursing journal *The Nursing Record/The British Journal of Nursing*, from 1893 to 1946, she staunchly advocated that nursing should be regulated and every nurse should be registered. She is considered to have contributed to phenomenal achievements in nursing's development (Griffon, 1995). She died on 13 March 1947.

### ACTIVITY 1.1

Find out more about the pioneers of nursing practice and identify their contribution to the development of nursing and nurse education.
You can start by accessing the UK Association for the History of Nursing at http://ukahn.org/wp/

We should not deny the fact that, while nursing was struggling for recognition, this aspect also reflects an earlier period in medicine where doctors had little recognisably organised training as such. The Medical Act of 1858 responded to a need for the public to be able to determine whether or not a doctor was qualified to practise and resulted in the inauguration of the General Medical Council. This professional body was (and remains to this day) charged with registering practitioners and ensuring that the public have access to that information (although this is now governed under the Medical Act of 1983). Following on from this, many recognised the logic for nurses to be registered in a similar fashion. The debate and will for this became more organised, especially after the beginnings of nurse training in 1860.

By 1880 the Hospitals' Association (HA) was in agreement that some form of nurse registration was a necessity and therefore voluntary registration was introduced. Ethel Bedford Fenwick (a member of the Matrons' Committee) passionately believed in professionalism and that nurses should be registered in a similar fashion to doctors. She set up the British Nurses' Association, which provided an alternative voluntary register that noted completion of a programme of study, but also more importantly aligned itself with a remit to protect the public.

The First World War provided the pivotal impetus for registration. Many women had answered a call to go and nurse which had, incidentally, raised the profile of nursing with the public. Women's role in society was changing and their contribution to working life while soldiers were away was generally noted and applauded. Meanwhile the College of Nursing was founded in 1916 (later to become the Royal College of Nursing). This organisation led and supported initiatives to further develop and raise nursing's profile and the need for a nursing register. In 1919 one MP (Major Barnet) was persuaded to propose a Private Members Bill which resulted in the Nurse Registration Act. This called upon the General Nursing Council to maintain and monitor a nursing register, as well as provide central guidance to inform nurse training programmes. It was replaced by the United Kingdom Central Council in 1983 and subsequently by the Nursing and Midwifery Council in 2002. All had similar duties in their role to maintain the register, provide educational guidance and ensure protection of the public. It is interesting to note that women still had no right to vote and nursing would not be officially recognised as a profession for almost another 100 years but at least they had registration and regulation.

The NHS was born in 1948 which again reflected the changes that war had brought to society. However, and despite the work of many groups, nurse education and the role of the nurse were slow to evolve. Graduate education for nurses was embryonic although several university medical schools began offering some form of nurse education at degree level. The University of Edinburgh offered the first degree in nursing in 1960 and the University of Manchester's Bachelor of Nursing degree soon followed. It was at the University of Manchester that the first Professor of Nursing was appointed – Jean Kennedy McFarlane, later to become Baroness McFarlane of Llandaff. Other 'experimental' courses were tried throughout the 1960s and 1970s, with some at degree and some at diploma level.

# The birth of modern nursing

Several reports during the twentieth century culminated in the Briggs Committee's remit to consider various concerns surrounding the methods, content and quality of nurse education and its interface with the NHS. Margaret Scott Wright was an influential member of this committee and the report that followed in 1972 recommended a step change: a move away from training towards professional education and the development of research into all aspects of education and nursing practice. After much wrangling the Nurses, Midwives and Health Visitors Act (passed in 1979) saw the beginnings of a modern-day nurse education.

Project 2000 was introduced in 1988 and diploma education for nurses was piloted in a number of schools prior to it being rolled out across Britain. Student nurses now had student status and were no longer employees of the hospital in which the School of Nursing was based. This created some challenges for nursing practice, but these were not insurmountable and many nurses at all levels engaged with this new approach to education with enthusiasm. Between 1990 and 2010 diploma and degree courses in nursing ran side by side, but in 2010 legislation was enacted to ensure that every nurse in England would be educated to degree level, reflecting previous changes already effected in Scotland, Northern Ireland and Wales, for both nursing and other allied health professions such as physiotherapy, radiography and occupational therapy.

## ——————— TWENTIETH-CENTURY PIONEERS IN NURSING ———————

**Lisbeth Hockey** was born Lisbeth Hochsinger on 17 October 1918 in Graz, Steiermark, Austria. In 1936, at the age of 18, she commenced her medical studies at the Karl-Franzens University of Graz. However, following the Nazi occupation of Austria in 1938 she left for England. Hockey was not able to recommence her medical studies in England for three reasons: she was a woman (and few British women went to university at that time); she did not speak English; and she had no money. British friends recommended nursing as an alternative and so Hockey began her training at the London Hospital in Whitechapel in 1939 (Mason, 2005: 2–5). Her importance to the nursing profession came from her natural desire to ask questions. However, during her training this was to cause her problems with those in authority:

> What intrigued me or alarmed me was the number of pressure sores and bed sores of course in those days. But what interested me more, was why some people did not get bed sores ... And I went to the sister one day and said, 'please explain to me why some patients have got bed sores and others didn't' seeing as I was interested in the ones that didn't, and she said, 'it's not your place to ask questions, go back and do your work'. (Hockey, 2001)

She was not put off, and after qualifying as a nurse she trained as both a district nurse and then a health visitor before becoming a tutor at the Royal College of Nursing. In 1971, Hockey became the Director of the first Nursing Research Unit at the University of Edinburgh (Weir, 2004). She was awarded her PhD on 3 December 1979 and on 4 December the same year was invested Order of the British Empire in recognition of her contribution to nursing research (Mason, 2005: 2). She died on 15 June 2004.

**Baroness Jean McFarlane** of Llandaff (Jean Kennedy McFarlane) was born on 1 April 1926. The youngest child of a large family, she did well at school and went to study sciences at London University. However, her voluntary work with people experiencing difficult life situations led her to undertake a nursing course at Manchester Royal Infirmary, and then later she qualified as both a midwife and health visitor. Her career in nursing saw her lead a project, sponsored by the then Department of Health and Social Security and the RCN (1967), to research nursing care in depth and provide evidence for quality care. McFarlane's role was to summarise the project and produce a literature review on 'The proper study of the nurse' (McFarlane, 1970). She returned to Manchester in the early 1970s to work with the Department of Community Medicine, her vision being that nurses' education should be of graduate standing and prepare them to work equally in a hospital or a community setting. This resulted ultimately in the development of a Bachelor's degree in Nursing with additional health visiting and district nursing qualifications. Her work was renowned on both the national and the international stage. McFarlane was awarded a chair in nursing at Manchester in 1974 – the first in England – and her subsequent work for the Royal Commission on the NHS led to her parliamentary seat in the House of Lords and further influence on a number of select committees. Although Baroness McFarlane died in 2012, her influence on people and undergraduate nurse education continues to evolve and respond to the dynamic world of healthcare provision.

**Margaret Scott Wright** (a contemporary of both Jean McFarlane and Lisbeth Hockey) enjoyed significant nursing and nurse management roles at St George's and the Middlesex Hospitals in London before embarking on a challenging career as a nursing researcher in both Edinburgh and several Canadian universities. Her clinical work spanned a period of immense development of the nursing role in care, the advance of technology in diagnostics and treatment, and a stronger dialogue between medical practitioners and nurses, which would evolve into clinical specialist nursing opportunities. Scott Wright was passionate about the development of nursing research because she believed it would enhance the quality of care provision by adding an academic rigour to the clinical nurse's expertise. She was also one of the first UK nurses to study for a Doctorate of Philosophy (1961) and in 1971 was awarded the first chair of nursing studies in Europe while at Edinburgh University. Her desire to see nursing research as a central theme in nurse education was helped by her role in the influential Briggs Committee which reported to government in 1972 and strongly supported the development of nursing research units across the UK. Her career finally took her to Canada where she continued to have international influence on the development of nursing research.

## So, what can we learn from our nursing history?

We can learn that nursing has, at its roots, nurture, caring, comfort and compassion, ministered by those committed to humanitarian values and often enduring significant hardship in the process. Several conflicts have given rise to ground-breaking innovations and discoveries in medical technology and treatment (as necessity has driven invention), and the evolution of nursing has taken place alongside these. As a result, advances in nursing practice, and more recently nursing research, have often followed the development of medical practice. One thing that we can be absolutely sure of is that as a nursing student you will study, learn, practise and develop your knowledge and skills in the light of new discoveries and treatments. Indeed, nursing in the future will surely be different from what it is today. However, in this regard we must advise some caution: we must be careful not to live in our history because this can distract us from the importance of our present and the potential for nursing's future. A healthy interest in events that have shaped the profession will often provide the impetus and courage to ensure that our nursing practice continues to evolve and can meet the needs of service users in a dynamic world.

- Are you able to identify your reasons for becoming a nurse?
- What is it that you wish to achieve?
- What skills and attributes do you feel you can offer the profession?

Keep a note of your answers to these questions because we shall revisit this topic later in the chapter.

## Where are we now?

Today, those aspiring to be professional nurses can access the benefits of established educational pre-registration programmes which are both validated and monitored by a professional body, the Nursing and Midwifery Council (NMC), and the Higher Education Institution (HEI) in which the course takes place. As new registrants launch their careers, learning continues. Nurses grow in knowledge and skill while experience, reflective practice, and professional discussion facilitate effective, compassionate care for patients and colleagues alike. Several strategies support this development: *Modernising Nursing Careers* (Department of Health, Social Services and Public Safety or DHSSPS, 2006) and *Preceptorship Frameworks* (Department of Health or DH, 2010a; NHS Wales, 2012; Willis Commission, 2012; Northern Ireland Practice and Education Council, 2013; NHS Employers, 2014; Cummings, 2016).

The role of the nurse has extended and nurses are now significant partners with other health professionals and service users in care provision. Increasingly, specialist nurses are the leaders of care and take on additional responsibilities in areas such as prescribing, implementing complex care interventions, and performing minor surgery and other invasive treatments. It is clear that as a profession we are facing an unprecedented rate of change. This is partly in response to the changing face of healthcare itself as we move towards a more community-based focus of care. However, it is also as a result of improvements in treatments and emergent technologies. We face targets and the competitive aspects of a free-market economy, which has been introduced to the NHS where it is almost impossible to put a price on the time you spend with a frightened patient waiting for uncertain news in an A&E, for example. We continue to face increased scrutiny from our service users and those who provide carer support. Increased media coverage has led to an atmosphere of alarm, ambiguity and a perception of neglect, especially in the context of ongoing chronic disease and end of life care. This lack of compassion and kindness was highlighted in its starkest form in the Francis Reports (DH, 2010b, 2013), which provoked a necessary period of professional introspection, an avowed reclaiming of our core values and the emergence of the seven principles of the NHS Constitution (NHS England, 2015), which will be explored and discussed in more detail later in the chapter.

It is our hope that as a registered nurse you will develop the knowledge, skills and confidence to enable you to provide high-quality, evidence-based nursing in a variety of settings. Furthermore, we hope that you will always be sensitive to the needs of those in your care, their families and/or carers, and to your multidisciplinary colleagues with whom you work and communicate in the provision of holistic care.

The parameters for your programme of study are laid down by the NMC in *Future Nurse: Standards of Proficiency for Registered Nurses* (NMC, 2018b). These standards provide a framework to which your university or higher educational institution (HEI) will add the appropriate knowledge and experience that will help you meet these essential requirements (see the Introduction to this book). During your studies you will undoubtedly learn about nursing theory and practice, anatomy and physiology in health and illness, psychology and communication, sociology, pharmacology, microbiology, health promotion and education, law and ethics. When applied to nursing these topics will form the building blocks that will then inform your practice. As you move through a number of practice placements you will begin to appreciate the diverse nature of adult nursing and the various specialist roles of those who work within it. There may well be some aspects that you will find more difficult to learn than others and some areas of practice where you will feel more at home. The point here is that you will be exposed to an essential variety of care settings that will facilitate your development and help you make decisions about where you will want to focus your practice when registered.

Your student experience will also be influenced by both local and national developments in policy and practice, for example National Service Frameworks, Clinical Guidelines or Plans for Care and/or Care Pathways (which will be referred to regularly throughout the chapters that follow).

Essentially then, wherever you undertake your learning, your placement will reflect the fact that contemporary adult nursing takes place in various settings where care is often delivered to a diverse client group. This might seem a tall order if you are new to a nursing programme, but you will bring knowledge and experience with you as you start a course of study, and gradually you will be encouraged and guided to build and extend that knowledge and understanding over the three years of your programme and beyond, thereby embarking on a lifelong learning journey.

This is where a professional portfolio or profile and your skills of reflective practice will prove invaluable. Completing a programme of study in a practice discipline such as nursing is akin to learning to walk up hills and mountains. When you first begin doing so the terrain is unfamiliar and you will find yourself concentrating on your feet so you don't fall over. Sometimes you will get out of breath if you try to climb too quickly or if you are trying to keep up with colleagues. At some point you will stop to catch your breath, turn around and admire the view, just in time to realise how far you have actually come. This then gives you the confidence to look up and out rather than down as the terrain has become more familiar. You will build sufficient stamina to keep going and face each new challenge. Occasionally, you will have to walk round or even down to be able to carry on climbing.

Professional practice can, on occasion, feel very similar to climbing a mountain, reliant as it is on self-awareness, resilience, resourcefulness and courage. All are necessary attributes in the pursuit of safe, self-aware nursing practice. Your professional portfolio or profile is a comprehensive record of your professional achievements and developing reflective skills. It is a requirement of registration with the Nursing and Midwifery Council that every nurse is able to demonstrate that they have met the requirements for practice and continuing professional development (NMC, 2017). Keeping a professional portfolio or profile will help you adopt a 'lifelong learning' approach to both your professional and your personal development in addition to supporting the revalidation process.

Within any profile it is important to provide evidence of that development. This evidence will help you demonstrate to others that you have achieved the required learning outcomes in practice. During your studies you will acquire both study and practice skills to prepare you for your role as a qualified nurse. These skills will include those that are necessary to become a reflective practitioner, i.e. a professional individual who challenges practice in a constructive and helpful way.

Hence your profile is a record of your development as a nurse throughout every aspect of your course. It is a means of demonstrating your ongoing achievement and recording your development throughout your course and beyond. It is also a tool to help you develop the skills of critical awareness, reflective practice, rational decision making and clinical judgement. In summary, your portfolio or profile is your showcase. It gives value to both the practical and the academic work you have completed.

Reflection is a process by which you can think about and achieve better knowledge and understanding of your practice, learning from your own experiences in order to improve the care you provide to patients. Reflecting on our experiences and interactions with others enables us, as caring professionals, to establish what we have learnt and the influence we may have had on others. The key message about reflection here is that it is purposeful and has meaning when it is undertaken and, just as with nursing practice, is constantly evolving. Reflection is often also referred to as reflexivity, acting as an internal monitor or check for an individual's ever-changing self (Todd, 2002: 62). As individuals we learn and evolve through education and a range of professional, personal and third-party experiences; this then influences our behaviours and actions. Reflexivity is an integral part of developing as an effective nurse and is crucial whether we are caring for a dying patient, someone who is suffering from an acute illness or a patient who is in need of additional support to manage a chronic condition.

Schön (1983) suggests that there are two types of reflective practice, reflection in action (in the moment) and reflection on action (looking back on the moment), and purports that experienced nurses are able to reflect while in action and if necessary change and adapt, whereas the novice reflects retrospectively. However, in reality it is likely that these actions occur simultaneously, partly due to the evolution of nurse training since the 1980s. Nursing students are now introduced to the concept of reflection and are encouraged throughout their course and professional life to apply reflexivity to their practice. Reflection is an active, purposeful act intended to make us challenge the nursing world around us. It is a lifelong process of learning about ourselves and how things that happen to us can be thought about, deliberated and acted on. This does not have to be a significant life-changing episode that you may have witnessed with patients (for example a terminal diagnosis); it may be something that has made you stop and consider the impact this has had on you.

There are many different models of reflection that can be used depending on your individual learning style and personal preference. One such example, is the Gibbs reflective cycle (Gibbs, 1988) illustrated in Figure 1.1 which describes reflection as a process with distinct steps, i.e. as a description of what happened and the feelings evoked, followed by your evaluation and analysis of the situation, concluding with a review of the situation, including consideration of what you might do differently and the provision of an action plan based on your learning and aspirations for your future practice.

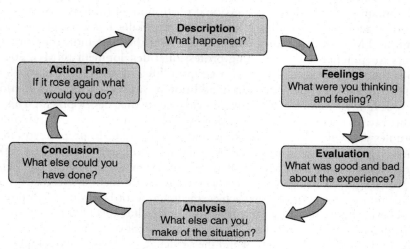

**Figure 1.1**   The Gibbs reflective cycle (1988)

By documenting in your student profile the things you have learned, the challenges you have faced (both the good and bad experiences encountered) and the wide range of people you have met in possibly heart-breaking circumstances, you will not only make a record of your student journey and provide evidence of your achievements, but also build your reflexive aptitude and a capacity for self-awareness which should help you engage more effectively in order to improve patient outcomes. The important thing is that you are able to learn from your experiences and apply what you have learnt to your future practice. By using reflective practice and your profile in this way you should be able to trace the development of your knowledge base and skills for practice, your clinical judgement and decision making, and your leadership and management approaches as you prepare to nurse adults irrespective of their age, health status, culture or disability. The ability to reflect upon practice in this way is something that we will revisit in subsequent chapters.

## 'Profession', 'professional' and 'professionalism'

Throughout this chapter we use the words 'profession' and 'professional' quite liberally. However, it is important to understand the difference between the two.

- What does being professional mean to you?
- Can you describe what professionalism means?

Entering or belonging to a profession means that you have undertaken a specific area of study (mainly at degree level), and the way in which you carry out your work is governed by a set of codes and standards that is regulated by legislation (law). As a professional, you have a certain level of autonomy and you are both responsible and accountable for all of your actions. Belonging to a profession affords a status; being professional describes how you conduct yourself in that status. 'Professionalism' describes a set of values and behaviours that influence not just what you do but also how and when you do it. Professionalism is also framed in terms of awareness, attitudes and behaviours and relates to having sufficient professional judgement to identify the attitude and type of behaviour that are appropriate in any given situation. This is a distinction that may sometimes be missed. In all of the caring professions, professionalism includes the ability to demonstrate the following values:

- Integrity;
- Honesty;
- Transparency;
- A sense of duty;
- Decency.

These are the values that will dictate how you should behave as a professional and therefore will have a direct impact on patient care. Indeed, being an accountable professional is the first platform of the NMC (2018b) proficiencies.

## ACTIVITY 1.2

1. Go to the Scottish Government website and access and read the Chief Nursing Officer (CNO) for Scotland's report below which focuses on professionalism: CNO for Scotland (2012), 'Professionalism in nursing, midwifery and the allied health professions in Scotland: a report to the Coordinating Council for the NMAHP Contribution to the Healthcare Quality Strategy for NHS Scotland' (available at: www.gov.scot/Publications/2012/07/7338).

Write down the key elements that are thought to be important and keep these handy. You will need to compare these later.

2. Now access the Health and Care Professions Council UK (HCPC) website and download the latest report focusing on 'Fitness to practise' cases referred to professional regulators (available at www.hcpc-uk.org.uk:publications/reportsindex).
3. Make a list of the type of cases the HCPC is likely to consider.
4. Access a copy of the subsequent study commissioned as a result of these findings by going to www.hpc-uk.org and go to 'research publications'. Download the *Professionalism in Healthcare Professionals* document (HCPC, 2011).

In the study outlined in the report on the Scottish Government's website above, you may notice a trend in cases linked to a broad range of behaviours which were distinct from technical capability and generally termed 'professionalism'. The subsequent study carried out by Durham University included students and educators from three different regulated health professions (paramedics, occupational therapists and podiatrists/chiropodists) and provides an excellent summary of what professionalism entails. It also puts this in the context of healthcare in terms of relevant examples.

The key findings of the study were that:

1. The concept of what professionalism is remains common regardless of the professional group, status or training route;
2. Regulations are considered to be basic guidance and signposting on what is appropriate and what is unacceptable behaviour (acting as a baseline for behaviour rather than a specification) (HCPC, 2011).

An appropriate set of moral values and personal qualities must be the foundation to which we would add specialist knowledge and clinical skills. The above study supports the view that it is both possible and desirable to 'be professional' before acquiring the necessary knowledge and skills to become a registered professional. This is particularly crucial in the context of healthcare students who, unlike many other undergraduate students, must be professional from day one because they must interact with patients, families and qualified healthcare professionals while on placements. Professionalism is the consequence of qualities that an individual brings to the profession – indeed many of those questioned in the study felt that this was an essential part of themselves. Yet how does this manifest itself?

Consider the examples in the following 'Stop and Think'.

The way in which we present ourselves is significant because it is the first impression people will get. What does it say about you if:

- You regularly turn up on time for lectures or shifts?
- You respond to a text during your first meeting with your practice assessor or supervisor?
- You often appear dishevelled and unkempt?
- You turn up to pre-arranged meetings with your supervisor or assessor having undertaken some preparation beforehand?
- You are sometimes rude or brusque?
- You listen carefully and act upon feedback?

How might a patient interpret each of the above behaviours in terms of the standard of care they will receive?

Obviously, there will always be the odd occasion when we are running late and even with the very best of intentions our plans can sometimes go wrong. However, turning up on time to meetings, lectures or shifts in practice is one way of demonstrating our ongoing commitment – to patients, colleagues and other professionals. Similarly, being rude to or about our colleagues gives a very poor impression to patients and their families, not only of ourselves as individuals but of the whole team providing care. Faulkner (1998) argues that those who find it difficult to communicate effectively with each other are less likely to be effective when interacting with patients and families. This is also demonstrated by HCPC UK (2011) who found that individuals who are professional have an innate sense of decency towards others and suggest that they are polite, courteous, non-condescending, and act honestly and with integrity.

## How do legal and ethical principles underpin our professional practice?

The law may be broadly defined as:

The system of rules which a particular country or community recognises as regulating the actions of its members and which it may enforce by the imposition of penalties. (*Oxford English Dictionary*, 2014b)

This is clearly reflected in *The Code* (NMC, 2018a: 18) where it states that, as a nurse:

- You should uphold the reputation of your profession at all times;
- You should display a personal commitment to the standards of practice and behaviour set out in *The Code*;
- You should be a model of integrity and leadership for others to aspire to.

This should lead to trust and confidence in the profession from patients, people receiving care, other healthcare professionals and the public.

As our professional roles develop alongside innovations in healthcare knowledge and practice, associated technologies and increasing public demand, Wheeler (2012: 3) reminds us that 'moral values guide our thinking and behaviour and impact on our ethical decision making in relation to caring'. Therefore, as a student of nursing you are a developing professional and it is essential that you understand *The Code* (NMC, 2018a) to which you ultimately aspire and how this relates to all aspects of your everyday life and work.

---

### ACTIVITY 1.3

Access and read the latest copy of the NMC *Code*, available at www.nmc.org.uk/standards/code.

- What do you consider to be the aims of *The Code*?
- Which elements do you consider to be the most important and why?

---

*The Code* (NMC, 2018a) is designed to ensure that your practice is safe and that you do not leave your actions open to challenge. However, you are also expected to explore topics such as moral values, ethical theories, attitude development, accountability, confidentiality, integrity and trust, to mention but a few. Each of these will underpin the relationships you form with service users, colleagues, the profession and society in general. Developing your knowledge base to include these aspects will help you increase your appreciation of how legal requirements affect your work and also be alert to situations where you should gain further advice and support.

If an understanding of the law helps us to have better understanding of what is considered to be legally right and wrong within the parameters of our nursing practice, then an appreciation of ethical principles helps us determine, through a process of structured reasoning, the morally 'good' course of action from the 'bad'. In both cases the perception of what is right and what is good will be influenced by your personal beliefs and values. For example, in a previous Stop and Think when asked to reflect on why you want to become a nurse, you may have considered that your desire is driven by your own moral compass, including your personal beliefs and values. Is this perhaps related to a belief in the centrality of integrity, compassion and a willingness to be kind and caring, and a wish to empathise with those in need? However, what happens if your impulse is not based on a willingness to care? What if you are not empathic or non-judgemental?

It is important for nurses to be open-minded and able to care equally for all individuals, irrespective of their illness, age, sexuality, race or religion. As an adult nurse you will be required to adhere to the ethical principles enshrined within *The Code* (NMC, 2018a), including the intention to do good, the insight to do no harm, the capacity to ensure justice, and the competence to promote dignity by respecting autonomy and affording participation and choice (Beauchamp and Childress, 2013). This is a complex and complicated process that relies on commitment and conviction, and will require discipline and an enduring capacity to explore your own impulses. You will need to foster an ability to justify and articulate your choices in terms of both your actions and your omissions. You will often be called on to balance your private understandings against public expectations and professional requirements, and to promote the best interest of individuals, society and the profession. You will need to accept shared professional parameters and role model professional values. You will also need to understand and be able to articulate your obligations to clients and colleagues alike.

It is vital to your own development – and more specifically to those in receipt of your care – that you are sure of the moral basis of your impetus to nurse. You may remember the answers you gave to the previous Stop and Think above. However, we would invite you to expand on these here and reflect upon the following questions:

- What informs your impulse to care?
- Why have you deliberately opted to work with individuals experiencing illness?
- How would you define nursing?
- What makes a good nurse and what kind of nurse do you want to be?
- As a conduit through which caring is facilitated, what skills do you possess/would you like to foster in order to best enact your nursing role?
- How might these skills be best secured and articulated?
- How can you give yourself the best chance of success?
- What are your goals?
- What are your sources of motivation and inspiration?

When reflecting upon how you might define nursing you may wish to consider the three definitions of nursing that have evolved over the last 150 years:

Nature alone cures … and what nursing has to do … is to put the patient in the best condition for nature to act upon him. (Nightingale, 1859)

The unique function of the nurse is to assist the individual – sick or well – in the performance of those activities contributing to health or its recovery (or to peaceful death) that he would perform unaided if he had the necessary strength, will or knowledge. And to do this in such a way as help him gain independence as rapidly as possible. (Henderson, 1960)

Nursing is the use of clinical judgement in the provision of care to enable people to improve, maintain, or recover health, to cope with health problems and to achieve the best possible quality of life – whatever their disease or disability until death. (RCN, 2014)

As a registered nurse you will inevitably face a range of ethical dilemmas during the course of your studies and indeed throughout your professional life. As the conduit of care, your moral compass will dictate your actions and inform your choices. Patients deserve to be nursed at all times by someone who is careful, compassionate and considerate. This calls for purposeful moral engagement combined with emotional intelligence based on a deliberate intention to place patients at the centre of all your care, a personal philosophy of nursing as privilege and the facilitation of candour in terms of truthfulness and transparency. We work in partnership with those we care for, fostering a deliberate shared-care ethos whereby we recognise the autonomy and inner resources of those we nurse.

The concept of moral engagement arises from social cognitive theory (Bandura, 1986, 1991) and requires you to stand firm in your moral behaviour, despite the possibility of peer or social pressure to act differently. This takes moral courage. Bandura suggests that a sure way to demonstrate this concept is through empathy. This means that you must accept responsibility for your behaviours and demonstrate a humane concern for others at all times. This ability to self-govern our behaviours ensures that we are able to consider best practice and best interest for those in our care.

In April 2015, the Criminal Justice and Courts Act made it an offence for 'an individual who has the care of another individual by virtue of being a care worker to ill-treat or wilfully to neglect that individual'. It relates to the conduct of the individual and applies to healthcare workers (such as nurses, doctors, dentists and the like) and exposes what that person did, or did not do, for the patient rather than specifically any harm caused. Offences under this and associated legislation extend to all patients irrespective of mental capacity or age. Griffith (2015) reports that neglect is said to occur where a healthcare worker does not do what is expected of them in relation to patient care provision, and can include omission of medication, incorrect recording of care or failing to assist a patient in difficulty. It is clear that nurses must be honest and truthful at all times and meet the standards of law and the NMC by understanding the need to follow good practice. Nurses must be able to justify the reasons for their actions and duty of care, and all verbal engagement and records must reflect their precise involvement in any care provision.

Emotional intelligence (EI) is defined by Vitello-Cicciu (2002) as the ability to perceive and regulate your own emotions and those of others in a way that positively influences communication, motivation and team work. Snowden et al. (2015) comment that, although elements of EI may be trait based, it can also be learned. The concept has gained popularity in a nursing context and appears to have links with quality of care provision, supports reflective practice and thus facilitates an increase in nurse resilience. Fernandez et al. (2012) explored the notion that higher levels of EI might link to increased performance and, although there are limited available studies as to whether EI can influence academic intelligence, Codier and Odell (2014) found a positive correlation between academic performance and EI in Year 1 student nurses. According to Goleman (1995) there are five integrated EI domains: self-awareness, self-regulation, motivation, empathy and social skills. An interesting longitudinal study from Snowden et al. (2015) found that previous caring experiences did not mean that EI was heightened but rather that over time specific strategies to support the development of EI were helpful. Most recently, Carragher and Gormley (2016) have explored the link between EI and leadership, demonstrating the importance of this quality to the promotion of effective and supportive leadership. We will be revisiting the importance of EI again in subsequent chapters.

Resilience is defined as an ability to adapt to, or recover from, change or challenging situations (McAllister and McKinnon, 2009) and where you learn new skills to address similar situations in the future. It originates from the Latin, *to rebound*. Nurses meet both joy and grief in their everyday work and must be able to respond to and support patients in joy and adversity. In addition, they must manage the demands of professionals working alongside the current constraints on the care provision workforce and regulatory changes. These challenges are complex and Hart et al. (2014) link the lack of resilience to increased stress, dissonance and the likelihood that healthcare workers will leave their profession for work of lesser emotional and ethical challenge. This requires nurse educators to be proactive in the facilitation of your learning and to include resilience as part of your professional and personal development. You may ask why this is important but, as Stephens (2013) suggests, you will inevitably meet new situations that challenge your existing views and beliefs, such that you must review the basis of your existing knowledge and be prepared to explore further. You will learn these skills, not just from a theoretical perspective but also during your practice learning together with clinical colleagues and via your reflections. Thomas and Revell (2016) suggest that this aspect of development will not just benefit you in the longer term but will help to create an environment in which your wish to learn will flourish.

# The 10 commitments of nursing: from 6 to 10

We have established that caring and compassion have been fundamental aspects of a nurse's role since nursing's inception, and that good moral values and personal qualities are central to who a person is and will ultimately directly impact on their behaviour towards others. You will note that the title of this chapter begins with values and is followed by knowledge and skills, which, in their entirety, underpin nursing practice and ultimately give rise to the best possible patient outcomes. Without the appropriate set of values and personal qualities, there is no foundation on which to add the building blocks of clinical skills, education, professional standards, codes and ethics.

In 2012, and in recognition of the importance of these values, the Chief Nursing Officer of England and the Director of Nursing at the Department of Health launched a new strategy (DH, 2012b) based on six core values (the 6Cs), which were adopted as a means to determine effective care. This followed similar standards previously outlined in Northern Ireland (DHSSPS, 2006, 2008). These include moral values, professionalism and aspects of dedication that are used to define the basis of good quality nursing care.

The key elements identified within this framework are outlined below (Figure 1.2):

- *Care*: the care we deliver helps the individual person and improves the health of the whole community. Caring defines us in our work. The people receiving care expect it to be right for them consistently throughout every stage of their life.
- *Compassion*: this is how the care is given through relationships based on respect.

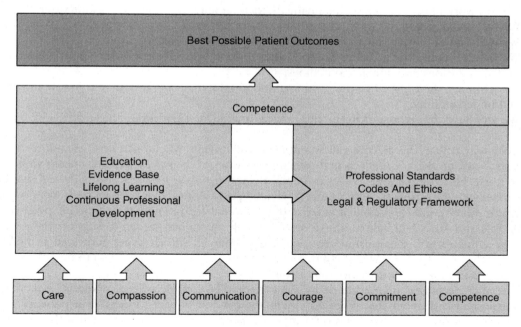

**Figure 1.2**  The 6Cs: the foundations of professional nursing practice

- *Communication*: this is central to successful caring relationships and effective team working. All successful interactions between individuals are based on good communication, which comes in many formats and encompasses multiple means, such as non-verbal, verbal and written.
- *Courage*: this relates to us as nurses having the courage to do the right thing for the people we care for, to speak up when we have concerns, and to have the personal strength and vision to embrace new ways of working.
- *Commitment*: commitment to our patients and populations is the cornerstone of what we do and we need to build on this to improve the care and experience of our patients.
- *Competence*: all those in caring roles must have the ability to understand an individual's health and social needs, and have the clinical expertise and technical knowledge to deliver effective care and treatments based on research and evidence. In 2015, 'candour' was an additional C added by the NMC and relates to 'a professional responsibility to be honest with patients when things go wrong'.

In 2016 Cummings, in her role as CNO for England, played a key role in the publication of *Leading Change, Adding Value*, which enhanced her concept of the 6Cs and introduced the 10 commitments as described here:

1. We will promote a culture where improving the population's health is a core component of the practice of all nursing, midwifery and care staff (health improvement);
2. We will increase the visibility of nursing and midwifery leadership and input in prevention;
3. We will work with individuals, families and communities to equip them to make informed choices and manage their own health;
4. We will be centred on individuals experiencing high value care;
5. We will work in partnership with individuals, their families, carers and others important to them;
6. We will actively respond to what matters most to our staff and colleagues;
7. We will lead and drive research to evidence the impact of what we do;
8. We will champion the use of technology and informatics to improve practice, address unwarranted variations and enhance outcomes;
9. We will have the right education, training and development to enhance our skills, knowledge and understanding;
10. We will have the right staff in the right places and at the right time.

As you may realise, the six core values and ten commitments, as outlined here, are not really new. They are based on the key fundamental principles of what have always been considered vital to the role of nurse. Florence Nightingale, for example, always tried to strive for accessibility and simplicity of expression and to stress the importance of enacting core values. However, perhaps there is now a need to be more specific and explicit in terms of what these are and how they underpin practice.

The 7Cs and 10Cs highlighted above resonate with the values needed to support the development of a therapeutic relationship. You will notice that all the elements enshrined in both are framed within *The Code* (NMC, 2018a), and all are used by nurses in tandem to help them refine their appreciation of the complexity that is nursing.

Remember, nothing you will ever do as nurses should be considered basic. Nursing is a complex and purposeful endeavour that relies on you as the conduit of care to meet your patients' needs. Everything you do as a nurse relies on a myriad of technical and interpersonal skills, which are themselves underpinned by multiple intelligences, including intellectual, moral, social and aesthetic ways of knowing and seeing the world.

---

### ⊡ ACTIVITY 1.4

Compare the 6Cs Framework and the 10 commitments outlined above with the principles outlined by the CNO for Scotland in Activity 1.2, the NHS Constitution (NHS England, 2015) and the Royal College of Nursing's *Principles of Practice* (RCN, 2011).

   You can access the NHS Constitution document at the following website: www.nhs.uk/choice intheNHS/Rightsandpledges/NHSConstitution/Pages/Overview.aspx

---

## Upholding the professional reputation of nursing

Thus far we have outlined the fundamental values and principles of nursing practice. However, let's now stop and think about contemporary nursing practice.

- What is the image of nursing today?
- How is the nursing profession perceived by patients, carers and/or members of the general public?

Follow the link as detailed below which will take you to the personal account of Christina Patterson, a well-known and respected journalist: www.bbc.co.uk/programmes/b010mrzt (this highlights a programme recorded for BBC Radio 4 (2011), entitled 'Care to be a nurse?', in which she describes her experiences while undergoing six operations for breast cancer over a period of eight years at different hospitals).

   While listening consider the following questions and make a note of your answers:

- What were the key issues here?
- Why do you think this happened?
- How did Christina feel?
- How does this account make *you* feel?
- As a nurse involved in Christina's care what would you have done differently?
- Were there any barriers – and if so – how might you have overcome them?
- What were the key positive nursing actions important to her?

*The Code* (NMC, 2018a) requires us to 'be open and honest, act with integrity and uphold the reputation' of our profession, and therefore it would be disingenuous if we did not acknowledge the gravity and extent of the challenges to the nursing profession's reputation over the last few years. Although it is important to recognise that in some areas there are excellent standards of nursing care we have to acknowledge the evidence that demonstrates that in other areas current opinion of the nursing profession is low. At this point should we perhaps look at events that have brought into question the professional reputation of nurses over the last few years? We need to try to work out why and how these events have been allowed to happen and then create a strategy of both reform and support to ensure that they will not do so again. One of the key aspects that Christina focuses on is a lack of care, compassion and 'basic human kindness'. Crucially, before Christina went into hospital the first time she wasn't worried about her care since she didn't think she would have to. Yet she experienced poor care consistently throughout her patient journey. Why was this? Where was the effective communication, care and compassion for her situation, the competence and commitment to provide the best evidence-based care and the courage to ensure that the nurses who worked with her understood her personal journey through ill health? As her case clearly demonstrates, somewhere along the way the nurses involved in the delivery of her care seemed to have lost sight of the art of nursing. This example indicates that vulnerability and patient status constitute universal features of the illness experience. Hallett (2012) considers a range of potential factors that may have contributed to Christina's poor experience, including:

- The changing emphasis towards more technical skills and knowledge;
- The shift in roles between what doctors used to have sole responsibility for and the extended role of the nurse;
- The professionalisation of the nursing role;
- The delegation of primary care to healthcare assistants;
- Bureaucracy and box ticking given priority over compassion;
- The wider social, economic and political factors.

Christina's account also adds to revelations from the Care Quality Commission's (CQC's) inspection of over 150 hospitals and care homes (CQC, 2013), the events at Winterbourne View Hospital (BBC, 2012; DH, 2012a), the Princess of Wales and Neath Port Talbot hospitals (Andrews and Butler, 2014) and the publication of the Francis Reports (DH, 2010b, 2013) leading to the abuse and 'appalling suffering of many patients' between 2005 and 2008 at the Mid Staffordshire Foundation NHS Trust.

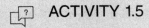 **ACTIVITY 1.5**

Access and read the following documents:

1. The Francis Report.
   You can find this information on the Executive Summary and recommendations at: www.midstaffs publicinquiry.com/report
2. Care Quality Commission (CQC), Nursing and Midwifery Council (NMC) and NHS Wales responses to the Francis Report.

You can find this information at the following websites:

- www.cqc.org.uk/content/care-quality-commission-response-francis-report
- www.cqc.org.uk/content/cqc-highlights-changes-following-francis-report
- www.nmc-uk.org/About-us/Our-response-to-the-Francis-Inquiry-Report

Make a list of all factors identified in each report.

The original report into events at Mid Staffs (DH, 2010b) noted that 'It was striking how many accounts related to basic nursing care as opposed to clinical errors leading to injury or death'. Jane Cummings (Chief Nursing Officer for England) noted that 'such poor care is a betrayal of all that we stand for' (DH, 2012b: 7). The Francis Report (DH, 2013) went on to highlight 290 recommendations for stakeholders to consider across a wide and enduring spectrum of concern including the neglect, negligence and abuse of individuals, along with a wide range of associated factors including organisational structures, staff shortages, management policies, bonus payments for managers and the imposition of targets devoid of any research evidence base. Nor did the CQC emerge from the Francis Report unscathed because it was clear that their criteria for inspection were not sufficiently robust. A response issued by the CQC (2013) acknowledged these shortcomings, highlighting a schedule of changes including the appointment of an Inspector of Hospitals, a more searching assessment process in profiling institutions and an expert base for their inspection teams. They also reaffirmed their remit to monitor the quality of healthcare environments for the people who matter most – service users.

Although the vast majority of nurses would find these behaviours and actions to be as abhorrent as they are incomprehensible, you will by now have recognised that nurses have a personal duty of care that includes obligations and promises to adhere to the standards as espoused within *The Code* (NMC, 2018a). This means that we are personally and collectively responsible and accountable for the decisions we make and the actions we take, regardless of the pressures or environment within which we are working. This therefore calls upon us to display courage and commitment, acting as advocates for our patients to ensure that we always act in their 'best interest'.

## The challenges to contemporary practice

At the outset of this chapter we outlined the challenges faced by nurses, whether they be in the nature of some of the very personal aspects of the work, the issues of gender, the fight for recognition as a profession, the emotional labour involved or the hardships of nursing during wartime. Some of these challenges remain ever present whereas others will change and evolve. Many of these are covered in more depth in later chapters but this chapter highlights some of the key issues facing nurses today. Perhaps the most significant challenge is that of public perception, namely the image of nursing and the prevailing culture of care within our profession.

Advances in technology and the changing emphasis in recent years on nurses becoming more technically specialised have been blamed in a number of quarters for the loss of care and compassion (Hallett, 2007; Pearcey, 2008; Law and Aranda, 2010). However, we should consider whether these two must be mutually exclusive. We would be failing ourselves and our profession if we did not maintain our competence and continue to develop as techniques and technology improve. Hallett (2007) also suggests that core values are constants whereas technology is a tool to be wielded in the services of health.

When people require any kind of medical intervention, it is the level of empathic and compassionate care they receive that makes the difference between a good and a bad experience: it is good communication (especially listening carefully), kindness, caring and empathy and not the technical intervention (which is almost taken as a given) that really make the difference. It is also clear that such values, qualities and behaviours are crucial to good nursing. In one study, Smith (2012) found that 44 different words or phrases were used by patients to describe 'ideal' and 'real' nurses. Interestingly, only six of these related to functional attributes such as efficient, observant and capable of doing their job. The caring and emotional aspects of nursing were clearly seen as distinct but complementary to and, more importantly, underpinning the functional aspects of everything we do as nurses. Kindness, helpfulness and patience were the attributes most frequently used. Talking, listening, showing interest and sympathy also featured heavily as aspects of the ideal nurse. It is clear how these attributes align closely with *The Code* (NMC, 2018a), 7Cs and subsequent 10 commitments (DH, 2012b; GMC/NMC, 2015; Cummings, 2016), but perhaps all of this is best expressed by one patient who concluded:

> A nurse has to be aware of the patient's condition and how to tackle it. She has to have a nursing manner which requires a lot of patience and forethought and to try and relieve pain and suffering not by medical means but by compassion. (Smith, 2012: 27)

Furthermore, perhaps as a result of wider access to the internet, the public are much better informed and have access to a huge amount of information and related data about their health. They will often have high expectations in terms of openness and transparency, and the right to be included and informed. As a result, as nurses we must work hard to keep our own knowledge up to date and ensure that our practice is firmly based on sound evidence. We must also demonstrate care and compassion not only in how we treat our patients and their families, but also in respecting their right to be involved in all the decisions affecting them. Respect, privacy and dignity should feature strongly in every aspect of our care delivery. We must ensure that we listen to their concerns, needs and wants, acting as patient advocates when required. This requires commitment to ensure that we are continually updating our knowledge and that we maintain our competency. It also requires good communication to ensure that we listen to people's concerns and answer their questions, making sure that we explain ourselves clearly and that we have been understood (a topic that will be focused on in more detail in subsequent chapters).

## Fitness to practise

Part of the NMC's role as a professional regulator is to maintain the professional register and ensure that the public are protected from poor practice. The NMC takes these aspects of their work most seriously in order to maintain the reputation of the profession and promote public confidence that nurses on the register meet the necessary standards of a competent practitioner. There are procedures in place to guide employers, colleagues and the public who wish to raise concerns about any nurse's fitness to practise and the NMC investigates these concerns thoroughly.

So, what does the term 'fitness to practise' mean? The current NMC guidance (NMC, 2016) states that a nurse who is fit to practise is one who has successfully completed an approved pre-registration education programme, is registered with the NMC and thereafter maintains that ability to practise safely and independently while following the professional code of practice as set out in *The Code* (NMC, 2018a). In practical terms this means that, as a nurse, you maintain appropriate standards of proficiency, ensure that you are of good health and good character, and that you adhere to the principles of good practice that are set out in the various standards, guidance and advice.

The notion of being suitably prepared by your educational programme to undertake the nurse registrant's role, and that you should have valid and current registration with the regulatory body, is really quite straightforward. Demonstrating that you are of good health and good character is closely linked to the ways in which you work and live and ensuring that these are aligned to *The Code* (NMC, 2018a).

### ⬚ ACTIVITY 1.6

Follow the links on the NMC website and read the current version of *The Code* and the information related to fitness to practise and good health and good character.

Make a note of any questions that occur to you as you read this and consider where or to whom you might go for help in answering your questions.

Some of your questions may well be 'How do I prepare for this responsibility?' or 'What happens if something occurs that means I question my own fitness to practise?'.

It is important that we explore this concept of 'fitness to practise' with you and what it means to be of good health and good character. You will soon appreciate that during your programme of study you will normally be well prepared to face the challenges of professional life and demonstrate the knowledge, skills, behaviours and standards of care that the public would expect from nurses.

During your programme of study there will be information and opportunities for discussion which will enable you to develop a better understanding of these concepts and recognise the implications for student nurses who fail to study appropriately and/or fail to abide by *The Code* (NMC, 2018a) to which you aspire. Although you are not expected to enter your pre-registration education with all the required professional attributes, it is important to ensure that you are made aware of these concepts, that you understand them, and that you grow in competence and confidence with regard to these skills alongside other areas of your development.

We will start with the concept of good health. You may wonder why demonstrating good health is an essential component of a nurse's fitness to practise. Clearly, if we are able to demonstrate that we lead a healthy lifestyle then the benefits of this are that we may be better able to guide those in our care. However, there will be occasions for all of us where we become temporarily incapacitated such that we are unable to work or study. In these circumstances our professional behaviour is to follow the relevant sickness and absence policies. There may be some conditions that challenge our ability to undertake our role safely and competently. At these times it is vital that we seek appropriate support in a timely way to make certain that we have the right help and that we do not endanger our colleagues or service users. Often it is not the event or incidence of ill health that becomes an issue but rather what we have done about it. Have we been honest with ourselves and others? Have we sought appropriate professional support and guidance?

The NMC (2018b: 8) proficiencies state that nurses must 'understand the professional responsibility to adopt a healthy lifestyle to maintain the level of personal fitness and wellbeing required to meet people's needs for mental and physical care'. How does this proficiency relate to the situations highlighted above?

How are we to interpret this competency perhaps in relation to going to work even though we are not really well enough?; a nurse living with diabetes not taking regular breaks for food or medication; a student who feels that they never have a hangover so they can drink heavily before going on duty. All these actions demonstrate a lack of insight into our health, wellbeing and professional obligations. Health issues can catch us all out.

- Should a nurse smoke or be over- or underweight?
- Should nurses at all times role model healthy behaviour?
- Are nurses policing or promoting health?

There are four main areas from which an individual's fitness to practise can be called into question. These are criminal behaviour, dishonesty, unprofessional behaviour and ill health (Ellis et al., 2011). Here you will see that honesty and integrity figure highly in the professional equation, i.e. our ability to know right from wrong and thus act appropriately.

In considering these four areas again it may be that some activities feel easier to identify than others: for example, harm to another person; stealing; misuse of or dealing in illegal substances; fraudulent activity; and the abuse of vulnerable people. These are unacceptable behaviours and ones that do not adhere to *The Code* (NMC, 2018a). However, by reading this chapter you should also be aware that unprofessional behaviours (e.g. ongoing poor time management, rudeness to service users or colleagues, breach of confidentiality, examination cheating or plagiarism, and bullying) are equally relevant.

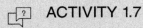

## ACTIVITY 1.7

Visit the NMC website and find a case presented to the Fitness to Practise Committee that related to out-of-work activities compromising their professionalism.

- How do you feel about these circumstances?
- Which circumstances were work related and which occurred in their own personal time?

Perhaps what is particularly significant here is the notion that what happens in your personal life is just as important as events in your professional, registrant and/or student life.

Whether you are a student or a registrant, sit back for a minute and think about the things you do in terms of email correspondence, being out with friends or engaging in online social media:

- How do you speak to people?
- Does this vary depending on who it is?
- Do you use a form of shorthand in text or on social media?
- Is this appropriate?
- Does it matter?

These are the sorts of questions you must be able to answer. Perhaps you can discuss this with fellow colleagues, teachers or line managers. As students we are able to seek advice and feedback from teachers and mentors to support our professional development and, since 2004, we have been asked as students to affirm that we are of good health and good character in line with the NMC Quality Assurance (QA) Framework requirements for pre-registration courses (NMC, 2017).

As registrants we also affirm our good health and character each year when our registration is renewed, and it is clearly stated in *The Code* (NMC, 2018a) that we have a duty to inform both our employer and the NMC of any concerns we have about our ability to practise safely or any involvement with the police as soon as possible after a concern has been highlighted. Do remember that any caution or conviction recorded by the police remains on your personal record for life and is viewed by employers through the Disclosure and Barring Service (further information about this service can be accessed at the following website: www.gov.uk/government/organisations/disclosure-and-barring-service).

What are the processes for investigating 'fitness to practise' in your school of nursing and how are these issues addressed in your programme of study?

Now visit www.nmc.org.uk/concerns-nurses-midwives/hearings and compare your university process with that of the NMC when investigating allegations of professional misconduct.

- What differences have you highlighted?
- Does your university process mirror that of the NMC?

Most students and registrants do not have their fitness to practise challenged in such a way that requires investigation and possible sanction. David and Bray (2009) acknowledge that the percentage of students investigated via these procedures is thought to be low. The reason for this is that, although each university is charged with having a 'fitness to practise' procedure for students, there is no central collation of the number of students investigated or the outcomes of such investigations. However, from half a million registered nurse and midwives less than 1% of registrants had concerns raised against them, meaning that a total of 5476 cases were investigated by the NMC in 2016–17 (NMC, 2017).

David and Lee-Woolf (2010) also point out that student nurses are still learning and therefore the seriousness of any given situation may vary dependent on the stage reached in the programme of study. However, it is necessary that you are aware of the potential pitfalls that can sometimes catch you unawares and you must not close your eyes to the subject. You should be careful to be self-aware and not self-righteous in respect of this concept, ensuring that by safe practice and reflective development you are able to recognise any problems or challenges to your practice and act appropriately. Similarly, as a registrant, although there is an expectation that you will adhere to *The Code* (NMC, 2018a), there is also an acknowledgement of varying degrees of experience that may impact on any allegation that questions your fitness to practise as a nurse.

Both student and registrant processes that examine fitness to practise have a number of sanctions that can be applied to any given situation. These can range from there being no case to answer, through varying levels of supervision or suspension, to a student's place on their course being withdrawn or a registrant removed from the register permanently. Whatever the outcome in relation to the sanctions applied, there must be robust evidence in support of any allegations made and the probability of the event reoccurring must be balanced against the sanction chosen.

In most cases – as either student or registrant – there will be evidence of mitigation to be considered alongside an allegation. It is important to realise that such mitigation can never condone an unprofessional action but it may be used to determine the outcome and level of sanction imposed.

> ### ⬚? ACTIVITY 1.8
>
> Explore the summary on professional behaviour which you will find on the NMC website https://www.nmc.org.uk/globalassets/sitedocuments/other-publications/enabling-professionalism.pdf
> Are you ready to be a professional?
> Now visit the section of the NMC website where professional practice hearings are recorded, then continue with the activity as it was. What do you think?

## The importance of evidence-based practice

We have acknowledged growing public awareness and the perennial challenge that nurses should be able to justify their actions. *The Code* (NMC, 2018a) also tells us to ensure that our nursing practice should be based on the best available evidence. Therefore, as adult nurses we must learn how to find this evidence and ascertain whether or not it is good.

Good, evidence-based, patient-centred care is vital to modern healthcare and will underpin the expertise and sensitivity of care strategies, thus demonstrating the quality of care provision (Emanuel et al., 2011). Evidence-based practice is an essential component in defining the efficacy of our nursing practice, though it is perhaps worthwhile realising that we will not find a research base for every aspect of care. However, the increasing breadth of knowledge and technology available to inform our decisions adds weight to the explanations of why we do what we do. Our knowledge base for nursing is influenced by knowledge from other disciplines such as the physical and social sciences, law and ethics. We must be able to work with these different elements and apply them to all the clinical situations we encounter.

The capacity to know what is the right thing to do in any nursing situation relies on our ability to explore the relevant and current knowledge in a certain area, to understand what that is trying to tell us, and for us to utilise our research appreciation skills to distil whether or not this knowledge can be applied to a particular situation. Although this is a tall order, we as professional nurses are committed to lifelong learning that will facilitate our clinical development over our working lives.

Therefore, during your programme of study or as a registrant you will be expected to learn and develop the skills of research appraisal (see Chapter 6). These will enable you to reflect critically on research worthiness and not only to understand the implications of research for nursing care but also to play your part in ensuring that appropriate research-based care strategies are implemented in practice.

## Developing your nursing skills

We all enter nursing with different levels of life experience and emotional maturity, and these can differ widely regardless of age. The concept of emotional intelligence is often associated with experiential learning and learning from the lessons of life, and this will evolve as we are exposed to more such experiences and gain experience in the nursing context (Bulmer Smith et al., 2009).

- Are you ready to practise nursing?
- Are you fit to practise?

Pause for moment and reflect on whether these questions are asking the same thing.

- How would you answer these questions if asked?

## Chapter summary

Throughout this chapter we have introduced you to the complexity of the nursing role and hopefully posed challenging questions that will help you to scrutinise your impulse to nurse and aspirations for your future nursing practice. We have drawn your attention to the evolution of nursing by highlighting significant events and people who have helped to shape the profession we have today. In so doing, we have asked you to reflect upon your motivation to nurse and your own philosophy on caring, and to that end we have explored some of the legal, moral and ethical issues that can challenge our fitness to practise. We have also discussed some of the challenges faced by nurses today and the tension that exists between the technical expertise of caring and its softer, yet vital skill counterpart – compassion.

As you begin your lifelong journey in the profession we trust that this chapter has helped you to share our passion for nursing, and has stimulated your interest to read and explore the concepts and issues highlighted in subsequent chapters of this book.

## Further reading

Cullum, N., Ciliska, D., Haynes, B. and Marks, S. (2013) *Evidence Based Nursing: An Introduction.* Chichester: Wiley.

Dimond, B. (2015) *Legal Aspects of Nursing.* Harlow: Pearson Education.

Goleman, D. (1995) *Emotional Intelligence.* New York: Bantam.

Hallett, C. (2014) *Veiled Warriors: Allied Nurses of the First World War.* Oxford: Oxford University Press.

Rafferty, A.M., Philipou, J., Fitzpatrick J.M. and Ball, J. (2015) *'Culture of Care' Barometer*, National Nursing Research Unit, London, Kings College.

Timmins, F. and Duffy, A. (2011) *Writing Your Nursing Portfolio: A Step by Step Guide.* Maidenhead: Open University Press.

## References

Alexander, Z. and Dewjee, A. (1984) *The Wonderful Adventures of Mary Seacole in Many Lands.* Bristol: Falling Wall Press.

Andrews, A. and Butler, M. (2014) *Trusted to Care. An Independent Review of the Princess of Wales Hospital and Neath Port Talbot Hospital at Abertawe Bro Morgannwg University Health Boards (Executive Summary).* Available at: http://gov.wales/topics/health/publications/health/reports/care (last accessed 8 April 2018).

Baly, M. (1997) *Florence Nightingale and the Nursing Legacy.* London: Whurr.

Bandura, A. (1986) *Social Foundations of Thought and Action: A Social Cognitive Theory.* Englewood Cliffs, NJ: Prentice Hall.

Bandura, A. (1991) 'Social cognitive theory of self-regulation', *Organizational Behavior and Human Decision Processes*, 50: 248–87. Available at: www.uky.edu/~eushe2/Bandura/Bandura1991OBHDP.pdf (last accessed 18 May 2018).

BBC Radio 4 (2011) *Four Thought Series 2: Christina Patterson: Care To Be A Nurse?* Available at: www.bbc.co.uk/programmes/b010mrzt

BBC (2012) *The Hospital That Stopped Caring*. Available at: www.bbc.co.uk/programmes/b01nqn4d

Beauchamp, T. and Childress, J. (2013) *Principles of Biomedical Ethics*, 6th edn. Oxford: Oxford University Press.

Bostridge, M. (2008) *Florence Nightingale: The Woman and Her Legend*. London: Penguin.

Bulmer Smith, K., Profetto-McGrath, J. and Cummings, G.G. (2009) 'Emotional intelligence and nursing: an integrative literature review', *International Journal of Nursing Studies*, 46: 1624–36.

Care Quality Commission (2013) *Care Quality Commission Response to Francis Report*. Available at: www.cqc.org.uk/content/care-quality-commission-response-francis-report (last accessed 18 May 2018).

Carragher, J. and Gormley, K. (2016) 'Leadership and emotional intelligence in nursing and midwifery education and practice: a discussion paper', *Journal of Advanced Nursing*, 73(1): 85–96.

Codier, E. and Odell, E. (2014) 'Measured emotional intelligence ability and grade point average in nursing students', *Nurse Education Today*, 34(4): 608–12.

Cummings, J. (2016) *Leading Change, Adding Value: A Framework for Nursing, Midwifery and Care Staff*. London: NHS England.

David, T.J. and Bray, S.A. (2009) 'Healthcare student fitness to practise cases: reason for referral and outcomes', *Education Law Journal*, 196–203.

David, T.J. and Lee-Woolf, E. (2010) 'Fitness to practise for student nurses: principles, standards and procedures', *Nursing Times*, 106(39): 23–6.

Department of Health (2010a) *Preceptorship Framework for Newly Registered Nurses, Midwives and Allied Health Professionals*. London: DH.

Department of Health (2010b) *Independent Inquiry into Care Provided by Mid Staffordshire NHS Foundation Trust, January 2005–March 2009*. London: HMSO. Available at: www.midstaffspublicinquiry.com (last accessed 18 May 2018).

Department of Health (2012a) *Transforming Care: A National Response to Winterbourne Hospital*. London: HMSO. Available at: https://assets.publishing.service.gov.uk/government/uploads/system/uploads/attachment_data/file/213215/final-report.pdf (last accessed 18 May 2018).

Department of Health (2012b) *Compassion in Practice: Nursing, Midwifery and Care Staff: Our Vision and Strategy*. London: HMSO.

Department of Health (2013) *Report of the Mid Staffordshire NHS Foundation Trust Public Inquiry*. London: HMSO. Available at: www.midstaffspublicinquiry.com (last accessed 18 May 2018).

Department of Health, Social Services and Public Safety (2006) *Modernising Nursing Careers: Setting the Direction*. Belfast: DHSSPS.

Department of Health, Social Services and Public Safety (2008) *Improving the Patient and Client Experience*. Belfast: DHSSPS.

Ellis, J., Lee-Woolf, E. and David, T. (2011) 'Supporting nursing students during fitness to practise hearings', *Nursing Standard*, 25(32): 38–43.

Emanuel, V., Day, K. and Diegnan, L. (2011) 'Developing evidence-based practice amongst students', *Nursing Times*, 107(49/50): 21–3.

Faulkner, A. (1998) 'The ABC of palliative care: communication with patients, families and other professionals', *British Medical Journal*, 316(7125): 130–2.

Fernandez, R., Salamonson, Y. and Griffiths, R. (2012) 'Emotional intelligence as a predictor of academic performance in first-year accelerated graduate entry nursing students', *Journal of Clinical Nursing*, 21: 3485–92.

Gibbs, G. (1988) *Learning by Doing, A Guide to Teaching and Learning Methods*. Oxford: Further Education Unit, Oxford Brookes University.

GMC/NMC (2015) *Openness and Honesty When Things Go Wrong: The Professional Duty of Candour*. London: GMC/NMC.

Goleman, D. (1995) *Emotional Intelligence*. New York: Bantam.

Griffith, R. (2015) 'Patient protection: ill-treatment and wilful neglect', *British Journal of Nursing*, 12 June 24(11). Available at: www.magonlinelibrary.com/doi/abs/10.12968/bjon.2015.24.11.600 (last accessed 15 May 2018).

Griffon, D.P. (1995) '"Crowning the edifice": Ethel Fenwick and state registration', *Nursing History Review*, 3: 201–12.

Griffon, D.P. (1998) '"A somewhat duskier skin": Mary Seacole in the Crimea', *Nursing History Review*, 6: 115–27.

Hallett, C.E. (2007) 'Editorial: a "gallop" through history: nursing in social context', *Journal of Clinical Nursing*, 16(3): 429–30.

Hallett, C.E. (2012) *Nursing: the lost art?*. Conference paper presented at the International History of Nursing Conference, Kolding, Denmark, 11 August.

Hart, P.L., Brebban, J.D. and Chesney, M. (2014) 'Resilience in nursing: an integrative review', *Journal of Nursing Management*, 22(6), 720–34.

Hawkins, S. (2010) *Nursing and Women's Labour in the Nineteenth Century*. London: Routledge.

Health and Care Professions Council UK (2011) *Research Report: Professionalism in Healthcare Professionals*. London: HCPC. Available at: www.hpc-uk.org/publications/index.asp?id=s11 (last accessed 15 May 2018).

Helmstadter, C. (1993) 'Old nurses and new: nursing in the London teaching hospitals before and after the mid-nineteenth century reforms', *Nursing History Review*, 1: 43–70.

Helmstadter, C. (1996) 'Nurse recruitment and retention in the 19th century London teaching hospitals', *International History of Nursing Journal*, 2(1): 58–69.

Henderson, V. (1960) *Basic Principles of Nursing Care*. London: International Council of Nurses.

Hockey, L. (2001) *Oral history interview by Jane Brooks in Edinburgh on 8 August 2001*. UK Centre for the History of Nursing and Midwifery, School of Nursing, Midwifery and Social Work, University of Manchester.

Law, K. and Aranda, K. (2010) 'The shifting foundations of nursing', *Nurse Education Today*, 30: 544–7.

Mann Wall, B. (1998) 'Called to a mission of charity: the sisters of St Joseph in the Civil War'. *Nursing History Review*, 6: 85–113.

Mason, K. (2005) *Dr Lisbeth Hockey, 1918–2004: Biography*. Available at: www.bmh.manchester.ac.uk/research/nursing-groups/uk-centre-for-the-history-of-nursing/publications (last accessed 18 May 2018).

McAllister, M. and McKinnon, J. (2009) 'The importance of teaching and learning resilience in the health disciplines: a critical review of the literature', *Nurse Education Today*, 29(4): 371–9. http://dx.doi.org/10.1016/j.nedt.2008.10.011

McFarlane, J.J. (1970) *The Proper Study of the Nurse*. London: Royal College of Nursing.

McGann, S. (1992) *The Battle of the Nurses: A Study of Eight Women Who Influenced the Development of Professional Nursing, 1880–1930*. London: Scutari.

NHS Employers (2014) *Simplified Knowledge and Skills Framework (KSF)*. Available at: www.nhsemployers.org/Simplified (last accessed 18 May 2018).

NHS England (2015) *The NHS Constitution*. London: DH.

NHS Wales (2012) *Preceptorship Foundation Policy for Newly Qualified Nurses*. Available at: www.wales.nhs.uk/sitesplus/documents/862/112PreceptorshipFoundationPolicyForNewlyQualifiedNursesv1.pdf (last accessed 18 May 2018).

Nightingale, F. (1859) *Notes on Nursing: What It Is and What It Is Not*. London: Harrison.

Northern Ireland Practice Education Council (NIPEC) (2013) *Preceptorship Framework for Nursing, Midwifery and Specialist Community Public Health Nursing*. Belfast: NIPEC.

Nursing and Midwifery Council (2016) *Health and Character Guidance for AEIs*. Available at: www.nmc.org.uk/education/what-we-expect-of-educational-institutions/good-health-and-good-character-for-aeis (last accessed 30 April 2018).

Nursing and Midwifery Council (2017) *Quality Assurance Framework*. Available at: www.nmc.org.uk/education/quality-assurance-of-education/qa-framework-for-education (accessed 30 April 2018).

Nursing and Midwifery Council (2018a) *The Code: Professional Standards of Practice and Behaviour for Nurses and Midwives*. Available at: www.nmc.org.uk/globalassets/sitedocuments/nmc-publications/nmc-code.pdf (last accessed 30 April 2018).

Nursing and Midwifery Council (2018b) *Future Nurse: Standards of Proficiency for Registered Nurses*. London: NMC.

O'Brien D'Antonio, P. (1993) 'The legacy of domesticity: nursing in early nineteenth-century America', *Nursing History Review*, 1: 229–46.

Oxford English Dictionary (2014a) Available at: http://dictionary.reference.com/browse/nurse (last accessed 15 May 2018).

Oxford English Dictionary (2014b) Available at: www.oxforddictionaries.com/definition/english/law (last accessed 15 May 2018).

Pearcey, P. (2008) 'Shifting roles in nursing: does role extension require role abdication?', *Journal of Clinical Nursing*, 17(10): 1320–6.

Reverby, S. (1987) *Ordered to Care: The Dilemma of America Nursing*. New York: Cambridge University Press.

Royal College of Nursing (2011) *Principles of Nursing Practice*. Available at: www.rcn.org.uk/professional-development/principles-of-nursing-practice (last accessed 2 May 2018).

Royal College of Nursing (2014) *Defining Nursing*. London: RCN. Available at: www.rcn.org.uk (last accessed 2 May 2018).

Schön, D. (1983). *The Reflective Practitioner: How Professionals Think in Action*. London: Temple Smith.

Smith, P. (2012) *The Emotional Labour of Nursing Revisited*, 2nd edn. Basingstoke: Palgrave Macmillan.

Snowden, A., Stenhouse, R., Young, J., Carver, H., Carver, F. and Brown, N. (2015) 'The relationship between emotional intelligence, previous caring experience and mindfulness in student nurses and midwives: a cross sectional analysis', *Nurse Education Today*, 35(1): 152–8. Available at: www.sciencedirect.com/science/article/pii/S0260691714003025 (last accessed 2 May 2018).

Stephens, T. (2013). 'Nursing student resilience: a concept clarification', *Nursing Forum*, 48(2), 125–33.

Thomas, L.J. and Revell, S.H. (2016) 'Resilience in nursing students: an integrative review', *Nurse Education Today*, 36: 457–62.

Todd, G. (2002) 'The role of the internal supervisor in developing therapeutic nursing'. In: D. Freshwater (ed.), *Therapeutic Nursing*. London: Sage, pp. 58–82.

Vitello-Cicciu, J.M. (2002) 'Exploring emotional intelligence: implications for nursing leaders', *Journal of Nursing Administration*, 32(4): 203–10.

Weir, R.I. (2004) *Educating Nurses in Scotland: A History of Innovation and Change, 1950–2000*. Penzance: The Hypatia Trust.

Wheeler, H. (2012) *Law, Ethics and Professional Issues for Nursing: A Reflective and Portfolio Building Approach*. London: Routledge.

White, R. (1978) *Social Change and the Nursing Profession: A Study of the Poor Law Nursing Service, 1848–1948*. London: Henry Klimpton.

Willis Commission (2012) *Quality with Compassion: The Future of Nursing Education*. Available at: www.macmillan.org.uk/documents/newsletter/willis-commission-report-macmail-dec2012.pdf (last accessed 1 May 2018).

# 2

# NURSING THERAPEUTICS

## CAROLINE JAGGER, HEATHER ILES–SMITH AND DIANNE BURNS

---

### CHAPTER OBJECTIVES

- Explain underpinning theories used to define a therapeutic approach in nursing;
- Identify key communication skills that assist in the development of a therapeutic relationship with all patients, clients and their families;
- Discuss the importance of person-centred care and how this can be achieved in practice;
- Assist you to recognise your duty of care and any actions that you may need to take in relation to the safeguarding of vulnerable adults.

---

The term 'nursing therapeutics' encompasses the therapeutic relationship that exists between nurse and patient, and the key elements that influence that relationship. Influencing factors include the notion of person-centred care and the use of systematic approaches in planning, implementing and evaluating nursing care provision. The application of effective interpersonal skills and an ability to critically reflect upon the care we have provided, along with consideration of the underpinning professional values and the legal and ethical frameworks outlined in Chapter 1, are also of the utmost importance.

Nursing therapeutics is not a new concept. It has been an integral part of nursing throughout history, although it has not always been clearly defined or its importance articulated in the nursing literature.

Throughout this chapter the concept of a therapeutic nurse–patient relationship and the associated concepts above will be explored in more depth. The overarching aim of this chapter is to define what we deem to be a therapeutic relationship, to identify the components of such a relationship, and to explore how this can be developed through the use of frameworks and reflection. Examples from practice will be used to highlight how a therapeutic relationship is established and maintained in practice.

## Related NMC proficiencies for registered nurses

The overarching requirement of the Nursing and Midwifery Council (NMC) is that all registered nurses must act in the best interests of people, putting them first and providing nursing care that is person centred, safe and compassionate. They must communicate effectively, act as role models for others and be accountable for their actions. Registered nurses must prioritise the needs of people when assessing and reviewing their mental, physical, cognitive, behavioural, social and spiritual needs (NMC, 2018a).

 **To achieve entry to the nursing register you must be able to**

- Communicate effectively using a range of skills and strategies with colleagues and people at all stages of life, and with a range of mental, physical, cognitive and behavioural health challenges;
- Understand the need to base all decisions regarding care and interventions on people's needs and preferences, recognising and addressing any personal and external factors that may unduly influence your decisions;
- Provide and promote non-discriminatory, person-centred and sensitive care at all times, reflecting on people's values and beliefs, diverse backgrounds, cultural characteristics, language requirements, needs and preferences, taking account of any need for adjustments;
- Demonstrate and apply an understanding of what is important to people and how to use this knowledge to ensure that their needs for safety, dignity, privacy, comfort and sleep can be met, acting as a role model for others in providing evidence-based person-centred care.

(Adapted from NMC, 2018a)

## Therapeutic relationships

A therapeutic relationship in nursing involves nurse and patient working in partnership to help speed up the recovery process and enhance the patient experience (Peplau, 1991). However, due to the complexity of disease processes and the human body's resourcefulness, it is important to acknowledge that patients may recover in spite of, rather than because of, what we do. Nevertheless, the therapeutic relationship enables us to maximise the likelihood that an individual will recover because we have helped them in some way.

There is no single definition of a therapeutic relationship. Likewise there is no single means of defining the role of a nurse, other than a fundamental wish to make a positive difference to the patient's or service user's life. However, there are numerous models detailing the key elements of a therapeutic relationship.

─────────── THERAPEUTIC RELATIONSHIP MODELS ───────────

**Travelbee's** (1966) human-to-human relationship model: 'caring involves the dynamic, reciprocal, interpersonal connection between the nurse and the client developed through communication and the mutual commitment to perceive self and other as unique and valued'.

**Watson** (1979) suggested that the therapeutic relationship is seen as a two-way reciprocal relationship between nurse and patient, and that each 'grows' and learns from the other. She considers the mind, body and soul to be interlinked, and describes ten factors that could provide a framework for nursing care: formation of an altruistic system of values; instillation of faith–hope; cultivation of sensitivity to self and others; development of a help–trust relationship; acceptance of positive and negative feelings; use of the scientific problem-solving method for decision making; promotion of interpersonal teaching–learning; provision for a supportive, protective and/or corrective mental, physical, sociocultural and spiritual environment; assistance with the gratification of human needs; and the allowance of existential–phenomenological forces.

**Benner** (1984) explained that the nurse should view the patient with an unconditional positive regard, also known as 'mutuality'.

**Peplau** (1987) identified three essential attitudes of the therapeutic relationship: genuineness, respect and empathy.

**Muetzel's** (1988) model of activities and factors in the therapeutic relationship includes intimacy, reciprocity, and a partnership between patient and nurse. Intimacy includes 'spirit' closeness, vulnerability and atmosphere, such as security and freedom, with dynamics such as control, contact and communication.

**S. Rogers** (1996) suggested five client-related outcomes of nursing presence: achievement of client goals; satisfaction with nursing care; comfort; growth; and enhancing care. These all encompass what is viewed as the therapeutic relationship.

**Sundeen et al.** (1998) suggested four key stages:

1. A pre-interaction stage: requires planning and includes a review such as patient notes, past medical history and social circumstances;
2. An orientation stage: first meeting with the patient laying down the foundation of the relationship where good communication is imperative. A 'contract' is developed and this can be either formal or informal: it is the foundation of the relationship;
3. A maintenance phase: both the nurse and patient are progressing towards the agreed goal, each of which involves good communication and leads to 'feelings' being exchanged;
4. A termination phase: the ending of the relationship.

---

A therapeutic relationship is considered to be two-way, with both the patient and the nurse positively benefitting from the experience (McKlindon and Barnsteiner, 1999). This falls within the notion of reciprocity, a theory underpinned by sociological concepts down the ages. Reciprocity can be defined as a positive act being returned via another positive deed between two individuals. Sociological studies have shown that such positive or 'kind' endeavours lead individuals to behave in a more friendly and cooperative way (Ernst and Gächter, 2000). A nurse's acts of kindness can give rise to feelings of wellbeing for both patient and nurse, which are likely to help build trust and aid the development of a positive therapeutic relationship. Muetzel (1988) developed a theory of partnership, intimacy and reciprocity that enveloped three circles with the patient at the centre (Figure 2.1).

Intimacy includes spirit closeness, vulnerability and atmosphere, such as security and freedom, encompassing dynamics such as control, contract and communication. Although Muetzel's theory may seem dated, it is still reflected in some government policies today. For example, the *No Decision About Me, Without Me* (Department of Health or DH, 2012) proposals are aimed at ensuring that patients and their families are involved in the decision-making aspects of care

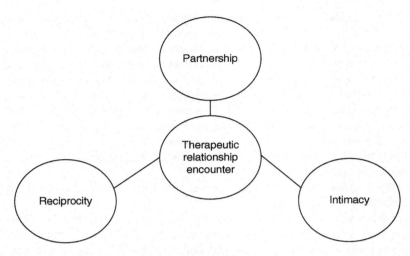

**Figure 2.1**   Meutzel's model of activities and factors in the therapeutic nurse–patient relationship. (Adapted from Meutzel, 1988)

provision. Similarly, an independent review of the use of the Liverpool Care Pathway (a multidisciplinary, patient-centred tool for all health professionals involved in the terminal stage of life) highlighted concerns about instances where relatives had not been informed of the decision to end active treatment and where care decisions were taken without the consent of the families involved (Neuberger, 2013).

The therapeutic relationship is concerned with both the science and the art of nursing and how we transfer our knowledge and skills into meaningful exchanges with patients, service users and carers. The science of nursing is conceptualised by a scientific understanding of the human body (including normality and symptoms) and knowledge of the latest medications, treatments and evidence-based care. Conversely, the art of nursing includes the practitioner's high levels of emotional intelligence, expert interpersonal and communication skills, and values-based care, which encompass notions of compassion, empathy, trust, dignity and respect. The ability to engage in judiciously intimate interactions with patients is a key part of the therapeutic relationship (Williams, 2001). Nursing is dependent on a thorough understanding of its science and a mastery of its art. Factors such as experience and additional learning will influence the ease with which you are able to build effective therapeutic relationships with your patients. Yet compassion, empathy, emotional intelligence and good communication skills are at times far more important than experience. Adult nursing requires commitment, intellectual intelligence, emotional intelligence and the inherent capacity to care.

## Moral dimensions of nursing care

By previously focusing on nursing history and the development of professional nursing in Chapter 1 you will have already explored the societal expectation that all nurses will possess characteristics associated with the strong moral virtues or values – sometimes being referred to by patients, the public and the media as an 'angel'. The expectation to do good, to be compassionate at all times, express empathy and sympathy, and treat patients and their families with dignity and respect – these qualities are a fundamental requirement of the adult nursing role. They lie at the heart of delivering good nursing care and are the foundation of a therapeutic relationship (Von Dietze and Orb, 2000).

Compassion is a complex concept and is often discussed alongside associated notions such as empathy, sympathy, respect and dignity (Dewar et al., 2011). In fact, it is often difficult to separate these concepts because they are all interconnected, resulting in ill-defined definitions of compassion. However, Schantz (2007) believes that compassion goes further than purely sympathy and pity, and involves actions to relieve distress. Other authors suggest that compassion is a basic human-to-human understanding, and a need to receive and give comfort and alleviate someone's suffering, distress or pain (Straughair, 2012). A great deal of emphasis has been placed on the integral part compassion plays in the delivery of good nursing care and effective therapeutic relationships by both government and professional bodies. Indeed, the NHS Constitution (DH, 2013), Northern Ireland's Strategy for Nursing and Midwifery (Department of Health, Social Services and Public Safety or DHSSPS, 2010), the Scottish Government's Quality Strategy (Scottish Government, 2010) and NHS Wales's Quality Delivery Plan (NHS Wales, 2012) all outline pledges that patients, service users and carers can expect to be treated with compassion, humanity and kindness by all healthcare professionals. Likewise, compassion is a consistent thread throughout the Nursing and Midwifery Council's Code (2018b) and Proficiencies (2018a).

Empathy, often described as 'the ability to walk in another's shoes', has also been widely accepted as an essential part of effective nursing care and is at the heart of the therapeutic nurse–patient relationship. Empathy is a key component of compassion and the therapeutic relationship. It is an essential attribute – not only to have an understanding of a patient's emotional state but also to have the ability to remain professional. Empathy is different from sympathy because sympathy is more emotionally charged (Peplau, 1987). According to Kunyk and Olson (2001), there are five conceptualisations of empathy:

1. A human trait;
2. A professional state;
3. A communication process;
4. A caring relationship;
5. A special relationship.

That is not to say that, when patients receive bad news, as a professional you should remain stoic and motionless, but as a nurse you will still need to be able to function and support patients and their emotional needs, having an ability to put the needs of patients above your own. Presence can also be linked with empathy because it entails sensitivity along with other traits such as holism, intimacy, vulnerability and the ability to adapt to unique circumstances. Finfgeld-Connett (2006) suggests that there are six features of presence:

1. Uniqueness;
2. Connecting with the patient's experience;
3. Sensing;
4. Going beyond the science;
5. Knowing;
6. Being with the patient.

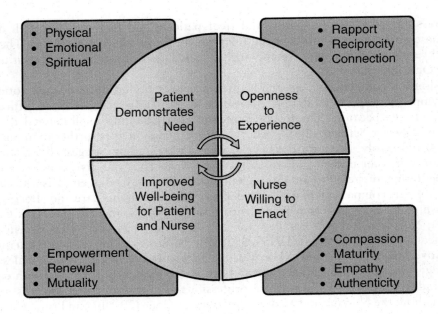

**Figure 2.2**  Presence model: implications for practice. (*Source:* Boeck, 2014)

Fredriksson (1999) argues that the value of presence lies in a nurse's ability to create a space where a patient can be in deep contact with their suffering, thereby allowing that patient to share with a caring individual and assisting the patient in finding their own way forward. S. Rogers (1996) suggests five client-related outcomes of nursing presence: achievement of client goals; satisfaction with nursing care; comfort; growth; and enhanced healing. The act of being present with a patient allows that individual to perceive a meaningful exchange. Boeck (2014) clearly illustrates the meaning and value of 'presence' in contemporary nursing practice (Figure 2.2).

The importance of reflective practice and emotional intelligence has already been established (see Chapter 1). The use of reflection enables a therapeutic relationship to be developed and sustained through the assessment of our behaviours and our impact on patient care. Goleman (1995) suggests that it is vital to recognise that personal qualities such as self-awareness, self-confidence, self-control, self-knowledge, personal reflection, resilience and determination are the foundation of how we behave.

## ACTIVITY 2.1

Access the following YouTube clip where Daniel Goleman explains his EI theories: https://www.youtube.com/watch?v=Y7m9eNoB3NU

- What personal qualities would you associate with emotional intelligence?
- How might you use these positively to develop therapeutic relationships with patients?
- Consider how emotional intelligence links to the concept of professionalism and the 6/7Cs framework.

As nurses our work is clearly set within a rollercoaster of human emotions whether these be fear, pain, sadness and despair, or, at the other end of the spectrum, joy, relief and hope. It is understandable that patients want empathic and emotionally competent nurses but it is equally clear that patients' perceptions suggest that these aspects are often lacking, along with effective communication skills (Williams and Stickley, 2010).

A defining quality in being able to establish a therapeutic relationship is the ability to recognise what others are feeling. Although this in part is being able to empathise, we must first recognise that there are some concerns or problems. As described below, in terms of communication, more than 90% of messages are transmitted non-verbally and as a result we must use our emotional intelligence to identify those feelings.

Activity 2.1 might have prompted you to include some of the following:

- Sensitivity;
- Awareness;
- Perceptive;
- Thoughtful;
- Anticipatory;
- Intuitive;
- In tune;
- Insightful.

You may also have noted that it is clear, from looking again at the core values of the 6/7Cs in the context of emotional intelligence and professionalism, that there are significant overlaps. Many of the values associated with one are also associated with the others, and thus are many sides of the same thing – the art of nursing that is so fundamental to the therapeutic relationship. It is often through the application of these attributes and skills that we can identify the real issues faced by our patients. By having a sensitive awareness and/or intuition, or by simply 'being interested', we can often pick up on something being wrong. Our own life experience of the same or similar situations enhances our ability to do this. However, previous experience in a similar situation that we have observed, reflected upon and learnt from also provides us with increasing perceptiveness or anticipation of what may occur. By listening carefully to what is being said, the tone or verbal expression that is used – and perhaps more importantly what is not said (along with facial expressions and body language) – can reveal more information to us.

## The importance of effective communication

It is widely accepted that words form only a small percentage of our communication (Hargie et al., 2004). Over 90% of communication is via non-verbal messages transmitted through our body language, tone and facial communication.

Reflecting on the role that we ourselves play in our interactions is integral to understanding how effective we are as practitioners at communicating with others. Awareness of our own values and beliefs and how these influence our behaviours can also lead to us being more attentive to patients' needs and help us to develop productive therapeutic relationships (we will revisit this concept again later in the chapter). To make our interactions with patients, service users and

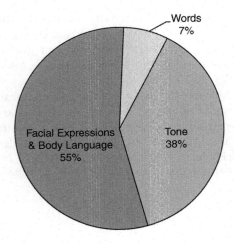

**Figure 2.3** It's not just what you say, it is very much how you say it

carers meaningful we must consider what we wish to achieve. For example, if we intend to advise how to take a medication, this is likely to be achieved by using a more formal, verbal interaction with written information supplied to aid concordance. How we transmit information that is meaningful and that our patients can process and understand is crucial to prevent misunderstanding, misinterpretation and confusion. This is dependent on our ability to combine non-verbal and the most appropriate verbal communication through the use of jargon-free language, coupled with active listening, questioning, clarification and summarising the conversation to ensure that we have been understood (Figure 2.3).

Active listening is defined by Mobley (2005) as the primary way of conveying empathy because it demonstrates that we are giving individuals our full attention. According to Webb (2011), active listening is important for several reasons. When people are worried they will often experience difficulties in communicating their ideas or problems clearly. It can help people who are in a stressful situation to get their ideas across so that their problems can be resolved more easily. Active listening is as much to do with body language as it is to do with verbal skills, and such skills are particularly useful when people are angry or highly emotional. The skills of active listening include the following:

- Attending and acknowledging, e.g. providing verbal or non-verbal awareness of the other person;
- Restating and paraphrasing, e.g. responding to the person using their basic verbal message;
- Reflecting, e.g. feelings, experiences or content that has been heard or perceived through cues;
- Summarising, e.g. bringing together feelings and experiences to provide a focus;
- Checking perceptions, e.g. are your perceptions and interpretations accurate?;
- Being quiet, e.g. giving the other person time to think as well as to talk.

## HILDA

Hilda, an elderly woman under your care in hospital, is very upset. She is both tearful and fractious. She has mislaid her wedding ring but she doesn't tell you because she doesn't want to trouble you. You think she is a little agitated because she is due to undergo an operation in the morning.

- Consider how you would respond to this situation.

Freshwater (2003: 93) asserts that 'One sigh may be communicating a lifetime of emotions'. Having picked up that something is wrong, we then have to engage and this can be achieved very simply. It is the emotionally intelligent practitioner who hears the sigh, makes eye contact, communicates understanding and demonstrates human care. This very basic human contact – achieved through engaging with the eyes together with perhaps a knowing look or a smile – could in that moment have the most profound and healing effect (Freshwater and Stickley, 2004).

As an emotionally intelligent nurse in this situation you would speak to Hilda and try to elicit the reason for her distress. You might also consider that there could be another reason behind this (other than the obvious one) and would then actively explore the possibility. One way of earning Hilda's trust and respect would be by demonstrating genuine interest and care or as C. Rogers (1961) describes it as 'being present'. Active listening requires a nurse to listen very carefully to what is being said so they are able to understand the position from the patient's point of view. More than this though, Egan (2017) argues that it also requires an ability to convey to the patient that they understand what has been said, not by repeating their words but to be present – psychologically, socially and emotionally.

Hilda is far more likely to open up to you if she knows she will be actively listened to. By taking the time and care to find out more you might learn, for example, that Hilda had lost her wedding ring and that her husband of more than 40 years had died only 3 months previously. You would therefore have a deeper understanding that the emotions expressed by Hilda were manifested in her raw grief. As an emotionally intelligent nurse you would perhaps use the whole spectrum of communication and interpersonal skills to allow Hilda to talk about and express her feelings and emotions, taking into account that she may be afraid of the impending surgery but that this has been compounded by the loss of her husband and now, further compounded, by not having the comfort of her wedding ring and all that it represented to her. Demonstrating this understanding could have a profound impact – even if the ring could not be found.

## Verbal communication

Communicating effectively through verbal discourse enables a nurse to establish whether a patient is confident and if they have understood what their care involves. This is clearly illustrated in the scenario below.

## HARSHA AND PETER

Harsha (the district nurse) is undertaking one of her weekly visits to her patient Peter. Peter's HbA1c (glycated haemoglobin) blood glucose readings have been consistently higher than normal over the past six months despite being prescribed medication to control his diabetes. Harsha suspects that this might be due to the fact that Peter has stopped taking his medication regularly.

In order to understand if Peter takes his medication at a certain time of day, in a certain way, or has stopped taking it altogether, further information is required. In nursing there are different purposes for our questioning and so we must use a series of open, closed or searching/probing questions. If we consider whether Peter is taking his medication as prescribed we may use closed questions such as 'Have you taken your diabetes medication today?'. This is factual and can be used in an emergency situation or to give structure to a conversation. However, leading questions are generally considered to be unhelpful because the question may prompt and influence the answer. This in turn may skew the information given by Peter when replying to the question. Open questions, on the other hand, are a way to allow him to give additional information. For example, asking Peter what time of day he normally takes his medication allows for further discussion. A searching or probing question would allow him time and help Harsha develop a deeper understanding of his perceptions. Therefore questioning in the right format is crucial to successfully communicating with patients and their carers.

## Questioning styles and active listening

The types of questions Harsha may use during her interaction with Peter about his medication may include closed or open questions such as the following:

Example of a closed question: 'Do you understand how to take your medication?' (Peter's response would probably be 'yes' or 'no'.)

Example of an open question: 'What do you understand about taking your medication?' Example of a searching question: 'How are you feeling today?'

Paralanguage is concerned with the way something is said such as the pitch and tone, and the softness or loudness of words, all of which can support or contraindicate what is being said (Thompson, 2011). Therefore it is important to consider not only what you are going to say but how you are going to say it. Of equal importance is the environment in which the communication takes place. The need to consider the scene for an interaction also plays a part in successful communication. In a study undertaken by Swayden et al. (2012), patients perceived that a doctor spent more time with them when they had sat down next to their bedside than when they had stood up, demonstrating how the perception of the time can be affected and lead to an increased satisfaction with the information received.

Non-verbal communication is concerned with anything that is communicated without the use of verbal language, such as the way we nod appropriately. In fact, Argyle (1988) suggested that non-verbal communication is up to five times more effective than verbal communication. During any interaction it is crucial that we consider how we are positioned in relation to a patient. Egan (2017) suggests using the acronym SOLER:

S = sit squarely in relation to the patient

O = in an open position

L = lean slightly towards the patient (at approximately 45°)

E = maintain eye contact

R = remain relaxed.

Applying the SOLER framework during a clinical interview when breaking bad news, or during any other communicative contact with patients and/or relatives, will help set the scene and put individuals at ease. If managed well it can also help us transmit empathy and compassion to those with whom we are interacting.

Can you think of a conversation you have had with someone who has not given you their full attention or there was a contrast between what they are saying and what they are doing?

- How did it make you feel?

Consider now dealing with a patient who feels that they have not been listened to:

- How could you make this different?
- How could the environment, your body language, vocabulary, pitch and tone, as well as the content of your conversation, affect the outcome of the situation?
- What could you do to show that you are attentive to their needs?
- How could you frame the interaction so that it helps to build a positive mutual relationship?

It may be that the inferences made through inflections in the voice or body language or the lack of eye contact were main elements that led to your dissatisfaction. Professional communication is a skill that can be enhanced by being aware of your own interactions: it differs from social communication because it is purposeful and ethical, and has boundaries. Good communication is an important component in any workplace and professional role. Moreover, in nursing, excellent communication and advanced interpersonal skills are crucial for successful interactions with carers, other healthcare professionals and patients. They are the bedrock for formulating and maintaining therapeutic relationships. However, unfortunately 21% of all written hospital complaints arise from communication difficulties (NHS Digital, 2017) and therefore the use of communication as an effective tool should never be underestimated. Recognising and actively listening to a patient can be very beneficial. By making every interaction with patients count, one small act of kindness or just being 'present' in the moment can make all the difference.

It is important to recognise that there are many potential barriers to effective communication. These include the following:

- Use of jargon, slang terms or abbreviations;
- Use of foreign languages, dialect or difficulties with speech;
- Sensory deprivation (i.e. blindness, deafness or difficulty hearing);

- Cultural differences;
- Emotional difficulties, anxiety or distress;
- Environmental issues (i.e. poor lighting, noisy environments or physical barriers).

## Anxiety and hospital admission

Admission to hospital is a major event in many patients' lives and can cause varying levels of anxiety as a consequence of fear of the unknown, fear arising from adverse media reports of poor hospital care and an awareness that hospitals can be dangerous places. In particular, there is potential for anxiety and fear when patients are admitted to hospital for elective surgery (Pritchard, 2011).

Pritchard (2011: 35) defines anxiety as 'an unpleasant state of uneasiness or tension that may be associated with hypertension and tachycardia'. An anxious patient may appear to be aggressive or demanding and require a lot of attention from nurses. High levels of nervousness and apprehension may also hinder the ability to understand or follow simple instructions (Pritchard, 2011).

Pritchard argues that all health professionals should be able to identify patients who are at risk of anxiety or depression and respond appropriately with effective and supportive care. For example, in adult nursing there is a professional responsibility to ensure that patients are adequately prepared for surgery both physically and psychologically. The provision of accurate information about what to expect during the pre- and postoperative periods has been found to contribute to reductions in anxiety (Pritchard, 2011).

What would you do to ensure that you could communicate effectively in the following scenarios:

- Asefa, a 26-year-old female refugee who doesn't speak English;
- Alice, a 40-year-old woman who is partially sighted and deaf;
- Bobby, a young man with a learning disability;
- Victor, an 85-year-old man with dementia.

All of the individuals above could face huge challenges because their situations or conditions can affect their ability to understand or use language to communicate effectively. In all circumstances it would be important to take into account their own preferred communication methods and background culture, dealing with each issue sensitively. Speaking clearly using short sentences – not giving too much information or asking too many questions – using simple vocabulary and avoiding jargon will help in most situations.

Ensuring that they have access to necessary aids and equipment (e.g. glasses or hearing aids) is also crucial. It might be necessary to request interpreter services or use other visual, auditory and tactile or signing methods to help individuals make effective use of alternative means of communication as appropriate to their needs. In Bobby's case, for example, he may require information concerning services and treatments in accessible formats, such as pictures, symbols, DVDs. The Royal College of Nursing (RCN, 2013) identifies the importance of communication in removing barriers to satisfactory use of healthcare services, and offer the following advice when caring for individuals with learning disabilities:

- Use simple language;
- Use pictures and photographs;
- Avoid abstract words or concepts.

Making reasonable adjustments to services requires the possession of knowledge of the health vulnerabilities that are specific to individuals, coupled with an assessment of the service user's communication abilities, views and preferences (Thomas and Atkinson, 2011). Thomas and Atkinson (2011: 35) suggest the following reasonable adjustments where applicable:

- Health passports: these documents contain an outline of the individual's health and illness history, health problems and treatments;
- Informed decision making: knowledge and appropriate use of the Mental Capacity Act 2005 (www.legislation.gov.uk/ukpga/2005/9/contents) to ensure that an individual makes their own decisions as far as possible, or decisions that are made on the individual's behalf are in that person's best interests;
- Liaison nurses (e.g. learning disability nurses or dementia specialist nurses): these professionals use their expertise to coordinate care and provide advice.

There is also some evidence to suggest that reminiscence therapy (making use of past experiences and life stories, or using prompts such as photographs, household and other familiar items from the past) could help improve communication with patients suffering from dementia, although more research is needed to determine which patients are most likely to benefit (Woods et al., 2018).

## ACTIVITY 2.2

Find out more about how you might effectively communicate with vulnerable patients by accessing the following websites:

1. www.alz.org/care/dementia-communication-tips.asp
2. www.mencap.org.uk/learning-disability-explained/communicating-people-learning-disability
3. www.actiononhearingloss.org.uk/live-well/communicate-well/communication-tips/tips-for-communicating-with-deafblind-people/

Now take a look at the accompanying website for this book and read the article: 'Culturally competent communication with refugees' (see Online further reading resource).

## The importance of cultural competence in nursing

Cultural competence can be defined as having the attitude, knowledge and skills necessary for providing quality care to diverse populations: ensuring that the needs of all patients and service users are addressed, irrespective of their ethnicity or cultural background (Seeleman et al., 2009). The term 'cultural competence' is often used to describe an ability to consider how social and cultural factors influence individual attitudes towards health and healthcare (Black and Purnell, 2002). At an interpersonal level, this includes having an ability to bridge cultural differences in order to build an effective therapeutic relationship. The key features of cultural competence are outlined by Saha et al. (2008) as follows:

The ability of the healthcare organisation to meet the needs of diverse groups of patients, for example:

- A diverse workforce that reflects the patient population;
- Healthcare facilities that are convenient for the community;
- Language assistance available for patients with limited English proficiency;
- Ongoing staff training regarding the delivery of culturally and linguistically appropriate services.

The ability of a healthcare provider to bridge cultural differences in interpersonal interactions and to build an effective patient relationship, for example:

- Exploring and respecting patient beliefs, values, preferences and their understanding of the meaning of illness;
- Building rapport and trust;
- Finding common ground;
- Being aware of own biases/assumptions;
- Being knowledgeable about other cultures;
- Being aware of disparities and discrimination affecting minority groups;
- Using an interpreter when needed.

The essence of cultural competence lies in a nurse's ability to see a patient as an individual. In that sense Saha et al. (2008) suggest that there is some degree of overlap between the two and, as cultural context and effective communication are relevant to the care of patients, cultural competence has the capacity to enhance patient centredness and improve quality for all patients, not just those from a different ethnic, racial or cultural background to our own.

Think carefully about how you might demonstrate cultural competence in your daily nursing practice:

- What will this involve?
- How does this influence the outcome of the care that you deliver?

First and foremost you will need the ability to learn about yourself (i.e. be self-reflective), a skill that is linked to emotional intelligence (Goleman, 1995).

Cultural awareness is defined as having the ability to acknowledge one's own culture, but also to recognise the potential for prejudice, bias and stereotyping. To recognise and reflect upon how our own culturally specific beliefs, customs and values influence not only our practice but also the behaviours of our patients and service users is crucial. Having the capacity to alter our behaviour in response to this deeper understanding is defined as cultural sensitivity. Matteliano and Street (2012) describe this as learning about different cultures and then adapting the way we deliver care to account for these differences.

It perhaps also goes without saying that you will need to draw on most of the skills outlined earlier by doing the following:

- Building trust and conveying unconditional positive regard by never making assumptions about cultural practices or beliefs and showing respect for a patient's support group (e.g. their family, friends, religious leaders);
- Asking questions about cultural practices in a professional and thoughtful manner if necessary;
- Addressing any communication or language barriers (e.g. using interpreter services if appropriate).

## Unconscious and conscious bias

Unconscious bias can happen when we make decisions or assumptions based on our own background, values, beliefs and experiences without realising it. There is evidence to suggest that healthcare professionals unfortunately exhibit the same levels of unconscious bias as the general population, and that such bias is likely to influence diagnosis, decisions about treatment and levels of care in some circumstances (Fitzgerald and Hurst, 2017). Conscious bias or explicit bias refers to the attitudes and beliefs that we have about individuals or groups at a conscious level. Stockwell (1972) concluded that people who behave in a certain manner (e.g. grumbling, complaining or otherwise demanding attention) could at times be considered by nursing staff to be difficult or unpopular (conscious bias). Certainly there may be times when some patients project challenging behaviour and this may be due to many complex reasons. It could be that they are in pain, anxious or distressed, that they may be incapacitated or that feel that they have a lack of control due to their illness. Nevertheless it is the nurse's role to reflect on their own behaviours and find a way to develop a therapeutic relationship and remain professional. Take a look at the following case scenarios. As you read through them, make a mental note of any feelings, thoughts and views that you are experiencing.

### ALICE

Alice (a 76-year-old patient) is admitted on to a busy medical unit for routine investigations. Several days after her admission she becomes more demanding, and in particular (especially during the nursing handover) keeps pressing the buzzer for various things she needs, for example she wants fresh water, her pillows are uncomfortable or the sheets are not 'sitting right' on the bed.

### ANDRE

Andre (a 42-year-old man) is admitted on to a surgical ward directly from theatre. Information given to the nurse at handover is that he has suffered deep lacerations from a knife injury. He has been placed in a side ward and his allocated nurse has taken baseline observations and completed a nursing assessment. He has many wounds to his abdomen and when checking his wound dressings the nurse asks Andre how he had sustained his injuries. Andre describes how he had opened his front door to be confronted by a man wielding a knife who then tried to stab him, resulting in the numerous lacerations. It transpires later that Andre had been stabbed by his brother for allegedly raping his young niece.

## VIVIENNE

Vivienne aged 35 is admitted to a busy surgical unit post-surgery to recover from injuries she sustained after an attempted suicide. Vivienne is currently in the process of transitioning from her birth identity to becoming female. She has had breast implants and hormone replacement, but is very unhappy and had been subjected to verbal and physical abuse due to her changing appearance. On admission she is very reluctant to speak other than to confirm the essential information, and when providing any information speaks very quietly.

How were your feelings, thoughts and views provoked by each of the scenarios above?

- How would you manage each situation?
- What are the challenges you would face?
- How would you develop a therapeutic relationship with patients who exhibit challenging behaviour or are unpopular? For example, would you be able to ensure your body language remained unchanged?
- How could the culture on the ward influence the reactions of members of staff to these patients?
- How might these affect each patient's recovery?
- How would you ensure that you are non-judgemental and engage with each of the patients above to ensure that each receives the best care?

C. Rogers' (1961) core condition of unconditional positive regard is simply having an attitude that enables us to be non-judgemental and always to act without bias or prejudice. In this way, the emotionally intelligent practitioner will not see or pre-judge any of these patients. Indeed, the NMC (2018b) makes it clear that all nurses must practise in a holistic, non-judgemental, caring and sensitive manner that avoids assumptions, supports social inclusion, recognises and respects individual choice, and acknowledges diversity. Where necessary you must provide the highest standard of practice and person-centred care possible at all times; in addition, you must put aside your own personal and cultural preferences when considering the needs of those in your care.

Certainly, there are many aspects of care to consider in each of the above scenarios, not just physical but also emotional and ongoing mental health. For example, some lesbian, gay, bisexual or trans patients (LGBTs) often feel discriminated against by healthcare staff. Many older LGBT patients avoid getting help for conditions due to fear (Steelman, 2018). It is essential that nurses are aware of their own implicit biases and prejudices because this can affect the way patients are perceived and can impact on the interaction and eye contact of a certain group of patients (Fitzgerald and Hurst, 2017). Indeed current legislation (The Equality Act 2010 – see www.legislation.gov.uk/ukpga/2010/15/contents) means that it is against the law to discriminate against a person on the grounds of age, disability, gender reassignment, race, religion or belief, sex, sexual orientation, and pregnancy or maternity. The Royal College of Nursing (2016, 2017) have produced some useful guidelines in relation to the care of LGBT patients, aiming to ensure that as nurses we can challenge stigma and address unlawful discrimination in healthcare.

# The use of therapeutic touch

Consideration should be given to the use of therapeutic touch as a means of non-verbal communication. There are formal ways of using touch (such as massage and Reiki), but the act of laying hands on a patient (such as hand holding) can also have a positive effect; it is a means of communication at a very basic human level. As children we are often nurtured and given lots of hugs by our parents and families. As adults, generally speaking, there are fewer opportunities to continue with this, with the loss of partners and grown-up children. The appropriate use of touch can cut through culture, race and nationalities, and help us to connect with patients. It can be considered a visible sign of caring (Busch et al., 2012), although as healthcare professionals it is important to remain cognisant of cultural differences, certain settings and particular circumstances where touch is not appropriate (Davidhizar and Giger, 1997). Muliira and Muliira (2013) propose the use of an acronym 'TOUCH' which should be considered before using a therapeutic touch:

- T: Talk to patients and identify preferences and comfort levels before touch.
- O: Observe a patient's verbal and non-verbal cues to guide their preference, such as avoiding eye contact.
- U: Understand and show understanding when touch is rejected.
- C: Care provider (e.g. if the same sex it is more acceptable to the patient).
- H: Handedness (e.g. touch with the right hand is preferred as some Muslim patients, believing the left hand is unclean).

Although Clark and Clark (1984) argue that empirical support for the use of therapeutic touch is weak some studies have shown that patients have benefited from the use of touch. These benefits can show a reduction in anxiety, a decrease in perceived pain, and a reduction in heart rate and blood pressure (Blankfield et al., 2001; Denison, 2004; Woods et al., 2005).

# Person-centred care

In recent years there has been a shift from the doctrine of the patient being at the mercy of healthcare professionals to one where the patient is now the centre of all decisions. Person-centred care (PCC) is considered the bedrock of good patient care and the opposite of disease- or task-based care, something that has been extensively implemented throughout nursing and medical history. PCC plays a key role in developing and maintaining a therapeutic relationship because it enables both patient and nurse to establish trust and understanding. Although there are numerous definitions of PCC and also differing terminologies for similar outcomes-based care, C. Rogers (1961) was one of the first to develop a form of PCC known as 'client-centred therapy'. This is not a technique but an approach based on a small set of core conditions that are required to facilitate therapeutic relationships, requiring high-level skills of emotion, intellect, attitudes and behaviour, which encapsulate the concept of emotional intelligence discussed earlier. These conditions are:

- Empathy;
- Unconditional positive regard;
- Congruence.

Unconditional positive regard is having an attitude that enables us to be non-judgemental and to act without bias or prejudice. Congruence relates to sincerity, genuineness and 'being present' in the relationship because you genuinely care. It is the difference between caring for the patient and caring about the person. Corbin (2008) describes this as putting caring into practice through behaviours that address the specific needs of patients by getting 'in touch' with the person behind the patient to discover and understand those needs.

The overarching goal of PCC is to include patients or service users in the assessment and planning of their care to meet their agreed physical and psychological needs, ensuring that they feel valued, listened to and included. This method elicits trust between the nurse and patient, and empowers the patient to make decisions about their own care and future health requirements, thereby fostering a productive therapeutic relationship. During PCC the locus of control or power between nurse or healthcare professional and patient is likely to be equally distributed (Parley, 2001). Conversely, disease- or task-based care involves a nurse delivering care according to a patient's disease or symptoms. In such cases, assumptions about a patient's requirements can often be made by those delivering care. Task-based care was constructed around Parsons' (1951) 'sick role', which theorised that a patient was dependent on a nurse, doctor or carer who was the most knowledgeable participant in the relationship. The power of the relationship was firmly within the remit of the healthcare professional and patients were often discouraged from asking about or questioning the care delivered by nurses or doctors. Historically, task- or disease-based nursing care was often delivered according to a nurse's schedule, focused around their need to 'get the job done' by the end of the shift rather than based on the needs of individual patients. This kind of care often involved the allocation of basic nursing care tasks as separate duties, with nursing staff focusing on a task or several tasks during their shift (such as observations, toileting, changing dressings, escorting patients to theatre). Unfortunately there are still elements of task-based nursing care visible in modern-day nursing, particularly where time pressures are prevalent.

In general PCC is the care model of choice in mainstream nursing, with its advantages leading to effective relationships between patients and healthcare professionals. However, although the approach is more challenging to implement when patients or service users have diminished cognitive abilities or reduced capacity, there is some evidence that patients do better. For example, Edvardsson and Innes (2010) conducted a literature review related to PCC in patients with dementia. This suggested that implementing PCC reduced agitation and patients appeared calmer.

PCC should be at the heart of what nurses do and care for all the patients in a non-judgemental way so that patients engage and feel included in their care.

---

### ACTIVITY 2.3

Access and read the following publications:

1. The Health Foundation (2014) Person-centred made simple. Available at: https://health.org.uk/sites/health/files/PersonCentredCareMadeSimple_0.pdf.
2. National Voices (2017) Person-centred care in 2017. Evidence from service users. Available at: www.nationalvoices.org.uk/publications/our-publications/person-centred-care-2017.

What could you do to ensure that all patients feel included in their care?

# Safeguarding vulnerable adults

It is the duty of every qualified nurse to promote patient safety and to recognise and assess people at risk of harm and situations that may put them at risk, ensuring that prompt action is taken to safeguard those who are vulnerable (NMC, 2018a, 2018b). An adult's capacity for self-care will be affected by their own personal circumstances such as physical ability, learning disability, mental health, illness and frailty, as well as factors within the local environment, personal strengths, and social contacts and support (DH, 2011). Harm or abuse may be physical, sexual, psychological, discriminatory, financial or neglectful in nature (DH, 2011). Nurses are in a key position to identify possible safeguarding concerns, for example when a vulnerable adult is admitted to hospital with unexplained injuries, or when a community nurse makes a home visit and suspects abuse within the family unit. In both cases local protocols and procedures will provide guidance on what action to take. Whatever the response, it is likely to involve a range of professionals and agencies. Local authorities hold statutory responsibility for the safeguarding of adults, but equally all staff working within health and social care settings have a duty of care to ensure the safety and wellbeing of their patients. That duty is outlined by key six principles outlined in The Care Act 2014 (see www.legislation.gov.uk/ukpga/2014/23/contents/enacted):

1. Empowerment: people being supported and encouraged to make their own decisions and informed consent;
2. Protection: ensuring support and representation for those in greatest need;
3. Prevention: taking action before harm occurs;
4. Proportionality: ensuring that any response is the least intrusive and is appropriate to the risk presented;
5. Partnership: working in partnership with other services and communities to prevent, detect and report neglect and abuse;
6. Accountability: accountability and transparency in safeguarding practice.

(Social Care Institute for Excellence, 2017)

As a registered nurse, you will need to ensure that you are familiar with procedures for safeguarding vulnerable adults in your area and also know whom to contact to express any concerns you might have. If you suspect the abuse of an adult, you should report your concerns to a more experienced colleague, who can refer the matter to the named nurse for safeguarding adults, who in turn can make a referral to social services. You must record your concerns – exactly what you observed and heard from whom and when. You should also record why this is of concern and what you did about your concerns. Good communication and record keeping are crucial. The Mental Capacity Act 2005 (see www.legislation.gov.uk/ukpga/2005/9/contents) provides a framework to empower and protect adults who may lack the capacity to make decisions for themselves. This might be as a result of an illness such as dementia, a brain injury, a learning disability or mental health problems. The Act aims to provide a balance between an individual's right to make their own decisions and their right to protection from harm if they lack such capacity. Accordingly every adult must be assumed to have capacity unless proved otherwise – you cannot assume someone lacks capacity on the basis of a diagnosis. If an adult patient in hospital needs continuous supervision, is not free to leave, and lacks the capacity to consent to treatment or care arrangements, extra safeguards may be needed. In England and Wales, the Deprivation of Liberty Safeguards (DoLS) or Liberty Protection Safeguards (LiPS) (additional amendments to the Mental Capacity Act) seek to provide legal permission to be able to restrict or restrain individuals if it is deemed to be in their own best interests.

### ⬚? ACTIVITY 2.4

Find out more about the Mental Capacity Act, the Deprivation of Liberty Safeguards and Liberty Protection Safeguards at the Social Care Institute for Excellence website: www.scie.org.uk/.

## Emotional resilience

It is very clear that compassionate care is central to nursing practice. As an adult nurse you will no doubt be faced with many challenging situations in the future, which you will need to reflect upon and then consider how these experiences might influence or change your future practice. As healthcare professionals we learn to put the needs of others before our own. Nurses will often spend their working day exposed to the emotional strain of dealing with people who are sick or dying, and those who have extreme physical and/or emotional needs. However, with an ever-increasing workload and an unprecedented demand on resources, nurses can often feel 'stressed' and begin to suffer from physical and mental fatigue. One American physician (Remen, 2006: 52) suggests that 'the expectation that we can be immersed in suffering and loss daily and not be touched by it is as unrealistic as expecting to be able to walk through water without getting wet'. This emotional strain, coupled with other stress factors inherent in the healthcare work environment, results in healthcare professionals being especially vulnerable to stress and burnout; this is more likely to occur when a nurse struggles with their work–life balance, job uncertainty, a lack of control in the workplace and feeling undervalued (Garrosa et al., 2011).

### ⬚? ACTIVITY 2.5

Access the following webpages and articles and then write down your answers to the questions that follow in 'Stop and Think':

1. www.compassionfatigue.org/
2. Wright. S. (2013) 'The differences between stress, burnout and compassion fatigue', *Nursing Standard*, 28(5): 34–5.

Who does compassion fatigue affect?

- How might we recognise it in ourselves and/or our colleagues?
- What are the contributory factors?

Access and take a look at the following document before considering what you can do to reduce the risks: www.compassionfatigue.org/pages/Top12SelfCareTips.pdf.

It is important to develop some strategies to cope with such stressors. Maytum et al. (2004) found that both short- and long-term coping strategies, such as taking part in self-care activities (e.g. going to the gym, walking and having a sense of humour and a positive mental attitude) were useful. Longer-term strategies included having an awareness of the various triggers and developing coping strategies, e.g. having both professional and personal supportive relationships.

Access the NMC (2018a) *Future Nurse: Standards of Proficiency for Registered Nurses* document, identifying all of the clinical competencies required of registered nurses.
Focusing particularly on effective communication skills, what do you need to do to ensure that you can develop your skills to meet the required competencies outlined?

## Chapter summary

Contemporary nursing practice demands an ability to build therapeutic relationships with all our patients. The development of an effective therapeutic relationship, and the ability to demonstrate empathy, compassion and caring, foster reciprocity and uphold the professional values of nursing are what remain central to the delivery of good nursing care. To do this well you will need to be able to communicate effectively with all your patients, putting them at the heart of your decision-making processes, listening to their views and involving them in decisions that are taken about their care (so long as they are willing and able to do so). In addition, the use of empathy and the 6/7Cs, encompassing care and compassion, is a vital element of nursing therapeutics that should be realised and put into practice by all nurses.

## Further reading

Arnold, E. and Underman-Boggs, K. (2011) *Interpersonal Relationships: Professional Communication Skills for Nursing*, 6th edn. St Louis, MO: Elsevier Saunders.

Egan, G. (2017) *The Skilled Helper. A Client Centred Approach*, 2nd edn. Belmont, CA: Brooks Cole Cengage Learning.

Freshwater, D. (2002) *Therapeutic Nursing: Improving Patient Care through Self Awareness and Reflection*. London: Sage.

NHS England North Designated Professionals for Safeguarding Adults (2017) *Safeguarding Adults (Pocket Guide)*. Available at: www.england.nhs.uk/wp-content/uploads/2017/02/adult-pocket-guide.pdf.

Skills for Health, Health Education England and Skills for Care (2015) *Dementia Core Skills Education and Training Framework*. Available at: www.skillsforhealth.org.uk/services/item/176-dementia-core-skills-education-and-training-framework.

Skills for Health, Health Education England and Skills for Care (2016) *Learning Disabilities Core Skills Education and Training Framework*. Available at: www.skillsforhealth.org.uk/services/item/660-learning-disabilities-cstf-download.

Skills for Health, Health Education England and Skills for Care (2016) *Mental Health Core Skills Education and Training Framework*. Available at: www.skillsforhealth.org.uk/services/item/525-mental-health-download.

## References

Argyle, M. (1988) *Bodily Communication*, 2nd edn. London: Methuen.

Benner, P. (1984) *From Novice to Expert: Excellence and Power in Clinical Nursing Practice*. Menlo Park, CA: Addison-Wesley.

Black, J.D. and Purnell, L.D. (2002) 'Cultural competence for the physical therapy professional', *Journal of Physical Therapy Education*, 16: 3–10.

Blankfield, R.P., Sulzmann, C., Geotz Fradley, L., Artim Tapolyai, A. and Zyzanski, S.J. (2001) 'Therapeutic touch in the treatment of carpal tunnel syndrome', *Journal of the American Board of Family Practice*, 14(5): 335–42.

Boeck, P.R. (2014) 'Presence: a concept analysis', *SAGE Open*, 4. doi:10.1177/2158244014527990. Available at: http://journals.sagepub.com.manchester.idm.oclc.org/doi/pdf/10.1177/2158244014527990.

Busch, M., Visser, A., Eybrechts, M., Komen, R., Oen, I., Olff, M., Dokter, J. and Boxma, H. (2012) 'The implementation and evaluation of therapeutic touch in burn patients: an instructive experience of conducting a scientific study within a non-academic nursing setting', *Patient Education and Counselling*, 89: 439–46.

Clark, P.E. and Clark, M.J. (1984) 'Therapeutic touch: is there a scientific basis for the practice?', *Nursing Research*, 33(1): 37–41.

Corbin, J. (2008) 'Guest editorial: is caring a lost art in nursing?', *International Journal of Nursing Studies*, 45: 163–5.

Davidhizar, R. and Giger, J.N. (1997) 'When touch is not the best approach', *Journal of Clinical Nursing*, 6: 203–6.

Denison, B. (2004) 'Touch the pain away: new research on therapeutic touch and persons with fibromyalgia syndrome', *Holistic Nursing Practice*, 18: 142–51.

Department of Health (2011) *Safeguarding Adults: The Role of Health Service Practitioners*. London: DH. Available at: https://assets.publishing.service.gov.uk/government/uploads/system/uploads/attachment_data/file/215714/dh_125233.pdf (last accessed 9 May 2018).

Department of Health (2012) *Liberating the NHS: No Decision About Me, Without Me*. London: DH. Available at: https://assets.publishing.service.gov.uk/government/uploads/system/uploads/attachment_data/file/216980/Liberating-the-NHS-No-decision-about-me-without-me-Government-response.pdf (last accessed 8 May 2018).

Department of Health (2013) *The NHS Constitution*. London: DH. Available at: www.gov.uk/government/publications/the-nhs-constitution-for-england (last accessed 9 May 2018).

Department of Health, Social Services and Public Safety (2010) *A Partnership for Care, Northern Ireland Strategy for Nursing and Midwifery 2010–2015*. Belfast: DHSSPS.

Dewar, B., Pullin, S. and Tocheris, R. (2011) 'Valuing compassion through definition and measurement', *Nursing Management*, 17(9): 32–7.

Edvardsson, D. and Innes, A. (2010) 'Measuring person centred care: a critical comparative review of published tools', *The Gerontologist*, 50(6): 834–46.

Egan, G. (2017) *The Skilled Helper. A Client Centred Approach*, 2nd edn. Belmont, CA: Brooks Cole Cengage Learning.

Ernst, F. and Gächter, S. (2000) 'Fairness and retaliation: the economics of reciprocity', *Journal of Economic Perspectives*, 14(3): 159–81.

Finfgeld-Connett, D. (2006) 'Meat-synthesis of presence in nursing', *Journal of Advanced Nursing*, 55(6): 708–14.

Fitzgerald, C. and Hurst, S. (2017) 'Implicit bias in healthcare professionals: a systematic review', *BMC Medical Ethics*, 18: 19.

Fredriksson, L. (1999) 'Modes of relating in a caring conversation: a research synthesis on presence, touch and listening', *Journal of Advanced Nursing*, 30(5): 1167–76.

Freshwater, D. (2003) *Counselling Skills for Nurses, Midwives and Health Visitors*. Buckingham: Open University Press.

Freshwater, D. and Stickley, T. (2004) 'The heart of the art: emotional intelligence in nurse education', *Nursing Enquiry*, 11(2): 91–8.

Garrosa, E., Moreno-Jimenez, B., Rodriguez-Munoz, A. and Rodriguez-Carvajal, R. (2011) 'Role stress and personal resources in nursing: a cross-sectional study of burnout and engagement', *International Journal of Nursing Studies*, 48(4): 479–89.

Goleman, D. (1995) *Emotional Intelligence*. New York: Bantam.

Hargie, O., Dickson, D. and Tourish, D. (2004) *Communication Skills for Effective Management*. Basingstoke: Palgrave.

Kunyk, D. and Olson, J.K. (2001) 'Clarification of conceptualizations of empathy', *Journal of Advanced Nursing*, 35(3): 317–25.

Matteliano, M.A. and Street, D. (2012) 'Nurse practitioners' contributions to cultural competence in primary care settings', *Journal of the American Academy of Nurse Practice*, 24(7): 425–35.

Maytum, J.C., Heiman, M.B. and Garwick, A.W. (2004) 'Compassion fatigue and burnout in nurses who work with children with chronic conditions and their families', *Journal of Pediatric Health Care*, 18(4): 171–9.

McKlindon, D. and Barnsteiner, J.H. (1999) 'Therapeutic relationship', *American Journal of Maternal and Child Health Nursing*, 5: 237–43.

Mobley, J. (2005) *An Integrated Existential Approach to Counseling Theory and Practice*. Lewiston, NY: Edwin Mellon.

Muetzel, P.A. (1988) 'Therapeutic nursing'. In A. Pearson (ed.), *Primary Nursing: Nursing in the Burford and Oxford Nursing Development Units*. Beckenham: Croom Helm, pp. 89–116.

Muliira, J. and Muliira, R. (2013) 'Teaching culturally appropriate therapeutic touch to nursing students in the sultanate of Oman: reflections on observations and experiences with Muslim patients', *Holistic Nursing Practice*, 27(1): 45–8.

Neuberger, J. (2013) *More Care, Less Pathway: A Review of the Liverpool Care Pathway*. Independent review of the Liverpool Care Pathway (Executive Summary). Available at: www.gov.uk/government/uploads/system/uploads/attachment_data/file/212450/Liverpool_Care_Pathway.pdf (last accessed 9 May 2018).

NHS Digital (2017) *Data on Written Complaints in the NHS 2016–17*. Available at: https://files.digital.nhs.uk/pdf/l/a/data_on_written_complaints_in_the_nhs_2016-17_report.pdf (last accessed 23–4 April 2018).

NHS Wales (2012) *Achieving Excellence: The Quality Delivery Plan for the NHS in Wales*. Cardiff: Welsh Assembly Government.

Nursing and Midwifery Council (2018a) *Future Nurse: Standards of Proficiency for Registered Nurses*. London: NMC.

Nursing and Midwifery Council (2018b) *The Code: Professional Practice and Behaviour: Standards of Nurses and Midwives*. London: NMC.

Parley, F. (2001) 'Person-centred outcomes: are outcomes improved where a person-centred care model is used?', *Journal of Intellectual Disabilities*, 5(4): 299–308.

Parsons, T. (1951) *The Social System*. London: Routledge & Kegan Paul.

Peplau, H.E (1987) 'Interpersonal constructs for nursing practice', *Nurse Education Today*, 7: 201–8.

Peplau, H.E. (1991) *Interpersonal Relations in Nursing*. New York: Springer. (Original work published 1952.)

Pritchard, M.J. (2011) 'Using the Hospital Anxiety and Depression Scale in surgical patients', *Nursing Standard*, 25(34): 35–41.

Remen, R.N. (2006) *Kitchen Table Wisdom: Stories that Heal*, 10th anniversary edn. London: Penguin.

Rogers, C. (1961) *On Becoming a Person: A Therapist's View of Psychotherapy*. Wiltshire: Redwood Books.

Rogers, S. (1996) 'Facilitative affiliation: nurse–client interactions that enhance healing', *Issues in Mental Health Nursing*, 17(3): 171–84.

Royal College of Nursing (2013) *Dignity in Healthcare for People with Learning Disabilities: Guidance for Nurses*, 2nd edn. London: RCN. Available at: www.rcn.org.uk/professional-development/publications/pub-004439 (last accessed 8 May 2018).

Royal College of Nursing (2016) *Caring for Lesbian, Gay, Bisexual or Trans Clients or Patients*. London: RCN.

Royal College of Nursing (2017) *Fair Care for Trans Patients*. London: RCN.

Saha, S., Beach, M.C. and Cooper, L.A. (2008) 'Patient centeredness, cultural competence and healthcare quality', *Journal of Natural Medicine Association*, 100(11): 1275–85.

Schantz, M. (2007) 'Compassion: a concepts analysis', *Nursing Forum*, 42: 48–55.

Scottish Government, The (2010) The *Healthcare Quality Strategy for NHS Scotland*. Edinburgh: The Scottish Government.

Seeleman, C., Suurmond, J. and Stronks, K. (2009) 'Cultural competence: a conceptual framework for teaching and learning', *Medical Education*, 43(3): 229–37.

Social Care Institute for Excellence (2017) *Safeguarding Adults*. Available at: www.scie.org.uk/safeguarding/adults/introduction/highlights#principles (last accessed 9 May 2018).

Steelman, E. (2018) 'Person-centred care for LGBT older adults', *Journal of Gerontology Nursing*, 44(2): 3–5.

Stockwell, F. (1972) *The Unpopular Patient. The Study of Nursing Care Project Reports*. London: Royal College of Nursing.

Straughair, C. (2012) 'Exploring compassion: implications for contemporary nursing, Part 2', *British Journal of Nursing*, 21(4): 239–44.

Sundeen, S.J., Stuart, G.W., Rankin, E.A.D. and Cohen, S.A. (1998) *Nurse–Client Interaction: Implementing the Nursing Process*, 6th edn. St Louis, MO: Mosby.

Swayden, K., Anderson, K., Connelly, L., Moran, J., McMahon, J. and Arnold, P. (2012) 'Effect of sitting versus standing on perception of provider time at bedside: a pilot study', *Patient Education and Counselling*, 86(2): 166–71.

Thomas, B. and Atkinson, D. (2011) 'Improving health outcomes for people with learning disabilities', *Nursing Standard*, 26(6): 33–6.

Thompson, N. (2011) *Effective Communication: A Guide for People Professions*, 2nd edn. Basingstoke: Palgrave Macmillan.

Travelbee, J. (1966) *Interpersonal Aspects of Nursing*. Philadelphia, PA: F.A. Davis.

Von Dietze, E. and Orb, A. (2000) 'Compassionate care: a moral dimension of nursing', *Nursing Inquiry*, 7(3): 166–74.

Watson, J. (1979) *Nursing: The Philosophy and Science of Caring*. Boulder, CO: University of Colorado Press.

Webb, L. (2011) *Nursing: Communication Skills in Practice*. Oxford: Oxford University Press.

Williams, A. (2001) 'A literature review on the concept of intimacy in nursing', *Journal of Advanced Nursing*, 33(5): 660–7.

Williams, J. and Stickley, T. (2010) 'Empathy and nurse education', *Nurse Education Today*, 30: 752–5.

Woods, B., OPhilbin, L., Farell, E.M., Spector, A.E. and Orell, M. (2018) 'Reminiscence therapy for dementia', *Cochrane Database of Systematic Reviews*, 3: CD001120. DOI 10.1002/14651858.CD001120.pub3.

Woods, D.L., Craven, R.F. and Whitney, J. (2005) 'The effect of therapeutic touch on behavioral symptoms of persons with dementia', *Alternative Therapies in Health and Medicine*, 11(1): 66–74.

# FUNDAMENTAL ASPECTS OF ADULT NURSING

## DIANNE BURNS, MARK COLE AND PENELOPE STAMFORD

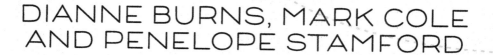

---

### CHAPTER OBJECTIVES

- Explain the concepts of informed consent, mental capacity and patient confidentiality;
- Describe how systematic approaches can be used to assess a patient's capacity for independence and self-care;
- Identify appropriate evidence-based assessment tools to determine the need for support and intervention in order to optimise mobility and safety;
- Make relevant links to core nursing skills;
- Outline the basic principles of infection control and wound care practices.

---

The previous chapter highlighted the importance of the nurse's ability to develop and build a therapeutic relationship with patients and their families. It also identified some of the key skills needed by nurses in order that they are able to communicate effectively with patients to identify their wishes and needs when planning care. Here we will begin to explore ways in which nurses can undertake a holistic nursing assessment, identifying more of the core nursing skills needed in order to be able to provide high-quality nursing care. It is perhaps important to point out here that we are not intending to provide specific instruction on how to carry out various clinical skills. There are plenty of other excellent resources that can help you with this aspect of your development. Instead, our intention is to utilise a series of activities and case scenarios to help you to consider some of the fundamental aspects of adult nursing practice. The chapter will also help to set the scene for Part 2 of this book, which will examine specific aspects of nursing and care provision that are commonly encountered when caring for adults and their families.

## Related NMC proficiencies for registered nurses

The overarching Nursing and Midwifery Council (NMC) requirement is that registered nurses must use information obtained during assessments to identify the priorities and requirements for person-centred and evidence-based nursing interventions and support. They must work in partnership with people to develop person-centred care plans that take into account their circumstances, characteristics and preferences (NMC, 2018a).

### To achieve entry to the nursing register you must be able to

- Understand and apply a person-centred approach to nursing care, demonstrating shared assessment, planning, decision making and goal setting when working with people, their families, communities and populations of all ages;
- Effectively assess a person's capacity to make decisions about their own care and to give or withhold consent;
- Understand and apply the principles and processes for making reasonable adjustments and best interest decisions when people do not have capacity;
- Demonstrate and apply knowledge of human development from conception to death; knowledge of body systems and homoeostasis, human anatomy and physiology, biology, genomics, pharmacology, and social and behavioural sciences when undertaking full and accurate person-centred nursing assessments to develop appropriate care plans;
- Demonstrate and apply knowledge of all commonly encountered mental, physical, behavioural and cognitive health conditions, medication usage and treatments when undertaking full and accurate assessments of nursing care needs and when developing, prioritising and reviewing person-centred care plans;
- Demonstrate the knowledge, skills and ability to act as a role model for others in providing evidence-based nursing care to meet people's needs related to nutrition, hydration and elimination;
- Recognise and assess people at risk of harm and the situations that may put them at risk, ensuring prompt action is taken to safeguard those who are vulnerable.

(Adapted from NMC, 2018a)

## Consent, mental capacity and confidentiality

In accordance with the NMC *Code* (2018b), a patient must give informed consent before any actions (including treatment, investigations or care) are provided. Informed consent means that, as nurses, we need to be able to provide patients with all the relevant accurate and truthful information in a way that they can understand in order to help them make an 'informed decision' about their care. Patients have the right to refuse or withdraw consent at any time. As a nurse we have to always act in our patients' best interests (NMC, 2018b). However, occasionally this might mean that we have to respect and support a patient's right to refuse care and treatment if they have the mental capacity to make that decision. Having mental capacity means having the ability to make your own decisions. The Mental Capacity Act 2005 (see www.

legislation.gov.uk/ukpga/2005/9/contents) aims to protect vulnerable adults who are not in a position to make decisions for themselves. In England and Wales, The Law Commission (2017) are seeking to amend this Act further to encompass the concept of the Deprivation of Liberty Safeguards (DoLS) with an overall revised approach: the Liberty Protection Safeguards (LiPS).

Furthermore, any information obtained within a nursing assessment or that relates to any aspects of their care must remain confidential. As a nurse or indeed any other healthcare professional we owe a duty of confidentiality to all of our patients. 'Information can only be shared with the patient's permission or when patient safety or public protection override the need for confidentiality' (NMC, 2018b: 8).

---

### 🔲❓ ACTIVITY 3.1

You can find out more by reading the documents outlined below:

Royal College of Nursing (2017) *Guidelines on the Principles of Consent*. Available at: www.rcn.org.uk/professional-development/publications/pub-006047 (last accessed 5 Oct 2018).

The Mental Capacity Act 2005. Available at: www.legislation.gov.uk/ukpga/2005/9/contents (last accessed 5 Oct 2018).

The Law Commission (2017) *Mental Capacity and the Deprivation of Liberty*. Available at: www.lawcom.gov.uk/app/uploads/2017/03/lc372_mental_capacity.pdf (last accessed 5 Oct 2018).

Mental Capacity Act (Northern Ireland) 2016. Available at: www.legislation.gov.uk/nia/2016/18/contents/enacted.

Scottish Government (2000) Adults with Incapacity (Scotland) Act (Short Guide). Available at: www.gov.scot/Publications/2008/03/25120154/1 (last accessed 5 Oct 2018).

NHS England (2016) *Confidentiality Policy*. Available at www.england.nhs.uk/wp-content/uploads/2016/12/confidentiality-policy-v3-1.pdf (last accessed 5 Oct 2018).

---

## Care planning

Care planning is a highly skilled process. Applying a systematic approach to care planning is a way of encouraging us to think clearly about what we do for patients and why we do certain things rather than carrying out nursing tasks in a ritualistic fashion. It also provides us with opportunities to plan, implement and evaluate care effectively, taking into account all the factors that can impact on health. The nursing process was first conceived by Orlando (1961) as a cyclical way of focusing on patient-centred nursing problems, setting agreed measurable and realistic goals intended to improve health. The modern-day process ASPIRE (Barrett et al., 2012) includes the following:

- Assessment: finding out what the patient can or cannot do;
- Systematic diagnosis: making a nursing diagnosis – identifying the health and nursing care needs of the patient;
- Plan: in discussion with the patient, coming to an agreement about how their identified health and nursing needs can be met, setting mutually agreed goals;

- Implement: delivering evidenced-based nursing interventions;
- Recheck: considering if the interventions selected are helping to meet the agreed goals;
- Evaluate: measuring and carefully documenting whether or not agreed interventions and approaches have been successful.

Following the evaluation of our nursing interventions the cycle begins again with a reassessment and evaluation of the effectiveness of any care undertaken in close collaboration with the patient. The cycle ensures that patient needs are constantly re-evaluated using the latest evidence-based care.

## Nursing assessment

The assessment of patient needs and their care requirements also involves the use of other nursing models. For example, the Roper Logan and Tierney model (Roper et al., 2000) encompasses 12 activities of daily living (ADLs) (Figure 3.1). ADLs are the fundamental activities that are required by an individual to manage basic physical needs. This framework or model can help us to structure a holistic assessment of patient need.

The ADL model is applicable to patients irrespective of the disease or problems they are experiencing. Using it allows us to gain valuable information relating to the level of help that may be required by the patient in order for them to enact day-to-day activities. However, care must be taken to ensure that the 'list' of ADLs is not merely used as a checklist. Instead, it should be incorporated within a person-centred approach to care planning, which involves the nurse and patient

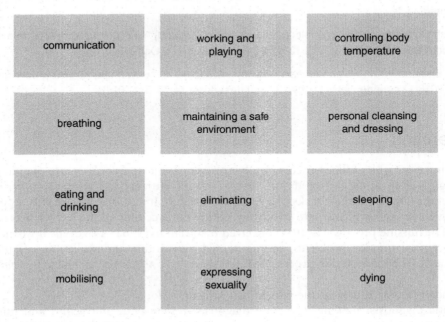

| communication | working and playing | controlling body temperature |
| breathing | maintaining a safe environment | personal cleansing and dressing |
| eating and drinking | eliminating | sleeping |
| mobilising | expressing sexuality | dying |

**Figure 3.1**  Activities of daily living

where possible setting short- and long-term goals for the actual and potential problems identified. However, although using a systematic nursing process and the ADL framework is useful, as you work your way through this chapter you will no doubt begin to recognise that one assessment tool will not always fit every situation; you may sometimes need to 'mix and match' additional tools and frameworks to ensure that the best approach is adopted, so that you can provide good quality, holistic nursing care. For example, the Instrumental Activities of Daily Living (IADL) scale (Lawton and Brody, 1969) was developed to assess more complex activities associated with independent living. According to Mlinac and Feng (2016), these activities are more sensitive to early cognitive decline because IADL function is usually lost before ADL capability. Gold (2012) suggests that assessing cognitive and functional capabilities in these areas helps to evaluate the impact of cognitive impairment in adults. Activities include:

- Ability to use the telephone or mail;
- Shopping and food preparation;
- House cleaning and home maintenance: personal laundry and performing domestic tasks to keep the living space reasonably tidy;
- Managing transportation: either driving or arranging other means of transport;
- Managing medications: being responsible for ensuring medication is taken correctly;
- Managing finances: paying bills or keeping track of income and expenditure.

- Will these models/frameworks successfully capture information that is needed?
- What other nursing models might be more suitable depending on the care setting?

It is important to remember that patients may not be able to fully address all of the above as a result of physical and/or mental illness or disability. For example, depression or anxiety can have a significant impact on a person's ability to self-care. Depression is described by Taylor and Ashelsford (2008: 49) as a 'medical condition involving changes in mood, appetite, sleep, thoughts and psychomotor activity' and can be a reaction to life events such as physical illness, bereavement, or problems with relationships or finances (Hardy, 2013). Three key symptoms include persistent sadness or low mood, loss of interest or pleasure, and fatigue or low energy, but may also include other associated symptoms, for example disturbed sleep, poor concentration or indecisiveness, low self-confidence, poor or increased appetite, suicidal thoughts or acts, agitation or slowing of movements, and guilt or self-blame. Alternatively, anxiety can present as restlessness and irritability, difficulty in concentration or withdrawal, making threats or demands (World Health Organization or WHO, 2016). Thus, as an adult nurse you will need to be alert for signs of depression or anxiety, and engage in accurate assessment as part of a therapeutic relationship with your patients.

What evidence-based tools are used in your placement areas to assess levels of patient anxiety and depression assessment? (e.g. Patient Health Questionnaire 9PHQ-9, Kroenke et al., 2001).

## RUTH

Ruth, a frail 77-year-old woman, is admitted to hospital accompanied by her daughter, although she lives alone. On admission she appears confused.

First of all, as Ruth initially appears confused, you would need to assess her capacity to make decisions about her own care and to give or withhold consent. In Ruth's case you would need to understand and apply the principles and processes for making reasonable adjustments and best interest decisions if you determine that she lacks mental capacity. If Ruth has capacity, you would seek her consent for treatment. You would offer constant reassurance, keeping her informed of what was happening. At the earliest opportunity you would take a full nursing history using a systematic approach, for example using the ADL and IADL frameworks outlined earlier as a guide.

- How would you assess Ruth's needs?
- What other frameworks or tools might help you in this process?
- What initial observations would you carry out?

We have already determined that Ruth will need a mental capacity assessment. Other additional assessments might include:

- A pressure ulcer risk assessment (e.g. Waterlow, 2008);
- A falls risk assessment (e.g. National Institute for Health and Care Excellence [NICE], 2013);
- A nutritional assessment (e.g. Malnutrition Universal Screening Tool [MUST], British Association for Parental and Enteral Nutrition, 2011);
- A depression and anxiety assessment (e.g. Patient Health Questionnaire 9PHQ-9, Kroenke et al., 2001);
- A Deprivation of Liberty Safeguard (DoLS)/Liberty Protection Safeguard (LIPS) Assessment.

## Making reasonable adjustments

It is more than 10 years since the MENCAP report (2007), *Death by Indifference*, relayed the stories of the avoidable deaths of six people with learning disabilities and raised concern about hospital care for people with learning disabilities. The stories include the sad case of a 43-year-old man (Martin) with a severe learning disability who was admitted to hospital following a stroke. Martin could not speak or swallow so speech and language therapists advised that he should not attempt to eat or drink and alternative feeding methods should be used. Apart from intravenous fluids, no other attempts were made to provide Martin with nutrition and he had no food for the 26 days he spent in hospital before his death.

The inadequacies in care that contributed to the deaths were attributed to a lack of concern for the individuals' disabilities. A subsequent Ombudsman's report found evidence in some cases of NHS trusts not making reasonable adjustments to the organisation and delivery of care in order to accommodate the special needs of these individuals (Parliamentary and Health Service Ombudsman, 2009). Common areas of concern included poor communication, poor partnership working and coordination, poor relationships with families and carers, a failure to follow routine procedures, poor management and a lack of patient advocacy. Unfortunately, more recently, the Leading Disabilities Mortality Review (LeDeR) programme (NHS England, 2017) has again reported similar findings with delays in treatment, gaps in service provision, organisational dysfunction, and neglect or abuse adversely affecting the health of individuals with learning disabilities.

## SEAN

Sean is 37 years old and has moderate learning disabilities. He lives at home with his parents who are his main carers, although the family has some help from outside agencies. Sean has been admitted to a surgical ward for exploratory surgery to investigate a possible cancer.

Make some suggestions about what 'reasonable adjustments' you might make to accommodate Sean's needs.

The above case scenario encourages you to consider how Sean and his family might cope with his acute admission to hospital and perhaps how you might make reasonable adjustments in order to improve the provision of care. You probably decided that an assessment of Sean's needs would be appropriate in order to apply your general knowledge to his specific and unique situation. It is important to note that, according to the Department of Health's (2013) Learning Disabilities Good Practice Project, one of the indicators of good practice is a 'capabilities approach'. This means focusing on Sean's strengths and what he can do rather than what he cannot do, and should also include a mental capacity assessment. According to Phillips (2012) other significant considerations would include assessing the effect on Sean of being in hospital. Hospitalisation is stressful for anyone but particularly so for people with learning disabilities (Doyle et al., 2016). Hospital routines often fail to cater for the needs of people with learning disabilities and staff tend to lack knowledge and experience of dealing with such patients (Phillips, 2012; NHS England, 2017). Reasonable adjustments may be needed to comply with the legal requirements of the Equality Act 2010 (see www.legislation.gov.uk/ukpga/2010/15/contents). Public Health England (2018) state on their website that reasonable adjustments entail:

making changes to services to ensure all are able to access. This may entail changes to building access, but also changes to policies and procedures and staff training …

Making reasonable adjustments requires possession of knowledge about the health vulnerabilities that are specific to an individual with learning disabilities, coupled with an assessment of that individual's communication abilities, views and preferences (Thomas and Atkinson, 2011). The Confidential Enquiry into Premature Deaths of People with Learning Disabilities (CIPOLD; Heslop et al., 2013) suggests the following reasonable adjustments to services:

- A mental capacity assessment each time a decision needs to be made, applied on the basis that sometimes individuals can make some decisions about their care but not others;
- Annual health checks: in order to monitor health and detect health problems early on;
- Summary care records: to ensure ease of finding and consulting information;

- Health action plans: these documents contain an outline of the individual's health and illness history, health problems and treatments;
- Informed decision making: knowledge and appropriate use of the Mental Capacity Act 2005 to ensure that an individual makes their own decisions as far as possible, or decisions that are made on the individual's behalf are in that person's best interests;
- Learning disability liaison nurse roles have now been established in a number of NHS trusts. Morton-Nance (2015) suggests that these professionals use their expertise to coordinate care and provide advice, and are best placed to support care within the acute setting.

The potential role of his parents is also another consideration. With Sean's permission, for example, how might they be encouraged to continue to help and support Sean during his hospital stay?

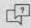 **ACTIVITY 3.2**

In 2018 Public Health England updated their guidance *Making Reasonable Adjustments for People with Learning Disabilities*. Take a look at the accompanying website for this book and access the Public Health England website to read more about what you can do to ensure that you enact these in your own role.

## Activities of daily living
### Breathing

Breathing is fundamental to life. It provides the cells in our body with oxygen and helps us to expel waste products. Without oxygen, our cells and tissues would begin to die after a few minutes. Where there is reduced oxygen intake (i.e. as a result of injury or disease), there is a risk of patients developing hypoxia (low oxygen levels in the tissues or cells) or hypoxaemia (low oxygen levels in the blood). The main causes of breathlessness are chronic lung diseases, such as chronic obstructive pulmonary disease (COPD), emphysema and chronic bronchitis which cause breathing difficulties characterised by the restriction of airflow. These can have a significant impact on a patient's ability to undertake normal daily activities because exercise capacity can be reduced, which often results in worsening health status and physical inactivity (van Helvoort et al., 2016).

### DANIEL

Daniel is a 65-year-old man with COPD who is admitted to hospital with a chest infection, accompanied by his daughter. He is breathless and finding it difficult to hold a conversation.
What knowledge and skills would you need to have to undertake a respiratory assessment?

The ability to undertake a full respiratory assessment requires a good understanding of the anatomy and physiology of the respiratory system. It might be quite obvious from looking at Daniel that he isn't very well. He may look warm and sweaty or perhaps pale and clammy. You would of course speak to him and offer constant reassurance. You would want to seek his consent to treatment and keep him informed of what was happening throughout. You could initially make him comfortable, perhaps propping him up with pillows if he finds it easier to breathe sat upright, and administer any initial treatment as prescribed. As he is quite breathless, with his permission you could try to gain as much information as possible from his daughter before consulting with him again once he is well enough to contribute.

In accordance with your own levels of competence, you would measure, record and interpret (i.e. recognise healthy ranges and clinically significant low/high readings) all baseline observations (i.e. respiration rate, pulse oximetry, peak flow, blood pressure, pulse, temperature, blood glucose levels) to detect signs and symptoms of physical ill health. You would undertake a whole-body systems assessment, focusing initially on his respiratory problems (which should include chest auscultation and interpretation of the findings), but then also a full assessment of his circulatory, neurological, musculoskeletal and cardiovascular systems, recording and reporting your findings accurately. You would also undertake venepuncture and cannulation and blood sampling, interpreting normal and common abnormal blood profiles and venous blood gases. If he has a productive cough, you would collect and observe his sputum, sending a sample to the laboratory for further analysis if needed. You might also take a urine sample to screen for abnormalities (e.g. leucocytes, blood, glucose, etc.). At the earliest opportunity (e.g. once he is more able) you would take a full nursing history using a systematic approach (e.g. using the ADL framework and/or other suitable assessment tools as a guide).

In accordance with the nursing process, you would assess the need for care interventions which would be agreed with Daniel and provided in accordance with current evidence-based guidelines and care pathways (NICE, 2018). You would closely monitor his progress, amending his plan of care in response to his progress and wishes.

**Other related clinical skills required for entry to the nursing register (NMC, 2018a) include**

- Responding to restlessness and agitation using appropriate interventions;
- Managing airway and respiratory processes and equipment;
- Managing inhalation, humidifier and nebuliser devices;
- Managing the administration of oxygen using a range of routes and best practice approaches.

## Nutrition and hydration

In order to keep healthy, warm and active, we need energy. The importance of good nutrition and hydration cannot be over-emphasised. Malnutrition is both a cause and an effect of ill health (NICE, 2012a). According to Manz and Wentz (2005), even mild dehydration can have a negative impact on health. Therefore, ensuring that the nutrition and hydration needs of patients are met is an important part of the nurse's role.

However, in order to be able to undertake a thorough nutritional assessment, a sound knowledge base is needed. This knowledge should comprise good understanding of related anatomy and physiology of the gastrointestinal system, the normal processes involved in the acquisition and assimilation of nutrients, the factors that can influence nutrition, and the effects of malnutrition on health and healing, for example. In order to manage a patient's nutritional needs effectively, a baseline assessment must first be undertaken and this should then be reviewed regularly. Once an assessment has been undertaken problems can be identified and a plan of care developed, implemented and evaluated.

- What factors might impact on an individual's ability to eat and drink?

The NICE quality standard for nutritional support in adults recommends that 'people in care settings are screened for the risk of malnutrition using a validated screening tool' (NICE, 2012a: 7). This suggests that all patients, irrespective of setting, should be screened. As an adult nurse you will undertake many of these assessments, often as part of the initial assessment or hospital admission process. It is therefore important that you understand the assessment tools you are using to ensure an accurate and appropriate outcome for the patient. One commonly used tool is the Malnutrition Universal Screening Tool or MUST (BAPEN, 2011). This is used in many hospitals across the UK and comprises five simple steps that identify whether a patient is at low, medium or high risk of malnutrition. The overall score is determined by body mass index (BMI), which will require you to measure the patient's weight and height; an assessment of unplanned weight loss in the past three to six months and how acutely ill the patient is in terms of poor nutritional intake for more than five days. Those individuals identified as low risk should have repeat screening – the regularity of this is determined by local protocol and is often influenced by where the patient is being cared for (e.g. annual screening is recommended for individuals over 75 living in their own homes). Those at medium risk should be observed, which involves documentation of their dietary intake for three days, with action taken after that. Those at high risk should be treated unless this is of no benefit to the patient, and includes referral to a dietician. In a very simple way, the MUST tool identifies level of risk and suggests basic actions to take.

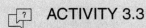 ACTIVITY 3.3

Access a copy of the Malnutrition Universal Screening Tool (MUST) (BAPEN, 2011) and familiarise yourself with it.

- Do you think this provides an adequate assessment of nutritional status?
- What other tools are available?

It needs to be acknowledged (as with all screening tools) that they are meant to be used as a guide only (together with your own knowledge and professional judgement). Following on from the assessment, regular monitoring should be undertaken. This may be as a result of the patient being identified as medium risk or on the recommendation of the dietician, and may involve the use of a food diary or fluid balance chart.

It is the nurse's role to ensure that patients receive adequate nutrition and hydration. As some patients may be unable to feed themselves, this requires assisting patients to eat and drink. Care may need to be taken with some patients due to swallowing difficulties, and advice from professionals such as the speech and language therapist about issues such as thickness of fluids will need to be adhered to. The nurse's role in health promotion and nutrition is vital here. In order to provide advice and support for a patient about their diet, you will need to be knowledgeable yourself. Of course, the dietician can provide additional in-depth information but it is beneficial to have some knowledge and awareness of what a healthy diet is, the impact of nutritional deficiencies, and some of the diet restrictions involved in conditions such as diabetes mellitus. Some patients will be unable to take nutrition orally. NICE (2006) provide guidance for the care of such patients in relation to enteral and parenteral nutrition. As nurses we need to ensure that patients who cannot take food orally (e.g. due to a swallowing impairment after a stroke or if a patient is unconscious) are adequately fed and hydrated.

Documentation (as with other aspects of nursing) is also vital in relation to fluid and nutritional management. Records of the administration of enteral and parenteral nutrition and intravenous fluids should be made, so that accurate calculations can be made about progress. This will include keeping accurate records of fluid balance (i.e. intake and output), regularly documenting assessment findings such as subsequent MUST scores, recording the patient's BMI, keeping food diaries, and noting any changes and amendments to patient management in the care plan.

**Other related clinical skills required for entry to the register (NMC, 2018a) include**

- Assisting with feeding and drinking and using appropriate feeding and drinking aids;
- Recording fluid intake and output, and identifying, responding to and managing dehydration or fluid retention;
- Managing nausea and vomiting;
- Inserting, managing and removal of oral/nasal/gastric tubes;
- Managing artificial nutrition and hydration using oral, enteral and parenteral routes;
- Managing the administration of intravenous (IV) fluids;
- Managing fluid and nutritional infusion pumps and devices.

## Elimination: bladder and bowel health

Bladder and bowel elimination are essential to maintain health. The urinary and gastrointestinal systems provide the ability to eliminate most of the body's waste products, maintaining the body's homoeostasis and ensuring effective excretion of toxins. However, an individual's ability to effectively eliminate waste products can be affected by various physical, psychological, sociocultural and/or environmental factors, or surgery. In order to be able to undertake a thorough assessment of elimination needs, you will need to have a good understanding of related anatomy and physiology of the gastrointestinal and urinary systems. Bowel and bladder problems can also affect fluid and electrolyte balance, hydration and nutrition.

When seeking a detailed elimination history from the patient, you will need to approach the subject sensitively, acknowledging the intimate nature of possible nursing interventions and ensuring that patient privacy and dignity are always respected. Health issues faced by some patients can include constipation, faecal impaction or diarrhoea, and urinary and faecal incontinence. It is important to identify any specific problems and toileting needs, accurately assessing not only the patient's capacity for independence and self-care but also determining the need for support and intervention (e.g. assisting with toileting or assessing elimination patterns to identify and respond to potential issues appropriately).

**Other related clinical skills required for entry to the register (NMC, 2018a) include**

- Collecting and observing urine, stool and vomit specimens, undertaking routine analysis and interpreting findings;
- Selecting and using appropriate continence products;
- Inserting, managing and removing catheters for all genders, and assisting with self-catheterisation when required;
- Managing bladder drainage;
- Administering enemas and suppositories, and undertaking rectal examination and manual evacuation when appropriate;
- Undertaking stoma care, and identifying and using appropriate products and approaches.

## Assisting with personal care

When considering best practice approaches for meeting the needs for care and support with hygiene and the maintenance of skin integrity, again it is important accurately to assess the person's capacity for independence and self-care before agreeing appropriate interventions. This would include assessing needs for help with washing, bathing, shaving and dressing, oral, dental, eye and nail care; identifying and managing any skin conditions (e.g. irritations, rashes or wounds and sores) and taking into account when onward referral to other members of the multidisciplinary team (MDT) is appropriate (e.g. dentist, podiatrist, tissue viability nurse). The Essence of Care (DH, 2010a) benchmarks state that personal hygiene is 'the physical act of cleansing the body to ensure that the hair, nails, ears, eyes, nose and skin are maintained in an optimum condition'. It also includes mouth hygiene, which is the effective removal of plaque and debris to ensure that the structures and tissues of the mouth are kept in a healthy condition. As an adult nurse you may encounter many patients who have pre-existing periodontal disease made worse by their current health status (Table 3.1).

**Table 3.1** At-risk groups: patients with pre-existing periodontal disease that is often exacerbated by current health status

| | |
|---|---|
| Dementia | Individuals receiving oxygen therapy or head and neck radiation |
| Frail elderly | Ventilated patients |
| Learning disabilities | Immunocompromised individuals |
| Palliative care | Poor mobility |
| Chemotherapy | Stroke |
| Delirium | Physical disability |
| Mental health | |

## ACTIVITY 3.4

Identify a care-dependent adult who might need assistance with their oral health.

- How often do they receive oral care?
- What equipment is used?
- How does this compare with the hospital policy?

You may be familiar with a criticism that the modern graduate nurse is 'too posh to wash'. This rests with the idea that delivering personal care can be an unpleasant, repetitive, 'mundane' task that involves physical hard work. However, personal care is an essential nursing responsibility that contributes to the comfort, safety, wellbeing and dignity of the individual. It also provides the nurse with an opportunity to assess the patient's activities and gain valuable insights into the appearance of the skin, hair, nails and mucous membranes which may be present in healthy and diseased states. The term 'skin integrity' refers to the skin being a sound and complete structure in unimpaired condition. As we age subcutaneous fat is diminished and the skin becomes thinner, drier and less elastic. Sebaceous and sweat gland activity is reduced, as is capillary blood flow. The cumulative effect of the ageing process is that skin becomes significantly more vulnerable to damage and there are delays in wound healing. Skin conditions, xerostomia (dryness), fissures (cracks) and pruritus (itching) are common in elderly people but often go unrecognised and untreated (Cowdell and Garrett, 2014). Alterations in the colour, moisture, temperature, texture, mobility and turgor of skin, and the presence of skin lesions can alert the nurse to an underlying pathology. Only when you have assessed and documented the condition of the patient's skin can you then formulate an appropriate care plan to maintain skin integrity.

There are a number of acute and chronic wounds that will breach the integrity of the skin. Three will briefly be considered here:

1. Pressure ulcers;
2. Leg ulcers;
3. Surgical wounds.

## Pressure ulcers

A pressure ulcer is defined as a 'localized injury to the skin and/or underlying tissue usually over a bony prominence, as a result of pressure, or pressure in combination with shear' (European Pressure Ulcer Advisory Panel, 2009). The most common anatomical sites are the sacrum and the heels. Severity varies from erythema to full-thickness skin loss, and incidence increases in elderly people. Although seen as largely preventable, there are about 2000 newly acquired pressure ulcers in NHS England each month (NHS Digital, 2015). Risk factors include:

- Significantly limited mobility (e.g. people with a spinal cord injury);
- Significant loss of sensation;
- A previous or current pressure ulcer;

- Nutritional deficiency;
- The inability of an individual to reposition themselves;
- Significant cognitive impairment.

A pressure ulcer risk assessment should take place for all patients admitted to hospital within six hours of their admission. They should be reassessed after a surgical or interventional procedure, or after a change in their care environment following a transfer (NICE, 2015). There are nearly 40 available risk assessment tools but in essence these are checklists that alert practitioners to the most common risk factors that predispose individuals to pressure ulcer development (Moore and Cowman, 2014). Completing a risk assessment allows the nurse to protect the patient's skin integrity through careful moving and handling techniques, regular repositioning, the use of pressure-redistributing devices, and the need for nutritional supplements and hydration.

### JOSEPHINE

Josephine is an 82-year-old woman who has been admitted from accident and emergency. She had a fall six hours ago and has sustained a fractured neck to the left femur. She is normally independent and in good health. Currently she is bedbound. You estimate that she has a below-average BMI, has dry skin and suffers occasionally from stress incontinence.

Complete a risk assessment using the approved tool in your current placement. What measures would you put in place to prevent pressure damage?

## Leg ulcers

Venous leg ulcers are a form of chronic wound characterised by skin loss below the knee on the leg or foot that remains unhealed after four weeks. They can affect one in 500 people in the UK and cost the NHS up to £400 million a year (Stanton et al., 2016). The incidence of leg ulcers rises with age and can take longer to heal in people from lower socioeconomic groups (Scottish Intercollegiate Guidelines Network or SIGN, 2010). Venous leg ulcers are caused by sustained venous hypertension that is exacerbated by obesity, immobility, a history of varicose veins and deep vein thrombosis. These patients endure numerous bio-psychosocial problems, which include pain, odour, sepsis, absence from work, loss of independence and social isolation. Patients with leg ulcers are often seen in the community, in their own home or in a specialist leg ulcer clinic. They may be admitted to hospital if experiencing secondary sepsis. Local wound care and graduated compression therapy that improves the microcirculation is the cornerstone of leg ulcer management (O'Meara et al., 2012). However, it is reported that many patients cannot tolerate, or do not adhere to, compression therapy.

- What are the reasons why someone might not tolerate compression therapy?
- As an adult nurse, what things would you take into account when managing this situation?

## Surgical wounds

The aim of postoperative wound care is to allow the wound to heal rapidly without complications, and with the best functional and aesthetic results. Due to the natural mass of microorganisms in the environment, it is not possible to achieve sterility in a typical healthcare setting. However, the principles of asepsis, to remove viable pathogenic microorganisms at the time of a high-risk procedure, is a more achievable aim and helps to protect the patient's portal of entry. Aseptic Non-Touch Technique has garnered approval throughout the NHS as a set of standardised practices and procedures that ensure only uncontaminated equipment, referred to as 'key parts' or sterile fluids, comes into contact with susceptible areas, called key sites during clinical procedures (Rowley et al., 2010).

The key components of Aseptic Non-Touch Technique are:

- Always wash hands effectively;
- Non-touch-technique is used at all times to protect key parts;
- Touch non-key parts with confidence;
- Take appropriate infective precautions.

Broadly, the risks of surgical wound infection can be separated into the preoperative period, the intraoperative period and postoperative period. A recent review (Harris et al., 2018) suggested that where possible the following 12 key risk factors should be identified and addressed in the preoperative period:

1. Obesity;
2. Malnutrition;
3. Smoking;
4. Hypertension and coronary artery disease;
5. Pre-existing body site infection;
6. Diabetes mellitus (poor glycaemic control);
7. Size and virulence of the microbial inocula;
8. General health and co-morbid disease processes, including medications that affect integrity of the individual's host defences;
9. Alcohol or substance use;
10. Physical activity and mobility limitations;
11. Previous complications with anaesthetic and surgeries;
12. Advanced age.

Important components of the intraoperative risks (during surgery) can include length of the procedure, whether it is 'clean' or 'contaminated', the methods used, how well peripheral perfusion is maintained, whether it is an elective or emergency procedure, and the presence of an implant. Delayed healing can take place in the postoperative period through dehiscence (the wound breaking open) and infection. As an adult nurse you should look for the following signs when you undertake a postoperative wound review: fever, haematoma, seroma, separation of wound edges and purulent discharge from the wound. NICE (2008) have made a number of recommendations for postoperative wound management, and this includes keeping wounds clean and debriding non-viable tissue. If wound infection is suspected, a specimen should be taken and empirical antibiotic therapy commenced on the basis of the suspected pathogen. Once the pathogen and sensitivity have been identified the antibiotic should be tailored as required.

# Patient mobility

The ability for patients to move around safely is important in order to prevent complications associated with inactivity or long-term bedrest (e.g. deep vein thrombosis, pressure ulcers/bed sores, constipation, loss of muscle strength and confidence). Any loss of mobility, even if for a short period, can have an untoward impact on a person's independence and health (Ness and Murray, 2009). In order to be able to undertake a thorough assessment of mobility issues a nurse will need to have a good understanding of related anatomy and physiology of the musculoskeletal and nervous system.

- What are the factors that can impact on an individual's ability to mobilise?

Your nursing assessment would need to determine whether your patient had any medical condition that might impact on their ability to mobilise safely (e.g. muscle weakness, poor vision or balance, low blood pressure or anxiety related to the risk of falling). You would need to assess any mobility restrictions or limitations on how far they could walk. You would also need to establish whether they needed any walking aids (e.g. walking stick, Zimmer frame) or specialist equipment (if any) to move around.

Although mobilisation can help patients regain or maintain function and reduce complications, unsafe or reduced mobilisation increases the risk of falls. Growdon et al. (2017) highlight the tensions faced by healthcare practitioners when considering the need to promote mobility while also preventing falls. Indeed, Kneafsey et al. (2013) point out that nurses will often focus on keeping people safe to prevent problems, rather than focusing on a rehabilitation goal. However, Growden et al. (2017) argue that promoting mobility may actually help to prevent injury sustained by falls, and therefore they question the common practice of immobilising patients for the sake of fall prevention. In consideration of these issues, any required and agreed interventions should be aimed at maximising mobility and independence while also maintaining patient safety, for example encouraging patients to move around as much as possible, referring to a physiotherapist to help agree a personalised mobility plan, providing required walking aids and teaching gentle exercises and techniques to move from bed to chair or wheelchair.

## ACTIVITY 3.5

Download a copy of the current NICE (2013) Guidelines for Falls Risk Assessment at: www.nice.org. uk/guidance/cg161.

Compare these with local guidelines and falls risk assessment policies that you have in your own placement setting. Are there any similarities or differences?

> **Other related clinical skills required for entry to the register (NMC, 2018a) include**

> - Using appropriate safety techniques and devices;
> - Using a range of contemporary moving and handling techniques and mobility aids;
> - Using appropriate moving and handling equipment to support people with impaired mobility.

## Resting and sleeping

Sleep plays an important role in our physical health. According to the National Heart, Lung and Blood Institute (NHLBI, 2011), sleep has a restorative function and helps to protect not only our health but also our quality of life and safety. Ongoing sleep deficiency can be linked to an increased risk of heart disease, kidney disease, high blood pressure, diabetes and stroke (NHLBI, 2011). Assessing and meeting the needs for care and support with rest, sleep and comfort involve making enquiries about the quality and duration of rest and sleep, identifying and addressing any factors that might adversely impact on this (e.g. noise, other disturbance, anxiety, depression, pain, etc.).

> ### ACTIVITY 3.6
>
> Go to the NICE website and identify/access relevant guidelines on the management of sleep disorders.
>    What actions can you take to help promote patient rest and sleep in your placement areas?

## Infection prevention and control

Healthcare-associated infection (HCAI) is a major patient safety concern that affects up to 6.4% of inpatients in acute NHS hospitals at any one time (Health Protection Agency, 2011). It is associated with significant morbidity and mortality (particularly if caused by multi-drug-resistant bacteria), protracted hospital stay and increased healthcare costs (Loveday et al., 2014). Reducing the burden of HCAI has become a key priority for the NHS (NICE, 2016). It is now a legal requirement for registered providers of health and social care in England to comply with a code of practice that makes explicit the way they develop and maintain high levels of infection prevention (Health and Social Care Act, 2008). There are comprehensive evidence-based guidelines produced by EPIC (Loveday et al., 2014) and NICE (2016), which underpin the Code of Practice, and these are complemented by the NMC's standards (NMC, 2018a), outlined below. These form the basis of this short section on infection prevention and control.

Meeting needs for care and support with the prevention and management of infection:

- Observe, assess and respond rapidly to potential infection risks using best practice guidelines;
- Use standard precautions protocols;

- Safely decontaminate equipment and environment;
- Safely use and dispose of waste, laundry and sharps;
- Use appropriate personal protection equipment including gloves and masks;
- Use evidence-based hand-washing techniques;
- Implement isolation procedures;
- Use effective aseptic, non-touch techniques;
- Safely assess and manage invasive medical devices and lines.

## Risk assessment and the cycle of infection

Contemporary acute healthcare placements can be understood as places where large numbers of sick people with weakened immune systems are placed close together. As a result of their pre-existing morbidities this often means an increase in invasive treatments that bypass the body's natural defences. To exacerbate this these treatments are often undertaken by busy staff, in environments of diminished resources. In order to observe, assess and respond rapidly to potential infection risks, the adult nurse needs to have some understanding of the interplay of the host, pathogen, healthcare workers and healthcare organisations that can result in HCAI. The 'chain of infection' (Figure 3.2) is a well-established model that captures the epidemiology of HCAI by taking what is known about the nature of microorganisms and describing how they can spread from one person to another. In short, a pathogenic microorganism must be present, and transmission will occur when it leaves its reservoir, or its common resting place, through a portal of exit; it is then conveyed by some mode of transmission, and enters a susceptible host through a portal of entry to cause an infection (Centers for Disease Control and Prevention or CDC, 2012). Many of the key principles of infection, prevention and control are based on targeting, and then breaking, the separate 'links' of the chain.

## Infectious agent

Microorganisms (often referred to as pathogens) that are responsible for HCAI are classified as bacteria, viruses or fungi. Gastrointestinal viruses such as norovirus, respiratory viruses, such as influenza, and fungal infections that cause oral thrush can all be problematic in healthcare settings. However, it is bacteria that are largely responsible for the incidence of HCAI (Khan et al., 2017). Paradoxically, bacteria also form an essential part of a human's microbiota and up to 1000 different

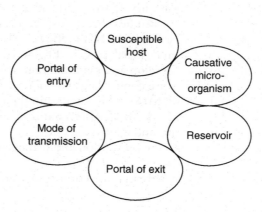

**Figure 3.2**  The six links within a chain of infection

species can be found colonising the upper respiratory tract, bowel, skin and female reproductive tract. Under normal circumstances this is part of a normal synergistic host–microbe relationship because bacteria aid digestion, produce essential vitamins and can create a microbial antagonism, whereby more benign species take up the space and nutrients that are required by more aggressive pathogens. However, when these bacteria grow beyond their normal range, as often seen in patients with suppressed immune systems, or begin to populate forbidden zones through medical devices, they become more invasive. As a nurse you cannot remove all bacteria but you can appreciate the conditions that allow them to thrive and how they build abnormal colonisations that result in infection.

## Standard precautions

Standard precautions (Table 3.2) refer to a cocktail of infection control practices that aim to minimise, and where possible eliminate, the risk of transmission of infectious agents from their natural reservoirs to a susceptible individual. They are named standard because they offer a basic level of care that should be used by all staff, in all care settings, at all times, for all patients regardless of their perceived or confirmed infectious status. Standard precautions particularly target the portal of exit and the mode of transmission as a nurse may become contaminated because they come into contact with the patient's excretions, secretions and skin scales.

Understanding the routes of transmission of infection helps to plan strategies to prevent cross-infection. There are four main routes as follows:

1. **Contact**: this is the most frequent mode of transmission and can be through direct physical contact with the patient or indirect though contact with equipment or the environment (e.g. meticillin-resistant *Staphyloccocus aureus* [MRSA]);
2. **Airborne**: through inhalation of light aerosol droplets that remain airborne for a long period of time and are breathed in (e.g. pulmonary tuberculosis, chickenpox);
3. **Faecal–oral**: hand-to-mouth transmission typically seen in enteric infections (e.g. *Campylobacter* spp., *Clostridium difficile*);
4. **Blood and body fluids**: this includes vertical transmission (mother to baby) or horizontal transmission (sharing needles, unprotected sex [e.g. HIV, hepatitis B and C]).

As living entities bacteria grow best when there is an ample supply of nutrients and water, an optimum pH, temperature and oxygen requirements. For these reasons the exact role that the inanimate environment may play in cross-infection can be difficult to quantify. Nevertheless, the fabric of a building, its furnishings and the medical equipment used on patients do become contaminated with hazardous

**Table 3.2** Standard precautions

Hand hygiene
Personal protective clothing
Safe handling of sharps
Cleaning and decontamination of equipment and the environment
The handling and disposal of healthcare waste
The handling and disposal of linen
The management of blood and body fluid spillages

substances, which are then handled and potentially passed on to a susceptible host. Decontamination is a generic term that refers to the removal of contaminants by a process of cleaning, disinfection or sterilisation. The precise method used will depend on the level of risk. So a surgical instrument entering a sterile body cavity would need to be sterilised to remove all microorganisms and their spores, whereas a blood pressure cuff that comes into contact with intact skin could be cleaned to remove contaminants to a safe level. In some cases a piece of equipment may not withstand a decontamination method and would be deemed a single-use item. Manufacturers of medical devices are legally obliged to provide information on how their devices should be decontaminated and this must be followed. If the instructions appear inappropriate or incomplete this should be reported to the Medicine and Health products Regulatory Agency (MHRA) as an adverse incident (MHRA, 2015).

Recently a coroner reported a case of cross-infection caused by poor decontamination of laryngoscope handles and their blades (MHRA, 2015).

- How do you think this equipment should have been decontaminated?
- How do you think it was decontaminated?
- What are the possible reasons for the variations?
- What risks does this pose to the nurse and the patient?

## Hand hygiene

As a result of the way we interact with our environment, we continually attract transient microorganisms on our hands. For this reason hand-mediated cross-infection is seen as a major contributing factor in the acquisition and spread of HCAI (Loveday et al., 2014). In 2009 the World Health Organization (WHO) developed the five moments of hand hygiene:

1. Before touching a patient;
2. Before clean/aseptic procedure;
3. After body fluid exposure risk;
4. After touching a patient;
5. After touching patient surroundings.

This was an attempt to identify key moments of hand hygiene and house them within a framework that was easy to learn, logical and applicable to a wide range of settings, and could be woven into the natural workflow of care (WHO, 2009). It has now been widely adopted as the standard expected of clinical staff.

### ACTIVITY 3.7

Next time you are in practice observe your colleagues performing hand hygiene.

- Did you think compliance would be the same across all five moments?
- Were you right?
- Can you explain the differences between moments?
- Now read page 86 of the WHO hand hygiene guidelines.

As the requirement for hand hygiene increases, the technique required to systematically remove all transient bacteria from the hand may deteriorate. Posters that demonstrate an approved technique are often present in clinical environments. As well as identifying a good technique, posters will show the parts that are frequently missed: the thumbs and finger pads. These can be a useful aide memoire to the nurse. Broadly speaking, there are three products that can be used to decontaminate hands: antiseptic solutions which are rarely necessary outside the confines of a high-risk environment or procedure; soap and water, which should be used when hands are visibly soiled, potentially contaminated with body fluids, or when caring for patients with vomiting or diarrhoeal illness; and alcohol-based hand-rub which is the preferred product after direct patient contact with hands that are not visibly soiled (WHO, 2009). The frequent use of some hand hygiene products may cause damage to the skin and alter normal hand flora. The increased colonisation of pathogenic microorganisms and reductions in hand hygiene seen in nurses with damaged skin can increase the risk of cross-infection. Damaged skin and sore hands should be reported to the occupational health department.

## Personal protective equipment

Personal protective equipment (PPE) is equipment 'that is intended to be worn or held by a person to protect them from risks to their health and safety while at work' (NICE, 2012b). Common examples include gloves, aprons, and eye and face protection. PPE fulfils two functions: to protect the nurse and to protect the patient. In making decisions about PPE the nurse will need to undertake a risk assessment. Primarily this involves asking three questions: What is the risk of contamination to the nurse? What is the risk of transmission of microorganisms to the patient or carer? What is the suitability of the equipment for the proposed use? Plastic aprons and gloves are the most commonly used pieces of PPE. Although the evidence is unclear on whether a nurse's uniform plays a significant part in cross-infection they do become heavily contaminated during clinical care. Plastic aprons offer some protection, as well protecting clothing from the splashing effects of blood or body fluids (DH, 2010b). Similarly gloves can provide a physical protective barrier that protects the nurse's hands when they come into contact with body fluids. There are many different types of gloves, sterile or non-sterile, latex, vinyl and nitrile. It is important that you are aware of the gloves that are available to you. You can then assess the task, take note of any allergies that may be present, for example to latex, before selecting the correct product. Aprons and gloves protect the patient by preventing the nurse from becoming an unwitting portal of exit because their hands and clothing may become contaminated through routine clinical care. Masks, goggles and visors are less common components of PPE, and tend to focus more on protecting the nurse. Facial protection guards the mucous membranes of the eyes, nose and mouth from aerosol-generating procedures, such as sputum induction, suctioning and bronchoscopy, or from splash, spray or splatter of blood and body fluids from a poorly controlled haemorrhage.

It is important that you wear the appropriate PPE when coming into contact with contaminated waste, linen or spills of body fluids. The aforementioned can all be contaminated with hazardous microorganisms, and need to be handled, disposed of or managed in a safe manner. You should be aware of the colour-coded system for the disposal of clinical waste and know how to locate water-soluble alginate plastic bags to remove soiled linen. Spills of high-risk body fluids should be removed as soon as possible. This may involve pre-treatment using hypochlorite granules. All healthcare facilities will have a policy on this. As an adult nurse you will frequently come into contact with sharp objects when performing procedures such as injections. Between 2004 and 2013, there were

4830 occupational exposures to blood or other high-risk body fluids reported in healthcare settings; 3396 were caused by a sharp object and 45% of these were experienced by nurses, midwives and healthcare assistants (Public Health England, 2014). Not only do these injuries constitute a major threat to healthcare workers' psychophysical wellbeing, but the true number is likely to be significantly higher because needlestick injuries are notoriously underreported.

## Aseptic non-touch technique

Due to the natural mass of microorganisms in the environment it is not possible to achieve sterility in a typical healthcare setting. However, the principles of asepsis, to remove viable pathogenic microorganisms at the time of a high-risk procedure is a more achievable aim and helps to protect the patient's portal of entry. Aseptic non-touch technique has garnered approval throughout the NHS as a set of standardised practices and procedures to ensure that only uncontaminated equipment, referred to as 'key parts' or sterile fluids, come into contact with susceptible areas, called key sites, during clinical procedures (Rowley et al., 2010). As stated earlier in the chapter, the key components of aseptic non-touch technique are:

- Always wash hands effectively;
- Non-touch technique is used at all times to protect key parts;
- Touch non-key parts with confidence;
- Take appropriate infective precautions.

Healthcare organisations that have standardised aseptic technique with aseptic non-touch technique report improved compliance with the core components of aseptic technique and associated reductions in the incidence of HCAI (Clare and Rowley, 2018). Aseptic non-touch technique is particularly targeted at the maintenance of susceptible body sites because the presence of intravenous catheters, urethral catheters, mechanical ventilation and surgical wounds exponentially increases the risk of HCAI. They do this by undermining a patient's anatomical barriers to infection, allowing bacteria to create abnormal colonisations and resistant biofilms that attach to medical devices. The standard precautions that have been already outlined, aseptic non-touch technique, hand hygiene, the use of PPE and a clean, managed environment, help to manage risk. Nevertheless, medical devices are frequently implicated in both local and systemic infections. To be able to observe, assess and respond rapidly to these challenges, nurses need to maximise the opportunities available to them. For example, there are risk assessment tools such as the visual infusion phlebitis (VIP) chart (Jackson, 1999) which allows a daily assessment of a vulnerable site, identifying early complications of phlebitis and prompt timely removal. Another idea that is gaining approval within infection prevention and control is the notion of patient empowerment. According to McGuckin (2016) patients want to be empowered and contribute to their own health, but to do this they need the nurse to communicate information to them in a way that they can understand and be convinced that this knowledge will actually give them a shared responsibility in their health.

- What opportunities have you seen where empowerment would help both the patient and the nurse to prevent and control HCAI?

## Isolation

Isolation is another practice that seeks to address a number of links within the chain of infection. Broadly there are two types of isolation: *source isolation* (barrier nursing) where the patient is the source of the infection and *protective isolation* (reverse barrier nursing) where the patient requires protection, for example if they are immunocompromised. Source isolation is more commonly encountered in practice and it has become a mainstay in the management of multi-drug-resistant organisms such as MRSA and enteric infections such as with *Clostridium difficile*. Source isolation is best carried out in a single room that has en-suite facilities and a handwashing basin. When demand for single rooms outstrips supply, patients with the same infection can sometimes be placed in the same part of the ward, and this is called cohort nursing. There are times when demand outstrips supply and difficult decisions have to be made with regard to allocation of resources. This is where you would use your knowledge of the cycle of infection and perform a risk assessment. So, for example, if you had two patients, one with MRSA and one with *Clostridium difficile*, who would you allocate the single room to? At this point you may require further information. If you discovered the MRSA was in a wound that was covered with an occlusive dressing, but the *Clostridium difficile* infection was associated with explosive diarrhoea, do you now have enough information to make a confident decision? It is important to note that, from a psychological point of view, it is the infectious microorganism that is being isolated and not the person. There is some evidence to suggest that patients who are in isolation are more likely to exhibit symptoms of depression, develop pressure ulcers, suffer falls and have longer lengths of stay (Chittick et al., 2016). Moreover, nurses have been shown to have fewer direct interactions with and perform fewer examinations on patients in isolation. It is important not to forget the human face of infection prevention and control.

## Compliance

Despite a strong evidence base to support the use of standard precautions, they are sometimes seen as basic, repetitive and small scale. Moreover the rewards for performing them in a regimented way are not always obvious. There might be times when you witness poor practice. A number of studies have demonstrated that healthcare workers are not always compliant with the five moments of hand hygiene. When they do wash their hands it may not be for the 10–15 seconds of vigorous rubbing recommended in the guidelines. Some may have a habitual preference for soap and water, despite campaigns that encourage the greater use of alcohol hand rub (AHR). AHR has been found to be quicker, more effective and kinder to hands. At times healthcare workers may don gloves when there is no contact with blood or body fluids, but continue to wear them between patients when they have become contaminated. They may place themselves at unnecessary risk by not adorning facial protection, even when they should, overfilling sharps containers and re-sheathing needles. Documentation might not always be complete and patients are often passive in their contribution to preventing HCAI. This is merely to state the challenges that the adult nurse faces in today's busy contemporary healthcare. There are enormous opportunities as well. Compliance may not be perfect but there has been a cultural change in the way the NHS manages HCAI. Cases of MRSA and *Clostridium difficile* infection have fallen significantly and these are testament to the excellent care that is taking place. Each NHS organisation will employ an infection control team and a nurse(s) will play a central role in infection prevention and control.

ACTIVITY 3.8

Find out who the infection control nurse is for your area.
Arrange a meeting to discuss the contribution you can make to preventing infection in vulnerable patients.

Related clinical skills required for entry to the
register (NMC, 2018a) include

- Safely decontaminate equipment and the environment;
- Safely assess and manage invasive medical devices and lines.

## Developing your clinical skills

The NMC (2018a) requires registered nurses to be proficient in a range of technical and non-technical patient-facing procedures, and list an extensive range of clinical skills that the adult nurse is expected to perform as part of their sphere of practice. However, clinical skills should not be viewed as task related, nor should skills be performed without critical thought. They should be seen as a vital part of caring for a patient and not in isolation. Indeed the NMC (2018a) stresses that all nursing procedures should be carried out as part of holistic patient care. Furthermore, as a registrant you will always need to ensure that you do no harm to your patients. Performing a clinical skill for which you do not have the appropriate education and recent experience may have a negative impact on the patient experience and the safety of their care.

## Simulation-based learning

Some would argue that the most valuable learning experiences take place in practice. However, Dewey (1933) suggests experience is only the raw material for learning. Therefore it is how you utilise the learning experience and what you do with it that matters. There are now many various ways to learn clinical skills and simulation-based learning is an acknowledged pedagogical approach (Hays and Singer, 1989; Rehmann et al., 1995; Cooper, 2015). Recognising the value of simulated learning the NMC (2018a) has acknowledged this method as an acceptable way to learn clinical skills. It is also noteworthy that the NMC has not suggested an upper limit in terms of hours attributed to learning by simulation, which could perhaps be interpreted as meaning that as much value is attributed to simulated learning by the NMC as to the learning that takes place in the clinical area. The adult nurse, at whatever stage in their career either as an undergraduate student or as part of established lifelong learning and revalidation of practice, should not underestimate the value of simulated learning, and it should never be seen as a poor imitation for clinical practice.

There are a number of advantages of simulation, for example being away from the clinical environment and being given the opportunity to experiment and try out clinical procedures in a safe environment, before being taking part in direct patient care, allows mistakes to be made while learning without anyone coming to harm (Lewis et al., 2012). In fact, there is now a wealth of literature supporting the value of simulation for teaching and learning clinical skills (Yuan et al.,

2012; Sundeler et al., 2015; Wighus and Bjork, 2018), and the evidence concludes that this approach meets the learning needs of students in relation to clinical skills.

## Fidelity and simulated learning

You are likely to see the term 'fidelity' connected to simulate learning. An early definition of fidelity is 'the degree of similarity between the training situation and the operational situation that is being simulated' (Hays and Singer, 1989: 50). That said, there are distinctions in the fidelity of a simulated experience. These are listed below:

- Low-limited interactivity (Wilson et al., 2005);
- Medium/intermediate-manikins with realistic sounds, e.g. breathing (Yuan et al., 2012);
- High fidelity: 'as much realism as possible' (Rehmann et al., 1995: 2), for example human-size manikins with physiological responses (Yuan et al., 2012).

The fidelity of your simulated learning experience will depend on the type of clinical skill and the availability of resources at the university or within the learning environment. It would be incorrect to assume that high-technological simulation is the optimum way to learn a clinical skill. Simulated learning can take place in a clinical skills laboratory, in a classroom, in the clinical area away from patient care or online. Nor should we underestimate the importance of reflective learning as an opportunity to reflect on undertaking a clinical skill. What is important, however, is that learning a new skill is aligned to learning objectives. These might be curriculum related (e.g. as an intended learning outcome of a particular module or unit of learning) or related to your own personal learning goals. Again, it is essential that learning the skill is not task orientated but that your learning and also the skill itself are very much central to a holistic model of nursing care.

---

### ACTIVITY 3.9

In each of your placement areas, you should be thinking about opportunities for developing your clinical skills and considering which clinical skills you wish to learn.

- Set yourself three learning objectives for each skill you wish to learn or develop;
- Take part in learning the clinical skill;
- Reflect on your learning in your portfolio. Have you met your learning objectives? If not what can you do to meet your learning needs?

---

## Chapter summary

It is crucial that nurses can deliver person-centred, evidence-based nursing care in a sensitive and compassionate manner. Systematic approaches to nursing care and the use of assessment frameworks and models offer us processes by which we can work closely with patients to plan individualised care pathways and guide the delivery of high-quality person-centred nursing care. However in order to be able to do so, our decisions need to be informed and underpinned by a good level of knowledge and understanding of the associated anatomy, physiology and pathophysiology, an understanding of the need to protect patient safety and an ability to integrate theory, simulation and practice.

# Further reading

Barrett, D., Wilson, B. and Woollands, A. (2012) *Care Planning: A Guide for Nurses*, 2nd edn. Harlow: Pearson.
Boore, J., Cook, N. and Shepherd, A. (2016) *Essentials of Anatomy and Physiology for Nursing Practice*. London: Sage.
Delves-Yates, C. (2015) *Essentials of Nursing Practice*. London: Sage.
Doherty, L. and Lister, S. (2015) *The Royal Marsden Manual of Clinical Procedures*, 9th edn. Chichester: Wiley.
Holland, K., Jenkins, J., Solomon, J. and Whittam, S. (2008) *Applying the Roper–Logan–Tierney Model in Practice*, 2nd edn. Edinburgh: Churchill Livingstone.
Moore, T. (2017) 'Observations and monitoring'. In T. Moore and S. Cunningham (eds), *Clinical Skills for Nursing Practice*. Oxon: Routledge, Chapter 7.

# References

Barrett, D., Wilson, B. and Woollands, A. (2012) *Care Planning: A Guide for Nurses*, 2nd edn. Harlow: Pearson.
British Association for Parental and Enteral Nutrition (2011) *Malnutrition Universal Screening Tool*. London: BAPEN. Available at: https://www.bapen.org.uk/pdfs/must/must-full.pdf
Centers for Disease Control and Prevention (2012) *Principles of Epidemiology in Public Health Practice*, 3rd edn. *An Introduction to Applied Epidemiology and Biostatistics*. Available at: www.cdc.gov/ophss/csels/dsepd/ss1978/lesson1/section10.html (last accessed 14 May 2018).
Chittick, P., Koppisetty, S., Lombardo, L., Vadhavana, A., Solanki, A., Cumming, K., Agboto, V., Karl, C. and Band, J. (2016) 'Assessing patient and caregiver understanding of and satisfaction with the use of contact isolation', *American Journal of Infection Control*, 44: 657–60.
Clare, S. and Rowley, S. (2018) 'Implementing the Aseptic Non Touch Technique (ANTT®) clinical practice framework for aseptic technique: a pragmatic evaluation using a mixed methods approach in two London hospitals', *Journal of Infection Prevention*, 19: 6–15.
Cooper, S. (2015) 'Simulation versus lecture? Measuring educational impact: considerations for best practice', *Evidence Based Nursing*, 19(2). Available at: http://dx.doi.org/10.1136/eb-2015-102221 (last accessed 14 August 2018).
Cowdell, F. and Garrett, D. (2014) 'Older people and skin: challenging perceptions', *British Journal of Nursing*, 23(12): S4–8.
Department of Health (2010a) *Essence of Care Benchmarks for Personal Hygiene*. London: DH.
Department of Health (2010b) *Uniforms and Workwear: Guidance of Uniforms and Workwear Policies for NHS Employers*. London: DH.
Department of Health (2013) *Learning Disabilities Good Practice Project*. London: DH. Available at: www.gov.uk/government/publications/learning-disabilities-good-practice-project-report (last accessed 13 May 2018).
Dewey, J. (1933) *How We Think: A Restatement of Reflective Thinking to the Educative Process*. Boston, MA: Heath.
Doyle, C., Byrne, K., Fleming, S., Griffiths, C., Horan, P. and Keenan, P.M. (2016) 'Enhancing the experience of people with intellectual disabilities who access health care', *Learning Disability Practice*, 19(6): 19.
European Pressure Ulcer Advisory Panel (2009) *Prevention and Treatment of Pressure Ulcers: Quick Reference Guide*. National Pressure Ulcer Advisory Panel, European Pressure Ulcer Advisory Panel and Pan Pacific Pressure Injury Alliance. Available at: www.npuap.org/wp-content/uploads/2014/08/Quick-Reference-Guide-DIGITAL-NPUAP-EPUAP-PPPIA.pdf (last accessed 14 May 2018).
Gold, D.A. (2012) 'An examination of instrumental activities of daily living assessment in older adults and mild cognitive impairment', *Journal of Clinical and Experimental Neuropsychology*, 34(1): 11–34.

Growdon, M.E., Shorr, R.I. and Inouye, S.K. (2017) 'The tension between promoting mobility and preventing falls in the hospital', *JAMA Internal Medicine*, 177(6): 759–60.

Hardy, S. (2013) 'Prevention and management of depression in primary care', *Nursing Standard*, 27(26): 51–6.

Harris, C., Kuhnke, J. and Haley, J. (2018) *Best Practice Recommendations for the Prevention and Management of Surgical Wound Complications.* Available at: www.woundscanada.ca/docman/public/health-care- ... Best practice recommendations for the prevention and management of skin tears. ... /public/555-bpr-prevention-and-management-of-surgical-wound-complications-v2/file (last accessed 14 August 2018).

Hays, R. and Singer, M. (1989) *Simulation Fidelity in Training System Design: Bridging the Gap Between Reality and Training.* New York: Springer.

Health and Social Care Act (2008) *Code of Practice on the Prevention and Control of Infections and Related Guidance.* London: Department of Health and Social Care.

Health Protection Agency (2011) *English National Point Prevalence Survey on Healthcare-associated Infections and Antimicrobial Use.* London: Health Protection Agency.

Heslop, P., Blair, P., Fleming, P., Hoghton, M., Marriott, A. and Russ, L. (2013) *Confidential Inquiry into Premature Deaths of People with Learning Disabilities (CIPOLD).* Bristol: Norah Fry Research Centre, University of Bristol. Available at: www.bristol.ac.uk/cipold (last accessed 13 May 2018).

Jackson, A. (1999) *IV Therapy and Care.* Rotherham General Hospital NHS Trust: A. Jackson.

Khan, H., Kanwal Baig, F. and Mehboob, R. (2017) 'Nosocomial infections: epidemiology, prevention, control and surveillance', *Asian Pacific Journal of Tropical Biomedicine*, 7(5): 478–82.

Kneafsey, R., Clifford, C. and Greenfield, S. (2013) 'What is the nursing team involvement in maintaining and promoting the mobility of older adults in hospital? A grounded theory study', *International Journal of Nursing Studies*, 50: 1617–29.

Kroenke, K., Spitzer, R.L. & Williams, J.B. (2001) 'The PHQ-9: validity of a brief depression severity measure', *Journal of General Internal Medicine*, 16(9): 606–13.

Law Commission (2017) *Mental Capacity and Deprivation of Liberty.* Available at: www.lawcom.gov.uk/app/uploads/2017/03/lc372_mental_capacity.pdf (last accessed 12 May 2018).

Lawton, M.P. and Brody, E.M. (1969) 'Assessment of older people: self-maintaining and instrumental activities of daily living', *Gerontologist*, 9: 179–86.

Lewis, R., Stachan, A. and McKenzie Smith, M. (2012) 'Is high fidelity the most effective method for the development of non-technical skills in nursing? A review of the current evidence', *Open Nursing Journal*, 6: 82–9.

Loveday, H., Wilson, J., Pratt, R., Golsorkhi, M., Tingle, A., Bak, A., Browne, J., Prieto, J. and Wilcox, M. (2014) 'Epic3: national evidence-based guidelines for preventing healthcare-associated infections in NHS hospitals in England', *Journal of Hospital Infection*, 86(Suppl 1): S1–70.

Manz, F. and Wentz, A. (2005) 'The importance of good hydration for the prevention of chronic diseases', *Nutrition Review*, 63(6 Pt 2): S2–5.

McGuckin, M. (2016) 'Patient and healthcare worker empowerment'. In P. Elliot, J. Storr and A. Jeanes (eds), *Infection Prevention and Control: Perceptions and Perspectives.* Boca Raton, FL: CRC Press, pp. 175–88.

Medicines and Healthcare products Regulatory Agency (2015) *Managing Medical Devices.* London: MHRA.

MENCAP (2007) *Death by Indifference: Following up the Treat me Right! Report.* London: MENCAP. Available at: www.mencap.org.uk/sites/default/files/2016-06/DBIreport.pdf (last accessed 13 May 2018).

Mlinac, M.E. and Feng, M.C. (2016) 'Assessment of activities of daily living, self care and independence', *Archives of Clinical Neuropsychology*, 31, 506–16.

Moore, Z. and Cowman, S. (2014) 'Risk assessment tools for the prevention of pressure ulcers', *Cochrane Database Systematic Reviews*, 5(2): CD006471.

Morton-Nance, S. (2015) 'Unique role of learning disability liaison nurses', *Learning Disability Practice*, 18(7): 30–4.

National Heart, Lung and Blood Institute (2011) *Your Guide to Healthy Sleep.* Bethesda, MD: NHLBI.

National Institute for Health and Care Excellence (2006) *Nutritional Support for Adults: Oral Nutritional Support, Enteral Tube Feeding and Parenteral Nutrition*. Available at: www.nice.org.uk/Guidance/cg32 (last accessed 12 May 2018).

National Institute for Health and Care Excellence (2008) *Surgical Site Infections: Prevention and Treatment* (updated 2017). London: NICE.

National Institute for Health and Care Excellence (2012a) *Nutrition Support in Adults (Quality Standard)*. Available at: www.nice.org.uk/guidance/qs24/resources/nutrition-support-in-adults-pdf-2098545777349 (last accessed 12 May 2018).

National Institute for Health and Care Excellence (2012b) *Healthcare-associated Infections: Prevention and Control in Primary and Community Care*. London: NICE.

National Institute for Health and Care Excellence (2013) *Assessment and Prevention of Falls in Older People*. Available at: www.nice.org.uk/guidance/cg161/evidence/falls-full-guidance-190033741 (last accessed 13 May 2018).

National Institute for Health and Care Excellence (2015) *Pressure Ulcers (Quality Standard)*. London: NICE.

National Institute for Health and Care Excellence (2016) *Healthcare-associated Infections (Quality Standard)*. London: NICE.

National Institute for Health and Care Excellence (2018) *Managing Exacerbations of COPD (Care Pathway)*. London: NICE. Available at: https://pathways.nice.org.uk/pathways/chronic-obstructive-pulmonary-disease (last accessed 12 May 2018).

Ness, V. and Murray, J. (2009) 'Mobilising'. In C. Doherty and J. McCallum (eds), *Foundation Clinical Nursing Skills*. Oxford: Oxford University Press, pp. 379–421.

NHS Digital (2015) Cited in National Pressure Ulcer Advisory Panel, European Pressure Ulcer Advisory Panel. London: Public Health England.

NHS England (2017) *The Learning Disabilities Mortality Review (LeDeR Programme) Annual Report*, December 2017. Bristol: Norah Fry Centre for Disability Studies.

Nursing and Midwifery Council (2018a) *Future Nurse: Standards of Proficiency for Registered Nurses*. London: NMC.

Nursing and Midwifery Council (2018b) *The Code: Professional Standards of Practice and Behaviour for Nurses and Midwives*. Available at: www.nmc.org.uk/globalassets/sitedocuments/nmc-publications/nmc-code.pdf (last accessed 30 April 2018).

O'Meara, S., Cullum, N., Nelson, E., et al. (2012) 'Compression for venous leg ulcers', *Cochrane Database of Systematic Reviews*, 11: CD000265.

Orlando, I.J. (1961) *The Dynamic Nurse–Patient Relationship: Function, Process And Principles*. New York: G.P. Putmans & Sons. [Reprinted, 1990, New York: National League for Nursing.]

Parliamentary and Health Service Ombudsman (2009) *Six Lives: The Provision of Public Services to People with Learning Disabilities*. Available at: www.gov.uk/government/publications/report (last accessed 13 May 2018).

Phillips, L. (2012) 'Improving care for people with learning disabilities in hospital', *Nursing Standard*, 26(23): 42–58.

Public Health England (2014) *Eye of the Needle: United Kingdom Surveillance of Significant Occupational Exposures to Bloodborne Viruses in Healthcare Workers*. London: Public Health England.

Public Health England (2018) *Reasonable Adjustments: A Legal Duty*. London: PHE. Available at: www.gov.uk/government/publications/reasonable-adjustments-for-people-with-learning-disabilities/reasonable-adjustments-a-legal-duty (last accessed 13 May 2018).

Rehmann, A., Mitman, R. and Reynolds, M. (1995) *A Handbook of Flight Simulation Fidelity Requirements for Human Factors Research*. Defense Technical Information Center. Technical report DOT/FAA/CT-TN95/46. Available at: www.dtic.mil/dtic/tr/fulltext/u2/a303799.pdf.

Roper, N., Logan, W.W. and Tierney, A.J. (2000) *The Roper–Logan–Tierney Model of Nursing: Based on Activities of Living*. London: Churchill-Livingstone.

Rowley, S., Clare, S., Macqueen, S. and Molyneux, R. (2010) 'ANTT v2: an updated practice framework for aseptic technique', *British Journal of Nursing*, 19(5): s5–11.

Scottish Intercollegiate Guidelines Network (2010) *Management of Chronic Venous Leg Ulcers*. Edinburgh: SIGN. Available at: www.sign.ac.uk/assets/sign120.pdf (last accessed 14 May 2018).

Stanton, J., Hickman, A., Rouncivell, D., Collins, C. and Gray, D. (2016) 'Promoting patient concordance to support rapid leg ulcer healing', *Journal of Community Nursing*, 30(6): 28–35.

Sundeler, A., Pettersson, A. and Burglund, M. (2015) 'Undergraduate nursing students' experiences when examining nursing skills in clinical simulation laboratories with high-fidelity patient simulators: a phenomenological research study', *Nurse Education Today*, 35: 1257–61.

Taylor, V. and Ashelsford, S. (2008) 'Understanding depression in palliative and end of life care', *Nursing Standard*, 23(12): 48–57.

Thomas, B. and Atkinson, D. (2011) 'Improving health outcomes for people with learning disabilities', *Nursing Standard*, 26(6): 33–6.

van Helvoort, H.A., Willems, L.M., Dekhuijzen, R., van Hees, H. and Heijdra, Y.F. (2016) 'Respiratory constraints during activities in daily life and the impact on health status in patients with early-stage COPD: a cross-sectional study', *NPJ Primary Care Respiratory Medicine*, 26: 16054.

Waterlow, J. (2008) *Pressure Ulcer Risk Assessment and Prevention*. Available at: www.judy-waterlow.co.uk/waterlow_score.htm (last accessed 12 May 2018).

Wighus, M. and Bjork, I.T. (2018) 'An educational intervention to enhance clinical skills learning: experiences of nursing students and teachers', *Nurse Education in Practice*, 29: 143–9.

Wilson, M., Shepherd, C., Kelly, J. and Pitzner, J. (2005) 'Assessment of low fidelity human patient simulator for the acquisition of nursing skills', *Nurse Education Today*, 25: 56–67.

World Health Organization (2009) *WHO Guidelines on Hand Hygiene in Health Care*. Geneva: WHO.

World Health Organization (2016) *International Classification of Diseases*, 10th revision. Geneva: WHO. Available at: http://apps.who.int/classifications/icd10/browse/2016/en#F34.0 (last accessed 12 May 2018).

Yuan, H., Williams, B. and Fang, J. (2012) 'The contribution of high fidelity simulation to nursing students' confidence and competence', *International Nursing Review*, 59: 26–33.

4

# INTERPROFESSIONAL AND MULTIDISCIPLINARY TEAM WORKING

## JEAN ROGERS AND SARAH BOOTH

---

### CHAPTER OBJECTIVES

- Define the terms multidisciplinary and interprofessional working;
- Reflect upon and identify the factors that contribute to the development of partnership and team work, considering how you can develop these skills;
- Identify and reflect upon factors that can prevent collaborative partnerships and team working;
- Explore strategies for overcoming the barriers to interprofessional working and consider how you can develop these skills;
- Explore the benefits of effective team working in the provision of effective healthcare and consider how you can apply these within a contemporary healthcare setting.

---

So far, the previous chapters have focused on the knowledge and skills required to be an adult nurse as well as the concept of safe and effective person-centred care. However, often good patient care cannot be provided or achieved by one individual: it takes a team of health and social care professionals to deliver truly effective, quality patient care. The aims of this chapter are therefore to explore how interprofessional and multidisciplinary working has the potential to impact positively on the health needs of patients and identify factors that contribute to the development of collaborative working partnerships.

## Related NMC proficiencies for registered nurses

The overarching requirement of the Nursing and Midwifery Council (NMC) is that all nurses must be able to play an active and equal role in the interdisciplinary team, collaborating and communicating effectively with a range of colleagues. They must work effectively across professional and agency boundaries, actively involving and respecting the contribution of others to ensure the provision of integrated person-centred care. They must know when and how to communicate with and refer to other professionals and agencies in order to respect the choices of service users and others, promoting shared decision making to deliver positive outcomes and coordinating smooth, effective transition within and between services and agencies (NMC, 2018a).

## To achieve entry to the nursing register you must be able to

- Demonstrate an understanding of the roles, responsibilities and scope of practice of all members of the nursing and interdisciplinary team, and know how to make best use of the contributions of others involved in providing care;
- Understand and apply the principles of partnership, collaboration and interagency working across all relevant sectors;
- Demonstrate the knowledge and confidence to contribute effectively and proactively within an interdisciplinary team;
- Demonstrate the ability to write accurate, clear and timely records and documentation;
- Effectively and responsibly use a range of digital technologies to access, input, analyse and apply information and data within teams and between agencies;
- Confidently and clearly share and present verbal, digital and written reports or information and instructions with individuals and groups when delegating or handing over responsibility for care;
- Demonstrate knowledge of when and how to refer people safely to other professionals or services for clinical intervention or support.

(Adapted from NMC, 2018a)

Throughout this chapter we will use real examples and case studies so that you can gain a wider perspective of interprofessional and multidisciplinary working. However, before exploring interprofessional and multidisciplinary working in more detail, it would be useful to consider what each term means.

- What do the terms 'multidisciplinary' and 'interprofessional' working mean to you?

Multidisciplinary working describes the mechanism by which holistic care for patients is ensured and a seamless service delivered across the boundaries of primary, secondary and tertiary care (Jeffries and Chan, 2004). However, it is about the task and not necessarily the collective working process so it does not imply collaboration. There are some distinct advantages and disadvantages to multidisciplinary working (Table 4.1).

Alternatively, Pollard et al. (2014: 13) define interprofessional working as 'the process whereby members of different professions and/or agencies work with each other and patients/service users, to provide integrated health and/or social care for the latter's benefit'. This is supported by

**Table 4.1**  Advantages and disadvantages of multidisciplinary working

| Advantages | Disadvantages |
| --- | --- |
| Patient receives better all-round care | Differing professions work together but keep their defined role (working in their silos) |
| All plans can be discussed so that all pros and cons can be considered | Takes more time to come to conclusions |
| More likely to provide comprehensive care and less likely that anything is missed | Information not always shared properly |
| Team members aware of progress in case anyone becomes ill | Communication can be a challenge |
| Best use of resources | Professional rivalry and mistrust |
| Reduces the number of people to whom the patient needs to relate | |

Day (2006: 9) who believes it is about 'professions relating to and among each other for the mutual benefit of those involved'. Similarly there are also some clear advantages and disadvantages to interprofessional working, which will be discussed later in the chapter.

Barrett et al. (2005) believe the prefix 'multi' indicates the involvement of personnel from different professions and does not imply collaboration, whereas 'inter' implies collaboration. Therefore, it is sensible to define collaboration.

- What does the term 'collaboration' mean to you?

Biggs (2006) defines collaboration as working together to achieve something that no profession could achieve alone. Barrett et al. (2005) agree and describe collaboration as a common purpose that develops mutually negotiated goals with agreed plans and procedures. Individual knowledge and expertise are brought together to facilitate decision making which is undertaken jointly with shared viewpoints from a number of professions for the benefit of patients. As Barrett et al. (2005) maintain, collaborative practice is the same as interprofessional working. The terms 'interprofessional' and 'multidisciplinary' are often used interchangeably and thus, for the purposes of this chapter, we will be using the term 'interprofessional working'.

## Background to interprofessional working

Interprofessional team working is a key objective in any contemporary health and social care setting. Working interprofessionally is seen by all professional bodies as essential for promoting effective patient care. However, it is not a new concept (Lavin et al., 2001) because team working has been an integral part of healthcare from the 1960s onwards (Baldwin, 1993). Before this, staff from various disciplines worked in distinct professional teams (silos) and had no real knowledge of what each other's roles entailed. This required multiple duplication of documentation, which often resulted in patients being asked for the same details over and over again. Patient care was also fragmented. Ongoing developments in approaches to service delivery frequently resulted in high levels of specialisation. Irvine et al. (2002) maintain this meant that it was not possible for any one professional to have the knowledge and skills to respond appropriately to patient need, particularly where the complex needs of communities or individuals are required.

- What do you think are the key strengths of interprofessional working?

One of the key strengths of interprofessional working is that the combined expertise of a range of health professionals is used to deliver seamless, comprehensive care to individual patients. The World Health Organization (2010) suggest that interprofessional collaboration is an essential component of satisfactory service delivery. Barrett et al. (2005) argue that the quality of service received is dependent on how effectively different professions work together. This is supported by Baker et al. (2006) who believe that the modernisation of healthcare delivery has initiated a move towards the collaborative delivery of care and that this effective team work links to more positive patient outcomes (Grumbach and Bodenheimer, 2004). The year 1997 saw massive and radical changes in health and social care policy with UK governments advocating collaboration and clear partnership working across the public sector, placing a strong emphasis on collaborative working and its importance in meeting patients' needs by bringing together health and social care professionals across a range of organisations. It was clear that in order for health service modernisation to be effective, robust and integrated professional working was required. In England this was promoted in the NHS Plan (Department of Health or DH, 2000a), a ten-year plan to reform practice that was instrumental in shaping the way we view and adopt interprofessional working today. Indeed UK healthcare provision has changed radically and rapidly in the last decade and this is reflected in political and policy decisions at all levels; regionally, nationally and internationally (Furlong and Smith, 2005).

## ☐? ACTIVITY 4.1

Within NHS settings, what recent changes are you aware of that have impacted on the delivery of patient care? Make a list of these.

Now access one of the following websites below and identify the relevant government health policy documents that highlight the changing context in which healthcare is delivered in your area:

**England**: www.gov.uk/government/organisations/department-of-health

**Scotland**: www.scotland.gov.uk

**Northern Ireland**: www.dhsspsni.gov.uk

**Wales**: www.wales.gov.uk

In England several documents highlight the changing context in which healthcare is delivered: these include *The NHS Plan* (DH, 2000a), *Modernising Nursing Careers: Setting the Direction* (DH, 2006), *High Quality Care for All: Next Stage Review* (DH, 2008) and the Berwick Report (DH, 2013). In addition, the Health and Social Care Act 2012 (see www.legislation.gov.uk/ukpga/2012/7/contents/enacted), Willis Commission Report (2012) and the Care Act 2014 (see www.legislation.gov.uk/ukpga/2014/23/contents/enacted) all highlight the changing context in which healthcare is delivered. These documents emphasise the increasingly busy environment in which care takes place; the constantly changing staff population; the growing use of technology; the increasing acuity of the patient population; an ageing population and the move to more community-based services with limited resource availability. It is expected that these changes will continue and there is now, more than ever, a realisation of the importance of holistic patient-centred care and a wider recognition that no one person has the knowledge and skills to deliver high-quality care (Atwal and Caldwell, 2005). Thomas (2005) also maintains that the active contribution of patients to the decision-making process will make working together truly collaborative. This has become more crucial than ever in the wake of highlighted examples of poor NHS care, for example in Bristol (DH, 2001), Alder Hey (The Royal Liverpool Children's Enquiry, House of Commons, 2001) and the Mid Staffordshire NHS Foundation Trust (Mid Staffordshire NHS Foundation Trust, 2013).

Socially and politically there is a demand for service-user involvement in planning and prioritising service delivery, with UK governments promoting the principle of choice for users and working in partnership. For example, in 2006 the Department of Health stressed the importance of effective interprofessional and multidisciplinary working when planning services for people with long-term needs (DH, 2006). The aim was to establish joint health and social care teams, using joint case notes and/or records to support people with the most complex needs, thereby ensuring that care was truly multidisciplinary. Indeed, there are some excellent examples where health and social care teams have been able to work effectively and collaboratively together, for example working with people with severe and long-term mental health problems in their own homes (Scottish Government, 2010). Other examples include work in intermediate care settings when addressing safeguarding concerns. Health and social care professionals working together, communicating and addressing the complex needs of the patients, as well as combining expertise, perspectives and resources, can form a common goal to restore, maintain and improve outcomes for patients. In Greater Manchester, the government have gone further, strengthening devolution to the Greater Manchester Combined Authority (GMCA) by devolving spending power of £6 billion worth of health and social care. Other areas (i.e. London, Cornwall, Liverpool and North East England) are likely to follow suit.

Reflect on the teams you have previously worked within.

- Has your experience been a positive or a negative one?
- Why do you think this might be?

Over the last decade significant progress has been made towards creating environments where interprofessional working can thrive and be a positive experience, but in some practice areas it appears this is not so easy to achieve (Hanson et al., 2008). There have been numerous examples where difficult interprofessional working has been reported (Glasby et al., 2008). Atwal (2002) argues this is because power, status, autonomy and expert knowledge have become challenges. Weiss and Welbourne (2008) agree, stating that the characteristics of some professions bring about distinct occupational identities and exclusionary market shelters (domination), which set occupations apart and often in opposition. Kell and Owen (2008) maintain that this is as a result of creating boundaries so tight that only one profession can deliver that activity (e.g. medicine), which can then make them static. This strong group bonding legitimises participants and ensures that they have negative attitudes to people outside of their group.

You may remember that in Chapter 1 we highlighted that, until late in the twentieth century, some groups – predominantly male occupations (e.g. medicine) – were identified as professions, with distinct characteristics of completing a course of education to at least graduate level, having autonomy and self-regulation and remaining free from managerial control. Alternatively, other predominantly female occupations (e.g. nursing and midwifery) were seen as semi-professions that in contrast received 'training' and were regulated and overseen by other occupational groups (Barrett et al., 2005). Kesby (2002) maintains that the current drive towards interprofessional working will help to give the semi-professions power to raise their status. Jeffrey and Trowman (2009), however, disagree and state that professions are losing their position of prestige and trust. Medicine and other professions are 'under attack'. The development of clinical commissioning groups (CCGs) has seen new NHS organisations set up to organise the delivery of NHS services in England underpinned by the Health and Social Care Act 2012 (see www.legislation.gov.uk/ukpga/2012/7/contents/enacted), thus giving other clinicians as well as GPs the power to influence commissioning decisions for their patients.

## HEALTHCARE PROVISION IN A PRISON SETTING

A large male prison sends prisoners with medical problems for scans on an individual basis to the local hospital. Only one prisoner at a time is able to attend for security reasons and has to be accompanied by a member of staff at a cost of £250 a visit. Therefore, waiting times for these patients are huge. There are also further problems in that prisoners have to be handcuffed, resulting in a high failure rate for scans (for security reasons the prisoners are not told in advance the day or time of the scan). This often means that they are not prepared properly, for example having eaten when they should not have done so. In response to the issues identified above, the prison service and CCG have developed a more collaborative approach to meet patient need. The local CCG commissioned a GP-led ultrasound team who now visit the prison once a week, working with and alongside the prison healthcare team, scanning seven or eight prisoners at any one time. This saves local money, improves efficiency and provides dignity for the prisoners (Tweedale, 2013), thus streamlining their care.

The above scenario provides a good example of how money can be saved in the NHS. However, it is about not just saving money but also utilising precious resources more efficiently and effectively in order to achieve a better standard of care for patients and their families. This may require greater involvement and collaboration between the private sector and charities as well as healthcare providers. On the other hand, media scandals such as the Shipman Enquiry (Smith, 2002), the Bristol Enquiry (DH, 2001), failures at the Mid Staffordshire NHS Trust (Mid Staffordshire NHS Foundation Trust, 2013), Morecambe Bay (Kirkup, 2015) and Liverpool Community Trust (Kirkup, 2018) have changed the public perception of professions, thereby increasing the number of lawsuits. The public have become much more knowledgeable through the increase in technology and education making knowledge more accessible. Sometimes, that knowledge is incorrect or limited and does not provide the full picture. It can therefore be much more challenging to negotiate and compromise with members of the public. This has had an effect on policy, creating turbulence where policy is formulated in order to achieve political goals, address systemic failings and produce rapid-fire responses to public disillusionment (Bradford, 2008). Healthcare professionals working within these environments are then left to make sense of new ways of working and demands, i.e. what they do and how they should go about it (Baxter, 2011).

List the reasons why people/patients may lose faith in the NHS.

- What effect do you think this might have on the healthcare professionals working within this service?

Across the UK poor interprofessional collaboration has been identified as a contributing factor in very high-profile cases with poor outcomes (DH, 2001, 2003; Laming, 2009; Mid Staffordshire NHS Foundation Trust, 2013). Following such criticisms people lose faith in the NHS because they are concerned with carelessness in services, long waits and poor communication. For health professionals this can cause disillusionment within the profession and lower morale. There are assumptions that interprofessional working will prevent such tragedies as well as poor practice, but as yet there is no real research or evidence to support this assumption. This is mainly due to the complex nature of the research, the funding available, and the collaboration needed across practice and **higher education institutions** (HEIs) (Barwell et al., 2013).

- There are some advantages to interprofessional working. What do you think these are?

The advantages to interprofessional working include:

- **Enhancing personal and professional confidence;**
- **Promoting mutual understanding** of all the professions and their roles;
- **Promoting interprofessional communication** and breaking down barriers to communication;
- **Recognising and respecting** each professional role and their contribution to patient care;
- **Contributing to job satisfaction**: working together in harmony makes working life much better;
- **Sharing information and knowledge** to provide improved decision making with regard to patient care (Spry, 2006);
- **Problem sharing**: as the old adage goes 'a problem shared is a problem halved'. Just talking through patient care problems with another professional colleague can sometimes help to provide the solution to a problem.

## SANJIT

Sanjit suffered a spinal injury and after many months of rehabilitation he was more or less ready to go home. Members of the multidisciplinary team had been involved in his care. Physiotherapists had got him to a stage where he could transfer himself from his wheelchair to a bed or toilet. The occupational therapist had assessed him as being able to make simple drinks and food. The nursing staff had ensured he remained motivated and had included his family in his care. Medical staff had monitored him and ensured that he had fully recovered and the pharmacist had ensured that his medication met his new needs. Sanjit was going on a home visit with a view to staying at home if all was okay. Two hours later he returned to the ward very subdued. The occupational therapist explained to the team that, when Sanjit arrived at his home, he was unable to get into the house as the doors were not wide enough; she also advised that it could take up to two weeks for the adaptation service to resolve this. One small thing was therefore keeping Sanjit in hospital and damaging his morale, which could affect his future. On further discussion one staff member suggested that she would contact the facilities staff and ask them for a favour. She rang them and explained the situation and they promised to carry out the alterations in the next hour 'although it was not part of their remit'. The occupational therapist agreed to stay on in order that Sanjit could be safely discharged as planned. The doors were widened and the patient was discharged that day much to his and the team's delight.

The case scenario above illustrates multiprofessional working at its best, with all disciplines working together to achieve streamlined quality patient care that helped Sanjit to return back to his own home as soon as possible.

## GEORGE

George was admitted to hospital after a stroke that resulted in him suffering a left-hand-side weakness and speech difficulties. A case conference was held to agree a discharge plan (attended by the social worker, occupational therapist, physiotherapist, speech and language therapist, member of the nursing team and a medical colleague). The physiotherapist was concerned that George's wife, Gloria, may not manage. The occupational therapist offered to carry out a home assessment visit before discharge to ensure that she could. The team devised a mobilisation programme to enhance George's mobility, a social work assessment to see if he needed any more help and a speech and language assessment to ensure that his nutrition remained at an optimum level. The speech and language therapist also helped Gloria to communicate with her aphasic husband. George was discharged home three weeks later.

- Referring to the above scenario, what do you think went well?
- What could have been improved and how?

This scenario displays good interprofessional working, although this could have been improved further by including George and his wife in the discussions. Service users and carers can offer a unique perspective on how a particular illness or disease affects them or their loved ones. It is therefore essential that interprofessional teams ensure that patients and carers are fully consulted and involved in decision-making processes about their care provision, and that their contribution to care planning, implementation and evaluation is meaningful.

Over the last decade healthcare policy in the UK and Scotland has been centred around patient empowerment, with service users/carers being at the centre of decisions made around their care (Scottish Government, 2010). One good example of that is patients with dementia who come into hospital with their own passport of care. In this case, the multidisciplinary team members who have been working with the patient clearly identify what they have been doing and what works or does not work for that particular patient. Patients are able to input their thoughts, feelings and needs about their care. This then allows staff to work to get the patient home in their optimal healthcare state.

## Team working

Working in health and social care settings usually involves some aspect of team working. Effective team working does not just happen when a team of people work together – in fact team work could be really poor in a group of people working together or could be really effective. Katzenbach and Smith (1993) define team work as a small number of people who have skills that are complementary and are committed to a common purpose, performance goals and approaches, generating synergy through their coordinated effort. Within a healthcare setting, team working is vital in delivering high-quality care. The best outcomes are achieved when professionals work and learn together as well as engaging in clinical audits and generating innovative ways of moving the practice and service forward.

Consider your current or recent placement and the teams you have worked in:

- Did the teams work well together or not?
- Why do you think this was the case?
- Try to identify all of the potential barriers to effective team working. How do you think these might be overcome?

In order to do this effectively there are some key factors that encourage team work (Reeves et al., 2009; Salas et al., 2009), including the following:

- *Personal commitment*: this comes from individuals who are committed to the success of the team and also requires that the leader of the team allow members to ask questions. In teams where this occurs, all members will have an idea about what best practice is and are not expected to go beyond their level of competence unsupported. An individual's weaknesses are minimised and their strengths maximised, thereby releasing their true potential.
- *A common goal or vision*: all teams need to develop a common goal or vision. When teams are working towards a common goal they are committed and this inspires team members to learn and gain confidence. In fact, within a healthcare team there may need to be two visions: one for the team and one for the organisation.

- *Clarity of roles*: team members need to be clear about their various roles within a team because this will maintain their motivation. It is also important that they are clear about the roles of the other team members. In today's environment, we are increasingly working with members from different organisations and professional groups. It is thought that this understanding encourages a team approach to patient need, where information and knowledge are shared to enable improved decision making about patient care (Spry, 2006). This will also encourage mutual trust and respect within teams.
- *Communication*: effective communication between team members is crucial for patient safety. It encourages joint problem solving and the provision of excellent interprofessional patient-centred care. The team should adopt two-way information giving rather than unidirectional pathways, thus ensuring that information is shared with the whole team.
- *Support*: the best teams work most effectively where there is a framework to support interprofessional working, although Pirrie et al. (1998) believe the degree of support can be variable.

---

### ACTIVITY 4.2

Consult the views of current members of the team in which you are working.

- What do they think are the advantages and disadvantages of team working?

---

There are some clear advantages to team working in a healthcare setting (Clements et al., 2007; Leggat, 2007). In the activity above your colleagues may have identified some or all of these:

- Improvements in the quality of patient care: when the team communicates effectively and works together as a unit the quality of patient care increases. They have a clear commitment to excellence of care. This increases coordination, especially in complex cases;
- Improvements in patient safety: if team work is effective the patient becomes an active partner in their own care. The patient is listened to and monitored and procedures are based on feedback. This has the potential to reduce medication errors and unnecessary procedures, thereby creating a safer environment for the patient;
- Improvements in staff satisfaction: teams that work efficiently and effectively brainstorm and problem solve together. The workload tends to be distributed more evenly and stress is reduced;
- Improvements in communication: because the team members regularly interact with each other they are able to contribute to the decision making in the team, thus making their shared goals and visions achievable;
- Improved knowledge of each person's role: a team working well together will learn about each person's role and limitations. This strengthens relationships and builds unity in the team;
- Enhanced reflection: efficient and effective teams regularly reflect on how they work together and how effective they are being;

- More innovative approach to work: a team that works well together can potentially be more innovative in their outlook. There is verbal and practical support for new ideas, thus moving the team forward;
- Improved problem solving: an effective team bounces ideas off each other. Each person offers their unique perspective on a problem and comes up with the best solution;
- Enhanced skills: no one person is the same as another and so teams need to use each person's unique skills to improve one other and be more productive in the future.

## Disadvantages of team working

As you can see there are many advantages to team working that are often talked about but there are some disadvantages here too (Day, 2006; Sims et al., 2014), including the following:

- Unequal participation: sometimes some members of the team will sit back and let others do most of the work. This can have an adverse effect by causing resentment, which can then cause conflict and affect morale;
- Members who are not team players: some people do not function well as part of a team and prefer to work alone. They can be excellent workers in the right situation but have difficulty fitting into a team, thus causing dissatisfaction and disharmony;
- A lack of constructive conflict: once a team works well together members may become reluctant to argue or dispute a point. If all conflict is avoided resentment can build up and team members can become lazy and apathetic, thus stifling creativity;
- Traditions and professional cultures: for some this can cause split loyalties between the team and their own discipline. Some team members may be reluctant to accept suggestions from other professions and become very defensive, particularly if they are used to assuming sole responsibility;
- Personality clashes: not all people can get on all of the time and personality clashes can occur. These can then cause unwanted conflict in a team and even split the team.

 You will no doubt have come across some of the barriers identified above in some of your practice placements. How do you think these could be overcome? (Before reading on note down your ideas.)

## Barriers to effective team working

While acknowledging that there are some real advantages to interprofessional working we must also admit that there are some real barriers. Lymbery (2006) maintains that not acknowledging barriers to interprofessional working is, in itself, a cause for failure, and that it is crucial to recognise all the stumbling blocks encountered. Some of the common barriers to interprofessional working might include the following:

- Suspicion of the motives behind collaboration (e.g. is this about improving patient care or is there a different agenda?);
- A lack of confidence in one's own professional knowledge base for fear of being wrong, e.g. a newly qualified nurse might not challenge a newly qualified doctor because of fears he or

she might be wrong and does not want to appear as if he or she is not sure what he or she is talking about;
- Traditional professional cultures, e.g. joint working is difficult where there are perceived status differences between occupational groups. Some practitioners view this as a threat to their professional status, autonomy and control when asked to participate in more democratic decision making;
- Mistrust of other professions due to a lack of knowledge leading to stereotyping;
- Lack of training and preparation to work in teams;
- Lack of shared values, visions and principles;
- Lack of investment on an individual, professional and organisational level.

## Overcoming the barriers

Barriers can be overcome with time and patience and by undertaking the following:

- Choosing the right members of the team: although this is not always possible in a healthcare setting, as far as is practicable this should be done. Some team players may have to move to another area if they cannot work in the team;
- Team building: allow time for the team to get to know each other and each person's role and unique contribution to the team. This allows team members to develop respect for each other;
- Develop an atmosphere of trust and respect in the team members: this takes time and effort, and actions speak louder than words;
- Ensuring clarity of team goals: members of the team need to understand the team's common goal and vision. These should include specific and measurable outcomes;
- Encouraging a supportive environment: make sure that all members are aware how their action or inaction might impact on their patients and other team members;
- Encourage debate and constructive challenges: this can help the team to keep improving and coming up with their own ideas. Mechanisms need to be developed to review goals and roles over time;
- Dealing with conflict: this needs to be dealt with and resolved right away otherwise it can prove detrimental to the team.

## Hub-and-spoke team model

The 'hub-and-spoke model' to facilitate student learning has been adopted in some placement areas to help raise awareness of the roles of other healthcare professionals and the importance of team working. This model includes the main practice area to which a student is allocated (the hub), the 'spokes' being the other disciplines that are associated with that specialty (Figure 4.1). This then guides students to whom they should contact to work with and also to begin to explore the team working for the patients within that placement and how this contributes to patients' experiences.

- How might you use the above model on your placement to help you develop key team-working skills?

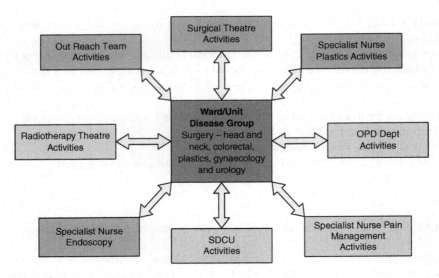

**Figure 4.1**  Hub-and-spoke model

Key skills that could be achieved by applying this model include:

- Developing a better understanding of the roles and responsibilities of other professionals;
- Building partnerships and therapeutic relationships through safe, effective and non-discriminatory communication;
- Working effectively across professional and agency boundaries, actively involving and respecting others' contributions to integrated person-centred care.

As a student nurse you could start by speaking to your mentor and exploring the other services or departments that are connected to that placement; in doing so you can really start to develop a deeper understanding of the roles of others. For example, if you are working on an elderly care ward, it would be useful to spend some of your time with the discharge coordinator. You can then reflect on their role:

- What is the discharge policy and how does it work in practice?
- Who do they need to liaise and collaborate with to ensure the discharge goes smoothly?

Under supervision you could then go on to plan a discharge of your own. This will help you become more confident and competent in your role and your future role as a qualified nurse.

## Integrating into teams

Wherever you are working it is essential that you try to integrate into the teams with which you will work as soon as possible. There are many challenges and opportunities in healthcare today. You will definitely need to plan and identify your experience and needs before you get to the placement, and once there it is a good idea to let your mentor/educator/practice supervisor know what these are.

As a student nurse (or even as a newly qualified nurse moving into another area of practice), consider how you might integrate into a new team.

- Who will be the members of the team?
- What could you do to enhance your integration into the team?

Here are some suggestions:

1. Do a little detective work and find out about the team you are joining before you get there. This might involve visiting the organisation's website or calling the placement area to ask them a little about themselves. If you are near enough, try to arrange to pop in for a short visit. This can often make a good first impression (though consideration should always be given to the demands on staff, particularly in a very busy environment!).
2. Once you are on the placement, find out who the key members of the team are and arrange to go and see them in collaboration with your mentor or practice supervisor. Refer to the hub-and-spoke model in Figure 4.1 and try to fill in the diagram as it relates to your placement area. This could help you identify relevant learning opportunities.
3. Be proactive rather than reactive because this really helps in the placement area. If you just stand around waiting to be told what to do you and with whom to meet, this will not make a good impression.
4. Know what you want to learn about the specialism and the team before you go on placement and also discuss this with your practice supervisor/assessor/mentor. So long as this plan meets the related learning outcomes of your placement, the team should help you achieve these.
5. Demonstrate a willingness to work as part of the team in all aspects of patient care.
6. Ask questions: learn as much as you can about all the professionals working to provide holistic patient care. Do not be afraid to ask any member of the team what they contribute to the care of the patient (no question is a silly question!).

## The importance of record keeping and team work

There is no denying that record keeping is crucial in healthcare and each member of a team has personal responsibility and accountability for good record keeping, including students (NMC, 2018b).

Patient record keeping is one of the most basic clinical tools that we can use to ensure that our patients receive the best possible care. This helps us communicate with each other and is essential for ensuring that an individual's assessed needs are met in a timely and efficient manner.

The principles of good record keeping apply to all types of patient records (e.g. electronic, hand-held or written) with the electronic patient record becoming more popular. The essential ability for healthcare professionals to be able to communicate effectively also demands that systems are developed that will allow this collaboration. O'Hanlon (2014) suggests that the related technology is the relatively easy bit. Much harder is navigating the legal framework around data sharing and this is where clinicians need clear policy direction to allow them to safely share medical information without fear of legal repercussions.

- **What can you do as a student nurse to ensure that you are involved in effective record-keeping processes?**

As a student it is important that you are involved in all aspects of record keeping. You will need to discuss with your practice supervisor/mentor the best ways you can do this within your placement. However, your record keeping should clearly differentiate between facts, opinion and judgements.

The way in which record keeping is undertaken is generally set out by the employer and in the past each discipline within a multiprofessional team would have maintained their own separate records. However, with an ever-increasing focus on improving the quality of care for patients, clinical governance is now a driver to maintaining and improving the delivery of quality care to patients. One of the main components of clinical governance is the use of high-quality systems to effectively monitor clinical care for clinical record keeping and the collection of relevant information (DH, 1998). This has led to many employers looking towards integrating their record keeping for all disciplines. The NMC (2018b) support the use of the same documentation within agreed protocols by all members of the team providing patient care because this can enhance collaborative working. The advantages of having one document for all patient notes are:

- Improved communication;
- Reduction in the duplication of information;
- Reduction in the recording of irrelevant data;
- Maintaining the continuity of a patient's journey;
- Encouraging deeper discussion about a patient and their care.

Electronic record keeping has now become more prevalent as national programmes for the use of information communication technology and electronic record keeping are introduced throughout the UK. Electronic records that are complete, integrated and legible offer added value because they can be accessed from multiple sites and used to generate risk alerts and prompts indicating that new information is available (Pullen and Loudon, 2006). This approach can sometimes cause issues for students in the practice area because they need to be able to obtain a password in order to access the systems. However paper records will not be made obsolete for some time and the principles of good record keeping must be adhered to regardless of how records are held.

## Confidentiality

Confidentiality is as crucial in record keeping, as it is in all aspects of healthcare and is identified in Article 8 of the European Convention on Human Rights (European Court of Human Rights, 1990). It is not acceptable for any member of staff, including students, to discuss patients or their care outside the clinical setting (e.g. in public where they could be overheard or on social media) or to leave records unattended where they could be seen. Patients need to be assured and have confidence in all staff that their data are protected. All of this is covered by the Data Protection Act 1998 (see www.legislation.gov.uk/ukpga/1998/29/contents) which governs the processing of information that can identify individuals. This is covered by legislation from common law and statute law. Common law refers to decisions made by a court of law; statute law is passed in parliament. Under these laws every patient can expect that any information given to a healthcare practitioner (including students) will be used only for the purpose given. It also encompasses a person's right to control access to their health information. Therefore if a relative were to ask for information on a patient, that patient would have to be consulted. In fact, confidentiality requirements also continue after the death of a patient.

Consider how a person's confidentiality can be breached.

- How might this occur?
- What would you do if you suspected that there had been a breach in confidentiality?

If you believe there has been a breach of a patient's confidentiality you must raise your concerns with someone in authority. A risk or breach of confidentiality may be a result of individual behaviour or organisational systems or procedures. *The Code* (NMC, 2018b: 14) is clear on this and states: 'Act without delay if you believe that there is a risk to patient **safety or public protection**'. We all have a professional duty to take action to ensure that the people in our care are protected, and failing to take such action could amount to professional misconduct. There are, however, certain circumstances where records can be disclosed.

## Disclosure

In all circumstances if at all possible, patients should be consulted and access to their records given with consent. They need to know why and with whom the information is being shared and give their consent freely. The only time that information about patients can be shared without consent is if it is in the 'public interest'. This includes the detection and prevention of serious crime and to prevent abuse or serious harm to others. As healthcare professionals we need to be aware that disclosures of this nature must be justified to the courts and the NMC, so clear and accurate decision trails, i.e. documentation, need to be kept. Contrary to popular belief, the police do not have an automatic right to access patients' records and must obtain a warrant to do so. However, if a person is at risk of serious harm then it is acceptable, but must be discussed with your management team and/or your union or NMC and patient consent should also be sought.

Record keeping in healthcare is a potential minefield. Therefore you need to ensure that you abide by *The Code* (NMC, 2015b) and the local policies of the organisation within which you are working.

## Interprofessional education

Humphries and Hean (2004) believe that the high-profile cases already mentioned previously highlight the need not only to move towards collaborative team working but also to review professional education and training in the UK, with a view to making this interprofessional as well as driving the interprofessional agenda within health and social care organisations.

At this point it is judicious to define and explore the concept of interprofessional education further because it does have an impact on interprofessional working. CAIPE (Centre for Advancement of Interprofessional Education, 2002: 19) define interprofessional education (IPE) as 'when two or more individuals from different professions within health and social care engage in learning from and about each other'. In the past nurses, doctors and allied health professionals (AHPs) were educated separately and there were no real opportunities for learning together. Therefore cohesive team working in everyday practice did not always occur. However, the delivery of the NHS's modernisation agenda requires interprofessional practice that is underpinned by robust and integrated working and learning (DH, 2000b, 2001).

The context of healthcare policy and the nature of healthcare itself have both had a major influence on educational developments in relation to interprofessional teaching and learning. The WHO began to promote IPE and, following their lead, some countries developed organisations that were dedicated to IPE. At the forefront in the UK is CAIPE (2007). Numerous other drivers include relevant professional bodies: the Nursing and Midwifery Council (NMC, 2018c), the Health Professionals Council (HPC, 2017) and the General Medical Council (GMC, 2015).

It is suggested that IPE should take place as early as possible to help break down the artificial walls that separate professional development programmes and reinforce the silo working that we know exists (Rafter et al., 2006; Barwell et al., 2013). Reynolds (2005) recommends this is best executed in practice placements and in higher education institutions (HEIs). In fact, it is recommended that interprofessional curricula be implemented where students from all disciplines can meet and collaborate before they enter practice settings so that they can build the basic values of working in interprofessional teams. The WHO (1988) argue that if healthcare professionals are taught together and learn to collaborate throughout their student years there is much more chance that they will work together in their professional lives. Lloyd-Jones et al. (2007) advocate that this will ensure practitioners are equipped with effective team-working skills to enhance patient care. This is supported by the Josiah Macy Foundation (2013), which believes that the face-to-face interaction of different professionals should help to prevent stereotyping and inform and challenge outdated beliefs. Although this is the ideal, it is not always possible in practice and can prove very difficult to achieve logistically.

## ACTIVITY 4.3

Reflecting upon your current and any previous placements, identify all of the potential/actual opportunities available to you for interprofessional learning:

1. Have these been arranged by your employing organisation or your educational provider?
2. Is there potential for you to be able to arrange individualised/bespoke/informal IPE for yourself (i.e. bespoke or experience days with other professionals)?

Write down/make a list of all the potential opportunities available to you. Discuss the practicalities and possibilities of these with your mentor/practice supervisor.

As an individual nurse you can often find creative ways for IPE to occur throughout your career so that you can continuously develop the skills you will need to work with other professions. Although IPE does takes place in practice on a day-to-day basis, Lloyd-Jones et al. (2007) maintain it is not easily recognised or acknowledged by staff. If it does occur it is usually very sporadic and ad hoc, with a lack of planning for specific experiences and a reliance on opportunistic experiences.

Miers et al. (2008) agree and also believe that even if staff do value the importance of IPE, they choose to prioritise profession-specific skills.

It is perhaps important here that we differentiate IPE from 'shared learning' (e.g. where professionals sit in the same lecture theatre). Recognising that some key skills that all health professionals could be taught together (e.g. communications skills, such as listening, gathering information and building a rapport with patients) would help students challenge discriminatory statements about other professions (Pecukonis et al., 2008). Yet IPE should also include the opportunity to collaborate, discuss and learn about each other with the aim being to improve patient care. The aims of IPE are to enhance the sharing of skills and knowledge across healthcare professions, which in turn allows for a better understanding of each other, sharing values and respecting each other's role. If this can be established then the quality and safety of patient care can be optimised. We have already seen in the high-profile cases identified earlier how poor healthcare team working and communication can have a very negative impact on patient outcomes.

IPE can work well if all professions can work together to make this happen (in both practice and academic settings). There are some excellent examples of how this works well within the UK (Oandasan and Reeves, 2005; Reeves et al., 2007).

## IPE

A community occupational therapist (OT) attends an 'Interprofessional Learning (IPL) Champions' Forum' (a forum that has been developed to enable IPL champions from all disciplines to meet together). Another member of the group (a podiatrist) shares information about some new drop-in sessions that she is holding in her area, and is surprised that the OT was unaware of these because the information has been distributed on flyers to all the clinics. However, the OT is based in another building that had not been included in the distribution. In addition, due to the hectic pace of NHS work, flyers and distribution information are often missed. The IPL Forum allows time for the podiatrist and OT to liaise and learn more about each other's services and remit, and the specific changes that are being implemented locally to improve patient care. The OT immediately starts to refer patients to the drop-in, which leads to much more timely treatment being provided for her patients. The podiatrist also becomes much more aware about the necessity for effective communication and the need to ensure that all appropriate colleagues are aware of any new services.

Whittington (2003) maintains that some centres are developing and piloting IPE programmes but acknowledge the difficulties because traditional classroom settings are known to be limited in what can be delivered and the setting often does not reflect the complexities that arise from interprofessional working. Nevertheless, there are some good examples of innovative teaching that do address this issue.

## Case examples

1. One university has developed a training ward at a local hospital to facilitate students from various disciplines to learn together. It was designed collaboratively as an innovative way of enabling different professions to work together in teams and develop their communication skills, learning about each person's role and responsibilities while caring for patients.

2. Another uses simulation scenarios (SIM) to encourage students from different professions to work together in problem solving complex patient issues. This is undertaken in the SIM suite where students can work together in a safe environment and make mistakes without causing any harm to patients. It involves recreating a real-life patient event so that learners can experience that event through use of a high-fidelity environment, thereby gaining new skills, knowledge and attitudes.
3. An IPL forum founded in partnership with a local mental health trust and the local council brings together key staff interested in education and learning where they can work towards integrated learning in practice. This involves having IPE champions at all levels in the organisation to help promote IPE in practice. The patient is seen as being at the centre of their care and the IPL forum promotes the importance of partnership working across all practitioners and their patients.

In some areas HEIs have yet to pursue IPE fully, possibly due to the organisational complexities involved. In the past some have argued that there has been a lack of research as to the effectiveness of IPE, suggesting that the cost, amount of labour required, lack of support and timetabling difficulties have helped to fuel this reluctance (Cooper et al., 2001). For example, even simple differences such as terms, length and different assignment requirements can often cause a problem and make it logistically very difficult to achieve. However, in the UK evidence is now growing for its implementation (Hammick et al., 2007; Lefebvre et al., 2007; Pollard and Miers, 2008; Josiah Macy Foundation, 2013).

In 2006, Health Education England (HEE) recognised the need for extra support for learning in practice and developed the role of the practice education facilitator (PEF). Scotland in 2009 also started to look at practice education in their paper *Delivering Care, Enabling Health* (NHS Quality Improvement in Scotland, 2009) and developing PEFs across Scotland. Wales has also developed a similar role (RCN Wales, 2016). Although initially slow to develop (Wright and Lindqvist, 2008) the role has been instrumental in the practice setting for supporting and managing practice-based multiprofessional student learning. As the PEF role has developed and the need for IPE has become more widely recognised, the role of the PEF has now expanded to assist and support mentors/educators, supervisors and students across all disciplines. Indeed some healthcare organisations have really embraced the notion of IPE and developed structures to support it.

More recently it has also been recognised that, as well as the need to work interprofessionally with other healthcare professionals within one area or organisation there is also a broad consensus about the importance of working across both acute and community settings, with a wider range of NHS, private and voluntary organisations working collaboratively to meet future patients' complex needs. The *Five Year Forward Review* (NHS England, 2014) describes a future that will see the NHS dissolving the classic divide between GPs and hospital care, and health and social care. Instead, the NHS will provide more integrated health and social care services which will empower patients to take more control over their own care and treatment. The review also calls for a radical upgrade in prevention and public health, recognising the crucial role that healthcare students can play within this important agenda. The increasing need for all healthcare students to gain valuable public health experience, together with the new models of integrated working across both health and social care services, has led to new opportunities for increased interprofessional working experiences for pre-registration students which could also play a crucial role in their public health exposure.

## IPE CASE STUDY: PROMOTING PUBLIC HEALTH

Public health experiences within placements are often ad hoc and dependent on the mindset of the practice supervisor/mentor. One organisation was keen to develop a new initiative that would strengthen, promote and formalise the public health experience for students, providing them with a deeper understanding of the wider issues involved when caring holistically for their patients. They developed an annual 'Public Health Conference' for healthcare students in collaboration with two local HEIs and a private healthcare organisation. The conference provided a more formalised opportunity for students from a range of professions to learn together about local public health services and explore their role in promoting health and signposting patients to services. This enabled the students to see public health in action and helped them link theory to real-life practice.

- What opportunities do you think public health might bring in relation to IPL for students?
- How do you think your own public health experience could be strengthened and formalised?
- When caring holistically for your patients, what do you think the wider issues might be in relation to public health?
- Do you think it is important for students from different professions to learn together?
- What do you think the key learning might be for students attending this conference?
- How do you think this conference might improve the care that students provide to their patients?

## IPE advantages and challenges

There are some key advantages to IPE including:

- Understanding the theoretical principles of team working and collaboration early in a student's career;
- Understanding all the roles involved in the patient experience;
- An ability to communicate appropriately and understand the language of different healthcare professionals;
- An understanding of the professional responsibilities, values and accountability of healthcare professionals in meeting the needs of patients;
- Being able to work effectively in an interprofessional team;
- Understanding how different professions make decisions about patient care;
- Understanding how IPE produces better team work, which in turn improves patient care;
- Removal of the fear of other professions;
- The ability to challenge professionals for the good of patient care.

There are also some challenges, including:

- Difficulty in mapping the curricula for different professions;
- Recognising that there needs to be a commitment from all stakeholders to effective planning of IPE;

- Recognising that time and opportunity need to be given for professions to address differences;
- Allowing for logistics and resource difficulties because learning in small groups is often labour-intensive and costly;
- A lack of evaluation of the IPE that has already been implemented; rigorous and robust evaluation is essential;
- A lack of preparation and support for the IPE teachers;
- A lack of student involvement in planning the IPE; Freeth et al. (2005) maintain students should be actively involved in steering their IPE.

Looking into the future of the healthcare service, Ramswammy (2010) believes that we must change the way we educate professionals and also change the milieu in which they work. Silo working and training cannot continue, and the development of an integrated interprofessional, multidimensional workforce is critical. For all of this to happen, team work is also crucial.

## Chapter summary

Interprofessional working and learning are not new concepts; however, it is obvious that they are essential to the future of healthcare and adult nursing. Indeed, the NMC (2018c) are clear that nursing students must be given opportunities and chances to learn with other professionals and as far as is reasonably possible with students from other professions. However, for this to occur, all professions need to show a commitment to learning and working together to provide the best high-quality patient care. This often involves breaking down traditional boundaries and barriers, and working flexibly. It also requires clear leadership and a commitment to ongoing collaborative education, all of which should help to build sustainable relationships with mutual understanding, respect and communication which occur through influencing and negotiating. This will involve breaking down hierarchical structures and taking a leap of faith and commitment in order to work proactively for true collaboration.

The key challenges have been identified here and the need for commitment to work through these challenges and develop effective policies is apparent (Barrett et al., 2005). For adult nurses team work is key and therefore every opportunity should be taken during the course of your programme to join in all team work activities.

## Further reading

Royal College of Nursing (2017) *Record Keeping: The Facts*. London: RCN.

Stockport IPL Champions Forum (2011) The IPL Toolkit for Educators and Mentors, Stockport IPL Champions Forum, Stockport (unpublished). The toolkit includes hints, tips, activities and ideas to help promote a minimal level of interprofessional working with students and ensure a collaborative approach. It can be used to help students in a practice setting develop interprofessional working skills. The ideas and activities can be used at the mentor's/educator's discretion and are not prescriptive. For further information contact the PEF team at Stockport NHS Foundation Trust (contact details available via the Trust website www.stockport.nhs.uk).

Virani, T. (2012) *Interprofessional Collaborative Teams*. Ontario: Canadian Health Service Research Foundation.

# References

Atwal, A. (2002) 'A world apart: how occupational therapists, nurses and care managers perceive each other in acute healthcare', *British Journal of Occupational Therapy*, 65: 446–52.

Atwal, A. and Caldwell, K. (2005) 'Do all health and social care professionals interact equally? A study of interactions in multidisciplinary teams in the United Kingdom', *Scandinavian Journal of Caring Sciences*, 19: 268–73.

Baker, D., Day, R. and Salas, E. (2006) 'Teamwork as an essential component of high reliability organisations', *Health Services Research*, 41(4): 1576–98.

Baldwin, D. (1993) *Development of Health Professionals to Maximise Health Provider Resources in Rural Areas. National Rural Health Association HRSA Contract*. Washington, DC: Bureau of Health Professions.

Barrett, G., Sellman, D. and Thomas, J. (2005) *Interprofessional Working in Health and Social Care: Professional Perspectives*. Basingstoke: Palgrave Macmillan.

Barwell, J., Arnold, F. and Berry, H. (2013) 'How interprofessional learning improves care', *Nursing Times*, 109(21): 14–16.

Baxter, J. (2011) *Public Sector Identities: A Review of the Literature*. Maidenhead: Open University Press.

Biggs, S. (2006) 'Interprofessional collaboration: problems and prospects'. In J. Day (ed.), *Interprofessional Working* (*Expanding Health and Social Care Series*, Wiggins, L., ed.). Cheltenham: Nelson Thornes.

Bradford, S. (2008) 'Practices, policies and professionals: emerging discourses of expertise in English youth work, 1939–51', *Youth and Policy*, 97(1): 13–26.

Centre for the Advancement of Interprofessional Education (2002) *Definition of Interprofessional Education*. Available at: www.caipe.org.uk/about-us/defining-ipe (last accessed 6 June 2014).

Centre for the Advancement of Interprofessional Education (2007) *Creating an Interprofessional Workforce: An Education and Training Framework for Health and Social Care*. London: CAIPE (supported by the Department of Health).

Clements, D., Dault, M. and Priest, A. (2007) 'Effective teamwork in healthcare: research and reality', *Healthcare Papers*, 7(Special Issue): 26–34.

Cooper, H., Carlisle, C., Gibbs, T. and Watkins, C. (2001) 'Developing an evidence base for interdisciplinary learning: a systematic review', *Journal of Advanced Nursing*, 35(2): 228–37.

Day, J. (2006) *Interprofessional Working*. Cheltenham: Nelson Thornes.

Department of Health (1998) *A First Class Service: Quality in the New NHS*. London: DH.

Department of Health (2000a) *NHS Plan: A Plan for Reform*. London: DH. Available at: www.nhs.uk/nationalplan.htm (last accessed 9 January 2014).

Department of Health (2000b) *A New NHS: Modern and Dependable*. London: HMSO.

Department of Health (2001) *Learning from Bristol: The Report of the Public Inquiry into Children's Heart Surgery at the Bristol Royal Infirmary*. London: HMSO.

Department of Health (2003) *The Victoria Climbié Inquiry*. London: HMSO.

Department of Health (2006) *Modernising Nursing Careers: Setting the Direction*. London: DH.

Department of Health (2008) *High Quality Care For All the NHS: Next Stage Review*. London: DH.

Department of Health (2013) *Berwick Report into Patient Safety*. London: DH.

European Court of Human Rights (1990) *Article 8 of the European Convention on Human Rights*. Available at: www.echr.coe.int/documents/convention_eng.pdf (last accessed 18 May 2018).

Freeth, D., Hammick, M., Reeves, S., Koppel, I. and Barr, H. (2005) *Effective Interprofessional Education: Development, Delivery and Evaluation*. Oxford: Blackwell.

Furlong, E. and Smith, R. (2005) 'Advanced nursing practice: policy, education and role development', *Journal of Clinical Nursing*, 14(9): 1059–66.

General Medical Council (2015) *Promoting Excellence: Standards for Medical Education and Training*. Manchester: GMC.

Glasby, J., Martin, G. and Regen, E. (2008) 'Older people and the relationship between hospital services and intermediate care: results from a national evaluation', *Journal of Interprofessional Care*, 22(6): 639–49.

Grumbach, K. and Bodenheimer, T. (2004) 'Can health care teams improve primary health care practice?', *Journal of the American Medical Association*, 291(10): 1246–51.

Hammick, M., Freeth, D., Koppel, I., Reeves, S. and Barr, H. (2007) 'A best evidence systematic review of inter professional education', *BEME guide No. 9, Medical Teacher*, 29(8): 735–51.

Hanson, A., Friberg, F., Segesten, K., Gedda, B. and Mattsson, B. (2008) 'Two sides of the coin: general practitioners' experience of working in multidisciplinary teams', *Journal of Interprofessional Care*, 22(1): 5–16.

Health Professionals Council (2017) *Standards in Education and Training*. London: HPC.

House of Commons (2001) *Royal Liverpool Children's Inquiry*. London: The Stationery Office. Available at: www.gov.uk/government/uploads/system/uploads/attachment_data/file/250914/0012_i.pdf (accessed 2 December 2014).

Humphries, D. and Hean, S. (2004) 'Educating the future workforce: building the evidence about interprofessional learning', *Journal of Health Services Research and Policy*, 9(1): 24–7.

Irvine, R., Kerridge, I., McPhee, J. and Freeman, S. (2002) 'Interprofessionalism and ethics: consensus in clash of cultures?', *Journal of Interprofessional Care*, 16: 199–210.

Jeffrey, R. and Trowman, G. (2009) '*Developing a performative identity*'. Paper presented at the European Conference on Educational Research: Theory and Evidence in European Educational Research, Vienna, Austria, 25–26 September.

Jeffries, N. and Chan, K.K. (2004) 'Multi-disciplinary team working: is it both hostile and effective?', *International Journal of Gynaecological Cancer*, 14(2): 210–11.

Josiah Macy Foundation (2013) 'Transforming patient care: aligning interprofessional education with clinical practice redesign: conference recommendations, 2013'. Available at: http://macyfoundation.org/docs/macy_pubs/TransformingPatientCare_ConferenceRec.pdf (last accessed 6 November 2017).

Katzenbach, J.R. and Smith, D.K. (1993) *The Wisdom of Teams: Creating the High-performance Organizations*. Boston, MA: Harvard Business Press.

Kell, C. and Owen, G. (2008) 'Physiotherapy as a profession: where are we now?', *International Journal of Therapy and Rehabilitation*, 15(4): 158–64.

Kesby, S. (2002) 'Nursing care and collaborative practice', *Journal of Clinical Nursing*, 11: 357–66.

Kirkup, B. (2015) *The Report of the Morecambe Bay Investigation*. London: The Stationery Office, William Lea Group.

Kirkup, B. (2018) *Report of the Liverpool Community Health Independent Review*. Available at: https://improvement.nhs.uk/news-alerts/independent-review-liverpool-community-health-nhs-trust-published/ (last accessed 21 March 2018).

Laming, W. (2009) *The Protection of Children in England: A Progress Report*. Norwich: HMSO.

Lavin, M.A., Ruebling, I., Banks, R., Block, L., Counte, M. and Furman, G. (2001) 'Interdisciplinary health professional education: a historical review', *Advances in Health Sciences Education: Theory and Practice*, 6(1): 25–47.

Lefebvre, H., Pelchat, D. and Levart, M.J. (2007) 'Interdisciplinary family intervention program: a partnership among health professional, traumatic brain injury patients, and caregiving relatives', *Journal of Trauma Nursing*, 14(2): 100–13.

Leggat, S.G. (2007) 'Effective healthcare teams require effective team members: defining team work competencies', *BMC Health Service Resources*, 7: 17.

Lloyd-Jones, N., Hutchings, S. and Hobson, S.H. (2007) 'Inter-professional learning in practice for pre-registration health: inter-professional learning occurs in practice – Is it articulated or celebrated?', *Nurse Education in Practice*, 7(1): 11–17.

Lymbery, M. (2006) 'United we stand? Partnership working in health and social care and the role of social worker in services for older people', *British Journal of Social Work*, 36: 1119–34.

Mid Staffordshire NHS Foundation Trust (2013) *Report of the Mid Staffordshire NHS Foundation Trust Public Inquiry: Executive Summary*. London: HMSO.

Miers, M., Rickaby, C. and Pollard, K. (2008) *Making the Most of Interprofessional Learning Opportunities: Professionals' and Students' Experience of Inter-professional Learning and Working*. Bristol: The Higher Education Academy and University of England.

NHS England (2014) *Five Year Forward Review*. Available at: www.england.nhs.uk/publication/nhs-five-year-forward-view (last accessed 5 January 2018).

NHS Quality Improvement in Scotland (2009) *Integration, Collaboration and Empowerment: Practice Development for a New Context*. Available at: www.healthcareimprovementscotland.org/previous_resources/policy_and_strategy/practice_development_framework.aspx (last accessed 5 January 2018).

Nursing and Midwifery Council (2018a) *Future Nurse: Standards of Proficiency for Registered Nurses*. London: NMC.

Nursing and Midwifery Council (2018b) *The Code: Professional Practice and Behaviour Standards of Nurses and Midwives*. London: NMC.

Nursing and Midwifery Council (2018c) Part 1: *Standards Framework for Nursing and Midwifery Education*. London: NMC.

Oandasan, I. and Reeves, S. (2005) 'Key elements for interprofessional education. Part 1: the learner, the educator and the learning context', *Journal of Interprofessional Care*, May, 21–38.

O'Hanlon, S. (2014) 'Data sharing: step out of the technological dark ages', *Health Service Journal*. [website]. Nov 2014. Available at: www.hsj.co.uk/technology-and-innovation/data-sharing-step-out-of-the-technological-dark-ages/5076581.article (last accessed 1 May 2018).

Pecukonis, E., Doyle, O. and Leigh Bliss, D. (2008) 'Reducing barriers to interprofessional training: promoting interprofessional cultural competence', *Journal of Interprofessional Care*, 22(4): 417–28.

Pirrie, A., Wilson, V., Elsegood, J., Hall, J., Hamilton, S., Harden, R., Lee, D. and Stead, J. (1998) *Evaluating Multidisciplinary Education in Health Care*. Edinburgh: SCRE.

Pollard, K.C. and Miers, M.E. (2008) 'From students to professionals: results in a longitudinal study of attitudes to pre-qualifying collaborative learning and working in health and social care in the United Kingdom', *Journal of Interprofessional Care*, 22(4): 399–416.

Pollard, K.C., Sellman, D. and Thomas, J. (2014) 'The need for interprofessional working'. In J. Thomas, K.C. Pollard and D. Sellman (eds), *Interprofessional Working in Health and Social Care, Professional Perspectives*, 2nd edn. Basingstoke: Palgrave Macmillan, Chapter 1.

Pullen, I. and Loudon, J. (2006) 'Improving standards in clinical record keeping', *Advances in Psychiatric Treatment*, 12: 280–6.

Rafter, M.E., Persun, I.J., Herren, M., Linfante, J.C., Mina, M. and Wu, C.D. (2006) 'A preliminary study of interprofessional education', *Journal of Dental Education*, 70(4): 417–27.

Ramswammy, L. (2010) 'Interprofessional education and collaborative practice', *Journal of Interprofessional Care*, 24(2): 131–8.

RCN Wales (2016) *Future of Nurse Education in Wales: Education Strategy*, RCN Wales leadership summit, Cardiff.

Reeves, S., Goldman, J. and Oandasan, I. (2007) 'Key factors in planning and implementing inter-professional education in healthcare settings', *Journal of Allied Health*, 36(4): 231–5.

Reeves, S., Goldman, J. and Zwarenstein, M. (2009) 'An emerging framework for understanding the nature of interprofessional interventions', *Journal of Interprofessional Care*, 23(5): 539–42.

Reynolds, F. (2005) *Communication and Clinical Effectiveness in Rehabilitation*. Edinburgh: Elsevier/ Butterworth Heinemann.

Salas, E., DiazGranados, D., Klein, C., Burke, C.S., Stagl, K.C., Goodwin, G.F. and Halpin, S.M. (2009) 'Does team training improve team performance? A meta-analysis', *Human Factors*, 50(6): 903–33.

Scottish Government (2010) *The Healthcare Quality Strategy for NHS Scotland*. Available at: www.gov.scot/resource/doc/311667/0098354.pdf (last accessed 1 May 2018).

Sims, S., Hewitt, G. and Harris, R. (2014) 'Evidence of collaboration, pooling of resources, learning and role blurring in interprofessional healthcare teams: a realistic synthesis', *Journal of Interprofessional Care*, 25(1): 20–5.

Smith, J., Chairman (2002) *The Shipman Inquiry: Death Disguised: First Report*. Norwich: HMSO. Available at: www.theshipmaninquiry.org.uk/firstreport.asp (last accessed 4 February 2014).

Spry, E. (2006) 'All together for health?', *Student British Medical Journal*, 14: 1–44.

Thomas, J. (2005) 'Issues for the future'. In G. Barrett, D. Sellman and J. Thomas (eds), *Interprofessional Working in Health and Social Care: Professional Perspectives*, 2nd edn. Basingstoke: Palgrave Macmillan, Chapter 17.

Tweedale, R. (2013) *Ultrasound Proves the Case for Prison Based Services*, Primary Care Commissioning (online). Available at: www.pcc-cic.org.uk/print/367424 (last accessed 18 August 2018).

Weiss, G.I. and Welbourne, P. (2008) 'The professionalisation of social work: a crossnational exploration', *International Journal of Social Welfare*, 17: 281–90.

Whittington, C. (2003) *Learning for Collaborative Practice with Other Professions and Agencies*. London: Department of Health.

Willis Commission (2012) *Quality with Compassion: The Future of Nurse Education*. London: Royal College of Nursing.

World Health Organization (1988) *Learning Together to Work Together for Health*. Geneva: WHO.

World Health Organization (2010) *Framework for Action on Interprofessional Education and Collaborative Practice*. Geneva: WHO.

Wright, A. and Lindqvist, S. (2008) 'The development, outline and evaluation of the second level of an interprofessional learning programme: listening to the students', *Journal of Interprofessional Care*, 22(5): 475–87.

5

# MEDICINES MANAGEMENT

## JULIE GREGORY AND CHARLOTTE MIDDLETON

---

### CHAPTER OBJECTIVES

- Identify the role of registered nurses in medicines management;
- Describe the processes required for medicines management and the associated skills;
- Consider some of the factors that may increase the risk of medication errors;
- Understand some of the legal and ethical issues relating to medicines management;
- Become aware of some of the developments of the registered nurse's role in relation to medicine management;
- Relate how pharmacological knowledge is applied to patient care.

---

## Introduction

This chapter will highlight the importance of medicines management, which is a complex and high-risk activity. Specifically, it will examine the processes of medicines management in relation to the registered nurse's role and responsibilities in ensuring the safety of patients in relation to medication.

Registered nurses are responsible for the effective and safe management of medication and as such, medicines management is a major aspect of professional practice (Kavanagh, 2017). Indeed, it is suggested that within a week approximately 16 hours of a registered nurse's clinical time is spent in the management of medicines (Leufter and Cleary-Houldforth, 2013).

## Related NMC proficiencies for registered nurses

The overarching requirements of the Nursing and Midwifery Council (NMC) are that all nurses must understand the principles of safe and effective administration and optimisation of medicines in accordance with local and national policies and demonstrate proficiency and accuracy when calculating dosages of prescribed medicines. They must be able to apply knowledge of pharmacology to the care of people, demonstrating the ability to progress to a prescribing qualification following registration (NMC, 2018a: 18).

**To achieve entry to the nursing register you must be able to**

- Carry out initial and continued assessments of people receiving care and their ability to self-administer their medications;
- Demonstrate the numeracy, literacy, digital and technological skills required to meet the needs of people in your care, to ensure safe and effective nursing practice;
- Demonstrate knowledge of pharmacology and the ability to recognise the effects of medicines, allergies, drug sensitivities, side effects, contraindications, incompatibilities, adverse reactions and prescribing errors, and the impact of polypharmacy and over-the-counter medication usage;
- Demonstrate knowledge of how prescriptions can be generated, the role of generic, unlicensed and off-label prescribing, and an understanding of the potential risks associated with these approaches to prescribing;
- Recognise the various procedural routes under which medicines can be prescribed, supplied, dispensed and administered, and the laws, policies, regulations and guidance that underpin them;
- Use the principles of safe remote prescribing and directions to administer medicines;
- Undertake accurate checks, including transcription and titration, of any direction to supply or administer a medicinal product;
- Demonstrate an understanding of how to identify, report and critically reflect on near misses, critical incidents, major incidents and serious adverse events in order to learn from them and influence their future practice;
- Exercise professional accountability in ensuring the safe administration of medicines to those receiving care.

(Adapted from NMC, 2018a)

## Background

In Chapter 4, we highlighted the importance of interprofessional working. This is particularly important when related to medicines management. To ensure that the medication taken by your patient is safe and effective, you will be required to work collaboratively with a team of healthcare professionals **and** the patient. Initially, a careful and detailed history and assessment of the patient are undertaken by a **prescriber** (usually but not always a doctor), before a written direction or prescription is produced. The **pharmacist** dispenses the medication after checking the accuracy of the prescription. Within a hospital setting the **nurse** may administer the medication to the patient with their consent. Self-administration of medicines has also been introduced to some hospital settings and obviously **patients** self-administer their medication at home.

An experienced registered nurse may make the administration of medicines appear straightforward, but it is not a mechanical task (White et al., 2010). Medication administration is complex, requiring knowledge of the patient's care and treatment plan (in addition to knowledge of the medication), thought, dexterity and exercise of professional judgement. The main responsibility of the registered nurse is to ensure that medicines are managed safely. This includes accurate interpretation of a prescription, knowledge of the reason for the medication and its action and usual dose. This is because registered nurses need to be able to question a possible mistake by the prescriber and when in doubt ask for advice or help.

The administration of medicines involves ensuring that the right medicine, correct dose and right route are used and that the medication is given to the right patient at the right time (Jones, 2009). Once all this has been completed, the nurse must record that the drug has been given or provide reasons for its omission and observe the patient's response (Greenstein and Gould, 2009; Kim and Bates, 2013). Registered nurses therefore need to have a comprehensive knowledge base and access to information to identify and prevent adverse reactions and errors associated with the management of medicines. This chapter aims to examine some of these aspects to ensure patient safety.

The NMC *Code* (2018b: 15) states that nurses should practise patient-centred care that effectively preserves safety. We must therefore reduce, as far as possible, any potential harm associated with our practice. One of the nurse's roles and responsibilities associated with medicine management is to safeguard against medication errors that could lead to patient harm (Cloete, 2015).

Medicines are potent substances that are used to promote health and to prevent, control and treat disease. They benefit individuals generally by saving and prolonging life, and enhancing lifestyles (Downie et al., 2008). They can also have potentially life-threatening effects on individuals if not correctly managed. Safely managing medicines is important for adult nurses because approximately 70% of the adult population take prescribed medication that increases to an estimated 80% of people over the age of 75 years (Baileff et al., 2012).

## Definition of medicines management

Medicines management encompasses the entire way in which nurses select, procure, provide, prescribe, supply, administer and review a patient's medicine. Optimal medicine management enables patients to get the maximum benefit from the medicines they need. This is achieved through concordance and teamwork, by placing the patient as the primary focus and by ensuring that nursing interventions are cost-effective, and that any associates risks are identified, communicated and carefully managed.

(Baileff et al., 2012: 379)

It is the system of processes and behaviours that determine how medicines are used by patients and by the NHS (Mason, 2008).

# The medicines management process and the registered nurse's role

## Nursing assessment

A medication or drug history should be obtained from the patient, or if necessary relatives and friends and/or the GP as part of the nursing assessment. This assessment should include which drugs are taken, doses and times, and any known allergies to medication. During this assessment the patient's experience and understanding of their medication is obtained. This is an important aspect of patient-centred quality healthcare and involves a two-way shared communication about their understanding of their medication (Kaufman, 2016), possible side effects experienced from their medication and any concordance issues, establishing possible reasons why they may have discontinued any medication. The drug history should include any over-the-counter medication, recreational drugs and herbal remedies (Greenstein and Gould, 2009). Patients do not always consider herbal remedies to be medication but the use of these substances may be related to a patient's current condition and they may interact with prescribed medication.

Eileen, a 54-year-old woman with poorly controlled asthma, complains of 'low mood and feeling tired all the time' to the practice nurse during her follow-up appointment at the asthma clinic. During her assessment, the practice nurse determines that Eileen has been self-medicating with St John's wort given to her by a friend. St John's wort is a herbal remedy that has been used to treat depression for hundreds of years, and can be bought from health food shops. It is not classed as a medication and is therefore not regulated; there is no recommended dose (Szegedi et al., 2005). The National Institute for Health and Care Excellence (NICE, 2009) do not recommend its use due to concerns including serious drug interactions, for example it can reduce the effectiveness of theophyllines (a medication sometimes taken by patients with asthma to help open the airways). It was therefore important for the nurse to discover she was taking St John's wort due to its potential interaction with her asthma medication. (St John's wort can reduce the effect of theophyllines, which may or may not be the cause of her increasing asthma symptoms.)

## Knowledge of the individual patient's care plan

Knowledge of the individual patient's care plan is necessary before administration of medication to determine where the prescribed medication relates to the treatment plan. This is important because a patient's condition may affect the action of the medication, for example reduced renal function slows the elimination of the medicine which could lead to an increased effect. The nurse may request a review of the patient by the prescriber as a result of their knowledge of the impaired renal function.

## Prescribing

Before a medicine can be administered it is prescribed and dispensed. Traditionally prescribing was the remit only of medical staff and the nurse's role was limited to the safe and reliable administration of medication. However, as nurses' roles have become more advanced (e.g. nurse-led clinics and services) they can, after additional education and preparation, prescribe medication. Prescribing enables the registered nurse to complete an episode of care to be delivered without referral to a medical practitioner.

The prescription must be legible to avoid any confusion, for example between drug names **oxybutytnin** (used for urinary frequency) and **oxycontin** (an opiate analgesic); they have similar names and could look similar if the prescriber's handwriting is poor but would lead to very different therapeutic effects. A prescription should be clearly written and contain the following:

- The name of the medicine;
- Dose and route of administration;
- Time;

- Signature of prescriber;
- Start date;
- Date when the medicine will be discontinued (though this is not always required).

Poor documentation is a common factor in drug errors. The use of computerised systems should lead to fewer errors as a result of poor handwriting. It is essential that you never accept illegible writing or unofficial abbreviations. You need to feel confident and be able to question a possible mistake made by a prescriber. When in doubt, always seek advice from a pharmacist or the original prescriber. Tact may be required when approaching the prescriber: basing your enquiry on the individual patient's care plan, their current condition, the reason for the prescription, knowledge of the drug, dosage, time and route of administration.

A pharmacist dispenses the medication once a prescription has been produced. The medication is checked to ensure that the dose is correct and the route appropriate and the directions have been made clear. At the same time the pharmacist will check expiry dates and that the packaging is intact and suitable for the person to whom it is dispensed (e.g. child-proof containers can be difficult to open for people with arthritic hands). They should provide labels with instructions about the safe storage of the medicine as well as directions on how to take the medication. In the community, pharmacists check details such as the patient's address to ensure that medicines are given to the correct patient.

As stated previously, administration of medication is a key aspect of a registered nurse's role and is one aspect of a collaborative process involving the prescriber, pharmacist and patient. It is complex and requires thought to prevent errors and harm to your patient and to promote therapeutic responses.

As a student nurse you need to be involved in medicines administration to learn this essential aspect of nursing practice. However, you must never administer a medication without supervision by a registered nurse (RN), not least because RNs are accountable for their action in the safe administration of medicines, which includes the delegation of this task to others. There are also many calculations involved in medicines management that may be fairly basic, e.g. calculating the number of pills required to make up the dose, or more complicated, e.g. when administering intravenous drugs that rely on the weight of the patient. As miscalculation results in drug errors, this is a key aspect of medicines administration.

- Do you have the mathematical skills necessary to undertake accurate drug calculations for a range of medications? If not, what can you do to ensure that you are able to safely calculate and administer medications?

Jones (2009) recommends the five 'rights' as principles to follow when administering medication:

1. The right patient (by checking their identification band if in hospital);
2. The right drug (this is particularly important when considering both generic and proprietary or trade names for drugs);
3. The right dose (this also includes checking that the dose prescribed is appropriate);
4. The right time (though drugs prescribed for 10am are not all administered at exactly 10am, it should be ensured that the drug is being administered at the correct time of day);
5. The right route (i.e. oral, intravenous, intramuscular, subcutaneous, etc.).

These are principles that on their own do not prevent errors and other factors can lead to errors which will be discussed later.

## ACTIVITY 5.1

Go to the Royal Pharmaceutical Society website at: www.rpharms.com.
Access their guidance document *Professional Guidance on Safe and Secure Handling of Medicines in all Settings.* Make a note of the processes and steps involved in administering medicines to patients.

Processes for the safe administration of medicines include ensuring that the patient is identified and the name on the prescription corresponds with the patient's details. This is because poor checking of the patient's identity can lead to error. In an inpatient setting all patients should wear a wristband containing identification information (National Patient Safety Agency or NPSA, 2005). This is checked and the patient should be addressed by name or asked to confirm their name to reduce the risk of administering the correct medication to the wrong patient. At the point of administration a final check is made to ensure that the patient does not have an allergy to the medication. Some medications, for example penicillin, can produce anaphylaxis, a serious allergic reaction that is potentially life threatening. Any known allergy should be recorded on the prescription chart as well as within the medical and nursing notes. Some hospitals use a red wristband to help alert staff to allergy status; this should not be relied on and allergy status must be checked before administration of a drug (Corben, 2009).

Once the medication has been administered, a clear and immediate record is made within the relevant documents and when medication has not been administered, the reason for this should be recorded and the relevant person informed of the omission.

There are many reasons for an error in administering medication. Two types of error have been described: **procedural error**, for example failing to check the patient's identity and **clinical error**, such as the wrong drug or dose (Westbrook et al., 2011).

Medication errors can lead to patient harm and should be avoided at all costs.

Distraction and interruption of the nurse during drug administration have been highlighted as one of the reasons for procedural errors (Connor et al., 2016). Interruptions have been implicated as potential contributory factors. Interventions aimed at reducing interruptions include marked quiet zones for preparation of medication; signage (requesting no interruptions); checklists with medicine procedures; and vests or tabards, sachets and lighted lanyards worn by nurses. However, a systematic review of seven studies examining the effectiveness of these interventions described the evidence as weak due to poor study design and low numbers of participants. Although the studies have suggested such interventions might demonstrate a reduction in the number of interruptions there is no evidence that they reduce the number of medication administration errors (Raban and Westbrook, 2014).

- In your practice placement, have you witnessed the nurse in charge of the medicines round wearing a red tabard or vest during medicine administration?

Pope (2002) suggests that this provides a visible symbol to increase awareness among other staff that the nurse is administering medicines, and acts as an effective reminder not to interrupt the nurse during drug administration and distract staff.

## ☐? ACTIVITY 5.2

Next time you are within a clinical setting and medicines are being administered, observe the process and make some observational notes on the following:

- The number of interruptions;
- Who made them;
- Was a red tabard worn? If so, did it seem to prevent and reduce interruptions?
- How did the nurse react to these interruptions?

The pressures of work related to other aspects of patient care means that nurses often feel rushed during the administration of medication and under pressure to complete the task (Cloo et al., 2013). This pressure may lead to shortcuts and a reduction in the required checks or a failure to ensure that the standards for the administration of medicines are maintained; this in turn may result in medication errors.

## Medication devices

A number of devices are available for use when administering medication and adult nurses need to have knowledge and training to ensure the correct and safe use of any such device. They include measuring pots and spoons for oral administration, syringes and needles for parental administration (injections), and oxygen masks and nebulisers for inhalation. The correct use of these devices is important to ensure that the accurate dose of medicines is administered, for example oral syringes (coloured purple) must be used for oral liquid medicines and not parental syringes which are used for injections.

Electronic devices, such as infusion and syringe pumps, may also be used to administer medication but should be used only after appropriate training. Before their use, such devices should be examined to confirm that they have been maintained appropriately (for example, there is usually a label on the device that indicates when the next service is required). Maintenance ensures accuracy because patient harm may result if, for example, medication is administered too quickly which could lead to serious consequences.

## ☐? ACTIVITY 5.3

Susan Smith, aged 30 years, has been admitted to hospital with an infected foot after standing on a drawing pin. She has been prescribed co-amoxiclav intravenously.

What do you need to know and check before administration?

| The medication (drug) | The patient | Aspects of IV administration |
| --- | --- | --- |
| | | |

In response to the activity above you should have included the following;

- **The medication:** dose, type of antibiotic, e.g. does it contain penicillin? Side effects of the medication. Check that the antibiotic powder is dry, the glass vial is intact and the expiry date has not passed. Nurses must have a working knowledge of the medications they administer. Co-amoxiclav contains penicillin. It is important for the nurse to be aware of this to check that Susan isn't allergic to penicillin because the consequences of this could be serious. The nurse should also be aware of the safe and appropriate dose of co-amoxiclav and an understanding of any side effects. This could be checked using the *British National Formulary* (BNF). The nurse should also undertake a visual check of the medication. For example, has the expiry date passed and does the packaging appear intact?
- **The patient:** check that she has consented to the medication administration, her name and date of birth (ensure correct patient) against the prescription, her care plan including any history of taking antibiotics in the past and any other prescribed medication. At the bedside check any known allergies. All patients need to provide informed consent before the administration of any medication. You will need to be certain of Susan's identity and should consult her care plan to check for allergies and other prescribed medications because some may be contraindicated.
- **Aspects of IV administration:** aseptic no-touch technique should be used. Check that an IV cannula is in place and that there is no sign of redness, swelling or pain at the cannula site. Reconstitute the medication, check which fluid to use and how much, give as a bolus or an infusion. An aseptic no-touch technique should always be used when administering intravenous medications. You should ensure that Susan's cannula is properly sited and secure.
- You must ensure that the co-amoxiclav powder is reconstituted with the correct volume of an appropriate diluent, in this case 0.9% sodium chloride.
- Although some medications may be administered intravenously as either an infusion or a bolus, others irritate the vein causing phlebitis or extravasation. It is therefore important for you to be aware of how to administer safely.
- You must continue to monitor the cannula site regularly for signs of erythema and oedema. This may indicate infiltration (whereby the tip of the cannula passes through the wall of the vein).

## Monitoring

Once the medication has been administered the patient is observed and assessed for any potential benefit and/or adverse effects of the medication.

As a student nurse you may be involved in this monitoring which will include taking physiological measures such as heart rate, blood pressure, respiratory rate and temperature. One specific example of monitoring is blood glucose levels; these are carefully monitored before and after insulin administration, which is given to regulate blood glucose for patients with diabetes. This is because blood glucose needs to be kept within specific parameters; if they are too high or too low the patient can become drowsy and/or unconscious.

---

### ⌨? ACTIVITY 5.4

Morphine is an opioid analgesic commonly used in the management of severe pain.

List the monitoring requirements of a patient following the administration of morphine and the reasons for the observations undertaken.

Nurses are expected to have knowledge of the common side effects of the medication they administer to be able to observe for potentially serious consequences. Most drugs have some effect that is not related to its therapeutic effect. Morphine, for example, reduces respiratory rate. If the dose administered is too high or the individual patient is sensitive to morphine this can, on rare occasions, lead to respiratory failure. Constipation is a much more common side effect of morphine, and morphine can also induce nausea and vomiting after administration. Antiemetics and laxatives are usually prescribed alongside morphine to prevent these side effects. An important aspect of the nurse's role is to monitor the patient to ensure that he or she obtains the pain relief required without these very unpleasant side effects.

An adverse drug reaction (ADR) is an unwanted or harmful reaction experienced by someone after the administration of a drug or combinations of drugs under normal conditions of use which is suspected to be related to the drug (Greener, 2014).

**Adverse drug events** are serious untoward reactions related to a medication; **anaphylaxis** is an example of an adverse event. Reporting of adverse events requires that the reaction and symptoms experienced by the patient must be documented in the patient's records and reported to the healthcare team. Within the UK a system of reporting of a suspicion of adverse reactions to medicines is known as the Yellow Card scheme and is available at http://yellowcard.mhra.gov.uk/the-yellow-card-scheme. Yellow Cards are also available in paper form in all copies of the BNF. The information gathered from 'Yellow Card Reports' made by patients and health professionals is continually assessed at the Medicines and Healthcare products Regulatory Agency (MHRA) by a team of medicine safety experts, comprising doctors, pharmacists and scientists who study the benefits and risks of medicines. A patient's reaction to a medication is individual and not predictable so side effects and an adverse event should not be confused with a medication error.

## Storage of medicines

Medicines must be stored according to the manufacturer's guidance. Most medicines are stored in coloured bottles or in foil strips to avoid exposure to light which may affect the chemical composition of the drug. To maintain their stability some medicines need to be stored at a specific temperature.

Within the hospital setting, all medications are stored in locked receptacles, cupboards, fridge, lockers and trolleys. Registered nurses are responsible for their safe storage and keeping the medicine keys on their person (Corben, 2009). Traditionally, a medicine trolley containing a stock of commonly used medicines has been used for their administration. The nurse wheels the trolley to each patient and administers medicines from it. Increasingly, however, individual medicine lockers at the side of the patient's bed space are used where each patient has their own stock of medicines. The introduction of the individual lockers is intended to reduce medication errors (Lawson and Hennefer, 2010). However, there does not appear to be any evidence to demonstrate a resultant reduction in errors. Therefore, there remains a need for identification checks, whether or not a trolley or a locker is used. It is also essential that the locker be checked after a patient has been discharged or transferred to ensure that the medicines have been removed.

Controlled drugs (CD) (for example, morphine) must be stored separately from other medicines in a specifically designed locker or cupboard which must be secured to a wall that cannot be accessed from outside, in line with the Misuse of Drugs Act 1971 (see www.legislation.gov.uk/ukpga/1971/38/contents). There is only one key available for an individual ward or unit CDs and it can be held only by a registered nurse, usually the senior nurse on duty.

## Communication

Teaching patients and providing explanations about their medication, its indication, dosage, times of administration, route and possible side effects are an important aspect of the nurse's role in both primary and secondary care in order to increase the likelihood of adherence to and concordance with the course of treatment (Greenstein and Gould, 2009). By explaining and demonstrating the correct administration of medication you can help to build your patient's knowledge of their medication and at the same time alert them to possible side effects. All opportunities should be used for teaching and when a patient is in hospital time needs to be found to incorporate this into the administration of medicines (Downie et al., 2008).

## Medicines management in the community

For nurses working in a community setting, the importance of educating patients is a high priority because the patients usually self-administer their medication. In order to aid adherence and concordance the patient and/or their relatives need to understand the reasons for the medication being prescribed and the possible consequences of not taking the medication as directed. The patient's ability to open containers and to remember when to take their medication may need to be assessed and monitored. Advice is also provided about storing medicines correctly and securely, for example kept out of the reach of children and other vulnerable groups. It is also important to monitor the effects and identify possible side effects or problems experienced by patients in the community.

## Legal and ethical aspects of medicines management

The Medicines Act 1968 (see www.legislation.gov.uk/ukpga/1968/67) regulates the production, testing and marketing of medical products. A licence is required for every medical product to ensure that it is administered appropriately and to achieve its best possible therapeutic effect. A licence is granted only once the safety and efficacy of the drug have been established, and that it is manufactured to the highest standards and has been tested and evaluated. The safety of the patient is always the prime consideration when a licence is granted (Downie et al., 2008).

## Categories of medicines

Patients can access medicines from different sources, which are divided into four categories (see box).

### LEGAL CATEGORIES FOR MEDICINES

- **General sales list** (GSL) medications are freely available to buy in many shops, for example cough medicines, paracetamol and antacids such as Gaviscon.

The advantages of the GSL are their convenience and it is a cost-effective way of obtaining simple medications without contacting a healthcare professional.

The disadvantage of GSL medications is that they may lead to other health problems. Ibuprofen is a non-steroidal anti-inflammatory drug (NSAID) that is freely available but can cause gastric ulcers with long-term use; NSAIDs may also cause renal damage and allergic reactions, including bronchospasm. NSAIDs can interact with many other medications such as warfarin (an anticoagulant).

- **Pharmacy** (P) medicines can be purchased only from a pharmacy or chemists shop where a pharmacist is available. The pharmacist supervises the purchase and will check for potential interactions and other problems, and also provide advice about potential side effects. They may also advise an individual to consult with a doctor if they feel it is necessary.
- **Prescription-only medicines** (POMs) can be obtained only with a written direction or prescription from a registered prescriber, traditionally a doctor, but more recently involving other healthcare professionals, including pharmacists, nurses and professionals allied to medicines (physiotherapists, podiatrists, etc.).
- **Controlled drugs** (CDs) are regulated by the Misuse of Drugs Act 1971. The ordering, dispensing, prescribing, storage and administration of these medicines are strictly monitored and controlled. Many of these medications are opiates, for example morphine.

---

The Misuse of Drugs Act 1971 relates to the licensing of the production, possession and supply of substances that may be misused. A number of changes were introduced after the enquiry into the deaths caused by Dr Harold Shipman (see Shipman Inquiry, 2001). These relate to the prescription, record keeping and destruction of CDs, mainly within community settings and are known as the Misuse of Drugs Regulations 2001 (see www.legislation.gov.uk/uksi/2001/3998/contents/made).

## Ethical aspects of medication management

When medication is prescribed and administered it should always be remembered that the patient should be respected; in particular their right to self-determination and autonomy should always be considered. The ethical principles of beneficence (to do good) and non-maleficence (to do no harm) should be at the forefront of every nurse's mind. The patient should always be at the centre of the management of their medication; they must be kept informed and treated as a partner, with an opportunity to be involved and make decisions about their medicines (Department of Health or DH, 2004). To ensure that patients make informed decisions relating to their medication, they should be involved in the production of a prescription and be provided with advice and information about both the benefits and any potential side effects of the chosen medicines. **Concordance** is the term used to suggest equal partnership and negotiation that occurs in the treatment process, rather than a patient being compliant or a passive recipient of treatment from a healthcare professional. Patients can decline the prescription and medication and as a nurse you will always need to respect their decision. You can try to persuade your patient by providing further information and explaining the consequences of omitting medication but should not coerce them or administer the medication covertly.

Covert administration of medication or disguising the medication in food or drink has long been an area of debate, centred around the notion that healthcare professionals can sometimes take on a 'paternalistic' approach when determining what is in a patient's best interest. However, if a patient can consent to or decline the medication, covert administration should *not* be attempted. If a patient is considered unable to understand or that they have been assessed as lacking capacity (Mental Capacity Act 2005 – see www.legislation.gov.uk/ukpga/2005/9/contents) their best interest needs to be considered before the decision to administer medication covertly is taken. This decision is made only when all other possible methods of administering the medication have been unsuccessful. An individual assessment of the patient is conducted and this includes relatives (or close caregivers) and members of the multidisciplinary team deciding if covert administration is in the patient's best interest. Support should be available to assist with the assessment and decision from local policy and guidelines.

## Incident reporting

When or if a medication error occurs it is important to be honest and report the mistake to ensure that action can be taken to minimise any harm that could occur as a result of the error. All medication administration errors and near-miss events (whereby incidents have not caused harm) should be reported to the National Reporting and Learning System (NRLS) database.

*The Code* (NMC, 2018b: 13) states that the nurse has a duty of candour, i.e. to be open and honest when things go wrong. Failing to act or denying that an error has occurred can not only harm the patient but would also lead to serious sanctions for the nurse. A number of referrals to the NMC misconduct hearings are related to poor documentation and attempts to change documentation in relation to medication errors. The charges made as a result relate to dishonesty rather than a medication error.

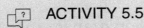

### ACTIVITY 5.5

Mr Malcom Jones, aged 72 years, is an inpatient on a medical ward. He takes a number of medicines that have been dispensed by the staff nurse, who has delegated their administration to you, a student nurse.

Mr Jones says he is 'fed up with taking all these tablets and doesn't want to take them this morning, thank you'.

What would you do?

What factors might you consider?

Who needs to be involved?

Where would you record this episode?

Initially in your response to the above activity you would try to persuade Mr Jones to take his medication by describing why each drug is necessary and any potential consequences of not taking the medicine. For example, atenolol is taken to lower blood pressure; if his blood pressure remains elevated cardiac problems could occur including a stroke. You would then need to consider if there are any other physical reasons for declining the medication, for example does he feel sick or is he having difficulty swallowing? You should always respect his decision to decline his medication, but, in doing so, consider if he has the capacity to make the decision. You would need to inform a qualified member of staff of his reluctance to take his medication. In addition, the pharmacist and doctor could look at his prescription and see if the medicines could be given at different times rather than all in the morning. Someone close to Mr Jones, for example his wife, may also be able to help persuade him to take his medication. If all else fails, the non-administration of his medication would be recorded on his prescription chart/sheet and in his nursing and medical notes according to local policy.

# Developments in medicines management

## Nurse prescribing

The introduction of nurse prescribing has been a gradual process, initially prompted by the findings of the Cumberlege Report (1986). The first nurse prescribers were district nurses and health visitors, qualifying in 1998 (Royal College of Nursing [RCN], 2012), although they were only allowed to prescribe a limited number of medicines. After robust reviews and evaluations (RCN, 2012; Weeks et al., 2016), this has now been expanded to include all registered nurses and since 2006, nurse prescribers have had access to all items in the BNF. The aim of nurse prescribing is to improve patient care, ensuring that all patients have equal and improved access to their medicines and to make better use of the nurse's skills (DH, 2006).

There are two categories of nurse prescribing: **nurse independent prescribing** (NIP) and **nurse supplementary prescribing** (NSP). The number of nurses registered as prescribers with the NMC in 2012 and 2017 is detailed in Table 5.1 and indicates increased numbers of nurse prescribers over this time.

- An **independent nurse prescriber (V200/V300)** can prescribe any medication within the nurse's area of competence, for its licensed use (DH, 2006), for example a clinical nurse specialist for diabetes prescribes insulin to a patient under her care.
- **Community practitioner nurse prescribers** are a subset of independent nurse prescribers. They are district nurses, health visitors (V100/V150) and school nurses who are qualified to independently prescribe certain medications from a limited formulary, including dressings and certain over-the-counter medications (RCN, 2012).
- **Supplementary prescribing** occurs in collaboration with the patient and their doctor. A diagnosis is made by a medical practitioner (doctor) and a treatment plan, which has been formulated as a clinical management plan (CMP), sets out the parameters within which the nurse/healthcare professional can adjust the prescription, for example the dose.

**Table 5.1**  The number of nurses registered as prescribers in 2012 and 2017

| Nurse prescriber | 2012 | 2017 |
|---|---|---|
| [V100] Community practitioner nurse prescriber | 3683 | 3747 |
| [V150] Community practitioner nurse prescriber | 1369 | 3075 |
| [V200] Nurse independent prescriber | 1460 | 1447 |
| [V300] Nurse independent/supplementary prescriber | 26,347 | 37,000 |
| Total | 62,859 | 72,990 |

**A patient group directive** (PGD) is a specific written direction for the supply or administration of a licensed named medication to a specific group of patients who may not be identified before presenting for treatment (NMC, 2010). As a student nurse you cannot administer medicines under a PGD even if supervised. The registrant using a PGD must be assessed as competent and identified by name within the document and must not delegate the administration of the specified medicine. An example of a PGD in the community is the administration of a vaccine. In secondary care they can be used to dispense analgesia, for example in day-case surgery and in Accident and Emergency departments.

## IV administration in community settings or patients home

The administration of medication intravenously, until recently, occurred only within a hospital setting – with an individual patient sometimes spending time in hospital where the only healthcare intervention was the administration of IV medicines. There have been significant developments in the provision of IV therapy in the community since 2000 (Baker and Lyden-Rodgers, 2016; O'Hanlon et al., 2017). Once it has been established that it is safe, medication can be administered three to four times a day in the patient's home by an IV therapy nurse team or by community nurses trained to deliver IV therapy (O'Hanlon et al., 2017). Antibiotics are the most common type of medication administered to systemically unwell patients experiencing, for example, a chest infection or cellulitis, cared for at home rather than in hospital. It may prevent a hospital admission or accommodate an earlier discharge, thereby reducing the risk of hospital-acquired infections and benefitting both the patients and the NHS (Baker and Lyden-Rodgers, 2016).

It is important that the required education and training be provided for nurses delivering the service to ensure required levels of evidence-based knowledge and skills needed to deliver a safe and effective IV therapy for patients in the community (Baker and Lyden-Rodgers, 2016; O'Hanlon et al., 2017). In such instances, nurses need to be competent in venepuncture and cannulation, administration of IV medicines and the management of vascular access devices (O'Hanlon et al., 2017). The service also requires multiprofessional working in liaising with a hospital, the GP, microbiologist and pharmacy.

## Self-administration of medicines in a hospital setting

People are prescribed and usually take their medication without supervision within the community. However, once they are admitted to hospital their medication is often taken away and a nurse provides the medicines as part of the ward or unit routine, which may not be the same as the patient's usual routine. This can sometimes leave the patient feeling that they have lost control or that the professionals do not trust or respect their abilities. Self-administration of medicines (SAM) schemes have been introduced into hospitals, but it is not consistent or widespread. The self-administration of medicines in hospital is described by the National Prescribing Centre (2008) as:

> a standardised approach to determining the ability of patients to take their own medication correctly and safely, increase the patients' knowledge and understanding of their medication and promote and maintain patient independence and autonomy.
>
> (Cited in Richardson et al., 2014)

> **Other related clinical skills required for entry to the NMC register (NMC, 2018a) include**
>
> - Administering injections using intramuscular, subcutaneous, intradermal and intravenous routes, and managing injection equipment;
> - Administering medications using a range of routes;
> - Administering and monitoring medications using vascular access devices and enteral equipment;
> - Recognising and responding to adverse or abnormal reactions to medications;
> - Undertaking safe storage, transportation and disposal of medicinal products.

- How can you ensure that you are proficient in the above clinical skills related to practice?

# Pharmacology: what do registered nurses need to know?

As a qualified nurse, you will be responsible and accountable for keeping your knowledge and skills up to date through continuing professional development and lifelong learning. You should use evaluation, supervision and appraisal to continuously improve your performance and enhance the safety and quality of patient care (Lawson and Hennefer, 2010). This includes constantly updating your knowledge and skills relating to medicine management because new medicines are constantly being developed. The NICE is a valuable resource for healthcare professionals found at www.nice. org.uk/mpc/index.jsp, and provides evidence for prescribing and access to the BNF. The underpinning knowledge nurses require includes the study of drugs or pharmacology and how they are used to treat medical conditions. Here we provide a basic knowledge of pharmacology, although more in-depth knowledge should be obtained elsewhere. An overview of the pharmacokinetics and pharmacodynamics of medicines with examples of commonly used drugs is included below.

**Pharmacokinetics** is concerned with how the body deals with a drug and relates to the absorption, distribution, metabolism and excretion of the drug (Greenstein and Gould, 2009). *Absorption* of a drug depends on the route of administration (Banning, 2007) (see Table 5.2 for different routes of administration and the speed of effect). It is important to know how quickly the medication is effective when monitoring a patient's reaction to it. Morphine can be administered parentally, intravenously, intramuscularly and subcutaneously; it can also be taken orally as a liquid or tablet, and therefore careful monitoring will need to be within seconds for an IV administration, up to 30 minutes if administered intramuscularly or subcutaneously, and 2 hours if orally administered.

The rapid effects of an intravenously administered drug are because the drug has direct access to the bloodstream. However, when drugs are administered via other routes they often have to cross membranes before they enter the circulation (Downie et al., 2008).

The most frequent route of administration is ingestion or orally (Figure 5.1). Orally administered drugs pass through the gastric or intestinal mucosa, to be absorbed by diffusion through the walls of the small intestine and into the bloodstream (Banning, 2007). The speed of absorption depends on the form the medication takes; liquid medication is absorbed quickly compared with tablets which need to be dissolved. Some tablets have a layer that delays or slows absorption (modified

**Table 5.2**  Route of administration and time to effect of the medication

| Route of administration | Time to effect |
| --- | --- |
| Intravenous | 30–60 seconds |
| Inhalation | 2–3 minutes |
| Sublingual | 3–5 minutes |
| Intramuscular | 10–20 minutes |
| Subcutaneous | 15–30 minutes |
| Rectal | 5–30 minutes |
| Ingestion | 30–90 minutes |

release) or are enteric coated to protect the gastric mucosa. When a patient has difficulties swallowing tablets it is important that they are not crushed because this may affect the absorption and/or alter the action of the drug. Always seek advice and help from a pharmacist when your patient has problems with swallowing tablets; they may be able to dispense an alternative form of the medicine. In older people delays in absorption may result from changes in gastric emptying, changes in pH and other factors including insufficiency in cardiac output (Banning, 2007).

*Metabolism* occurs after the absorption of the drug. After absorption from the small intestine it is transported in the blood to the liver where it is broken down or metabolised. This is known as first-pass metabolism. Patients with liver disease may have difficulties in metabolising drugs, resulting in delays in its action. Metabolism ensures that the drug reaches the circulation and can be carried or *transported* to the site of its action, such as the heart, the brain, etc.

*Distribution* of a drug in the bloodstream occurs when some of the drug metabolite binds with proteins found in the bloodstream and becomes inactive. Unbound drugs are free to move in the blood and to cross the plasma membranes to the tissues where they exert their effect (Downie et al., 2008). In a poorly nourished person an increased effect of the drug may occur because of low albumin levels and high levels of unbound drugs. The binding of a drug to proteins can also be affected by polypharmacy (multiple drugs) because the drugs compete for the same binding sites (Downie et al., 2008). Poor nutrition and polypharmacy are common in older people and you will need to be aware that there may be an increase in drug potency and to vigilantly monitor this. NSAIDs such as diclofenac have a 50% binding capacity at therapeutic levels and in low plasma protein (poor nutrition) it displaces warfarin from its binding sites, allowing more free or unbound warfarin to exert its biological effect, increasing the risk of bleeding (Banning, 2007).

*Excretion* is the removal of the drug from the body. The body's way of dealing with drugs is to try to get them out of the body as soon as possible through further metabolism and excretion (Greenstein and Gould, 2009). The kidneys, specifically the glomeruli in the kidneys, are the most common route for excretion of drugs and their metabolites. Some drugs are eliminated unchanged without metabolism and others need to be changed or metabolised in order to be eliminated (Downie et al., 2008). Factors affecting the excretion of a drug include its fat solubility, the acidity of urine and the health of the kidneys. It is important that a useful level of the drug in the bloodstream be maintained. The speed of metabolism and excretion (or the length of time a drug stays in the body) means that the dose of a drug needs to be repeated at different times to ensure that it has the desired effect (Greenstein and Gould, 2009).

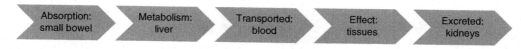

**Figure 5.1**  Diagram of basic life cycle of a drug taken orally

**Pharmacodynamics** is the term used to describe the way the drug exerts its effect by producing a physiological response in the body or controlling the changes that result from a disease (Greenstein and Gould, 2009). Some drugs or medicines act by replacing or substituting a substance such as ferrous sulphate for iron deficiency anaemia.

Enzymes are made up of proteins that speed up a chemical reaction and some medication blocks or inhibits enzymes. An enzyme inhibitor drug attaches itself to a particular enzyme to inhibit or stop the reaction. NSAIDs, such as ibuprofen, are an example of an enzyme inhibitor; they act by preventing the production of inflammatory chemicals known as prostaglandins through the inhibition of an enzyme cyclooxygenase (Downie et al., 2008).

Electrolytes within the body are carefully controlled to maintain homoeostasis. Specific electrolyte channels are found on cells and tissues; they permit the transportation of certain electrolyte ions into cells (Downie et al., 2008; Lawson and Hennefer, 2010). Muscles have electrolyte channels that allow only calcium to enter causing the muscle to constrict. Some drugs affect the transport process of electrolytes. A calcium channel blocker, such as nifedipine, is used to treat high blood pressure by occupying the calcium channel thereby preventing constriction of blood vessels and lowering the blood pressure (Lawson and Hennefer, 2010). One of the ways in which insulin works is to promote the transportation of glucose into cells which results in the lowering of blood glucose (Downie et al., 2008).

Some medications exert their effect by interacting with receptors which are found embedded in the plasma membrane of cell walls to assist in the chemical communication within the cell; they act as part of the regulation of the cells' activity. A receptor agonist drug mimics the effects of a neurotransmitter or hormone or alters the physiology of the cell by binding to the receptor (Downie et al., 2008). Morphine is an example of an agonist drug that binds to specific opiate receptors found mainly in the spinal cord and the brain, producing its analgesic effects. An antagonist drug binds with the receptor site and acts by inhibiting or blocking the agonist (Downie et al., 2008). Naloxone is a drug that competes with opiate receptors to block morphine and is used clinically to reverse the effects of opiates.

Synapses are found within the nervous system; they are the gaps between nerve fibres, muscles or glands. A neurotransmitter is released to activate the next nerve fibre or stimulate a muscle or gland into the desired action. Drugs can act as a neurotransmitter or inhibit the neurotransmitter. Salbutamol acts as a neurotransmitter to signal the dilatation of constricted airways in acute asthma. Ondansetron inhibits serotonin (a neurotransmitter) in the chemotrigger zone in the brain to control vomiting (Lawson and Hennefer, 2010).

Chemotherapy drugs act by interfering with cell growth and division to destroy rapidly dividing tumour cells. Unfortunately they also destroy normal cells; the ideal drug would selectively target the cancerous cells (Downie et al., 2008).

In infectious disease antibiotics and antiviral drugs affect the microorganisms causing the infection. Penicillin for example inhibits the synthesis of the bacterial cell walls and erythromycin inhibits bacterial protein synthesis. Nystatin acts by increasing the permeability of the invading organism's cell wall (Downie et al., 2008).

> **ACTIVITY 5.6**
>
> In order to help you to continue to build on your knowledge and skills, identify at least *10 of the common drugs and medications* used on each of your placements.
>
> Make a note of the aims of each treatment, drug strengths or concentrations, routes of administration, potential side effects and interactions.
>
> Keep a record of these in your portfolio or profile, adding to your list each time you undertake a new placement.

## Chapter summary

This chapter has provided an overview of the role and the skills an adult nurse requires in relation to medicine management and pharmacology. It is not intended to be a substitute for practical experience and student nurses will participate actively in most aspects of medicine management, especially the administration of drugs in clinical practice.

The administration of medicines is a key element of a registered nurse's role and involves a great deal of their time. The safe storage, use of medical devices, communication and monitoring of the patient's reaction to medicines are aspects of medicine management that are a nurse's responsibility. Nurses possess knowledge of the patient, their care plan and the role of the medication in relation to the care plan. They need to understand the pharmacology of the drugs they administer, the possible adverse effects and drug interactions that may occur. Ensuring that legal and ethical aspects of medicine management are adhered to and that professional standards and local policy are followed should ensure that medication errors are avoided.

## Further reading

*British National Formulary* (BNF) contains all licensed medications available, indications for use and potential side effects, as well as sections listing interactions with other drugs.

Local medicine administration/management policies will provide a practical application of how the information in this chapter is used in everyday practice.

## References

Baileff, A., Davis, J. and Davey, N. (2012) 'Managing medicines'. In I. Bullock, J. MacLeod-Clark and J. Rycroft-Malone (eds), *Adult Nursing Practice. Using Evidence in Care*. Oxford: Oxford University Press, pp. 378–95.

Baker, A. and Lyden-Rodgers, M. (2016) 'IV antibiotic therapy in the community: clinically effective and cost effective', *British Journal of Nursing*, 25(2): S4–8.

Banning, M. (2007) *Medication Management in Care of Older People*. Oxford: Blackwell Publications.

Cloete, L. (2015) 'Reducing medication errors in nursing practice', *Cancer Nursing Practice*, 14(1): 29–36.

Cloo, J., Johnson, L. and Manias, E. (2013) 'Nurses medication administration practices at two Singaporean acute care hospitals', *Nursing and Heath Sciences*, 15: 101–8.

Connor, J.A., Ahern, J.P., Cuccovia, B., Porter, C.L., Arnold, A., Dionne, R.E. and Hicket, P.A. (2016) 'Implementing a distraction-free practice with red zone medication safety initiative', *Dimensions of Critical Care Nursing*, 35(3): 116–24.

Corben, V. (2009) 'Administration of medicines'. In L. Baillie (ed.), *Developing Practical Adult Nursing Skills*, 3rd edn. London: Hodder, Chapter 4.

Cumberlege, J. (1986) *Neighbourhood Nursing: A Focus for Care* [Cumberlege Report]. London: Department of Health.

Department of Health (2004) *Building a Safer NHS for Patients: Improving Medication Safety*. London: DH.

Department of Health (2006) *Improving Patients' Access to Medicines: A Guide to Implementing Nurse and Pharmacist Independent Prescribing Within the NHS in England*. London: DH.

Downie, G., Mackenzie, J., Williams, A. and Hind, C. (2008) *Pharmacology and Medicines Management for Nurses*, 4th edn. Edinburgh; Churchill Livingstone.

Greener, M. (2014) 'Understanding adverse drug reactions: an overview', *Nurse Prescribing*, 12(4): 189–95.

Greenstein, B. and Gould, D. (2009) *Trounce's Clinical Pharmacology for Nurses*, 18th edn. Edinburgh: Churchill Livingstone.

Jones, S.W. (2009) 'Reducing medication administration errors in nursing practice', *Nursing Standard*, 23(50): 40–46.

Kaufman, G. (2016) 'Medicine optimisation: priorities and challenges', *Nursing Standard*, 30(30): 53–9.

Kavanagh, C. (2017) 'Medication governance: preventing errors and promoting patient safety', *British Journal of Nursing*, 26(3): 159–65.

Kim, J. and Bates, D.W. (2013) 'Medication administration errors by nurses: adherence to guidelines', *Journal of Clinical Nursing*, 22(3–4), 590–8.

Lawson, L. and Hennefer, D.L. (2010) *Medicines Management in Adult Nursing*. Exeter: Learning Matters.

Leufter, T. and Cleary-Houldforth, J. (2013) 'Let's do no harm: medication errors in nursing part 1', *Nurse Education in Practice*, 13: 213–16.

Mason, A. (2008) 'New medicines in primary care: a review of influences on general practitioner prescribing', *Journal of Clinical Pharmacy and Therapeutics*, 33(1): 1–10.

National Institute for Health and Care Excellence (2009) *Depression in Adults*, NICE clinical guideline. London: NICE.

National Patient Safety Agency (2005) *Wristbands for All Hospital Inpatients Improved Safety*. Safer Practice Notice 11. London: NPSA.

National Prescribing Centre (2008) *Service Improvement Guide: Self Administration of Medicines in Mental Health Trusts*. Liverpool: National Prescribing Centre.

Nursing and Midwifery Council (2010) *Standards for Medicines Management*. London: NMC.

Nursing and Midwifery Council (2018a) *Future Nurse: Standards of Proficiency for Registered Nurses*. London: NMC.

Nursing and Midwifery Council (2018b) *The Code: Professional Standards of Practice and Behaviour for Nurses and Midwives*. London: NMC.

O'Hanlon, S., McGrail, P. and Hodgkins, P. (2017) 'Community intravenous therapy provision', *Nursing Standard*, 31(28): 45–53.

Pope, T.M. (2002) 'The effect of nurses use of focused protocol to reduce distraction during medicine administration' (Dissertation), Houston, TX: Texas Women's University. [Cited in Cloo, J., Johnson, L. and Manias, E. (2013) 'Nurses' medication administration practices at two Singaporean acute care hospitals', *Nursing and Heath Sciences*, 15: 101–8.]

Raban, M.Z. and Westbrook, J.I. (2014) 'Are interventions to reduce interruptions and errors during medication administration effective? A systematic review', *British Medical Journal Quality & Safety*, 23: 414–42.

Richardson, S.J., Brooks, H.L., Bramley, G. and Cloeman, J.J. (2014) 'Evaluating the effectiveness of self-administration of medication (SAM) schemes in the hospital setting: a systematic review of the literature', *PLoS ONE*, 9(12): e113912. doi:10.1371/ journal.pone.0113912.

Royal College of Nursing (2012) *RCN Factsheet: Nurse Prescribing in the UK*. London: RCN.

Shipman Inquiry (2001) *The Regulation of Controlled Drugs in the Community*. The Shipman Inquiry, Fourth Report. Available at: webarchive.nationalarchives.gov.uk/20090808160142 or www.the-shipman-inquiry.org.uk/fourthreport.asp (last accessed 18 May 2018).

Szegedi, A., Kohen, R., Dienel, A. and Kieser, M. (2005) 'Acute treatment of moderate to severe depression with hypericum extract WS 5570 (St John's wort): randomised controlled double blinded trial', *British Medical Journal*, 330(7490): 503–6.

Weeks, G., George, J., Maclure, K. and Stewart, D. (2016) 'Non-medical prescribing versus medical prescribing for acute and chronic disease management in primary and secondary care'. Available at: http://cochranelibrary-wiley.com/doi/10.1002/14651858.CD011227 (last accessed 18 April 2018).

Westbrook, J.I., Rob, M.I., Woods, A. and Parry, D. (2011) 'Errors in administration of intravenous medications in hospital and the role of correct procedures and nurse experience', *British Medical Journal Quality & Safety*, 20(12): 1027–34.

White, R.E., Trbovich, P.L., Easty, A.C., Savage, P., Trip, K. and Hyland, S. (2010) 'Checking it twice: an evaluation of checklists for detecting medication errors at the bedside using a chemotherapy model', *BMJ Quality & Safety*, 19 August. Available at: http://qualitysafety.bmj.com/content/qhc/early/2010/08/16/qshc.2009.032862.full.pdf (last accessed 18 April 2018).

# EVIDENCE–BASED PRACTICE AND THE IMPORTANCE OF RESEARCH

## ANN WAKEFIELD AND NICOLA OLLEVEANT

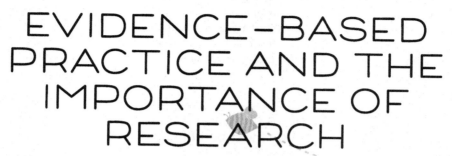

---

### CHAPTER OBJECTIVES

- Explore the origins of evidence-based practice, define what is meant by the term, and examine why it is important in today's healthcare systems;
- Develop the 'right' clinical question after identification of a problem;
- Search and retrieve evidence;
- Identify and appraise different types of evidence;
- Consider how to utilise and apply evidence-based practice within the healthcare environment;
- Evaluate the impact of using evidence in clinical practice, outlining the barriers to and enablers of implementation.

---

This chapter will explore the origins of evidence-based practice, define what we mean by the term 'evidence-based practice', and explore how to go about searching, critiquing and synthesising the literature. We will then consider how to implement evidence-based principles into clinical practice by examining some strategies that can be employed to encourage nurses to use evidence as part of their everyday work. In so doing we will investigate some of the barriers to nurses using evidence-based principles and explore how these might be overcome. The aim of this chapter is to help you nurture your ability to appraise evidence critically and make informed decisions about the care you administer. We also intend to support the development of critical appraisal skills so that you can decide if the evidence available is based on robust research principles.

# Related NMC proficiencies for registered nurses

The overarching requirements of the Nursing and Midwifery Council (NMC) are that all nurses must act in the best interests of people, putting them first and providing nursing care that is person centred, evidence based, safe and compassionate. They act professionally at all times and use their knowledge and experience to make evidence-based decisions about care. Registered nurses continually reflect on their practice and keep abreast of new and emerging developments in nursing, health and care (NMC, 2018a: 7).

 **To achieve entry to the nursing register you must be able to**

- Demonstrate an understanding of research methods, ethics and governance in order to critically analyse, safely use, share and apply research findings to promote and inform best nursing practice;
- Demonstrate the knowledge, skills and ability to think critically when applying evidence and drawing on experience to make evidence-informed decisions in all situations;
- Demonstrate the numeracy, literacy, digital and technological skills required to meet the needs of people in their care to ensure safe and effective nursing practice;
- Safely demonstrate evidence-based practice in all skills and procedures;
- Demonstrate the ability to accurately process all information gathered during the assessment process to identify needs for individualised nursing care, and develop person-centred, evidence-based plans for nursing interventions with agreed goals;
- Understand how the quality and effectiveness of nursing care can be evaluated in practice, and demonstrate how to use service delivery evaluation and audit findings to bring about continuous improvement.

(Adapted from NMC, 2018a)

# Background: the origins and purpose of evidence-based practice

It may come as a surprise to know that many researchers consider Florence Nightingale to be the first 'nurse' to have used evidence to improve patient outcomes way back in the 1850s. After her experience in the Crimean War, Nightingale was asked to oversee the management of the barrack hospital in Scutari, Turkey, which was known for its extremely unsanitary conditions. It was there Nightingale critically examined how the environment influenced health and ultimately patient outcomes. Hence, Nightingale utilised statistics to help her generate the evidence she needed to enable her to understand and predict patient morbidity and mortality (Nightingale, 1992; Aravind and Chung, 2010; Mackey and Bassendowski, 2017).

Contemporary evidence-based practice has its origins in evidence-based medicine, which emerged in the early 1970s. At this time Cochrane, a UK epidemiologist, found patients were not getting the care they needed so undertook a randomised controlled trial to compare usual care with care based on evidence. Not only did patients receiving evidence-based care achieve better outcomes, but also the practice they received was better (Mackey and Bassendowski, 2017).

In contrast, modern evidence-based nursing practice only really started to manifest from the 1990s onwards. Evidence-based nursing practice is in effect a decision-making process used to optimise patient outcomes, improve clinical practice and ensure accountability in nursing (Canadian Nurses Association, 2002). According to French (1999), tacit knowledge (that which is already known or taken for granted) is an important part of implementing evidence-based practice. Hence, when practitioners use evidence-based practice they invoke a problem-solving approach to the delivery of clinical practice and completion of administrative duties by integrating a systematic search for and critical appraisal of the most relevant evidence to answer a burning clinical question, via the incorporation of their own clinical expertise, patient preferences and personal values (Melnyk et al., 2014). Consequently evidence-based practice encourages nurses to assess the available research, clinical guidelines and other information sources based on high-quality findings to apply the results found to their clinical practice (American Academy of Medical and Surgical Nurses Association, 2017).

## What is evidence-based practice and why is it important?

Evidence-based practice has been defined as the conscientious use of current best evidence when making decisions about patient care (Sackett et al., 2000). As indicated in Figure 6.1 evidence-based practice is a way for nursing and indeed nurses to minimise the theory-to-practice gap. Therefore, evidence-based practice can also be defined as a problem-solving approach to 'clinical decision-making that incorporates a search of the best available literature and latest evidence, clinical expertise and assessment, and patient preference values within a context of caring' (International Council of Nurses, 2012: 6).

From the 1990s onwards, there has been an increase in the use of research to improve health and healthcare services, thereby turning evidence into everyday practice. Thus, by incorporating

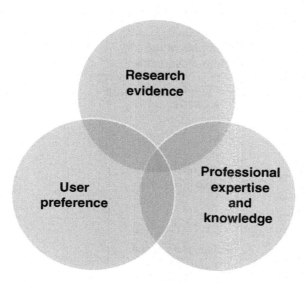

**Figure 6.1**  The relationship between theory and practice can be achieved when practising from an evidence base

evidence into practice uncertainties can be minimised when engaging in clinical decision making. Hence, nurses can now choose from a series of alternatives rather than basing their practice on tradition, as has been highlighted in Chapter 7.

 Go back to the International Council of Nurses' definition of evidence-based practice and note down why you think each of the elements has been listed: best available literature, clinical expertise and assessment, together with patient preferences and values, are all important components of evidence-based practice.

## Identifying different types of evidence

The knowledge you need in order to gain greater understanding about what you are doing as nurses and why can be generated from three main sources (Table 6.1):

1. Empirical research;
2. Clinical expertise;
3. Patient values.

## Empirical research

The 'gold standard' form of research under the empirical research umbrella is considered to be the randomised controlled trial – this form of research is employed in quantitative research studies when the researcher wants to evaluate the effectiveness of an intervention.

**Table 6.1**  Potential sources of evidence

| Type | Examples of the evidence sources | Generated by |
|---|---|---|
| Empirical research | Qualitative<br>Quantitative<br>Mixed methods | Empirical research<br>Curiosity<br>Questioning practice<br>Critical thinking<br>Reflection |
| Clinical expertise | Expert opinion<br>Clinical guidelines | Research<br>Trial and error<br>Formal learning<br>Conferences<br>Reflection |
| Patient values | Patient preferences<br>Attitudes<br>Beliefs<br>Choice | Action research<br>Questioning<br>Listening to patients<br>Communication |

Randomised controlled trials (RCTs) are part of the positivist, deductive paradigm. In other words, the researcher uses logical reasoning to understand and make sense of their findings. If conducted correctly RCTs help to minimise bias because the results are not prejudiced by any direct involvement from the researcher. For example, if the RCT is double blinded (i.e. neither the researcher nor the participant knows who is receiving what intervention), nothing should occur by chance and any change should normally occur only as a result of the intervention. As a consequence, RCTs are akin to experiments, and for this reason they are considered to have greater significance in terms of their position on the evidence hierarchy than other forms of evidence, as outlined below. Experimental designs without randomisation such as cohort, case–control or case report-based studies are still part of the quantitative paradigm but constitute lower levels of scientific evidence. For more details about the quantitative hierarchy of evidence, see Evans (2003) in 'Further reading' at the end of the chapter.

Nevertheless, not all research questions can be answered through positivist, deductive or what is often referred to as quantitative research strategies. Healthcare is not straightforward; rather it is embedded within personal, environmental, cultural and social dimensions and, as a consequence, quantitative approaches are not appropriate strategies to apply when exploring such elements of the person or their environment. For this reason, interpretative approaches are needed to explore how knowledge is socially constructed by an individual or group of individuals. Thus, qualitative research explores people's experiences, or their feelings, to generate understanding and meaning of their world, in a bid to uncover how people engage in interactions with others and how they make decisions, or how and why they live their lives in the manner chosen.

Qualitative researchers are therefore interested in gaining insight into the complexities of human behaviour rather than establishing cause and effect. The types of research approach used to generate this form of evidence might include ethnography, grounded theory, naturalistic enquiry, phenomenology, case study and a general, qualitative, descriptive design. Hence, rather than experimental, survey- or questionnaire-based data that you would use in quantitative studies, data collection in qualitative research is likely to include individual face-to-face or telephone interviews, focus groups, diary recordings, oral histories and/or observations. Hierarchies for qualitative evidence are less well used, although study rigour remains an important consideration. For more details about qualitative hierarchy of evidence, see Daly et al. (2007) and, for more details about rigour in qualitative research, see Baillie (2015) in 'Further reading' at the end of the chapter.

### ▣? ACTIVITY 6.1

Challenge yourself by reading more about qualitative research and thinking about how this might be conducted. Read the texts that we have suggested on our accompanying website about case studies, ethnography, general descriptive qualitative designs, grounded theory, naturalistic enquiry or phenomenology. Compare these with the texts on randomised controlled trials and survey research, also on the website, and write down what you think the advantages and disadvantages of using each type of research might include.

Potential reading related to this activity can be found on our accompanying website. However, you might like to find your own reading materials to see if you can use the databases effectively and also to see if you can source your own robust materials.

Increasingly, studies that draw on more than one methodological approach are becoming more prolific as the complexities of human behaviour impact on different aspects of healthcare. An example of this might include an individual's compliance with their treatment. For example, it is no use producing the best-ever cancer drug that will kill off all the cancer cells, only for patients to refuse to comply with the treatment because the side effects are so unbearable. For this reason, many drug trials that are based on RCTs also include a qualitative element, whereby researchers interview patients about their experiences of taking the drug and the impact of any side effects. This type of approach to research is called the mixed method approach, and some would argue this enables the researcher to gain a more complete picture of the phenomenon in question (Brannen, 2005). Others, however, would counter this comment, arguing that such research only amplifies the weaknesses of both approaches (Tariq and Woodman, 2013).

What do you think are the values of mixed methods research? Have a look at what others have had to say about this form of research and then write down the reasons why mixed methods is a useful strategy to employ.

### Mixed methods research

Creswell, J.W. and Clark, V.L.P. (2007) *Designing and Conducting Mixed Methods Research.* Wiley online library.

Schoonenboom, J. and Johnson, R.B. (2017) 'Wie man ein Mixed Methods-Forschungs-Design konstruiert' (How to construct a mixed methods research design), *KZfSS Kölner Zeitschrift für Soziologie und Sozialpsychologie*, 69(2): 107–31. Available at: https://link.springer.com/content/pdf/10.1007%2Fs 11577-017-0454-1.pdf.

Tariq, S. and Woodman, J. (2013) 'Using mixed methods in health research', *JRSM Short Reports*, 4(6): 2042533313479197.

Now write a list of all the possible limitations of mixed methods research.

## Clinical expertise

Clinical expertise can be based on research; however, it is often based on the clinicians' observations of many cases and comparisons of different people's outcomes. This accumulated wealth of knowledge, based on non-research-based forms of evidence, also needs to be taken into account when engaging in and implementing evidence-based practice. These forms of evidence might source evidence or information from case studies, conferences or discussion papers, and government reports. Consequently, Sackett et al. (1996) argue the clinician's 'proficiency and judgement' gained from university, continuing education and clinical practice experience should be taken into consideration when making patient care decisions. However, clinical expertise, although important, cannot be used as the sole basis for 'informing evidence-based practice' and with it your clinical decision making. (We will elaborate on this aspect in more detail in Chapter 7.)

## Patient values

Patient values and preferences can be defined as: 'The collection of goals, expectations, predispositions, and beliefs that individuals have for certain decisions and their potential outcomes' (Guyatt et al., 2015: 12). It is patients who benefit from care delivered by those who can interpret research findings, understand an individual's unique circumstances, and then work with that person to construct a plan of care that will be in their best interest, however the person defines it. Hence, without the incorporation of clinical expertise and patient preferences, best evidence could be used indiscriminately, so patients may choose not to comply with the treatment plan or the treatment may not be the most appropriate intervention for that particular individual, and so it may be ineffective. However, had the clinician consulted the patient to find out their values and preferences, the treatment may not have been considered in the first place and an alternative intervention selected instead. See Figure 6.2 to see the potential relationship between evidence, clinical expertise and patient preference and the impact these three components may have on improving patient outcomes.

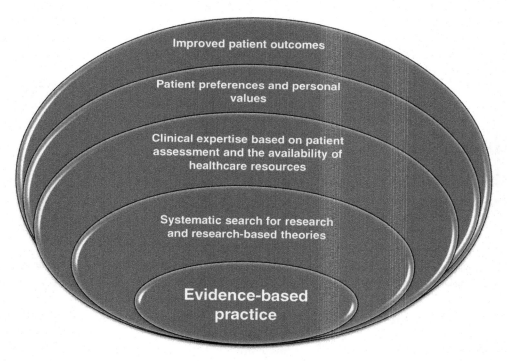

**Figure 6.2**   The relationship between evidence-based practice, clinical expertise, patient preference and its potential to improve patient outcomes

## Hierarchy of evidence

The evidence hierarchy is a form of ranking based on how robust (accurate and non-biased) a study may be. Hence, the evidence hierarchy can be considered as a pyramid with systematic reviews and other types of review, focusing on empirical research sitting at the top of the hierarchy with other forms of evidence located further down the hierarchy, depending on how reliable, valid, credible and trustworthy the data emerging from such evidence sources may be considered, as illustrated in Figure 6.3. However, before we continue we would like to draw your attention to the difference in systematic reviews, meta-analyses and meta-synthesis, so that you know what each of these terms refers to.

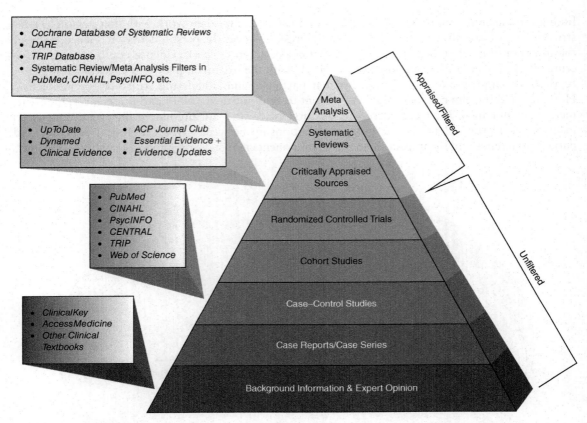

**Figure 6.3**   Hierarchy of evidence. (Adapted from Porzsolt et al., 2003. © 2001–2017, The Board of Regents of the University of Wisconsin System)

*Systematic review*: this is a specific type of literature review to generate a synthesis of the available literature. The Cochrane Collaboration has produced a handbook to guide people in how to undertake a systematic review of interventions, edited by Higgins and Green (2011), which outlines key features of all systematic review methodologies. Hence, a systematic review has:

- Clearly stated objectives underpinned by a set of predefined eligibility criteria to help you decide which studies to include in the review;
- An explicit, reproducible methodology;
- A systematic search that attempts to identify all studies that would meet the eligibility criteria;
- An assessment of the validity of the findings of the included studies, for example through the assessment of risk of bias;
- A systematic presentation, and synthesis, of the characteristics and findings that have been drawn from the included studies so that a set of conclusions and recommendations can be highlighted for future reference and development.

*Meta-analysis*: this is the use of statistical methods to combine and summarise the results generated by two or more or even a series of independent studies (Glass, 1976). By combining data generated from relevant studies that focus on the same issue, then meta-analyses can provide you with a more accurate estimate of the effects of healthcare than you could achieve if you drew data from an individual study. Hence, by combining data from a variety of related studies you can increase the statistical power of the data generated as part of a collective, rendering it more robust (Higgins and Green, 2011). For more information on statistical power, see Porter (2018) in 'Further reading'.

*Meta-synthesis*: this is an intentional and comprehensive approach to analysing data drawn from several qualitative studies. Meta-synthesis allows you or researchers to identify a specific research question, and search, select, appraise, summarise and combine the evidence from qualitative studies to then address the research question set. This process uses rigorous qualitative methods to synthesise existing qualitative studies to construct greater meaning through an interpretative process. For more information on meta-synthesis see Erwin et al. (2011) in 'Further reading'.

As you can see from Figure 6.3, the hierarchy of evidence largely encompasses quantitative methods. Hence, the hierarchy as presented would imply that qualitative research is less valuable than quantitative forms of research. However, as we have already pointed out in the section related to mixed methods, qualitative research can play a vital role in healthcare by helping us to understand better the people we are dealing with on a daily basis. Hence, we need to exercise some degree of caution when considering what research evidence to draw on, particularly when searching the databases for evidence on which to base our practice. If we focus on only one type of study we are unlikely to gain a full understanding of the topic or the phenomenon we want to examine in order to administer the best possible care.

We are now going to encourage you to have a look at how we might go about generating robust evidence on which to base our practice.

Reflect on the concept that all three components of evidence base practice are equal, namely research, clinical expertise and patient preferences. Compare this notion with the ideas presented in the evidence hierarchy. Does the hierarchy imply the research element has greater import over the other two? Should this be the case? Why do you think that? Write your ideas down and share them with your peers.

## Steps involved in evidence-based practice

Arguably evidence-based practice comprises six interrelated steps which incorporate the examination and application of robust research within clinical practice as outlined below and in Table 6.2.

## Developing the 'right' clinical question after identification of a problem

As we engage in clinical practice, questions constantly arise in our mind, given that we are curious about the world we encounter and the patients we nurse. Consequently, we often ask ourselves how something can be improved or why something happens or does not work. Or we might ask what would happen if things had been done differently. The type of question we ask will dictate which research approach we adopt to answer it. For example, if you wanted to ask descriptive, comparative or relationship-based questions you would need to use a quantitative approach to

**Table 6.2** Evidence-based practice in six steps

| | |
|---|---|
| **Assessing the patient** | Frequently when assessing a patient a question might arise where you want to answer why or how something happens, works (or not), or something has simply piqued your interest such that you want to find out more |
| **Asking the (right) question** | When asking a question it needs to be well constructed so that it addresses what you are interested in finding out |
| **Acquiring the evidence** | Within this context it is vital that you gain access to the best and most appropriate resources such as the most appropriate databases or documents to help you conduct a thorough search in order to generate the evidence you need to appraise, and establish how robust that information might be |
| **Appraising the evidence** | To be sure that the evidence you have found is appropriate you need to consider whether it is valid (sound or credible) and applicable (can be used or transferred into tangible clinical practice) |
| **Applying the evidence** | At this point the evidence needs to be incorporated into clinical practice by combining it with your own or the team's clinical expertise and aligning it with your patients' preferences |
| **Evaluating the impact of evidence in practice** | Evaluating the impact of evidence-based practice could involve you undertaking more research to find out how successful the change in practice has been, so that in effect a new question is generated and the process recommences |

generate the answers. Alternatively, if you wanted to ask exploratory, predictive or interpretive questions then you would adopt qualitative approaches to your data gathering. Table 6.3 gives a brief overview of what aspect each type of question addresses.

**Table 6.3** Types of research question

| | Type of question | Definition of what each type of question addresses |
|---|---|---|
| **Quantitative questions** | Descriptive | This type of question is used to describe something such as why a particular dressing is used to heal a wound |
| | Comparative | This type of question is used to explore the difference between two concepts or variables, e.g. why one dressing is used over and above a different form of wound dressing or why one drug is better than another |
| | Relationship based | This type of question looks as how one variable influences another, e.g. how might rest and/or elevation of a limb assist in healing a leg ulcer |
| **Qualitative questions** | Exploratory | Although similar in nature to the descriptive questions outlined above, exploratory questions are used in qualitative work to try to gain greater understanding about the topic of interest. An example of this might be to explore why individuals do not comply with their medication regimen. Or what forms of care a person might want to receive if they had a choice and why that might be |
| | Predictive | This type of question does as the name suggests. It tries to predict why a person would take a particular course of action |

| Type of question | Definition of what each type of question addresses |
|---|---|
| Interpretive | This type of question tries to gather feedback about a particular issue or topic and as such might seek to make sense of events such as why and/or how nurses organise their work in the way they do. Alternatively such questions might attempt to establish how acceptable a particular form of treatment is and why that might be |

Consequently, how you actually frame your question is a key element of evidence-based practice, as we will explore in the next section.

## Asking the right question

In order to find the most relevant, robust and reliable evidence it is essential to ask the **right** clinical question, which is grounded in practice.

Questions can be developed in a variety of ways:

- Undertaking or reviewing the research literature;
- Questioning your own or others' clinical expertise and practice;
- Reviewing patient experiences and examining patient feedback.

To help you develop your question you need to ensure it meets the following five criteria, namely the question should be:

1. Clinically relevant;
2. Contemporary;
3. Clear and simple;
4. Consistent with the needs of the patient, carer or service;
5. Manageable.

Let us use a sample question to look at how best to ask the right question in more detail. If we take the following question:

> What impact does case management have on health-related quality of life and patient satisfaction for cancer survivors?

In essence you could frame it as either a quantitative or a qualitative question depending on what focus you want to adopt. However, when engaging in evidence-based practice it is usual to adopt a formal framework or structure to help you focus your question and generate key terms. One of the frameworks you can use is referred to as the PICO (Springett and Campbell, 2015) or PICo framework (Joanna Briggs Institute, 2014).

PICO stands for:

P   patient, problem or population

I   intervention

C   comparator or control

O   outcome

whereas PICo stands for:

P    population

I    area of interest

Co   context

Let us have a look at how you can use both frameworks to address the question identified (Table 6.4).

**Table 6.4**   Quantitative question broken down using the PICO framework

| Element of the framework | Clinical question |
| --- | --- |
| P | Cancer survivors |
| I | Case management |
| C | Impact on health-related quality of life |
| O | Patient satisfaction |

What impact does case management have on health-related quality of life and patient satisfaction for cancer survivors?

Now let us see what happens if you apply the same question to the PICo framework (Table 6.5).

**Table 6.5**   Qualitative question broken down using the PICo framework

| Element of the framework | Clinical question |
| --- | --- |
| P | Cancer survivors |
| I | Case management |
| Co | Impact on patient satisfaction and health-related quality of life |

## Searching the evidence

If you are going to be successful when searching and retrieving the evidence on which you need to base your practice, you must be able to identify what literature has been written previously about the topic. However, in order to be able to retrieve robust evidence about a particular topic, you must first generate a comprehensive set of search terms to enter into the database(s) which will help you to identify quickly what data is available related to your chosen topic. Hence, you need to start by formulating a comprehensive set of alternative words or terms that best capture or describe the main concepts you have identified in your question. So let us explore this in more detail.

In Tables 6.6 and 6.7 we have identified each element of the PICO/PICo framework that corresponds to our question, and then applied the appropriate element of our question to the corresponding element of the PICO/PICo seen under the 'Clinical question' heading. Next we have identified alternative terms that correspond with the original question under the 'Potential search terms' heading. By adopting this approach we can enter as many terms as possible that reflect what we want to explore in the database(s), so that we can be sure that we are accessing all the possible research that has been published to date. The reason we need to identify alternative terms is because researchers do not always use universal words or expressions to describe a particular phenomenon; so, by looking for as many relevant key words as possible, we can ensure that we capture all the relevant papers that have been published related to the topic.

**Table 6.6** Generating key words using the PICO framework

| Element of the framework | Clinical question | Potential search terms |
|---|---|---|
| P | Cancer survivors | Cancer survivors or cancer patients |
| I | Case management | Case management or case management model of care or case management model |
| C | Impact on health-related quality of life | Impact or effect or influence or outcome or result or consequence Health-related quality of life (HRQoL) or quality of life (QoL) |
| O | Patient satisfaction | Patient satisfaction or patients' experiences or patients' perceptions or patient attitudes |

**Table 6.7** Generating key words using the PICo framework

| Element of the framework | Clinical question | Potential search terms |
|---|---|---|
| P | Cancer survivors | Cancer survivors or cancer patients |
| I | Case management | Case management or case management model of care or case management model |
| Co | Impact on patient satisfaction and health-related quality of life | Impact or effect or influence or outcome or result or consequence |
| | | Health-related quality of life (HRQoL) or quality of life (QoL) |
| | | Patient satisfaction or patients' experiences or patients' perceptions or patient attitudes |

So far we have talked only about the PICO/PICo framework; however, there are other equally appropriate frameworks that you can use to help you generate key words and organise your search effectively, depending on what the focus of your search is. These frameworks include the following: SPIDER (Cooke et al., 2012), SPICE (Booth, 2006), ECLIPS(E) (Wildridge and Bell, 2002) and BeHEMoTH (Booth and Carroll, 2015). Although we have not discussed each framework in detail here, there are dedicated texts linked to each of these alternative frameworks which are given in the references at the end of the chapter.

What is the value of using other frameworks to structure a question to define precisely what you want to find out? Reflect on the value of using more detailed frameworks and the additional complexities this may generate. Discuss with your peers the pros and cons of limiting searches depending on what you are searching the literature for.

## ACTIVITY 6.2

Try to generate a question for yourself that reflects what you want to look at in practice and apply it to one of the frameworks we have listed.

## Acquiring and retrieving the evidence

Once you have generated your search question, you need to use a database, or preferably several databases, to access the most relevant articles (sometimes referred to as papers or hits), so that you can then review them and establish if they are relevant to your research or are appropriate sources of evidence on which to base your practice. The articles accessed need to be based on sound sources of evidence, so you need to look for research-based evidence in what are termed academic databases because these will enable you to access peer-reviewed journal papers, which should be your main sources of evidence to draw on and help you generate your review.

## Academic databases

An academic database is essentially a computer program that has been instructed to collate information in an organised manner, after your search criteria have been entered into the search box. Hence, academic databases enable you to access peer-reviewed journal articles, conference proceedings, newspaper articles, government and legal reports, patents and books in a timely manner. In effect, a database can be compared with a sophisticated electronic filing system (Oxford Dictionaries, 2018). However, there are many databases to choose from and you will need to decide which are the most appropriate to help you to access the type of information you think you require. Table 6.8 lists some of the databases relevant to nursing and healthcare. However, if you are going to generate the most comprehensive search possible, you will usually need to access more than one database.

**Table 6.8** Examples of database information related to nursing and healthcare

| Database | Type(s) of information held in the database |
| --- | --- |
| AgeLine | Ageing, economics, public health and policy |
| ASSIA (Applied Social Sciences Index and Abstracts) | Health, social services, psychology, sociology, economics, politics, race relations and education |
| British Nursing Index (BNI) | UK nursing and midwifery |
| CINAHL (Cumulative Index to Nursing and Allied Health Literature) | Nursing and allied health |

| Database | Type(s) of information held in the database |
|---|---|
| The Cochrane Library | Systematic reviews and meta-analyses of high-quality medical research |
| DARE (Database of Abstracts of Reviews of Effects) | Systematic reviews |
| DOAJ (Directory of Open Access Journals) | Open access scientific and scholarly journals |
| EMB Evidence-Based Medicine Reviews | Best evidence about medical decision making |
| Embase Biomedical Database | Biological and pharmacological data |
| Health Technology Assessment Database | Health technology assessments worldwide |
| Medline | Medicine, dentistry and nursing-related topics |
| PsycINFO | Behavioural sciences and mental health |
| PubMed | Health, medicine, nursing, audiology and biology |

Reproduced with the permission of *Nursing Standard*.

---

### ACTIVITY 6.3

Using Table 6.9 as a template, list what you think might be the advantages and disadvantages of using each of the databases listed, to help you choose the most appropriate database for your particular task.

Table 6.9  Advantages and disadvantages of using different databases

| Name of database | Advantages | Disadvantages |
|---|---|---|
| ASSIA | | |
| CINHAL | | |
| Cochrane library | | |
| EMBASE | | |
| MEDLINE | | |
| PsycINFO | | |
| PubMED | | |

## Inclusion and exclusion criteria

Once a clear set of search terms has been developed you next need to develop a set of clear and robust inclusion and exclusion criteria so if we return to our question:

**What impact does case management have on health-related quality of life and** patient satisfaction for cancer survivors?

we might set the following inclusion criteria, in other words, when we have found our papers and start to review them they must address the following issues, namely the paper must:

- Focus on cancer survivorship:
  - and be related to any form of cancer patient;
  - associated with patients from any age group or gender;
- Focus on patients who have been exposed to case management processes as part of their cancer management plan;
- Address issues concerned with health-related quality of life;
- Address the impact of case management on the patient and their quality of life.

We can also add in additional limiters to focus the papers we review even further; this might include the following, namely that the papers must be:

- Published in the English language only;
- Published in the last 10 years only;
- Based only on empirical research;
- Available in full text only.

The exclusion criteria will be all those features that fall outside the inclusion criteria, for example, papers related to cancer that do not address survivorship, and do not address case management or health-related quality of life, and also fall outside the additional limiters set.

    However, you need to be aware that placing limiters on the type of text you uncover means that you could potentially miss papers or other sources of evidence that are important to your search. Nevertheless, if you are undertaking the search process for an undergraduate dissertation or review of a particular topic, placing limiters on the types of text you uncover will make the process more manageable. In contrast, if you were undertaking a systematic review, then full text limiters would not be appropriate because you would need to access as many of the papers that had been written as possible to gain a holistic view of the topic.

## Boolean operators

An additional way to refine your search is to use Boolean operators to identify the logical relationship(s) between terms. In order to retrieve the most relevant information you need to link key concepts or keywords together; you can do this with the use of the terms OR, AND, NOT. These terms are the most commonly used; however, another abbreviation you can include is ADJ, which looks for terms that are near to or similar to the term you want (see Table 6.10 below for more detail). For more details see also EBSCO help searching with Boolean operators (see 'Useful websites').

## Truncations

A further way in which you can improve your search is to use what are called truncations; these are symbols that are used to represent different types of endings for the same word. For example, if you are searching for something related to nurses or nursing, rather than entering both

**Table 6.10**  Using Boolean operators

| Boolean operator | Use | Example |
| --- | --- | --- |
| OR | Either one term or another is present | Depression OR Mood disorders |
| AND | Both key words are present | Depression AND Anxiety |
| ADJ | Finds near or adjacent terms | Childhood ADJ Trauma |
| NOT | To specify a term that should not be present | Books NOT Internet |

terms into the database you could use a truncation sign; this is usually represented by the dollar sign ($), although some databases use other signs such as (#). If we go back to our nurse example, if we enter nurs$ into the database it will pull up all variations of the word, including nurse, nurses, nursing, nursery. As you can see if we want to look only at papers related to nursing, using the truncation symbol we can also pull up papers that are not related to the topic, in this case nursery, so truncations need to be used with caution. Although truncations can help you capture multiple variants of a term, allowing you to broaden your search, they can make it too broad by adding in unwanted or inappropriate terms. For more details, see EBSCO help using wildcards and truncations in 'Useful websites'.

## Wildcards

A further tool you can use is the wildcard symbol, which allows you to search for words that mean the same but are spelt differently, e.g. behavior and behaviour; by inserting the wildcard symbol into your search term you can ensure that you capture all variations of the term you are looking for. Wildcards can be used in two ways: first as a substitute for one letter (#), e.g. analy#e to find analyse and analyze, and, second, as an additional letter (?), e.g. behavio?r to find behavior and behaviour.

### ☐? ACTIVITY 6.4

Try entering a term that relates to a question you might want to ask and identify what difference it makes to the number and quality of hits you generate when you use the wildcard and/or truncation tools.

## Medical subject headings: 'MeSH' headings

The final tool that you can use to help you search the databases is the thesaurus function or MeSH terms function. Databases have different sorts of tools to help you find alternative terms or words that you can use to help you broaden your search and are present in most, if not all, databases (Jones and Smyth, 2004; Hek and Moule, 2006).

MeSH, or 'medical subject headings' to give it its full title, comprises a list of over 26,000 terms that precisely describe the content of medical documents (such as journal articles). The MeSH vocabulary is a distinctive feature of the Medline database produced by the National Library of

Medicine (NLM). The NLM indexers examine articles and other publication types and assign specific MeSH headings to a paper that most appropriately describe what it is about, to help you identify more precisely the most suitable papers you need for your search.

Consequently, MeSH headings make searching the evidence more relevant. For example, if you were to enter the word 'aids' into a keyword search in Medline, you would retrieve all articles where the word 'aids' is used; this would include terms such as AIDS, hearing aids and clinical aids as an example. However, if you were to undertake a MeSH search it would map the word 'aids' to the term 'acquired immune deficiency syndrome' (the MeSH heading) and limit the search to that particular medical condition. Hence, MeSH terms may make your searches more relevant, because they allow you to focus your search by research topic.

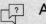 ACTIVITY 6.5

Using the Medline database, enter a term you have used as part of your question into the search section; first of all use a free text search and see what results you obtain. Now do the same thing, this time using the MeSH filter, and compare the two searches to see what has changed and whether the information you generate is more relevant to what you want to achieve.

## Running a search of the databases

Bearing in mind all we have said so far you should now be ready to run your own search, so in the case of our original question we could enter the following terms into the database(s) to see what sorts of papers we can generate (Figure 6.4):

What impact does case management have on health-related quality of life and patient satisfaction for cancer survivors?

 ACTIVITY 6.6

Enter the terms we have identified in Figure 6.4 into a database. We used CINHaL Plus; however, you might choose to use Medline or another database to which you have access. To narrow the search down further, we limited the texts to: full texts, published in English from 2008 to 2018. Then to narrow the search down further still, we limited the texts generated, by stipulating that the terms outlined had to appear in the exact major subject heading list and the papers had to have been published only in academic journals.

You might want to try different combinations of limiter to see what impact your actions have on the accuracy of your results and the number of hits (i.e. texts/papers) you generate.

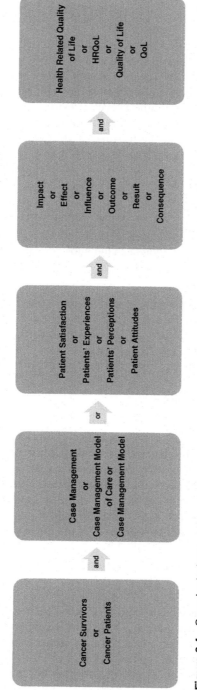

**Figure 6.4** Search strategy

# Identifying and appraising the different types of evidence/literature

Once the evidence has been retrieved you will need to make a decision about what evidence is the most relevant, reliable, robust and appropriate to use to help you answer your clinical question. Assessing the evidence can be limited by various factors including time and database availability. Practical resources to support evidence-based practice are continually evolving and as health professionals we should always look at the highest level of evidence available.

The first part of appraising the evidence is to sift the papers you have located in order to identify the most appropriate and relevant evidence to answer your question. This involves a four-stage process as identified in Table 6.11.

**Table 6.11** Literature-searching filters

**Preliminary literature-filtering process**

**Title.** Look at the title to decide whether it addresses the subject matter you are interested in

**Abstract.** Read the abstract in full to compare its content with the topic and your inclusion and exclusion criteria to see if the article addresses these

**Full text.** Read the full text to compare the content with the topic, purpose of the study, and your inclusion and exclusion criteria to see if the article meets all your requirements

**Type of article.** In this final stage, you will need to decide if the article is what you want. For example, if you want to use only empirical research data in your review

Adapted from Wakefield (2014).

It is often useful to critique papers as part of a team or with a second person to help to ensure that you have drawn robust conclusions about the papers you have found and the strength of the evidence you have sourced. The more accurate your critique the more confident you can be of the accuracy, relevance and applicability of your clinical decision to use the evidence you have sourced. However, if you are undertaking a review for an academic piece of work for your degree, you are not able to critique the papers you have found as part of a group because you could be in danger of being accused of academic malpractice in the form of collusion, so how might you achieve a robust assessment and critique of the papers on your own? Write down your thoughts and discuss them with your peers.

## Critiquing the literature

Once you have decided which papers you are going to keep then you need to critique them in order to see if they are robust and sound evidence on which to base your practice. The best way to do this is to use a critiquing tool; these tools can either be generic or specific. Generic checklists are not designed to appraise one particular type of research design (Moule et al., 2017). In contrast, however, there are several specific tools designed to critique different sorts of research, for example the Critical Appraisal Skills Programme (CASP) has developed a series of checklists that can be downloaded for free from their website, which address the following type of studies: systematic reviews, RCTs, qualitative studies, case–control studies and cohort studies, as well as economic evaluation, clinical prediction and diagnostic checklists.

The Joanna Briggs Institute also produce checklists that can be downloaded which address the following forms of study: case–control studies, case reports, case series, cohort studies, diagnostic test accuracy studies, economic evaluations, prevalence studies, quasi-experimental studies (non-randomised experimental studies), RCTs, systematic reviews, text and opinion papers, analytical cross-sectional studies and qualitative research.

As you can see there is considerable overlap between the types of tools produced by both organisations; however, neither provides tools that help you to appraise mixed methods studies critically. Pluye et al. (2011) from McGill University have designed a tool that is specifically for mixed methods reviews called the mixed methods appraisal tool (MMAT). The checklist was developed to provide a quality appraisal tool for quantitative, qualitative and mixed methods studies including systematic mixed studies reviews (Pluye and Hong, 2014).

---

### ACTIVITY 6.7

Choose two papers from your search and undertake a critique of both of these using an appropriate tool.

---

## Applying the evidence

Applying the research-based evidence to your practice is the next step to implementing evidence-based nursing practice. However, before we discuss how you might try to apply evidence to practice, we are first going to explore some of the barriers to implementing evidence-based practice so that you might consider some innovative ways in which your peers and your clinical colleagues could be stimulated and motivated to consider making evidence-based practice an integral part of their everyday considerations when engaging in clinical interventions.

### Barriers to implementing evidence-based practices within the clinical context

Multiple barriers have been identified as prohibiting the incorporation of evidence into clinical practice (Grol and Wensing, 2004). The following list is not exhaustive, but it offers some insight into why evidence does not always get translated into practice:

- Lack of time;
- Lack of mentoring or training;
- Lack of skills;
- Lack of confidence;
- Lack of perceived value of evidence-based practice;
- Lack of access to the best evidence; and
- Lack of administrative support.

(Melnyk et al., 2004; Pravikoff et al., 2005; Saunders et al., 2016)

## Lack of time

In the current healthcare climate there is often precious little time to breathe, let alone read, so nurses frequently do not engage in reading to improve or change their practice. More importantly, trying to implement change on your own is of little value because change management needs to have an impetus behind it; hence, you need a cadre of like-minded individuals to support you in your endeavour. Moreover, having one person do all the work is not realistic because it is too much for one person to implement change or to motivate others to engage in evidence-based practices, as opposed to those who base their practice on tradition and do not challenge practice.

## Lack of mentoring or training

As with any other skill the factors needing to be taken into consideration when implementing evidence-based practice also need to be learned. Hence, it is vital that team members have some form of training in how to search for, critically appraise and synthesise the literature so that evidence-based practitioners draw only on robust high-quality evidence. For this reason, you need to be aware of how to appraise research so that you can be sure you chose the best evidence to take forward for implementation in practice.

## Lack of skills

Many nurses do not have the skills to be able to critique the available evidence, so they need to be taught these skills to become proficient in critically appraising the research they find in order to change their practice in accordance with the latest evidence.

## Lack of confidence

Some nurses have the skills, yet doubt their abilities, so, in this case, it is important to encourage those individuals to make a contribution to any debate about practice and the sorts of changes you might want to invoke, taking into account everyone's views. It is important to have these inclusive discussions at clinically based meetings and in practice areas, so that change is a negotiated process that everyone agrees to in order to make the change happen.

## Lack of perceived value of evidence-based practice

Sometimes nurses may perceive evidence-based practice as simply another fad that needs to be implemented to keep managers or patients happy. However, it is important to provide such individuals with strong evidence to show them how and why evidence-based practice, as opposed to practice based on tradition or 'what we have always done', is more robust and likely to bring about more positive outcomes for patients.

## Lack of access to the best evidence

This element might be more difficult to overcome if there are strong firewalls in place to protect data and restrict access from rogue outside influences. Hence, it is vital that strong links are made with either the local higher education institute or a relevant medical library site in a bid to facilitate access to databases and web-based resources. In this way access to the best available evidence can be better facilitated.

## Lack of administrative support

Administrative support may not seem to be important. However, if you want to be able to access research papers and disseminate them among the team, then having to spend time copying documents would not be a good use of your time. Hence, you will need to negotiate with the ward manager or matron how you might gain access to the necessary resources. Alternatively, if you have access to institutional log-ins to journals via an organisation, hospital or educational institution you may be able to facilitate gaining electronic access to your selected articles.

# Utilising and applying evidence-based practice within the healthcare environment

Knowing how to use and apply research-based evidence is now a vital part of the nursing role; this is clear from *The Code* (NMC, 2018b: 9) under the heading 'Practise effectively' whereby nurses are expected to:

> assess need and deliver or advise on treatment, or give help (including preventative or rehabilitative care) without too much delay and to the best of your abilities, on the basis of the best evidence available and best practice. You communicate effectively, keeping clear and accurate records and sharing skills, knowledge and experience where appropriate. You reflect and act on any feedback you receive to improve your practice.
>
> (NMC, 2018b: 9, Clause 6: Practise effectively)

Consequently, in the final aspect of this chapter, we are going to explore how research-based evidence can be used in practice. For most of you reading this text, the type of evidence with which you will come into contact will be based on research undertaken by others, because many of you will not have undertaken original research as part of your undergraduate programme. In view of this, the evidence you use will be the work of others and for that reason we are going to explore how research can be championed in the clinical area by you as students and by clinical staff in the form of mentors, supervisors or coaches.

## Using evidence in practice

There are many ways in which evidence can be used in practice; the following are some examples of how you can do this;

- Developing an information library;
- Ward-based research seminars;
- Journal clubs;

## *Developing an evidence-based information library for students and clinical staff*

One of the ways you can help others to take note of research would be to formulate an evidence-based information library which could be located on an educational notice board on your ward. In order to generate your mini-library of evidence on which to base practice, you need to locate and review a small number of papers that are contemporary, relevant and research based about a topic that is relevant to the cases or patients you encounter on the ward.

As part of the above process you need to be able to rationalise why you have:

1. Identified the particular papers you have decided to include in your mini-library;
2. Targeted particular journals from which draw your papers;
3. Chosen specific limits to restrict the number of papers sourced;
4. Chosen to develop your mini-library of up to 10 papers for one of the following groups:

   - Students;
   - Registered nurses;
   - Patients;
   - Carers.

In addition you also need to articulate how you know the papers you have sourced are high quality and robust, based on sound research-based evidence. Did you use the tools we suggested earlier in the chapter to help you decide which papers to choose or did you choose them on the basis of the first 10 papers you found? Which approach is the most effective to use and why?

Write down your rationale and discuss this with your peers.

## *Ward-based research seminars*

Research seminars offer an opportunity for small groups of ward-based staff to learn with and from each other about a particular topic or patient group. Although these capture only a small number of people and may need to be run more than once to capture a larger group, they are, nevertheless, a useful way of stimulating conversations about research in a dedicated time-frame, so individuals can stop and think about what they are doing as part of their practice and why. As students you may ask the ward manager if you can run such an event because this will help to consolidate your learning in practice and also help you to understand better the research process and how evidence can be applied to practice. Engaging in such activities also stimulates discussion and questions practices that might be outdated or simply need to be refreshed.

## *Journal clubs*

Integrating evidence-based practice awareness, critical thinking skills and critical evaluation of the current research literature, and applying it to patient care can be facilitated best via the use of journal clubs (Lucia and Swanberg, 2018). In essence, journal clubs are an extremely useful tool that can be used to encourage individuals not only to engage in dialogue with and between peers, but also to actually read about research and appraise its quality for themselves. Journal clubs have been shown to positively impact on the development of evidence-based practice, knowledge and skills (Mohr et al., 2015; Harris et al., 2011).

You have been asked by the ward manager to run a journal club for the staff on your ward. How might you go about organising such an event? Write down your thoughts before moving on to the next section of the text.

## HOW TO RUN A JOURNAL CLUB

Although organising a journal club is not difficult, it is not just an excuse for a chat with your peers and colleagues. Hence, you need to give some serious thought to how you might go about arranging and running such an event. What follows is a brief outline of the considerations you need to take into account based on the suggestions offered by Russell et al. (2011) as outlined below:

Ten steps to success

### Step 1: *Select a leader*

This should be someone who is committed to the process because this person will need to review the paper or papers you have selected to discuss in considerable detail before the session takes place.

### Step 2: *Create goals*

This aspect is vital because it cements what you want to achieve. For example, the journal club can range from a forum designed simply to help people learn how to critique research articles, to reviewing the evidence to support a change in practice.

### Step 3: *Identify the audience*

This can be members of a unit, ward, department or particular specialty.

### Step 4: *Select a time and place to meet*

This could be once a month during lunch time in a hospital conference room or it could be weekly, based on the ward and just be for staff locally rather than from across the institution.

### Step 5: *Partner with your clinical library to select articles to review*

Connect with the clinical library to help select the most appropriate articles and provide additional training in relation to critiquing skills.

### Step 6: *Create forms for summarising/analysing your articles*

Share these in advance of the meeting.

### Step 7: *Market and promote your journal club*

Put up posters or send out email invitations.

*(Continued)*

(Continued)

    Step 8: *Hold your first meeting*

Encourage and motivate your participants to provide discussion and remember to invite a clinical librarian because this person may be able to help out when you get stuck, so that you do not shoulder all the responsibility of running the session on your own.

Step 9: *Evaluate your journal club*

At each session gather feedback from participants; this can be via either handouts or email-based surveys.

Step 10: *Make adjustments, if necessary*

Depending on your survey results, consider making changes to the sessions in response to what has been said.

# Evaluating the impact of the evidence in practice

So far we have discussed why evidence-based practice is an increasingly important part of contemporary nursing, given that it enables you to base your practice on the best available evidence, thereby minimising risk and promoting patient safety. However, it is not appropriate to simply accept the evidence, implement best practice and continue with that practice recommendation. It is vital that we evaluate whether the evidence is as robust as it claims to be or if improvements to that evidence need to take place. Hence, it is important for us to undertake evaluation studies to make sure that the evidence is still relevant or to engage in action research projects to see whether patients and carers feel the evidence-based practice is acceptable and fits with their personal values, preferences and philosophies. Potential ways in which you could evaluate the worth of having implemented evidence-based practice would be to engage in evaluation or outcomes-based research, or undertake an action research project. In the final section of this chapter we offer you a brief overview of how you might go about undertaking each type of study.

## Evaluation and outcomes-based research

Evaluative research is undertaken to assess the worth or success of something: a programme, a policy or a project. Social evaluation is not a method or technique like social surveys or participant observation. It is an increasingly common form of applied social research. What distinguishes evaluation research from other types of research is its purpose: in other words it is action oriented and often used to support or introduce a change in practice (Clarke and Dawson, 1999).

In nursing the focus of evaluation research is often on patient care and the ways in which it is delivered. Therefore outcomes will usually be determined by measuring the impact of an intervention, practice or policy. Different approaches to undertaking evaluation research can be implemented, depending on what is being evaluated and measured. These include goal-oriented approaches, which would be used to measure the extent to which an intervention has achieved specific goals or objectives. Economic evaluations are used to calculate the costs of resources and the benefits arising from these whereas utilisation-focused evaluations explore how every aspect of a project is used to determine the answers about a practice, policy or intervention. Consequently, a variety of research methods can be used in evaluation research, including quantitative, qualitative and mixed methods approaches. For more information on evaluation research, see Barlow (2004) in 'Further reading'.

## Action research

Action research involves healthcare practitioners conducting a systematic investigation into their own practice and as a consequence it is seen as a 'hands-on' participatory approach to research. Action research is primarily focused towards improving practice; hence the purpose of undertaking the research is to bring about change in a specific context (Parkin, 2009). Action research can often be seen as a cyclical process, beginning with the identification of a problem, planning actions, observing and finally reflecting on the outcomes. Nevertheless, the process still may not be completed at this point and may continue to until a complete understanding of what is being investigated is fully understood or what is being investigated is achieved. Action research is therefore reliant on both participatory and collaborative working in order to generate change and new knowledge. In nursing, action research is often about improving standards and generating new knowledge, grounded in the reality of practice. For more information on participatory action research (PAR), see MacDonald (2012) in 'Further reading'.

### ACTIVITY 6.8

What have you remembered? Test yourself.

Are you able to write a brief synopsis of what you have read without referring back to the content? For example, could you define what evidence-based practice encompasses? Could you formulate a robust search strategy? Can you remember how to identify best evidence to answer a research question? Why might evidence not be implemented in practice?

Write your answers down and then go back over the content of the chapter to see how much you have remembered.

## Chapter summary

In this chapter we have discussed where evidence-based practice emerged from, what we mean by evidence-based practice and how to develop robust, clinically based questions. We then examined how you could search and retrieve the evidence effectively. Subsequently we explored how you could appraise the evidence generated by quantitative, qualitative and mixed methods research, as well as outlining the barriers to implementing evidence-based practice. In addition we demonstrated how you might go about utilising and applying evidence-based practice within the healthcare environment. Finally, we explored how you might approach evaluating the impact of using evidence in clinical practice.

## Useful websites

Centre for Evidence Based Medicine, Oxford: www.cebm.net.

EBSCO help searching with Boolean operators: https://help.ebsco.com/interfaces/EBSCO_Guides/EBSCO_ Interfaces_User_Guide/Searching_with_Boolean_Operators.

EBSCO help using wildcards and truncations: https://help.ebsco.com/interfaces/EBSCO_Guides/EBSCO_ Interfaces_User_Guide/Using_Wildcards_and_Truncation.

Students4bestevidence.net: www.students4bestevidence.net.

TRIP database, Liberating the Literature: www.tripdatabase.com.

## Further reading

Baillie, L. (2015) 'Promoting and evaluating scientific rigour in qualitative research', *Nursing Standard*, 29(46): 36–42.

Barlow, A. (2004) 'Evaluation research: using comprehensive methods for improving healthcare practices', *Evidence-Based Midwifery*, 2(1): 4–8.

Claydon, L.S. (2015) 'Rigour in quantitative research', *Nursing Standard*, 29(47): 43–8.

Daly, J., Willis, K., Small, R., Green, J., Welch, N., Kealy, M. and Hughes, E. (2007) 'A hierarchy of evidence for assessing qualitative health research', *Journal of Clinical Epidemiology*, 60(1): 43–9.

Erwin, E.J., Brotherson, M.J. and Summers, J.A. (2011) 'Understanding qualitative metasynthesis: issues and opportunities in early childhood intervention research', *Journal of Early Intervention*, 33(3): 186–200.

Evans, D. (2003) 'Hierarchy of evidence: a framework for ranking evidence evaluating healthcare interventions', *Journal of Clinical Nursing*, 12(1): 77–84.

Harvey, M. and Land, L. (2017) *Research Methods for Nurse and Midwives. Theory and Practice*. London: Sage, Part 1, Chapters 4, 5 and 6.

MacDonald, C. (2012) 'Understanding participatory action research: a qualitative research methodology option', *Canadian Journal of Action Research*, 13(2): 34–50.

Mantzoukas, S. (2008) 'A review of evidence-based practice, nursing research and reflection: levelling the hierarchy', *Journal of Clinical Nursing*, 17(2): 214–23.

Mays, N. and Pope, C. (1995) 'Rigour and qualitative research', *British Medical Journal*, 311(6997): 109–12.

Porter, K.E. (2018) 'Statistical power in evaluations that investigate effects on multiple outcomes: a guide for researchers', *Journal of Research on Educational Effectiveness*, 11(2): 267–95.

Thomas, E. and Magilvy, J.K. (2011) 'Qualitative rigor or research validity in qualitative research', *Journal for Specialists in Pediatric Nursing*, 16(2): 151–5.

Welch, C. (2018) 'Good qualitative research: opening up the debate'. In *Collaborative Research Design*. Singapore: Springer, pp. 401–12.

## References

American Academy of Medical and Surgical Nurses Association (2017) *What is Evidence Based Practice?* Available at: www.amsn.org/practice-resources/evidence-based-practice (last accessed 18 May 2018).

Aravind, M. and Chung, K.C. (2010) 'Evidence-based medicine and hospital reform: tracing origins back to Florence Nightingale', *Plastic and Reconstructive Surgery*, 125(1): 403–9.

Booth, A. (2006) 'Clear and present questions: formulating questions for evidence based practice', *Library Hi Tech*, 24(3): 355–68.

Booth, A. and Carroll, C. (2015) 'Systematic searching for theory to inform systematic reviews: is it feasible? Is it desirable?', *Health Information & Libraries Journal*, 32(3): 220–35.

Brannen, J. (2005) 'Mixed methods research: a discussion paper'. NCRM methods review papers, NCRM/005. Available at: http://eprints.ncrm.ac.uk/89/1/MethodsReviewPaperNCRM-005.pdf A(last accessed 12 August 2018).

Canadian Nurses Association (2002) *Evidence-based Decision-making and Nursing Practice*. Available at: www.nurseone.ca/~/media/nurseone/page-content/pdf-en/ps63_evidence_based_decision_making_nursing_practice_e.pdf?la=en (last accessed 18 May 2018).

Clarke, A. and Dawson, R. (1999) *Evaluation Research*. London: Sage.

Cooke, A., Smith, D. and Booth, A. (2012) 'Beyond PICO: The SPIDER tool for qualitative evidence synthesis', *Qualitative Health Research*, 22(10): 1435–43.

French, P. (1999) 'The development of evidence-based nursing', *Journal of Advanced Nursing*, 29: 72–8.

Glass, G.V. (1976) 'Primary, secondary, and meta-analysis of research', *Educational Researcher*, 5(10): 3–8.

Grol, R. and Wensing, M. (2004) 'What drives change? Barriers to and incentives for achieving evidence-based practice', *Medical Journal of Australia*, 180(6 Suppl): S57.

Guyatt, G., Jaeschke, R., Wilson, M.C., Montori, V.M. and Richardson, W.S. (2015) 'What is evidence-based medicine?' In G. Guyatt, D. Rennie, M.O. Meade and D.J. Cook (eds), *Users' Guides to the Medical Literature: A Manual for Evidence-based Clinical Practice*, 3rd edn. New York: McGraw-Hill Education, pp. 7–14.

Harris, J., Kearley, K., Heneghan, C., Meats, E., Roberts, N., Perera, R. and Kearley-Shiers, K. (2011) 'Are journal clubs effective in supporting evidence-based decision making? A systematic review', *BEME Guide No. 16, Medical Teacher*, 33(1): 9–23.

Hek, G. and Moule, P. (2006) *Making Sense of Research: An Introduction for Health and Social Care Practitioners*, 3rd edn. London: Sage.

Higgins, J.P.T. and Green, S. (eds) (2011) *Cochrane Handbook for Systematic Reviews of Interventions*, Version 5.1.0. London: The Cochrane Collaboration. Available at: http://training.cochrane.org/handbook.

International Council of Nurses (2012) *Closing the Gap: From Evidence to Action*. Available at: www.icn.ch/publications/2012-closing-the-gap-from-evidence-to-action/ (last accessed 18 May 2018).

Joanna Briggs Institute (2014) *Reviewer's Manual*. Adelaide: Joanna Briggs Institute, University of Adelaide. Available at: http://joannabriggs.org/assets/docs/sumari/reviewersmanual-2014.pdf (last accessed 14 August 2018).

Jones, L.V. and Smyth, R.L. (2004) 'How to perform a literature search', *Current Paediatrics*, 14(6): 482–8.

Lucia, V.C. and Swanberg, S.M. (2018) 'Utilizing journal club to facilitate critical thinking in pre-clinical medical students', *International Journal of Medical Education*, 9: 7–8.

Mackey, A. and Bassendowski, S. (2017) 'The history of evidence-based practice in nursing education and practice', *Journal of Professional Nursing*, 33(1): 51–5.

Melnyk, B.M., Fineout-Overholt, E., Fischbeck Feinstein, N., Li, H., Small, L., Wilcox, L. and Kraus, R. (2004) 'Nurses' perceived knowledge, beliefs, skills, and needs regarding evidence-based practice: implications for accelerating the paradigm shift', *Worldviews on Evidence-Based Nursing*, 1(3): 185–93.

Melnyk, B.M., Gallagher-Ford, L., Long, L.E. and Fineout-Overholt, E. (2014) 'The establishment of evidence-based practice competencies for practicing registered nurses and advanced practice nurses in real-world clinical settings: proficiencies to improve healthcare quality, reliability, patient outcomes, and costs', *Worldviews on Evidence-Based Nursing*, 11(1): 5–15.

Mohr, N.M., Stoltze, A.J., Harland, K.K., Van Heukelom, J.N., Hogrefe, C.P. and Ahmed, A. (2015) 'An evidence-based medicine curriculum implemented in journal club improves resident performance on the Fresno test', *Journal of Emergency Medicine*, 48(2): 222–9.

Moule, P., Aveyard, H. and Goodman, M. (2017) *Nursing Research: An Introduction*, 3rd edn. London: Sage, Chapters 5, 14, 15 and 21.

Nightingale, F. (1992) *Notes on Nursing: What It Is, and What It Is Not*. Philadelphia, PA: Lippincott Williams & Wilkins.

Nursing and Midwifery Council (2018a) *Future Nurse: Standards of Proficiency for Registered Nurses*. London: NMC.

Nursing and Midwifery Council (2018b) *The Code: Professional Standards of Practice and Behaviour for Nurses and Midwives*. London: NMC.

Oxford Dictionaries (2018) *English Oxford Living Dictionaries*. Oxford: Oxford University Press. Available at: https://en.oxforddictionaries.com/definition/academic (last accessed 18 May 2018).

Parkin, P. (2009) *Managing Change in Healthcare: Using Action Research*. London: Sage.

Pluye, P. and Hong, Q.N. (2014) 'Combining the power of stories and the power of numbers: mixed methods research and mixed studies reviews', *Annual Review of Public Health*, 35: 29–45.

Pluye, P., Robert, E., Cargo, M., Bartlett, G., O'Cathain, A., Griffiths, F., Boardman, F., Gagnon, M.P. and Rousseau, M.C. (2011) 'Proposal: a mixed methods appraisal tool for systematic mixed studies reviews'. Available at: http://mixedmethodsappraisaltoolpublic.pbworks.com (last accessed 26 April 2018).

Porzsolt, F., Ohletz, A., Thim, A., Gardner, D., Ruatti, H., Meier, H., Schlotz-Gorton, N. and Schrott, L. (2003) 'Evidence-based decision making: the six step approach', *BMJ Evidence-Based Medicine*, 8(6): 165–6.

Pravikoff, D.S., Tanner, A.B. and Pierce, S.T. (2005) 'Readiness of U.S. nurses for evidence-based practice', *American Journal of Nursing*, 105(9): 40–51; quiz 52.

Russell, C., Bean, K.B. and Berry, D. (2011) '*How to develop a successful journal club*', International Transplant Nurses Society. Available at: http://itns.org/images/Membership/Chapters/Journal_Club_Guidelines.pdf (last accessed 12 August 2018).

Sackett, D.L., Rosenberg, W.M.C., Mur Gray, J.A., Haynes, R.B. and Richardson, W.S. (1996) 'Evidence based medicine. What it is and what it isn't', *British Medical Journal*, 312: 71–2.

Sackett, D.L., Strauss, S.E., Richardson, W.S., Rosenberg, W. and Haynes, R.B. (2000) *Evidence Based Medicine: How to Practice and Teach EBM*, 2nd edn. Edinburgh: Churchill Livingstone.

Saunders, H., Vehvilainen-Julkunen, K. and Stevens, K.R. (2016). 'Effectiveness of an education intervention to strengthen nurses' readiness for evidence-based practice: A single-blind randomized controlled study', *Applied Nursing Research*, 31: 175–85. Available at: https://doi.org/10.1016/j.apnr.2016.03.004.

Springett, K. and Campbell, J. (2006) 'An introductory guide to putting research into practice', *Defining the Research Question Podiatry Now*, 26–8. Available at: www.researchgate.net/publication/237406765/download.

Tariq, S. and Woodman, J. (2013) 'Using mixed methods in health research', *JRSM Short Reports*, 4(6): 2042533313479197.

Wakefield, A. (2014) 'Searching and critiquing the research literature', *Nursing Standard*, 28(39): 49–57.

Wildridge, V. and Bell, L. (2002) 'How CLIP became ECLIPSE: a mnemonic to assist in searching for health policy/management information', *Health Information & Libraries Journal*, 19(2): 113–15.

# CLINICAL DECISION MAKING

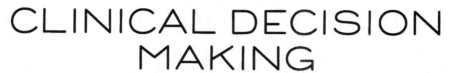

## MARY COOKE

---

### CHAPTER OBJECTIVES

- Determine how the decision-making process can be implemented with compassion, skill and safety, while promoting patient dignity, health and wellbeing;
- Critically review the components of specific theories and discuss the relevance of clinical decision-making theory to practice;
- Identify relevant sources of information and knowledge that can be used to inform the decision-making process;
- Recognise the importance of sharing the decision-making process with service users, carers, families and other professionals;
- Reflect upon and identify key areas for personal development to improve your own decision-making and problem-solving abilities in practice.

---

This chapter will explore the underpinning theories related to clinical judgement and decision-making processes used by nurses in healthcare settings. We will focus on key issues for nurses in managing complexity and critically review the determinants that often have an impact on the clinical decision-making processes. The chapter will include a critical consideration of higher-order intellectual skills associated with clinical (diagnostic) reasoning, empirical (diagnostic) judgements and the outcome for discerning clinical decision making. Furthermore, we will consider the role stress plays in making decisions, and the evidence for the beneficial aspects of stress in this context. The aim of this chapter is to help you nurture your ability to appraise knowledge (use information) critically to form a basis for the decisions you make. The chapter also intends to support the development of clinical judgement and decision-making skills for the effective delivery of nursing care.

# Related NMC proficiencies for registered nurses

The overarching requirement of the Nursing and Midwifery Council (NMC) is that registered nurses must take the lead in providing evidence-based, compassionate and safe nursing interventions, working in partnership with people, families and carers to evaluate whether care is effective and the goals of care have been met in line with patient wishes, preferences and desired outcomes (NMC, 2018a).

---

 ## To achieve entry to the register as an adult nurse you must be able to

- Understand the need to base all decisions regarding care and interventions on people's needs and preferences, recognising and addressing any personal and external factors that may unduly influence your decisions;
- Work in partnership with people to encourage shared decision making, in order to support individuals, their families and carers to manage their own care when appropriate;
- Demonstrate the knowledge, skills and ability to think critically when applying evidence and draw on experience to make evidence-informed decisions in all situations;
- Demonstrate resilience and emotional intelligence and be capable of explaining the rationale that influences your judgements and decisions in routine, complex and challenging situations.

(Adapted from NMC, 2018a)

---

# Background

Daily, we face momentous decisions with important consequences; from the time we wake each day, during the process of getting to our clinical workplace, lecture, library or study rooms, to the time we decide that the day's activities are completed or key issues remain for us to face another time. These decisions include what to wear or eat, whom to contact and what our priority is for the achievement of the day – or to leave for our 'to do' list. Fortunately we have never had better access to information and expertise although this data deluge has become a double-edged sword. Which sources of information are credible? How can we separate the 'signal' from the 'noise'? Whose advice do we trust?

We face decisions with important consequences throughout our lives. We become aware of each difficult and challenging issue and problem, and we are the person who has sole responsibility for solving it. Some individuals have even measured such things. For example, according to Douglas (2011) we have to make up to 10,000 trivial decisions every day and 227 are just about food (Wansink and Sobal, 2007). Wrong decisions about such issues as whether to have tea or coffee or what type of bread we prefer for the sandwich we eat at midday don't often matter too much – we can always decide to have something different the next time. However, decisions about an assignment, our finances or our health options are frequently faced and wrong choices here can affect our degree, make us poorer or lose us our job. If those decisions relate to others (e.g. our family, parents, children, the organisation where we work, colleagues or indeed the patients we are assigned to care for) these can irreversibly affect the direction of their lives too, imminently, for days, months and years. So, what is an important personal decision you will be making in the near future?

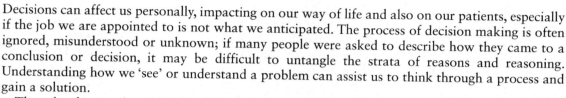

Consider where you would like to work for your first and second jobs when you qualify.

- When do you think is the best time to consider looking for places to apply?
- Are you relying on your peers to decide when?
- Do you think there's going to be much competition for the job you'd like?
- Why do you think you should consider two jobs this early in your career?

Decisions can affect us personally, impacting on our way of life and also on our patients, especially if the job we are appointed to is not what we anticipated. The process of decision making is often ignored, misunderstood or unknown; if many people were asked to describe how they came to a conclusion or decision, it may be difficult to untangle the strata of reasons and reasoning. Understanding how we 'see' or understand a problem can assist us to think through a process and gain a solution.

The role of nurses has shifted to become more task and detail focused as a result of revisions to *The Code* (NMC, 2018b), now embedded in UK nursing culture. Continual evolution of such policy and rules of professional practice indicates the interrelationship of government, patients and healthcare staff as colleagues who tend to manage such transitions in approaches with care, compassion for peers and dignity. This continuous relationship offers an opportunity to consider how decisions made by nurses in managing complexity in clinical situations require them to review critically the key determinants of the process and outcomes or consequences of decisions. There is also a consideration of the effectiveness of policy on roles and clinical outcomes, and how nurses balance the difference with their decision making.

Hertz (2013) describes how our emotions, feelings, moods and memories affect our choices and how these contribute to the way in which we understand our environment – either at work or study – in making key choices at given times. She draws on personalised discussions to develop ways in which the current environment inhibits as well as informs our ability to think smartly and choose solutions wisely.

One of the first activities you may have completed in Chapter 1 was 'Why did you become a nurse?'. Ask yourself this again and reflect upon the decision you made. Think about what led you to make this decision.

- What factors did you consider?
- What were the alternatives?
- Were there any major factors that led to your final decision?

Write down your answers.

Making decisions often involves choosing an option from a range of alternatives. In this case your decision may have been influenced by:

- A conscious choice;
- Rational thinking;
- A discussion with others in your family, or a partner who may be affected by this choice of career;
- Your motivation by assuming you would be able to positively affect other people and their lives.

In one study, first-year students undertaking non-medical health professional programmes identified altruism and professional values as rewards that decreased over time (Miers et al., 2007). Alternatively, nurses who had graduated seven years previously stated that their main source of motivation and satisfaction was focused on 'helping' and the 'people-centredness' aspects of nursing work (Robinson and Bennett, 2007). It seems that most nurses want to nurse because they inherently care about others. Perhaps, then, the recent reports highlighted in previous chapters of poor workplace practices and disastrous outcomes for patients' health – often through mismanaged processes – offer a backdrop as to the key reasons why we should aim to improve our critical understanding of situations and the people in them. These contextual factors influence clinical decision making. Hoffman et al. (2004) indicated that education and experience have a positive effect on nurses in their study because of the ways in which the interrelationships of values, knowledge, clinical setting and stress play a part in predicting outcomes of decisions.

## Clinical decision making

Thompson and Dowding (2002: 1721) define the clinical decision-making process as 'choosing between alternatives'. Standing (2010: 8) goes a little further and suggests that:

> clinical decision making is a complex process involving observation, information processing, critical thinking, evaluating evidence, applying relevant knowledge, problem-solving skills, reflection and clinical judgement to select the best course of action which optimizes a patient's health and minimizes the potential for harm.

Clearly then the clinical decision-making process is complex and will often involve the use of problem-solving skills. However, these two are distinct concepts. Problem solving involves working through the details of a problem in order to generate a solution, although this usually involves making decisions too. Both clinical decision making and problem solving require the use of higher-order cognitive skills such as critical thinking and reasoning, and the ability to analyse and synthesise information. Therefore, the two concepts are often discussed together and both are integral to a nurse's role.

Newly qualified nurses may have little confidence in such skills, and could find the decisions taken by more experienced colleagues confusing, becoming apprehensive about being expected to care for people on their own. For example, two newly qualified military graduates in an emergency department describe their experiences, and consider the emotions they felt, the benefits of previous nursing experience, and the importance of reflection and support from more experienced colleagues (Fullstone and Hall, 2017).

As nurses we are responsible and accountable for the professional decisions we make (NMC, 2018b). The importance of providing good quality, evidence-based nursing care and the growing emphasis on public accountability mean that we have to be able to justify our nursing interventions and approaches, which in turn calls for a good level of understanding of both the supporting evidence and the decision-making processes that inform our actions. Working in partnership with patients, their families/carers and other healthcare professionals demands that we are transparent and able to provide a good rationale to support the choice of patient-centred care we deliver. Thompson et al. (2013) also suggest that effective clinical decision making by nurses has the potential to assist in the efficient allocation of resources, promote health gains and benefits, and prevent patient harm.

## So how do nurses make clinical decisions?

One of the original critical nursing decision makers who pursued a notion of nursing care delivery that was not in keeping with the culture of the time was Florence Nightingale. In 1859 Nightingale realised that nurses needed to work with the universal 'laws of nature', which expressed 'uniform relations of simultaneity and succession, in which one mode of being is observed to exist to another' (Nightingale, 1859: 73). She recognised that illness caused similar patterns of physiological and sometimes psychological distress or discomfort in all people who had similar symptoms, which formed a clinical diagnosis. She acknowledged that a condition or illness had a noticeable process from start to finish, in which nurses could intervene or interrupt and potentially improve their patient's chances of survival or reduce their distress and pain.

Nightingale gathered the information related to the disease/condition process and collated it into a logical and structured framework as seen below:

- *Its beginning*: similarities in the presenting symptoms of a condition;
- *Its constitution* or nature: similarities in the condition or the effect of symptoms on the individual;
- *Its history*: adaptations of the individual in their reaction to the condition (e.g. infection or trauma) or the disease to circumstances of specific intervention and the patient's environment of care;
- *Its tendency or future*: the present is a definite preparation or prediction for a definite future. Nightingale indicated that, because there was data on several incidences of the disease or condition, there was information on the prediction for such outcomes from selected interventions for nursing care. She then considered that 'nursing has to put the patient in the best condition for nature to act upon him' (Nightingale, 1859: 75).

This early version of nursing practice has developed our understanding of how information about patients (e.g. the regular observations and reporting of changes resulting from nursing and medical interventions in a patient's ongoing condition) contributes to the decisions that are discussed with the patient or carer and health team. Henderson (1966: 15) based her thinking about nursing care and decision making on Nightingale's concept of nursing practice to state that:

> the unique function of the nurse is to assist the individual, sick or well, in the performance of those activities contributing to health or its recovery . . . that he would perform unaided if he had the necessary strength, will or knowledge.

To summarise, it seems that Nightingale was suggesting that the role of the nurse is to care for patients until they can care for themselves. In order to do this effectively, however, as we have already outlined in Chapter 3 we need to be able to elicit the nursing needs of patients and plan care strategies that aim to support them in achieving their goals. This will require decisions to be made about the plan of care and negotiated agreements that will enable us to carry out such plans. Ideas about how clinical decisions should be made have emerged and changed over time.

## Contemporary decision-making theories, models and frameworks

In more recent times, Standing (2010: 8) suggested that there are three main theories used to underpin the decision-making process in nursing:

1. *Normative* (systematic–positivistic): rational, logical scientific, evidence-based decisions (risk assessments, etc.), information processing;
2. *Descriptive* (intuitive–humanistic): as proposed by Dreyfus and Dreyfus, Benner, Carper, etc.;
3. *Prescriptive*: the use of frameworks or guidelines that have been designed to assist in the application of principles, which lead to enhanced decision tasks (e.g. nursing process, NICE guidelines, etc.). These can be linked to Nightingale's and Henderson's concepts of nursing above.

These theories, models and frameworks help us to think about how we can critically identify and collect appropriate data, consider priorities from key information and predict outcomes from the use of selected material to form a decision. Many of these date back to the 1970s when research into management in health and social sciences was beginning to become important in the USA due to the rise in administration and costs of the diverse private health systems. Early theorists include Dreyfus (1979), Elstein et al. (1978), Benner (1982), Carnevali et al. (1984) and Phaneuf (2008). Theories based in UK systems also occur from the 1950s, such as Lewin (1951) which has been adapted for use in healthcare decision making. This chapter will focus upon a number of theories, models and frameworks which have been used by nurses and can therefore be applied to a clinical nursing setting.

## Normative theories

Traditionally rationalists take the view that reason is the primary path to knowledge and understanding, using deductive or inductive logic. These principles are based on the following premises.

*Deductive logic* is a means of reasoning from a set of premises (assumptions) to a conclusion that can be logically inferred from these. An example here is, if you see a person has had a surgical operation, then they may have a wound of some type and this must be treated aseptically to prevent infection. You may assume that all patients who have been to the operating theatre will have a wound that needs aseptic dressings. With deduction you can provide absolute proof of your conclusions, given that your premises are correct. The premises themselves, however, remain unproven and unprovable. They must be accepted at face value, by faith or for the purpose of exploration. An example of an idea you could explore related to this concept of assuming facts is 'Do all operations in an operating theatre occur under aseptic conditions?'.

*Inductive logic* is the result of reasoning from specific instances to a general conclusion that is broader than what can logically be inferred from those instances. In the process of induction you begin with some data and then determine what general conclusion(s) can logically be derived from this data. In other words, you determine what theory or theories could explain the data. For example, you may note that the probability of becoming obese is greatly increased if at least one parent is obese, and from that you conclude that obesity may be inherited. That is certainly a reasonable hypothesis given the data. However, you might also consider that induction does not prove that the theory is correct. There are often alternative theories that are also supported by the data.

For example, the behaviour of the obese parent may cause the child to be obese and not genetic factors. What is important in induction is that the theory does offer a logical explanation of the data. To conclude that the parents have no effect on the obesity or size or lifestyle of their children is not supportable, given the data, and would not be a logical conclusion.

Think about your experiences in specialised surgical wards or units:

- Do all patients who attend theatre for an operation have equipment for a venous access *in situ* when they return?
- Do all operations occur under aseptic conditions?
- Do all patients who have been to theatre for an operation have open wounds?
- (Probably your answers to these questions will start with 'Well on some occasions they do' and you can list these, and 'On other occasions they don't' and you can list those also.)
- What does this mean for your deductive skills and therefore your decision making about such patient groups?

(Note: consider whether your analysis of these patient outcomes – based on your assumptions of the interventions the patient has undergone – are inductive or deductive.)

A second more contemporary theory we will consider here is based historically on work by Elstein et al. (1978) and can be described as an 'information-processing model' which incorporates an understanding of how doctors undergo their rational decision making based on information processing and clinical reasoning. Doris Carnevali (a nurse) together with Mary Thomas, adapted this way of critical reasoning to form decisions related to nursing interventions (Carnevali and Thomas, 1993). Their theory follows a clear administrative process so that accurate data (information) is used to make a decision and the decision-reasoning process is then recorded for future use. Specific headings are used which develop an audit trail of processes. The diagnostic reasoning process integrates observation and critical thinking to assign meaning in a nursing assessment. Carnevali applied her theory to clinical practice as nurses took on more administrative roles and needed to understand how the process of decision making occurred. Her model or framework attempts to explain the thinking or intellectual processes that underpin effective clinical judgements and clinical decision making. She describes several stages in the decision-making process:

1. The *collection of pre-encounter data about the client/family* would include information gathered by word of mouth, such as the nurse-to-nurse handover either at the bedside or by telephone before the patient's admission; the person's health records or notes would also form part of the assessment; and from there assumptions, generalisations and considerations become important in the value judgement about certain clients.
2. Assuming the patient is then introduced to the nurse, in a clinical setting, the next level of decision making is considered: *entry to the assessment situation*. The nurse takes an initial overview and determines the level of priority setting among other patients/clients and the current demand on resources. The nurse considers strategies for further data collection if necessary and the patient's own role in their assessment. This means that the nurse will judge whether and if the

patient is mentally or physically fit to participate in the necessary discussion required for such an admission into the system.

3. After the initial encounter with the patient, a *further collection of data* then takes place. This may entail screening or be problem oriented (e.g. determined by a client's presenting situation, and their immediate and secondary presenting needs, for example whether the patient has family present, or whether they require encouragement to mobilise, take note of diet and require dressings or specific treatments). The level of need (to ascertain the resource requirements of the ward or unit because of the admission of this person) becomes nursing's critical judgement. Prioritising is never an exact science. However, when making such decisions a nurse should rely on evidence taken from previous similar clinical situations and personal insights – what many nurses would consider to be 'instinct'.

4. *Pivotal cue clusters* are selected according to what is considered to be the greatest urgency or importance (priority) and the subsequent assessment of other cue clusters.

5. *The retrieval of possible diagnostic explanations* allows a nurse to consider moving from general to specific information that underpins their decision. In addition the considerations of competing or alternative diagnostic explanations are included and a secondary assessment, diagnosis from further test results or observations, for example, will indicate the diagnostic choices.

Carnevali defined this model of decision making as a means of understanding the stages in decisions based on clinical systems, and in doing so identified the need for sound evidence-based information on which to make a decision.

Return to the example of the assumptions made about what patients will need as they return from an operation:

- How will you know which equipment (if any) will be coming back with the patient when they return from an surgical procedure?
- How will you decide which equipment to place by the bed area in preparation for the patient returning from their surgical procedure?
- When your patients needing interventions have been to their therapy sessions (e.g. scan, blood transfusion, tissue sampling, stress management for hypertension):
  - How will you decide to let them have quiet time for self-reflection?
  - How will you decide when to use nursing as a therapeutic intervention for 'normal' conversation, or in assisting the patient to practise their therapeutic work, e.g. breathing exercises?

Four decades ago Elstein analysed how doctors decide the ways in which decisions are made about the interventions patients will have, diagnosis of conditions and plans for care. He based his findings on research with expert physicians who considered their decision making to be based on intuition and derived from years of accumulated knowledge and experience. Other researchers have reviewed and used the model since, for example, Tanner et al. (1987) who found they used a five-stage cognitive strategy – hypothetico-deduction:

1. *Cue recognition*: acts as an alert to the nurse, often in partnership with the patient;
2. *Cue acquisition*: searching for information (initial assessment) – considering sources of information and 'the patient encounter';
3. *Hypothesis generation*:

   ○ identifying possible problems (initial diagnoses) – from cues identified in first stage,
   ○ can be affected by knowledge and experience;

4. *Cue interpretation*: gathering more data to accept or reject identified problems (diagnostic reasoning). Allows initial hypotheses to be revisited. Assessment is viewed as ongoing process;
5. *Hypothesis evaluation*: choosing among alternatives (diagnostic reasoning, nursing diagnosis, treatment decisions). How well do data fit with decision alternatives? In partnership with the patient? (Nowadays we would expect this to be in collaboration with the patient.)

This model can be explained in Figure 7.1.

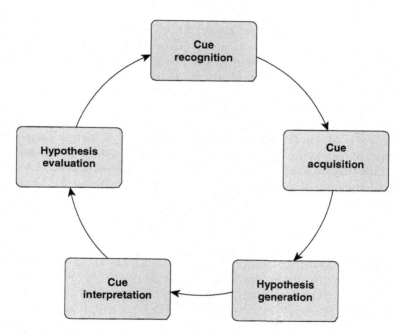

**Figure 7.1** A hypothetico-deductive approach to clinical decision making (Tanner et al., 1987). (Reproduced with permission of Wolters Kluwer)

## NAZIRA

Nazira is a staff nurse in the accident and emergency department. She uses a 'triage' system for collating information about patients and is able to make a decision about the priority of individual needs for specific interventions and care or treatment.

*(Continued)*

(Continued)

By utilising a simplistic triage decision tree based on a patient's initial observations (an ABDCE approach: A – airway, B – breathing, C – circulation and haemorrhage control, D – disability and neurological assessment, and E – exposure and environment), she is able to prioritise patients in need of immediate intervention.

When the receiving nurse (or triage nurse) continues with the assessment, he or she can ascertain the patient's heart rate, blood pressure, temperature, circulating oxygen levels and respiration rate, in addition to the stated reason for the person's visit to the department (e.g. their 'mechanism of injury'). Algorithms (or decision trees) arise from each decision pathway that are designed to provide standardised interventions adaptable for each individual need. Treatment options and decisions can then be made according to the physiological or psychological state of the patient.

Early Warning Scores (EWSs) (see Chapter 13) can be used to assist in the detection of deterioration in a patient's physical condition (McGauhey et al., 2007). Vital signs directly demonstrate a patient's current physiological state. The defining characteristics of the patient presentation data are sought in order to compare the current information against previous assessments of the same health problem, using the same scoring system in patients with similar symptom patterns. Subtle signs of deterioration can be seen in regular and timely recordings. The appropriate care can then be determined so that morbidity is reduced or death is avoided.

Clinical Decision Making Support Systems (computer software designed to assist in decision-making processes) are based on this theory and have been used in many clinical areas (e.g. to aid diagnosis, and improve patient outcomes in disease management, prescribing and calculating risk). Information obtained from individual patients is matched to a computerised knowledge base that allows pre-designed software algorithms to generate recommendations based on specific patient data (Amit et al., 2005). However, frameworks such as these assume that each decision-maker's thought processes are systematic and rational and logical (or normative), and that they will measure the same data in the same way. Yet research has clearly demonstrated the inability of healthcare professionals to correctly interpret or act on recorded data – most commonly underestimating the seriousness of the clinical data they have recorded (Thompson et al., 2004, 2005). If data are collected but not interpreted correctly the decisions that are taken are not rational or logical due to the lack of reasoning. Recent tragic examples of this misinterpretation of cues and data collected by health professionals are reported in the Francis Report (Department of Health or DH, 2013). Here we find the limitations of the inductive theory in practice.

## Descriptive theories

The empirical or (sensory) experiential approach takes the view that experience is the primary path to knowledge and seeks to describe the processes used by nurses when making clinical decisions. The intuitive–humanistic model outlined by Benner (1982) is based on the work of Dreyfus and Dreyfus (1986), and raises awareness of differences in the way decisions are made by nurses who have comparable years of experience in clinical practice and decision making. Benner (1982) identifies that nurses use their experiential learning to gain insight into clinical judgement and, as a result, can improve patient outcomes. Phenomenology, as a method of defining 'knowing what and knowing how', helps to describe these processes of decision making based on clinical learning

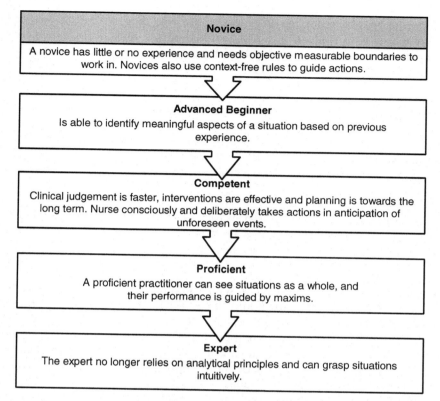

**Novice**

A novice has little or no experience and needs objective measurable boundaries to work in. Novices also use context-free rules to guide actions.

**Advanced Beginner**

Is able to identify meaningful aspects of a situation based on previous experience.

**Competent**

Clinical judgement is faster, interventions are effective and planning is towards the long term. Nurse consciously and deliberately takes actions in anticipation of unforeseen events.

**Proficient**

A proficient practitioner can see situations as a whole, and their performance is guided by maxims.

**Expert**

The expert no longer relies on analytical principles and can grasp situations intuitively.

**Figure 7.2**   From novice to expert (Benner, 1982). (Reproduced with the permission of Wolters Kluwer)

through understanding. The various stages of the evolution from novice to expert decision makers (defined by their use of knowledge) are described by Benner in Figure 7.2.

*Intuition*, identified in the realm of expert nursing, is often described as a 'gut feeling', 'insight' or 'instinct' (Benner, 1982). However, critics of Benner's thinking and research would suggest that this is merely 'custom and practice', arguing that clinical behaviour that takes place without assessing the differences between patient needs, or current research evidence, or analysing the depth of a complex patient condition, equates to a nurse who is not engaged with their role or the patient's needs.

Authors have considered several perspectives on this theory since Benner's original publication. Payne (2015) has described a middle-range theory of intuitive decision making in nursing, created by comparison and difference found through the Benner model of synthesis of skill acquisition, and Damasio's somatic marker hypothesis (Damasio, 1996). The 'somatic state' is proposed to be equivalent to what Benner identified as intuition. For example, when a nurse is faced with a decision, intuition, if developed, is a somatic state that creates a measurable physiological biasing signal (skin conductive response) that helps in making an advantageous decision. Reflecting back to Hoffman et al. (2004), the transitions in evidence to support the ways in which decisions are taken by nurses with differing levels of experience confirm further the importance of education, knowledge, experience and the clinical setting, which involves levels of stress to activate nurse intuition and emotive feeling. The theory that experienced nurses make fewer errors in decision making is supported by them reporting differences in the way they make decisions, and how stress affects them compared with student or newly qualified nurses. Specifically, when compared with new graduate nurses, experienced expert nurses report greater use of intuitive decision making (Traynor et al., 2010; Pretz and Folse, 2011).

Think back to a recent shift you completed in the clinical setting.

Consider your interaction(s) with a specific patient or their carer/relative where you know you made a difference (e.g. there was a positive change in the patient's response and their condition improved).

Write down the events and describe in detail your responses during that interaction. Now have a short break before you read your description again.

- What was it that happened?
- How did you make the decisions that caused the difference in the patient or their care/family member?
- Are the thought processes/decision processes you used illustrated by any of the elements identified in Benner's novice to expert continuum (see Figure 7.2)?

Other theorists have considered the ways in which nursing is accomplished and how decision making aids the care process. Phaneuf (2008) describes the decision-making process using key factors that form the basis for understanding what is needed to make a decision. She considers that essential knowledge in nursing and an ability to apply critical thinking skills are needed to make judgements, which are made by using a critical assessment of situations, people, systems and rules. This information is gained throughout the years of educational development and training as a student and confirmed by qualification. Clinical experience is then valued externally by judgements made about cause and effect, the impact of nursing interventions and the outcomes of decisions made about care. This means that public acknowledgement of nursing ability is considered and reflected in nursing roles as designated by governments. Policy clearly has an impact on the way nurses are perceived as change makers in healthcare. Phaneuf goes further in her demonstration of nurse decision making. She suggests that empirical information is used to make decisions (evidence-based nursing care) and that this stems from data perceived by the senses and not necessarily from the literature, publications or theoretical understanding (Figure 7.3). Experienced nurses are able to pick up non-verbal data and information subconsciously, and use this to assist in making insightful decisions. However, Phaneuf does not consider the length of time a nurse has been in clinical practice and whether this defines their level of ability. She determines a nurse's capacity for intellectual thought as the guiding feature of clinical decision making.

Further levels of clinical decision making are dependent on the nurse's conceptualisation of the problem or solution. The ability to make a decision arises by associating the available empirical data and synthesising the information. Nurses rationally consider the data, the framework of care, and the value of the outcome of the range of decisions to be selected, and then make a decision arising from critically assembling such information and by responsibly applying the various long- and short-term impacts of each part of the decision, analysed in terms of the individual, the unit of care delivery and the organisation.

Returning again to the example above, where you 'made a difference' to the care of your patient, you will have no doubt recognised that in a clinical setting there is often a huge amount of information to process in a short amount of time. Cioffi (1997) suggests that nurses who are

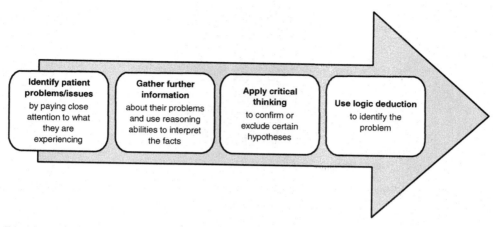

**Identify patient problems/issues** by paying close attention to what they are experiencing

**Gather further information** about their problems and use reasoning abilities to interpret the facts

**Apply critical thinking** to confirm or exclude certain hypotheses

**Use logic deduction** to identify the problem

**Figure 7.3** Clinical judgement: an essential tool in the nursing profession. (Adapted from Phaneuf, 2008)

more experienced can prioritise such complex sets of information, re-analyse them and then consider the synthesis of the decision. The use of certain identified and specific cues to ascertain a decision around all the bio-psychophysiological perspectives of the patient's case has been described as heuristics in an attempt to explain intuition. Often referred to as 'rules of thumb', these are used to describe the actions of experienced people who solve complex problems by undercutting or taking 'short cuts' to define the complexity of a situation, analysing the key facts and then determining the preferred outcomes. The nurse requires some years of consistent experience to be able to recall the usual presentation of patterns with particular conditions and compare the presenting patient's condition against any differences between them and other known cases – including the expected and actual progression points of the patient. However, one limitation of this theory is that it assumes that, even though the nurse encounters different people, they will all have similar sets of problems that require a simplistic set of solutions. It could also be argued that this is not strictly decision making because decisions require an analysis of the facts which may differ with each encounter. Instead, it reduces individualised decisions towards the nurse's past experience and makes assumptions that patient differences can be factored into 'silos' of solutions. Similarities can be synthesised between this factor-based model and Benner's intuitive model. Therefore, by that very fact, you may consider that nurses who have many years' experience could be considered as either safe or perhaps unsafe in their decision making if we were to employ these theoretical analyses. Recent research indicates that patient expectations and priorities are not always the same as those identified by nurses or other professionals. So decisions and their outcomes should be negotiated between all the people involved (Cooke and Thackray, 2012).

Alternatively, Carper's (1978) model (Figure 7.4) illustrates the interconnections between the creative processes and the social/political processes for determining the credibility for each pattern of thinking or decision making about care to be given in clinical practice.

As processes for forming understanding are engaged, knowledge (as the basis for an assessment of a patient and their care) takes the form of an integrated whole. Each set of processes is distinct for individual nurses' and patients' patterns of knowing, but these draw on and contribute to the processes within the whole patterns of knowing. This framework forms one of the first links

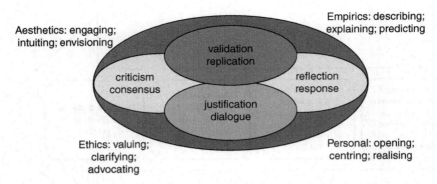

**Figure 7.4** Carper's (1978) interconnected 'patterns of knowing'. (Reproduced with the permission of Wolters Kluwer)

between the nurse and patient relationship for assessing and planning care progressions. As each nurse brings their past experiences to each patient encounter, the processes described in this theory/model/phenomenon are always likely to differ a little or a lot. For example, consider one of your earlier exercises where you were asked to think about patients who had been to the operating theatre. One nurse may consider ethics (using their moral compass to decide which outcome is preferable) to be more important in a specific case or patient care outcome; another may consider empirics as more important (the evidence for deciding how to deliver care or the known predictive outcomes of care based on past research). Ask yourself which element or pattern of knowing is more important when deciding how to assist a patient recovering from an operation such as a clinical termination of a pregnancy?

- Consider a recent time you were in practice and looking after a specific patient. Think about what the patient wanted and how they communicated their desires and needs to you.
- Now consider what your thoughts were about what the patient wanted or needed to happen.

You no doubt considered whether you had been asked to arrange for these needs previously, when you learned how to interpret the patient's needs and understand how best to follow them, and if you had then it would be easier to repeat the process. However, if this were a new experience for you then assumptions or experiential deductions would have to be made. You would be comparing your known experiences with the unknown experiences, reasoning that some things you know about and others are new to you. The patient and their family rely on your duty and commitment to care as well as your compassion, competence and courage to undertake the tasks. They assume that inductively you make opportunities to learn from every encounter by engaging in the ways in which nurses communicate with their responsibilities.

Carper's theory on nurses' 'ways of knowing' helps to unpick these processes and offers the understanding that decisions are complex and often made in complex situations. Carper sets out the sections of knowing, suggesting that decisions and actions depend on nurses' reflection and responses to common actions in order to respond to patients' needs; validity is sought from evidence and the repetition of actions that then form agreed and expected 'professional' decisions which arise from commonly expressed needs. There may have been critical review of the decisions and actions expressed via dialogue and thus justified by agreement, but now there is a consensus of opinion on the action to be taken.

In summary, Benner (1982) considers that decisions are made intuitively. That is the understanding and interpretation of patient needs are honed from experience and knowledge is developed by nurses who are active learners in practice. This aspect of developing decision making over time is not necessarily considered by Carper (1978). However, Carnevali et al. (1984) defend the need to record the process of decisions so that each stage is accurately determined by the repetitive collection of data. All of these theories can be seen to have a conceptual contribution to a discussion about decision making.

Over time, professional nurses develop their own intuitive theory about care and/or the responses they can safely make to specific patient needs as they work consistently in a specialism. Often nurses will avoid cases they have had little experience of, knowing it will take time to develop such knowledge. Such selection inevitably reduces the quality of nursing care delivered and limits a nurse in their understanding of the breadth of care required in a diverse population. There is, as a result, little control over professional judgement unless the audit and re-audit of clinical practices and outcomes can determine measures of patient-related outcomes, clinical guidance protocols and local policies that control the clinical setting. Indeed, there is little research or evidence to underpin these 'ways of knowing' other than an implicit understanding of practice. There is also an assumption that all individuals can develop a reflective ability and are then able to clearly articulate their intuitive judgements.

Later in the chapter we will consider the above theories in relation to the notion of evidence-based practice. Table 7.1 provides a useful overview of different theories relating to how nurses understand or know what decision to make.

However, it appears that nurses tend not to apply any of these theories or models exclusively. Instead, Hamm (1988) suggests clinicians will often use a combination of approaches. Using the cognitive continuum framework outlined in Figure 7.5, he suggests that the mode of cognition used by a nurse is determined by the task in hand, along with the information and time available. Cognition is viewed along a continuum ranging from analytical thinking at one end of the spectrum to intuition at the other end. The framework is further divided into six modes of cognitive practice. Hamm (1988) suggests that most clinicians (including nurses) make decisions around the cognitive modes 5 and 6 (peer-aided or system-aided judgement).

## Evidence-based nursing and clinical judgement

Evidence-based decision making is a prescriptive approach used by nurses to inform clinical decisions and choices. It involves actively combining knowledge gained from a variety of sources (e.g. own clinical expertise, patient preference, research evidence), which is then applied in order to deliver evidence-based care within the context of available resources (Thompson et al., 2004). The ability to carry out this process successfully demands a capacity to locate, retrieve and critically appraise appropriate evidence, then plan care and adapt accordingly to ensure care is individualised and patient centred (i.e. the clinical judgement process).

Drawing on data from two large UK studies, Thompson et al. (2004) outline the types of clinical decisions made by nurses in acute and primary care settings, highlighting the variety and complexity of decisions required by nurses (see Table 7.1).

**Table 7.1** Types of clinical decisions made by nurses in acute and primary care settings

| Decision type | Example of clinical choices/decisions |
|---|---|
| **Intervention/effectiveness** Decisions that involve choosing between interventions | *Choosing* a mattress for a frail elderly patient |
| **Targeting** This is a subcategory of intervention/ effectiveness decisions outlined above. It involves choosing patients who will benefit most from this type of intervention | *Deciding* which patient should get antiembolism stockings |
| **Timing** Involves choosing the best time to deploy the intervention | *Choosing* a time to commence asthma education for newly diagnosed patients |
| **Referral** Involves choosing a service to which the patient may be referred for ongoing or specialist treatment | *Choosing* to refer a patient with a leg ulcer for medical intervention rather than nursing management |
| **Communication** Focuses on choosing ways of delivering information to and from patients, families and other healthcare professionals | *Choosing* how to approach cardiac rehabilitation following acute myocardial infarction for an elderly patient who lives alone with her family nearby |
| **Service organisation, delivery and management** Decisions which are related to service configuration or processes of service delivery | *Choosing* how to organise handover so that communication is most effective |
| **Assessment** Deciding that an assessment is required and/or choosing what mode of assessment to use | *Deciding* to use the Edinburgh Postnatal Depression screening tool rather than a 'Patient Health Questionnaire-9' (PHQ-9) |
| **Diagnosis** Classifying signs and symptoms as a basis for a management or treatment strategy | *Deciding* whether thrush or another cause is the reason for a woman's sore and cracked nipples |
| **Information seeking** Choosing to seek (or not to seek) further information before making a further clinical decision | *Deciding* that a guideline for monitoring patients who have had their ACE inhibitor dosage adjusted may be of use, but *choosing* not to use it before asking the advice of a more senior or experienced colleague |
| **Experiential, understanding or hermeneutic** This relates to the interpretation of cues in the process of care | *Choosing* how to reassure a patient who is worrying about a cardiac arrest after having witnessed another patient arresting |

(Adapted from Thompson et al., 2004). Available at: www.evidencebasednursing.com

Reflect upon all of the clinical decisions nurses have been involved in on one of your recent shifts (decisions either you or your mentor/practice supervisor have made):

- Do they fall into each of the categories outlined above?
- Are there any that do not fall into the above categories? If so, why not?
- Try to identify the cognitive processes involved in each of the decisions that you identified above (you may wish to discuss this with your mentor/practice supervisor too).
- What information, knowledge and skills were needed in order to be able to make a decision effectively?
- Were decision processes influenced by patients and/or their family members or other healthcare professionals? If so, how?

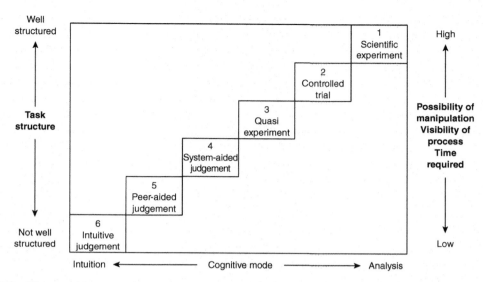

**Figure 7.5**   The cognitive continuum (from Hamm, 1988)

Clinical decisions should be based on accurate judgements, which are determined after consideration of all of the information cues available. Here we can incorporate the oft-quoted thoughts of Theodore Roosevelt, 'in any moment of decision the best thing you can do is the right thing, the next best thing is the wrong thing, and the worst thing you can do is nothing' (taken from 'What is decision making?', *Beginner's Guide*, 21 September 2005, para 2: http://beginnersguide.com/executive-coaching/decision-making/what-is-decision-making.php [last accessed 20 September 2014]).

From these two considerations we can begin to understand that one of the key qualities of decision making, leadership or management is personal awareness. As student nurses you are expected to participate in structured critical reflection during the three years' education towards qualifying. From there onwards the art of reflecting in and on practice should become second nature, especially as you will be required to submit reflective assessments of decisions made in your work for revalidation every three years (for further information on this process see Chapter 16).

Reflective exercises (such as the ones included throughout this book) aim to guide you in identifying and challenging your own assumptions, values and beliefs. This may lead you to alter your rationale or means of making decisions based on your previous assumptions of others, your own strengths and personal development. As you become more successful in analysing your reflections both 'on practice' and 'in practice' (Schon, 1991), your reflections and interpretations of learning throughout life become more apparent and your beliefs in self and others are deepened.

In further applying the essence of the key theories or models of decision making, we move towards the processes of collection, analysis and organisation of information methodologically in order that it can be tested, compared, assimilated and used in structured planning for decisions. The systematic (sequential, historical or hierarchical) collection of data or information is important. But so is the knowledge that the information is of a good quality, based on fact and incorporating all who are involved in making the decision – the 'stakeholders'. Therefore the methodology of facts or data collection is important and defines the quality of the decision eventually made.

Cognitive and practical expertise is the professional understanding that knowledge is generated by an ability to critically appraise good quality research and evaluate the strength of all the evidence available. In the previous chapter, we described the use of Critical Appraisal Skills Programme (CASP) when considering literature and its analysis.

Indeed, a prime objective of the Department of Health is that research and development become integral to healthcare so that clinicians, managers and other staff find it a natural process to rely on research in their day-to-day decision making, and in ensuring that the implementation of longer-term strategies of planning service delivery are based on sound evidence. The rationale behind this policy and its strategic implementation was the critique that strongly held views based on belief rather than sound information have exerted too much influence in healthcare in the past (DH, 1991).

The Centre for Reviews and Dissemination (CRD) and the Cochrane Collaboration are organisations that fund reviews and meta-analyses of published research to determine the overview of several results and qualify (as well as quantify) the validity and reliability of the individual results. The view or consensus is that the RCT is the 'gold standard' of research evidence. A well-conducted experiment is considered theoretically the best way of determining the effectiveness of particular interventions for specific conditions. The CRD also reviews qualitative research and funds overviews of published research papers that answer similar questions (systematic reviews).

Many organisations, including professional bodies and agencies, such as the National Institute for Health and Care Excellence (NICE), the Scottish Intercollegiate Guidelines Network (SIGN) and the Guidelines and Audit Implementation Network (GAIN), issue evidence-based guidelines for practitioners that are usually distillations of research findings focusing on specific treatments and compilations of current best practice as offered by the clinical authors. This 'evidence' of research-based practice is audited in clinical practice to define 'best' or most effective practice by all health professionals.

Outcomes of various national and local audits can be found in the National Audit Office website (www.nao.org.uk). You may recall from Chapter 6 that the frameworks for developing research questions to establish evidence for best practice include the PICO technique (Huang et al., 2006). In addition, an increasingly important method of interpreting the outcomes of clinical interventions, which include nursing interventions reported in research papers, is patient-reported outcomes measures (PROMs), whereby the results of trials use quality measures designed by patients on whom the trial intervention is tested to understand how useful the outcomes are.

### ☐? ACTIVITY 7.1

Find out more about the national organisations responsible for publishing evidence-based clinical guidelines by accessing the following websites below:

- NICE (England and Wales): www.nice.org.uk/guidance;
- SIGN (Scotland): www.sign.ac.uk;
- GAIN (Northern Ireland): www.gain-ni.org;
- PROM (NHS England): www.england.nhs.uk/statistics/statistical-work-areas/proms.

As an adult nurse you need to be able to understand and appraise research, apply relevant theory and research findings to your work, and identify areas for further investigation. Developing a good understanding of the current evidence will also enable you to participate in clinical debates as an equal with other healthcare professionals, knowledgeable patients and carers. The ability to make logical evidence-based arguments and also defend them if challenged not only will help you to justify your clinical decisions, but also should help you to improve your own knowledge and understanding of the evidence base that supports practice, addressing gaps in your personal knowledge and also those of others. Understanding your own beliefs and values through the use of reflection supports the notion that we, as professionals, will work in partnership with others (including patients) and will carefully, with courage, challenge illogical or unethical beliefs or practices.

With reference to the illuminating theory of Carper (1978), nurses are also required to become creative in their practice (i.e. 'think beyond the box'). This enables us to respond to everyday challenges in the clinical environment, enabling and empowering colleagues as well as individual patients as required. The process of discussion and debate about care often raises issues of complexity in decision making. However, astute nurses who develop an understanding of 'the world view', 'whole picture' or consideration of an issue or series of issues objectively inevitably develop decision-making skills that will enable them to make sound clinical decisions using the resources available. Consideration of these factors will help you to identify and promote new ways of working to address the diverse needs of your patient population.

One of the main foci of nursing judgement is an assessment of the unique situation of the patient/client/service user. This involves the perception of qualitative distinctions in a patient, picking up on differences that are reported by the patients themselves. Focusing on the patient has important implications for how decisions about treatment are made (Thompson and Dowding, 2002). In fact, nurses who make decisions or organise care packages and pathways without considering the service user and their family or support systems are ignoring 30% of the resources available in the decision-making process. The service user/patient/carer/family/public forms one of the major groups associated with patient care and delivery of services, with the other two groups being the managers (policy makers) and healthcare professionals. The 6Cs (first outlined in Chapter 1) provide us with a framework that we can use to negotiate positive outcomes with our patients.

Relating the 6Cs to the decision-making process and considering examples from your practice experiences, reflect upon the ways in which you were able to make decisions that made a positive change to a patient and/or their family.

Using short reflective 'bullet points' as outlined below, indicate the process of change that occurred:

- How the person/patient (or you) recognised the problem;
- How the problem had occurred;
- What you or the person/patient wanted as an outcome;
- How you planned to change or use a nursing intervention to alter the situation;
- Consider the resources you used or included to help you make your decision.

Now identify which of the 6Cs you brought into your decision-making process when deciding what you were going to do and how you did it. Make links to these on the bullet points you produced for the above activity.

- What difference did your decisions make to the overall outcome?

In carrying out this activity you may have considered that care can be experienced as a carer or as the person (or other) being cared for. This phenomenon could be considered philosophically and may be used tangibly as a function, a means of management, attentiveness or doing good. Decisions made about care should be based on compassion and the competence of the carer. Compassion is a personal consideration, often based on leniency or pity for the 'other', and determined by the question 'How would I feel if that were me?', whereas competence is a measurable ability to complete a task or participate in a role. Delegation is included in this, because we should understand the competency of the person to whom we delegate in order that the standard of care is the same as if we were to perform the role ourselves (we will revisit this aspect of care provision again in more detail in Chapter 8).

Compassion should drive the considerations of how nurses manage decisions around patient care with and for patients and their carers. Future research and evaluation will indicate the success of nursing compassion and assist in developing new cultural norms of care. Courage is not always assumed in a nurse. Most nurses would not consider themselves courageous or brave – perhaps they may see themselves as performing care under duress, or in favour of the patient against the rules of the organisation – but they would assume they could communicate and are committed. 'Whistleblowing' as a decisive action that takes courage comes to mind as in a patient or colleague advocate role. However, many student nurses' reflective analyses are taken from examples of a lack of communication, or misinterpretations, arising from poor understanding of a situation or thought or action. A commitment to expressing courage is therefore understood, in the context of nursing and caring, to be associated with perseverance, or a personal promise to perform a duty.

It is clear that solving problems using critical analysis of the evidence, as well as ensuring that we involve patients (and other healthcare professions as necessary) in the clinical decision-making process, calls upon the development of various sophisticated higher-order thinking skills needed by nurses to ensure that clinical decisions are evidence based and intellectually as well as factually justifiable, and address the individual needs of patients in their care.

## Involving patients in decision-making processes

It is understood that there are three key groups of people who interact in the health systems of the UK. These are (1) health professionals, (2) managers or policy developers, and (3) patients and carers, or service users. Since around 1980 in the UK, government policy has developed the processes by which service users and carers have become involved in managing health services (as members of trust boards), by reviewing healthcare (through the complaints services), or by participating in reviews of service delivery and planning health services, in research, in oversight panels and in consultations of planned change. Clinical partnerships (patients and health professionals) in decision making about care options have been enacted between patients and their carers, GPs and senior clinical nurses for several decades. Another method of case-based decision making is when medical staff (consultant or GP) and those in physiotherapy, occupational therapy and other therapy services come together with social services and sometimes community service managers, and the patient and their family, to hold a case conference. This is an important phase in the care process and is specific to deciding the outcome or investment of provision for individual patients or whole families who need not only healthcare interventions, but also support from mental health, social care, and perhaps child (school nurses) and adult field specialists where public health (health visitor) nurses may be involved. The involvement of the patient and their family is key during these processes, because their understanding of the problem is important, as well as of the proposed solution. The patient as the focus of care has to agree to participate in the solution so that a wider context of support can be implemented.

# BILL

Bill, an 81-year-old man, lives on his own since separating from Josie, his wife of 60 years. He has increasing symptoms of dementia, and has a diagnosis of cancer of the prostate and acute kidney disease (AKD). He is a farmer – no longer working – and lives in a large, poorly renovated house on the farmland. He self-manages his care until now.

Josie is Bill's estranged wife. She lives in sheltered accommodation and has a long-term diagnosis of chronic obstructed pulmonary disease (COPD); she is alcohol dependent and has intermittent relapses of depression. She self-manages her affairs and care.

Bill and Josie have three children, two males (Ed and Phil) and a female (Janet). Ed is married and lives in the USA. He doesn't visit much, but is in weekly contact with his siblings by phone. Philip lives in Scotland. He is married, works in a highly paid job and has split away from his birth family because they are too demanding. Janet lives alone in England. She does not work, is obese and has diabetes. Janet has two children: Charlotte is 19 years old and studying at university to be a nurse and DannyLee 16 years old, a drug user currently in rehabilitation.

Bill wants to live at home and stay there because he thinks he will lose his house if he is taken to live away in a nursing home, or in hospital. A case conference has been called to decide what care can be provided in Bill's home setting and what nursing interventions are available in the skills of the current district nursing and public health nurse teams (health visitors). A screening exercise needs to be carried out (set against continuing healthcare criteria) funded jointly between Social Services and the National Health Service, both of which prefer the other to take on the cost of this care contract. The panel will assess primary healthcare need in a local area and whether this should be provided at home or in a nursing home. The family decision has to be by competent adult members of the family who can actively support the decision made.

A crisis is looming. Bill has become less able to self-care while living on his own. He has cancer of the prostate which has now metastasised to his brain, and he has become incontinent of urine, needing a catheter. A case conference for capacity assessment is necessary to decide Bill's future:

- Gain Bill's consent to have care outside of hospital;
- Decide Bill's long-term residency (where he will live) and how it will be funded;
- What care services Bill will need, and his future regarding his current treatment.

---

In order to make the decision, all the health and social care service commissioner representatives have to be present, with the family, to make the decision about the future care for Bill. The outcome is important because the NHS and Social Services will jointly fund the care. So a full medical and social support assessment has to be conducted to consider the cost of care and assess how close to end of life Bill is. This is important because there is more funding for care costs in the last three months of life. The panel decision has to be made jointly with the consent of the family members, some of whom do not have capacity (such as his estranged wife Josie) or locality (Ed in the USA has no UK contribution to care costs to assess), and a decision has to be made by scoring whether Bill has the capacity to consent to any decision made with him, or on his behalf.

Here is a list of possible health and social care professional support you could decide to include in supporting Bill to be self-managing at home, which is his wish:

- Catheter care and regular physical assessment;
- Physiotherapist for mobility;
- Speech and language therapist to maintain communication;
- Podiatrist for foot care as Bill is over 80 years;
- Dentistry: Bill still has most of his own teeth and mouth care in patients with cancer is important;
- Macmillan nursing services for end of life care;
- A medical calculation on life expectancy by the consultant;
- Help with washing and dressing (activities of daily living) and feeding, moving, and handling and emptying of commode, etc.;
- Transport to and from GP and hospital clinic appointments, and day care – this is funded up to £120 per day (in 2018);
- Welfare benefits for social care are funded up to supporting ref these funds are only available for three months at end of life.

Take some time out to think about what your decisions would be on the panel, and why you have decided this.

The burgeoning problem for health- and social care in the coming decades in societies all over the world will be the cost of care for people such as Bill and his family, some of whom are already unable to care for him and others who do not want to take responsibility to care for him. This is such a large problem it is often called a 'wicked problem' because it is so complex and affects so many people and organisations that there is no simple solution.

## What can you do to develop your clinical decision-making skills?

Barriers to effective clinical decision-making processes in practice include a heavy workload, a lack of time, a lack of skills and understanding, and a lack of confidence (Mayer, 1992; Thompson et al., 2001; Majid et al., 2011; Fullstone and Hall, 2017). However, Gillespie and Paterson (2009) would argue that a useful framework should be adopted to support the development of decision-making processes by novice nurses who can help overcome at least some of these barriers. They suggest that the Situated Clinical Decision Making Framework can be used to guide reflection on decision-making processes in practice, and help foster the development of knowledge, skill and confidence in decision-making processes (Figure 7.6):

*Knowing the profession*: relates to the ability to acknowledge and incorporate relevant principles, values and standards of nursing, and to use these to inform the decision-making process.

*Knowing the self*: highlights the importance of being able to reflect on your own strengths and limitations, skills, experience, competence and learning needs, and to be willing to seek help and support if needed.

*Knowing the case*: reflects the use of knowledge and understanding of related sciences (e.g. pathophysiology and the typical patterns of health, disease and illness, patient responses and predicted outcomes), and the ability to apply this knowledge to the decision-making process.

*Knowing the patient*: involves focusing on the patient's physiological state and being aware of the patient's baseline data and the patterns within their physiological responses to treatment.

*Knowing the person*: builds on the concept of the therapeutic relationship and involves acknowledging that every patient's experience of health and illness is unique, as is their capacity to inform the clinical decision-making process.

Using the above approach may also help you ensure that you utilise the nursing process as it was always intended: as a tool to plan individualised patient care rather than to apply standardised care plans without the critical, analytical approach needed in order to adopt a more person-centred approach (Benner et al., 1996).

## ACTIVITY 7.2

Consider what you need to do in order to enhance your own decision-making abilities and develop the skills you need to make safe and effective clinical decisions (Table 7.2).

- How will you ensure that you are able to enhance your critical thinking skills?
- What will this involve?
- What additional help and support might you need?
- How and where can you access this?

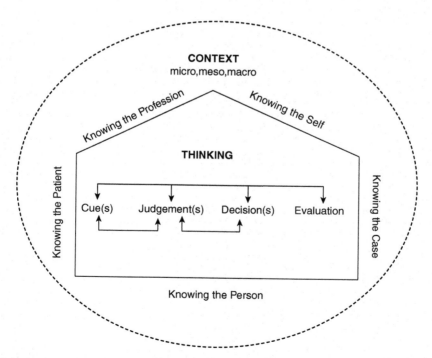

**Figure 7.6**  Schematic representation of the Situated Clinical Decision Making Framework (Gillespie and Paterson, 2009) (reproduced with permission of Wolters Kluwer)

**Table 7.2**  Top tips to ensure safe and effective clinical decision making

| DO | DON'T |
| --- | --- |
| Gather, critically review and collate all relevant information prior to making a decision | Try not to allow decisions to be made to build up and accumulate; make decisions as you go along |
| Use the available information to the best of your ability | Avoid basing decisions on 'the way things are always done here' |
| Take time to consider the pros and cons of the issue being dealt with | Make snap decisions, rush, pre-empt or jump to conclusions |
| Delay or revise a decision as you feel necessary – trust yourself and do not be afraid to do this | Make decisions for the sake of making them; avoid wasting your time making decisions that don't have to be made |
| Think creatively and 'outside the box' | Feel that there is a right or wrong decision; decisions are choices among alternatives |
| Remember that any decision you make will have ramifications and consequences which could impact on a wide range of individuals and situations | Procrastinate or be forced or coerced into making a decision |
| Seek additional help and support from more experienced colleagues if necessary | |

Adapted from Peate, I. (2006) *Becoming a Nurse in the 21st Century.*

## Chapter summary

This chapter has focused on some of the various theories, frameworks and models that seek to explain how nurses act and react when deciding how to manage complexity in clinical settings. We have examined key determinants that will often impact on clinical decision-making processes and have explored ways in which the 'art' of nursing knowledge implementation can be addressed. We have also outlined the higher-order intellectual skills associated with a critical appraisal of knowledge (using information), clinical (diagnostic) reasoning and empirical (diagnostic) judgements, and provided some examples of how you can develop these in order to ensure that you can make effective clinical decisions in practice.

## Useful websites

You can find more information on Critical Appraisal using Systematic Approaches (CASP) at www.casp.uk.net. The Department of Health provides an index of index of authoritative, evidence-based information from trustworthy and accredited sources: www.evidence.nhs.uk.

## Further reading

Standing, M. (2011) *Clinical Judgement and Decision Making for Nursing Students*, 2nd edn. London: Sage.
Thompson, C. and Dowding, D. (2002) *Clinical Decision-Making and Judgement in Nursing*. Edinburgh: Churchill Livingstone.

# References

Amit, X., Garg, A.X., Adhikari, N.K.J., McDonald, H., Rosas-Arellano, M.P., Devereaux, P.J., Beyene, J., Sam, J. and Haynes, R.B. (2005) 'Effects of computerised support systems on practitioner performance and patient outcomes: a systematic review', *Journal of American Medical Association*, 293(10): 1223–38.

Benner, P. (1982) 'From novice to expert', *American Journal of Nursing*, 82: 402–7.

Benner, P., Tanner, C.A. and Chelsa, C.A. (1996) *Expertise in Nursing Practice: Caring, Clinical Judgement and Ethics*. New York: Springer.

Carnevali, D.L. and Thomas, M.D. (1993) *Diagnostic Reasoning and Treatment Decision Making in Nursing*. Philadelphia, PA: Lippincott.

Carnevali, D.L., Mitchell, P.H., Woods, N.F. and Tanner, C.A. (1984) *Diagnostic Reasoning in Nursing*. Philadelphia, PA: Lippincott.

Carper, B.A. (1978) 'Fundamental patterns of knowing in nursing', *Advances in Nursing Science*, 1(1): 13–23.

Cioffi, J. (1997) 'Heuristics, servants to intuition, in clinical decision making', *Journal of Advanced Nursing*, 26: 203–8.

Cooke, M. and Thackray, S. (2012) 'Differences between community professional and patient perceptions of COPD treatment outcomes: a qualitative study', *Journal of Clinical Nursing*, 21(11–12): 1524–33.

Damasio, A.R. (1996) 'The somatic marker hypothesis and the possible functions of the prefrontal cortex', *Philosophical Transactions of the Royal Society of London Series B: Biological Sciences*, 351(1346): 1413–20.

Department of Health (1991) *Research for Health: A Research and Development Strategy for the NHS*. London: HMSO.

Department of Health (2013) *Report of the Mid Staffordshire NHS Foundation Trust Public Inquiry*. London: HMSO. Available at: www.midstaffspublicinquiry.com (last accessed 26 March 2015).

Douglas, K. (2011) 'Decision time: how subtle forces shape your choices', *New Scientist*, 14 November: 38–41. Available at: www.newscientist.com/article/mg21228381.800-decision-time-how-subtle-forces-shape-your-choices.html (last accessed 17 March 2015).

Dreyfus, H.L. (1979) *What Computers Can't Do: The Limits of Artificial Intelligence*, revised edn. New York: Harper & Row.

Dreyfus, H.L. and Dreyfus, S.E. (1986) *Mind over Machine: The Power of Human Intuition and Expertise in the Age of the Computer*. Oxford: Basil Blackwell.

Elstein, A.S., Shulman, L.S. and Sprafka, S.A. (1978) *Medical Problem-solving: An Analysis of Clinical Reasoning*. Cambridge, MA: Harvard University Press.

Fullstone, M. and Hall, O. (2017) 'Military preceptees' journey in the emergency department', *Emergency Nurse*, 25(8): 28–30.

Gillespie, M. and Paterson, B.L. (2009) 'Helping novice nurses make effective clinical decisions: the situated clinical decision-making framework', *Nursing Education Perspectives*, 9(3): 165–70.

Hamm, R.M. (1988) 'Clinical intuition and clinical analysis: expertise and the cognitive continuum'. In J. Dowie and A. Elstein (eds), *Professional Judgement: A Reader in Clinical Decision Making*. Cambridge: Cambridge University Press, pp. 78–105.

Henderson, V. (1966) *The Nature of Nursing*. New York: The Macmillan Company.

Hertz, N. (2013) *Eyes Wide Open: How to Make Decisions in a Confusing World*. London: Harper-Collins.

Hoffman, K., Donoghue, J. and Duffield, C. (2004) 'Decision-making in clinical nursing: investigating contributing factors', *Journal of Advanced Nursing*, 45(1): 53–62.

Huang, X., Lin, J. and Demner-Fushman, D. (2006) 'Evaluation of PICO as a knowledge representation for clinical questions', *AMIA Annual Symposium Proceedings*, 359–3. Available at: www.ncbi.nlm.nih.gov/pmc/articles/PMC1839740 (last accessed 14 August 2018).

Lewin, K. (1951) *Field Theory in Social Science: Selected Theoretical Papers* (D. Cartwright, ed.). New York: Harper.

Majid, S., Foo, S., Luyt, B., Zhang, X., Theng, Y., Chang, Y. and Mokhtar, I.A. (2011) 'Adopting evidence-based practice in clinical decision making: nurses' perceptions, knowledge, and barriers', *Journal of the Medical Library Association*, 99(33): 229–36.

Mayer, R.E. (1992) *Thinking, Problem Solving, Cognition*, 2nd edn. New York: W.H. Freeman & Co.

McGauhey, J., Alderdice, F., Fowler, R., Kapila, A., Mayhew, A. and Moutray, M. (2007) 'Outreach and early warning systems (EWS) for the prevention of intensive care admission and death of critically ill adult patients on general wards', *Cochrane Database of Systematic Reviews*, 3: CD005529. doi:10.1002/14651858. CD005529.pub2.

Miers, M.E., Rickerby, C.E. and Pollard, K.C. (2007) 'Career choices in healthcare: is nursing a special case? A content analysis of survey data', *International Journal of Nursing Studies*, 44(7): 1196–209.

Nightingale, F. (1859) *Notes on Nursing: What It Is and What It Is Not*. London: Harrison, 75. (Reprinted 1970.)

Nursing and Midwifery Council (2018a) *Future Nurse: Standards of Proficiency for Registered Nurses*. London: NMC.

Nursing and Midwifery Council (2018b) *The Code: Professional Standards of Practice Behaviour for Nurses and Midwives*. London: NMC.

Payne, L.K. (2015) 'Toward a theory on intuitive decision making in nursing', *Nursing Science Quarterly*, 28(3): 223–8.

Peate, I. (2006) *Becoming a Nurse in the 21st Century*. Chichester: Wiley.

Phaneuf, M. (2008) *Clinical Judgement: An Essential Tool in the Nursing Profession*. Available at: www.infiressources.ca/fer/Depotdocument_anglais/Clinical_Judgement%E2%80%93An_Essential_Tool_in_the_Nursing_Profession.pdf.

Pretz, J. and Folse, V.N. (2011) 'Nursing experience and preference for intuition in decision making', *Journal of Clinical Nursing*, 20: 2878–89.

Robinson, S. and Bennett, J. (2007) *Career Choices and Constraints: Influences on Direction and Retention in Nursing*. London: King's College, Nursing Research Unit.

Schon, D. (1991) *The Reflective Practitioner: How Professionals Think and Act*. Aldershot: Avebury.

Standing, M. (ed.) (2010) *Clinical Judgement and Decision Making in Nursing and Interprofessional Practice*. Berkshire: Oxford University Press.

Tanner, C., Padrick, K., Westfall, U. and Putzier, D. (1987) 'Diagnostic reasoning: strategies for nurses and nursing students', *Nursing Research*, 36: 358–63.

Thompson, C. and Dowding, D. (2002) *Clinical Decision-making and Judgement in Nursing*. Edinburgh: Churchill Livingstone.

Thompson, C., McCaughan, D., Cullum, N., Sheldon, T., Thompson, D. and Mulhall, A. (2001) *Nurses' Use of Research Information In Clinical Decision Making: A Descriptive and Analytical Study, Final Report*. London: NCC/SDO.

Thompson, C., Cullum, N., McCaughan, D., Sheldon, T. and Raynor, P. (2004) 'Nurses, information use, and clinical decision making: the real world potential for evidence-based decisions in nursing', *EBN Notebook*. Available at: www.ebn.bmj.com (last accessed 23 September 2014).

Thompson, C., McCaughan, D., Cullum, N., Sheldon, T. and Raynor, P. (2005) 'Barriers to evidence-based in primary care nursing: why viewing decision-making as context is helpful', *Journal of Advanced Nursing*, 52(4): 432–44.

Thompson, C., Aitken, L., Doran, D. and Dowding, D. (2013) 'An agenda for clinical decision making and judgement in nursing research and education', *International Journal of Nursing Studies*, 50: 1720–6.

Traynor, M., Boland, M. and Niels, B. (2010) 'Autonomy evidence and intuition: nurses and decision making', *Journal of Advanced Nursing*, 66(7): 1584–91.

Wansink, B. and Sobal, J. (2007) 'Mindless eating: the 200 daily food decisions we overlook', *Environment and Behavior*, 39(1): 106–23.

# LEADERSHIP AND MANAGEMENT
## DIANNE BURNS

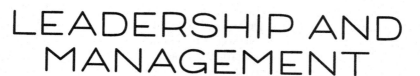
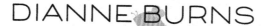

## CHAPTER OBJECTIVES

- Encourage consideration of your own identity as a leader and reflect upon the potential impact of personal resilience and emotional intelligence on your own leadership styles and approaches;
- Critically explore various leadership and management philosophies, styles, skills and approaches, and consider the extent to which these can be adopted in order for you to make a positive impact on multiprofessional care delivery;
- Explain the difference between 'risk aversion' and 'risk management', and apply effective strategies for risk assessment and management in order to provide a safe and healthy environment for patients, staff and visitors.

So far in this book we have focused on the knowledge, understanding and skills required by a registered nurse in order to assess the needs of patients and deliver evidence-based care effectively in a variety of settings. Yet this is not enough; being able to manage the delivery of care, coordinate team activities, delegate care tasks and supervise the work of others is an essential part of every registered nurse's role and there is an increasing expectation that nurses will take on more leadership roles in the future (The King's Fund, 2011).

The aim of this chapter is to introduce you to a selection of leadership and management theories, models, styles and approaches that can be applied within any contemporary healthcare setting. The activities in this chapter are designed to help you reflect upon the importance of leadership and management skills, recognising areas for personal development in order to help you successfully lead healthcare teams in the future.

# Related NMC proficiencies for registered nurses

The overarching requirement of the Nursing and Midwifery Council (NMC) is that all nurses must provide leadership by acting as a role model for best practice in the delivery of nursing care. They are responsible for managing nursing care and are accountable for the appropriate delegation and supervision of care provided by others in the team including lay carers. They play an active and equal role in the interdisciplinary team, collaborating and communicating effectively with a range of colleagues. They assess risks to safety or experience and take appropriate action to manage those, putting the best interests, needs and preferences of people first (NMC, 2018a: 19).

 **To achieve entry to the nursing register you must be able to**

- Demonstrate an understanding of how to make best use of the contributions of others involved in providing care;
- Exhibit leadership potential by demonstrating an ability to guide, support and motivate individuals, and interact confidently with other members of the care team;
- Understand the principles of effective leadership, management, group and organisational dynamics, and culture, and apply these to team working and decision making in order to safely and effectively lead and manage the nursing care of a group of people;
- Demonstrate appropriate prioritisation, delegation and assignment of care responsibilities to others involved in providing care;
- Apply an understanding of the differences between risk aversion and risk management and how to avoid compromising quality of care and health outcomes;
- Understand and apply the principles of health and safety legislation and regulations and maintain safe work and care environments;
- Demonstrate the ability to identify and manage risks and take proactive measures to improve the quality of care and services when needed;
- Demonstrate the ability to accurately undertake risk assessments in a range of care settings using a range of contemporary assessment and improvement tools;
- Understand the interrelationship of safe staffing levels, appropriate skills mix, safety and quality of care, recognising the risks to public protection and quality of care, and escalating concerns appropriately;
- Demonstrate an understanding of how to identify, report and critically reflect on near misses, critical incidents, major incidents and serious adverse events in order to learn from them and influence your future practice;
- Understand the principles and application of processes for performance management, and how these apply to the nursing team;
- Demonstrate the ability to challenge and provide constructive feedback about care delivered by others in the team;
- Support others to identify and agree individual learning needs and provide encouragement in a way that helps them to reflect on and improve their practice;
- Demonstrate effective coordination and navigation skills through conflict, applying appropriate confrontation, negotiation and de-escalation strategies.

(Adapted from NMC, 2018a)

# Background

The main purpose of leadership and management in healthcare settings is to maintain and improve patient care. This can be challenging when healthcare provision is constantly changing and there are a wide variety of competing factors to consider: an ageing and increasingly culturally diverse population; continuous pharmacological, technological and surgical advances, coupled with demands to meet government quality targets while also coping with rapid patient turnover; maintaining patient safety, managing risk and containing rising costs in current financial climates. All of these are very complex challenges. Added to this is evidence of serious deficiencies in care that have undermined public confidence and where leadership deficits have been clearly highlighted (Francis, 2013; Kirkup, 2015, 2018). Consequently, there are increasing calls for stronger leadership that not only positively influences the quality of patient care but also promotes a caring and compassionate culture (Cummings and Bennett, 2012; NHS Improvement, 2016; West and Chowla, 2017; West et al., 2017). It is clear that healthcare organisations need strong successful leaders and managers who have the ability to inspire and motivate others to achieve desired goals (The King's Fund, 2012, 2014; NHS England, 2014; Rose, 2015; Care Quality Commission, 2017).

So what exactly are we talking about when we refer to 'management' and 'leadership' and what part, if any, do 'followers' play?

- What do the terms 'leadership', 'management' and 'followership' mean to you?

Often leadership and management are viewed as being the same thing. However, some would argue that they are in fact distinct entities, albeit with some area of overlap. Most would agree that nurse managers and leaders are equally important and necessary to ensure that desired goals are successfully accomplished – although the focus of each of these roles may be different.

*Management* is mostly about processes. Huber (2010: 5) defines management as 'the co-ordination of resources through planning, organising, co-ordinating, directing and controlling to accomplish specific institutional goals and objectives'. Put simply, managers focus on systems and structure. A manager's role is based on authority and influence. Managers are usually formally appointed to a designated position, although you could argue of course that the role of any qualified nurse involves some aspect of management, particularly when directing the work of support staff or coordinating the delivery of patient care. Good management relies heavily on maintaining effective systems and involves ensuring that employees meet organisational goals and objectives; in essence managers maintain stability (Huber, 2010). More specifically a nurse manager's role 'combines responsibility for the daily delivery of care and the physical environment in which care is delivered with managerial responsibility of those who deliver the care (the nursing team) and a responsibility for those who receive that care' (Royal College of Nursing or RCN, 2009: 4). This role often involves:

- Coordinating patient care activities and supervising clinical care provision;
- Implementing new organisational policies and directives;
- Managing human resources such as recruitment, off-duty rotas, sickness and absence management and disciplinary procedures;
- Meeting government and organisational targets;

- Ensuring quality and maintaining patient safety: setting standards for care, data collection, audit and service improvement;
- Undertaking budgetary and resource management and control.

Furthermore, nurse managers are legally and professionally accountable for the decisions they make. They have a duty of care to ensure the safety of patients, visitors and other staff within their sphere of influence. This involves making sure that there are adequate resources available (including safe staffing levels) to deliver patient care and that these are used effectively according to the approved standards of care (Dimond, 2015). However, this does not detract from the fact that each registered nurse is also personally accountable for the actions and omissions of their own practice (NMC, 2018b).

*Leadership*, on the other hand, is mostly about behaviour. It can be an informal role rather than an officially designated position and, as such, can occur spontaneously in any group. In order to influence others leaders will often rely on their personal character and attitude to develop good interpersonal relationships. Described by Huber (2010: 4) as 'a complex and multi-dimensional process of influencing people to accomplish goals', leaders focus primarily on people. Although leadership may be considered from a number of different perspectives, a widely accepted view is that it is an interactive event based on human relationships and can best be described as the ability to inspire confidence and encourage followers to follow, collaborating effectively in order to enthuse and motivate others to create and innovate (Kouzes and Posner, 2017). Moreover, leadership is necessary at all clinical levels and is not an activity reserved for those in positions of authority.

Leadership and *followership* behaviours are closely related because each of these affects the other. Being a follower is as important as being a leader because without followers a leader would have no one to lead. Followership is also just as complex and multifaceted. Carsten et al. (2010) suggest that a follower's behaviour can be passive (e.g. obediently following direction with reduced responsibility taking), active (e.g. speaking up and making suggestions or verbalising ideas) or proactive (e.g. challenging the status quo for the good of the organisation). Chaleff (2009) suggests that the most effective followers are the ones who have initiative and can think for themselves. Therefore, competent and committed followers are a valuable asset to be nurtured, developed and valued by every aspiring leader. A leader should always have an understanding of the interests, ideas, attitudes and motivation of potential followers, and an ability and desire for their followers to release their potential.

In management, leadership and followership behaviours (Table 8.1), power is also closely linked. According to Bass (1990) power is the underlying force for all social exchange. This falls into two broad categories – personal power or positional power (French and Raven, 1960) – each of which can be utilised in order to influence others. Some managers may rely heavily on positional power whereas most leaders will rely primarily on personal power.

The personal power of followers is thought to be based on being effective communicators, sharing relevant information and sustaining strong relationships with others.

Although managers, leaders and followers all have different power bases, they may use similar strategies (Table 8.1), skills and attributes to achieve their goals. Indeed a leader, manager and follower may be one and the same person playing different roles at different times. Whichever role is adopted in any given circumstance, it is clear that managers, leaders and followers need to work together to improve the quality of patient care and the working environment.

Each of us will have preferred leadership, management or followership behaviour and style, and it would be useful at this stage to perhaps reflect upon the type of leader or manager you want to be.

**Table 8.1**   Leaders, managers and followers

| Leaders | Managers | Followers |
|---|---|---|
| Informal role | Formally designated role | A member of an informal group or formal team |
| Personal power (Expert/ Referent) based on ability to influence | Positional (Legitimate/Reward/ Coercive) power based on assigned position | Information/Connection power based on ability and choice of whether to cooperate and collaborate effectively with leaders/managers |
| Focus on people | Focus on processes, systems and structure (achieving organisational objectives by planning, organising, supervising, negotiating, evaluating and integrating services) | Support managers, leaders and other team members |
| | | Contribute to creating a comfortable and safe working environment |
| Influence, motivate, inspire and energise followers | Direct and control followers, ensuring adherence to policies and procedures | Follow the directions of managers |
| | | Cooperate and collaborate with leaders and managers |
| Focus on the future. Visionary – they identify future goals and show the way forward. Innovate and create | Focus on the here and now. Responsible for maintaining quality and managing resources. Maximise output and productivity | Focus on agreed tasks |
| An achieved position | An assigned position | A chosen position |
| Do the right thing | Do things right | Carry out agreed tasks |
| Do not need to be a good manager to be a good leader | Need to be a good leader to be a good manager | Good followers can be leaders, managers or neither! |

*Source*: Adapted from Barr and Dowding (2012).

Gaining a deeper understanding of your own preferences should help you identify areas for development in order to become a more effective manager, leader and follower in the future.

The activities suggested below should help you identify your own preferences. It is a good idea to try to be honest with yourself rather than focusing on what you think is the right or wrong answer.

## ACTIVITY 8.1

Using one of the leadership assessment instruments (accessible via links on our accompanying website), identify your own preferred leadership and followership approaches.

Now, take the time to reflect upon your preferences. Think back to your own positive and negative experiences of leadership and followership. How do you think your own experience has informed your views?

# What are management theories?

Management theories first arose during the nineteenth century at the time of the Industrial Revolution when the focus was on looking at ways to improve productivity, efficiency, and the relationship between managers and employees (Fayol, 1916). Theorists attempt to describe the role and function of managers and how they engage with employees in order to achieve organisational goals. It is thought that, by developing a greater understanding of how to efficiently manage situations and people, we can achieve better outcomes while simultaneously maintaining or improving levels of productivity. There are many different management theories and it is beyond the realms of this chapter to discuss all of these in any depth. What follows is a very brief summary of management theory development.

*Human relations theory* promotes the idea that people want personal fulfilment, good social relationships and to be an accepted member of a group (Mayo, 1949). The main principle of this theory is the belief that individuals cannot be coerced and forced to do things that they consider unreasonable – willing participants are needed.

*Theory X and theory Y*: McGregor (1960) explored the motivation of workers and their attitude to work, suggesting that by understanding these two aspects managers could develop a better understanding of how their own viewpoints of human behaviour influence their chosen management approach (e.g. theory X people dislike work and need to be directed and controlled because they want security rather than responsibility, and theory Y people like work, are self-motivated and accept or seek responsibility).

*Contingency theory*: some suggest that a manager's or leader's effectiveness is dependent on the match between leader/manager style and the setting or situation (Fiedler, 1967) and describes styles that are task or relationship motivated (Northouse, 2012).

*Situational theory* focuses on the idea that the effectiveness of a leader's/manager's style will be influenced by the situation itself, and that as a basic principle managers/leaders will need to consider the situation alongside the competence and commitment of staff when making a decision. This approach has both directive and supportive dimensions and each of these will need to be applied according to what is required in any given situation. The essence of this approach suggests that leaders need to match their approach to follower readiness (Blanchard et al., 1993).

*Systems theory* supports the idea that to be effective, organisations need to consider a complex network of numerous factors and the interplay of structure, people, technology and the environment (e.g. the provision of excellent patient care is dependent on the effective integration of effort across departments and disciplines). It is argued that changing one part of the system will affect the whole system because each system is a set of interrelated parts designed to achieve common goals (Senge, 1990). It is worth noting that systems theory has been seen by some as a way of understanding management needs within the NHS (Goss, 2015).

*Chaos theory* draws on the emerging science of complexity in an attempt to explain the unpredictable nature of organisations such as the NHS and the limitations associated with trying to organise a complex system into a 'manageable' state using rule-based frameworks (Tuffin, 2016).

# What are leadership theories?

Leadership theories attempt to enhance our understanding of the desired characteristics and specific qualities, skills and approaches that are considered helpful in distinguishing a successful leader from a follower. By developing a greater appreciation of successful leadership approaches we can

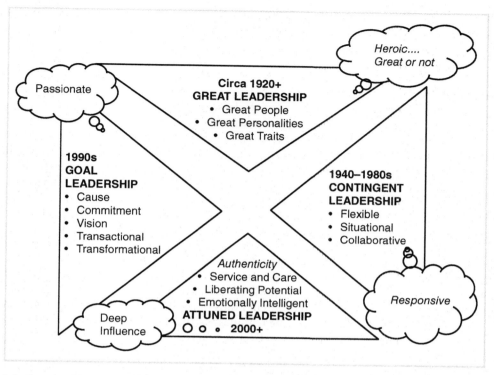

**Figure 8.1**  Leadership perspectives. (Adapted from Northouse, 2012)

use our influence as leaders to improve not only patient care but also the working environment for ourselves and others.

In general, leadership theories will vary according to:

- The emphasis placed on the personal characteristics of a leader;
- The effect of a leader on organisational functioning and culture;
- The emphasis placed on the leader and group behaviour (social interaction processes). (See Figure 8.1.)

'Great man' or trait theories are based on the belief that leaders possess exceptional qualities that influence the way a person leads (Bass, 1990). Over the years numerous research studies have attempted to identify key traits and skills, although there is still no complete agreement on the desired characteristics or skills. In one evidence-based review, West et al. (2015) suggest that desired leadership traits and skills include the following:

- High energy level and stress tolerance;
- Self-confidence;
- An internal locus of control (e.g. a belief that what happens around you is more under your control than the control of external forces);
- Emotional maturity (linked to the concept of emotional intelligence);
- Personal integrity;

- Socialised power motivation (use of power to achieve organisational objectives and to support the growth, development and advancement of those they lead);
- Achievement orientation;
- Low need for affiliation.

However, critics argue that a trait approach fails to take into account the influence of organisational culture and negates the part that social class, gender and race inequalities play in the opportunity for leadership development. Behavioural theories focus on the actions of effective leaders and how they behave (Hersey and Blanchard, 1988; Marquis and Huston, 2006). The current NHS Healthcare Leadership Model (NHS Leadership Academy, 2013) identifies what it believes to be the desired behaviours and attributes of leaders in healthcare – suggesting that both trait and behavioural theories still influence current thinking. For example, these are often reflected as desired attributes within some person specifications and job descriptions.

A recognition of the more complex nature of the phenomenon of leadership resulted in the development of contingency theories that examined leader characteristics and behaviour in the context of situational parameters. Contingency theories focus on the match between a leader's style and situational variables. Situational theories, on the other hand, attempt to explain how leaders adapt their leadership behaviours according to the situation. Fiedler (1967), for example, concluded that no one particular leadership style met the needs of every situation. Hersey and Blanchard (1988) suggest that different situations demand different kinds of leadership and that leaders should adjust their leadership styles in accordance with the readiness of their followers.

Functional theories suggest that leadership effectiveness is dependent on the relationship between the leader and a group (Adair, 2009). They focus on how leadership supports the function of the organisation to carry out work and relates to a leader's source of power and influence over others (e.g. how various roles relate to the organisational functions to meet the needs of the organisation), task needs, needs of the team, needs of the individual and effects on group behaviours.

### ACTIVITY 8.2

Access this short YouTube video clip, which provides a useful succinct overview of ten leadership theories: www.youtube.com/watch?v=XKUPDUDOBVo.

## Leadership and management styles

Leadership and management styles can be described as 'different combinations of tasks and relationship behaviours which are used to influence others to accomplish goals' (Huber, 2010: 6). Healthcare organisations are often very complex and the varied nature of the work involved, along with the diverse nature of the workforce, has led to calls for the adoption of alternative approaches to the traditional top-down (autocratic) methods of leadership and management. Models of 'shared/distributed' or 'collective' leadership are now considered to be much more appropriate

(West et al., 2014). The NHS Leadership Academy (2013) suggests that effective leaders need to be able to work through others – supporting, motivating and encouraging followers to achieve objectives, and empowering them to use their skills effectively, recognising their achievements and thereby creating an engaged workforce. The demand for more openness within organisations is also growing. The 'ethical' leadership framework encourages leaders and managers to take account of key ethical principles when making decisions and to use their authority or influence for the common good. Ciulla (2003), for example, recommends that a leader's focus should always be to do the right thing, in the right way for the right reason. The authentic leadership approach emphasises the importance of building honest relationships with followers by valuing their contributions and behaving ethically and transparently. Servant (Greenleaf, 1977) and spiritual leadership models emphasise the 'caring' principle (Northouse, 2012) in which leaders demonstrate care and compassion and are sensitive to the needs of others. Mindful leadership is considered as an approach by which to improve personal and professional effectiveness and overall organisational productivity (Rowland, 2017), particularly when leading and managing change (we will explore this in a little more detail in Chapter 9). Emotionally intelligent (EI) leadership approaches (Goleman et al., 2013; Stein, 2017) focus primarily on how we are able to manage our own emotions in order to handle relationships with others effectively.

Looking closely at the literature around leadership and management styles it is possible to identify the similarities and how they overlap. A number of commonly observed leadership and management styles are outlined in Table 8.2.

The evidence-based healthcare leadership model (NHS Leadership Academy, 2013) provides an outline of nine 'leadership dimensions', calling on future healthcare leaders to consider these when seeking to identify personal strengths and areas for development:

- Inspiring a shared purpose;
- Leading with care;
- Evaluating information;
- Connecting the service;
- Sharing the vision;
- Engaging the team;
- Holding to account;
- Developing capability;
- Influencing for results.

It is clear that there are various styles of leadership. However, the most effective leaders of today are likely to be those who can recognise that one leadership style is not necessarily better than another. Historical leadership styles do not always meet the needs of today's workforce, therefore leadership has had to evolve to match a growing sense of democracy and independence in the workforce. The current complexity and philosophy of healthcare provision today also emphasise the need for effective leadership at all levels. In order to achieve optimum patient outcomes, enhance nurse satisfaction and maintain healthy work environments, as a leader you will need to be able to recognise various factors that will influence your chosen leadership style – adapting and adopting a range of leadership styles where possible, depending on the demands of the situation. Leaders who perform well tend to be highly visible and thrive on collaboration and network building. Approaches that emphasise the view that leadership is something that is shared by multiple

**Table 8.2** Leadership and management styles

| Leadership Style | Advantages/Strengths | Disadvantages/Weaknesses |
| --- | --- | --- |
| *Laissez-faire* Leaders exert minimal influence and take a 'hands-off' approach (e.g. try to please everyone and therefore takes a non-directive or inactive approach – leaving the followers to decide upon the actions needed themselves). | Groups of fully autonomous and independent care providers working together can feel empowered to make decisions. | Can often result in a lack of direction (chaotic, frustrating, disheartening and unproductive), particularly where there is disharmony or a clash of work ethic values amongst team members. |
| *Autocratic/Authoritarian/Transactional* Top-down approach (controlling, directing, goal/target setting). Use of recognition and reward incentives to influence motivation. Transactional leaders focus more on tasks (e.g. dominate and make all decisions without allowing for the views of others to be considered). | Can be very efficient in certain situations (i.e. emergencies). Focuses upon the ability of leader/manager to monitor and correct subordinates. | Stifles creativity, fosters dependence, submissiveness and loss of individuality. Very little/limited collaboration and delegation. Shared values are not communicated. This can create discontent, hostility and even aggression amongst group members or followers. |
| *Democratic* Leaders work with and guide rather than direct followers. *Transformational* Based on the idea that leaders motivate others to perform by encouraging a shared vision and changing their perception of reality (e.g. shares the decision-making and planning processes as well as responsibility for their implementation). | Increased job satisfaction for followers (followers feel more motivated to get involved, empowered). | Takes more time and effort to execute effectively. |

individuals at all levels within the organisation (McKee et al., 2013) are those that will encourage distributed leadership (Lucas and Buckley, 2009; Hardacre et al., 2011; The King's Fund, 2012).

## Developing your leadership potential

Self-awareness is considered an integral attribute of a good leader (Goleman et al., 2013). Indeed, some argue that leadership training programmes will not produce good quality leaders because leadership qualities cannot be developed merely by learning about different approaches; some are in fact 'a state of being' (Rowland, 2017). Goleman et al. (2013) and Stein (2017) suggest that a more sustainable solution involves developing leaders with 'emotional intelligence'. They argue that the way that we manage ourselves is a central part of being an effective leader, and suggest that it is important to recognise that personal qualities, such as self-awareness, self-confidence, self-control, self-knowledge, personal reflection, resilience and determination, are the foundation of how we behave.

---

### ACTIVITY 8.3

Access the short video clip below:

www.youtube.com/watch?v=nyxnpHknKUU

After you have viewed the clip and reflected on your own current practice, how do your emotions currently influence your leadership practice? Try to think of some examples from your own workplace.

Now, click on the link below and complete the short quiz 'How emotionally intelligent are you?': www.mindtools.com/pages/article/ei-quiz.htm.

---

How did you do? What areas (if any) do you need to work on (i.e. self-awareness, self-regulation, motivation, empathy, social skills)? What could you do to improve your scores in these areas? What could you do differently to embody an 'emotionally intelligent' leadership approach?

Good leaders are also resilient. They can bounce back quicker from setbacks or adversity, and keep the team moving in the right direction. Personal resilience is arguably the most important resource for coping well during challenging times, enabling us to see things more clearly and solve problems more effectively. The American Psychological Association (2018) has discovered that several factors modify the negative effects of adverse life situations. Strong relationships at home and work that provide care and support, create trust, and offer encouragement and reassurance are critical to developing resiliency. Additional factors associated with resilience include the capacity to make realistic plans and carry them out, having self-confidence and a positive self-image, developing communication and problem-solving skills, and the capacity to manage strong feelings and impulses. Table 8.3 below suggests how you can enhance your leadership behaviour.

---

### ACTIVITY 8.4

How resilient are you?

Click on the web address below to access and complete a self-assessment questionnaire focusing on resilience. (You will need to complete registration for the 'Good Day at Work' network but this will then give you access to the free questionnaire and your own detailed confidential i-resilience report: www.robertsoncooper.com/iresilience/#free-for-individuals.)

Resilience skills are practical and can be developed and used to help us adapt our natural style and tendencies.

---

At this stage, you may also want to take some time to stop and think about the kind of difference you want to be able to make as a manager or leader. What additional areas/skills/attributes do you think you need to develop in order to make yourself a better leader/manager/follower in the following scenarios?:

- An emergency situation (e.g. dealing with a patient who has suddenly collapsed);
- Implementing a new way of working.

**Table 8.3**  Enhancing your leadership behaviour (Northouse, 2012)

| Trait/Behaviour | Suggested activity |
| --- | --- |
| Intelligence | Keep well informed, read widely about topical issues |
| Confidence | Develop a clear understanding of what is required. This will help you feel more confident when identifying and using future opportunities to take on leadership roles (e.g. leading a student discussion or speaking out in group work activities, volunteering, serving on committees and interest groups). Getting involved in all of the above activities can help boost your confidence |
| Charisma | You may or may not be a naturally charismatic or outgoing person. Nevertheless, by demonstrating that you are competent and can clearly articulate your goals, that you have strong values and high expectations, that you can encourage and show confidence in the ability of others – inspiring and exciting others with your ideas – will motivate others to follow |
| Determination | Know where you are going and how you intend to get there. Show initiative, be persistent, proactive and persevere; give direction to others if needed |
| Sociability | Make an effort to establish pleasant, social relationships. Try to be friendly and outgoing, courteous, tactful and diplomatic, kind, thoughtful and supportive to others in the group (e.g. make others feel included) |
| Integrity | Be open with others. Always act honestly and be loyal and dependable |

**Table 8.4**  The six pillars of character (Northouse, 2012)

| Ethical principles | Six pillars of character – suggested behaviour |
| --- | --- |
| Veracity and fidelity | Trustworthiness: being open and honest, representing reality as fully and completely as possible. Keep promises. This element also links to professional integrity (e.g. adhering to high moral values and professional standards) and confidentiality (in relation to personal or private matters) |
| Justice | Try to be non-judgemental, treat everyone equally and fairly, respecting and valuing their views and ensuring that you do not use followers as a means of meeting your objectives rather than their own. Encourage informed decision-making processes of the group based on a sound knowledge and understanding of issues. Involves using morally appropriate actions to achieve goals. Give credit to others when deserved |
| Autonomy | Responsibility and freedom of choice (e.g. accept responsibility for the actions you take as a leader) |
| Non-maleficence | Care for others to avoid harm. Caring leadership behaviour links to the notion of servant leadership outlined by Greenleaf (1977) and highlights the requirement to be attentive to the needs of others (e.g. establish goals that all parties can mutually agree to and assist others to develop emotional resilience) |

| Ethical principles | Six pillars of character – suggested behaviour |
| --- | --- |
| Beneficence | Develop good citizenship by making decisions that promote the common good of 'doing the right thing'. Develop collegiality and share goals. Leaders as servants focus on the followers' needs in order to help them become more autonomous and knowledgeable (Barr and Dowding, 2012), mentoring/teaching, team building, empowering others. Demonstrating compassion involves listening deeply to others in order to try to understand things from their perspective (Greenleaf, 1977) |

Similarly the six pillars of character in Table 8.4 outline how you might exhibit an ethical leadership approach in practice (Northouse, 2012).

As previously identified, being a member of an effective team means that you will often be required to shift between leadership and followership positions within the team, depending on your expertise, level of contribution and the overall goal. Engaged followership is also crucial in determining successful outcomes. The *Five Dimensions of Courageous Followership* (Chaleff, 2009) outlined in Table 8.5 also provide a useful framework when considering areas for developing your followership skills.

**Table 8.5** Five dimensions of courageous followership (Chaleff, 2009)

| | |
| --- | --- |
| The courage to assume responsibility | Know what you are expected to do and how you will achieve it. Take personal responsibility for completing (or not) the agreed tasks. Utilise effective communication skills to keep the leader and other team members fully informed |
| The courage to serve | Followers do not serve leaders. Rather, followers and leaders each serve a common purpose by supporting agreed decisions and shared values – creating a relationship of trust and support. Offer encouragement to the leader when necessary and help to communicate the leader's vision to others throughout the organisation. Cooperate and work energetically with others to achieve the agreed common goal<br>Provide timely and accurate feedback to the leader and other members of the group |
| The courage to participate in transformation | Make time and effort to consider what skills and attributes you will need to develop in order to transform the leader–follower relationship |
| The courage to challenge | This does not equate to being argumentative and unreceptive. However good followers should not be afraid to constructively challenge the leader when necessary. Be courageous and voice your opinion when it really matters to challenge current thinking or leadership decisions that you believe are misguided or unethical. Providing accurate feedback on plans will help to ensure that the leader has the necessary information to make critical decisions |
| The courage to take moral action | Be honest and trustworthy. Demonstrate a 'courageous conscience'. You should always seek to carry yourself with integrity and self-respect<br>If you do not morally agree with a leader's approach or agenda then this is the time to stand up for what you believe is the right thing to do. Leaving the group/team or even whistle-blowing is one option that may need to be exercised rarely |

# Leading and managing people

The provision of safe, high-quality, compassionate patient care is an essential priority for any nurse. However, it is not possible to achieve this alone. In Chapter 4, we identified the skills required to be able to work effectively within teams and also explored the facilitators and barriers of effective team work. When leading interprofessional teams, nurses have to be able to offer supportive and empowering leadership to others within their sphere of influence. This involves providing clarity, encouragement, support and feedback, so that others are not only able to practise safely but are also empowered to innovate and introduce new and improved ways of working. Collaborative team working is an important contributor to the quality of healthcare provision. Research evidence suggests that good team leadership is a determinant of high-quality care and positive patient outcomes (West et al., 2003; Wong and Cummings, 2007; Wong et al., 2013). The leaders of healthcare today will also have to acknowledge the need to work together with other professionals and health support workers in order to deliver high-quality care across traditional boundaries as the complexity of care increases (West and Lyubovnikova, 2012).

# Delegating responsibly

Every registered nurse needs to be able to coordinate work activities and delegate care to co-workers and other members of the team (NMC, 2018a). This requires a variety of skills, such as the ability to communicate clearly and directly, and provide instructions, explanations, support, guidance and feedback. However, nurses are sometimes reluctant to delegate to others, either because they lack the confidence to do so or because they fear that the task will not be carried out properly. Indeed, to ensure that the quality of patient care is not compromised you should delegate only those tasks that you know others can manage. The most effective leaders and/or managers are those who can build a culture where all the members feel valued and will flourish irrespective of their role.

> Delegation is the process by which you (the delegator) allocate clinical or nonclinical treatment or care to a competent person (the delegatee). You will remain responsible for the overall management of patient care and are accountable for your decision to delegate. You will not be accountable for the decisions and actions of the delegatee.
>
> (National Leadership and Innovations Agency for Healthcare, 2010: 3)

*The Code* (NMC, 2018b) sets out clear expectations that a registered nurse needs to meet when delegating care to others. It is important to remember that as a registered nurse you will remain legally and professionally accountable for the decision to delegate care and for the overall management of care delivery.

To ensure that you always delegate safely and effectively, you should always take into account the context of the situation, rather than just focusing on the task alone. When delegating care to others you will need to consider (RCN, 2017a; NMC, 2018c):

- The stability of the person being cared for;
- The knowledge, skills, abilities and standards of proficiency (e.g. nursing associate colleagues) of the delegatee and whether they are willing to accept responsibility for undertaking and completing the task;

- The complexity of the task being delegated and whether the delegatee has the authority (via national guidance, organisational policies and protocols) to perform the task;
- The expected outcome of the delegated task;
- The availability of resources to meet those needs.

On occasion the points above might be difficult to ascertain, particularly if you are working in unfamiliar surroundings or with unfamiliar people. Therefore, you should check that this person fully understands what is required and expected of them. You will also need to provide clear information and instruction (verbal, digital or written), and direction and supervision where necessary (NMC, 2018c). Once the task has been completed you will also have to check that it has been carried out satisfactorily (NMC, 2018c) and offer appropriate constructive feedback, identifying areas for improvement if necessary. You will need to ensure that the necessary documentation has been completed by the appropriate person, and countersign this only if you have witnessed the activity or can validate that it took place (RCN, 2017b).

However, delegating work to others can sometimes be difficult, particularly when staffing levels are low, or when the delegated task is considered unpleasant due to a fear of causing conflict (Hasson et al., 2013). Later in the chapter we will be exploring how such conflict can be dealt with appropriately.

## ACTIVITY 8.5

The following video clip produced by the Royal College of Nursing provides an overview of accountability and the responsibilities of all team members (qualified and unqualified) when delegating care to others:

www.youtube.com/watch?v=S-veLUO4ZQQ

Obviously, the potential range of tasks you could delegate to someone else is considerable. However, following professional guidance frameworks (e.g. NMC, 2018b, 2018c; RCN, 2017a, 2017c) can help you to decide whether or not delegation is appropriate. You may also want to reflect upon other factors that might impact on your delegating ability. For example, is your ability hampered by a lack of confidence in either your own abilities or in the abilities of others, a fear of losing your authority or control, wanting to avoid risk or merely a lack of ability to provide clear direction to others?

Improving your own delegating abilities:

- What tasks might you consider delegating to other members of staff in what situations?
- What might influence your ability to delegate effectively?
- What strategies or skills could help you further develop your delegating abilities?

## Creating a learning culture

Delegating care appropriately will help you to make the best use of contributions from other team members and can also be an effective way of developing the skills and abilities of others. As we have already highlighted, contemporary leadership approaches should be less about 'command and control' and more about supporting individuals with their own development, empowering them to identify and address their own learning needs (The King's Fund, 2011). Offering support and guidance in this way will also help to foster team work and collaboration (Huber, 2010). Coaching and mentoring styles of leadership provide a valuable opportunity to assist colleagues to reflect upon their own practice and performance, identifying potential for improvement.

- What are the similarities and differences of mentoring, training and coaching?
- What skills might you use and how would these differ depending on your approach?
- How might you use each of these approaches to help colleagues improve their own practice?

Table 8.6 below outlines the main similarities and differences of mentoring, coaching and training.

## Clinical supervision

Clinical supervision is 'a formal process of professional support and learning which enables individual practitioners to develop knowledge and competence, assume responsibility for their own practice and enhance consumer protection and safety of care in complex situations' (NHS Management Executive, 1993). Participation in clinical supervision as a process is considered to be helpful in setting the tone, values and behaviours of individual practitioners within an organisation (Care Quality Commission, 2013). Indeed, you could argue that the processes involved in professional revalidation (NMC, 2017a) are underpinned by similar principles in the interests of maintaining and improving standards of care in professional practice. There is growing evidence to suggest that the use of clinical supervision is associated with effectiveness of care with enhanced patient health outcomes (Snowden et al., 2017) and improved levels of confidence, team working, skill development and accountability (Cutliffe et al., 2018).

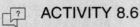

### ACTIVITY 8.6

Find out more about the use of Clinical Supervision in the workplace.

NHS Education for Scotland provide a useful overview of Clinical Supervision and a toolkit for how it can be implemented and utilised in the workplace. You can access this via the following website:

www.flyingstart.scot.nhs.uk/learning-programmes/safe-practice/clinical-supervision/

The Royal College of Nursing (2012) has developed a useful framework to help create a learning culture for older workers (Figure 8.2) although you could argue that this could equally be applied to all members of the team, irrespective of age.

**Table 8.6** Mentoring, training and coaching

| | Mentoring | Training | Coaching |
|---|---|---|---|
| Focus | Focus is on career and personal development | Typically narrow in focus | Focused on identifying and achieving specific goals |
| Source of expertise | Mentor is usually more experienced and qualified than the 'mentee' (often a senior person in the organisation who can pass on knowledge, experience and open doors to otherwise out-of-reach opportunities) | Trainer possesses skills or knowledge that students lack | Coachee: a coach does not need same background or experience – could be a superior, subordinate or peer |
| Relationship | Ongoing 1:1 relationship that can last for a long period of time. The relationship between mentor and mentee is more long term and takes a broader view of the person | Typically temporary, though could involve working with individuals or teams | Tends to be a short-term intervention. A collaborative relationship between both parties – one in which both sides work to reach an agreed destination. Could involve working with individuals or teams |
| Goal | Help at point of need, development of individual guidance and advice | To transfer information and knowledge and to support the attainment of specific skills | To improve an individual's performance. Unlock individual potential enabling coachee(s) to transform the quality of their working or/and personal lives |
| Agenda | Set by the mentee, with the mentor providing support and guidance to prepare them for future roles | Defined by trainer and intended learning outcomes | Typically set by the individual, but in agreement/consultation with the coach |
| Stakeholder | Other stakeholders may be involved | Other stakeholders usually involved | Other stakeholders may be involved |
| Setting | Can be more informal and meetings can take place as and when the mentee needs some advice, guidance or support | Generally well structured | Generally more structured in nature and meetings are scheduled on a regular basis |
| Approach | Based on personal experience | Provide targeted learning experiences | Ask powerful questions to tap into individuals' vision, wisdom and directed action in service of self-identified agenda |

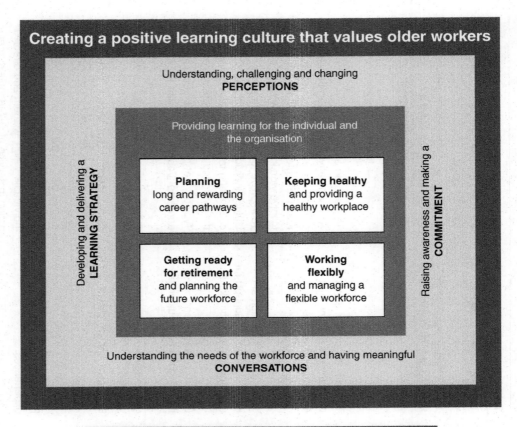

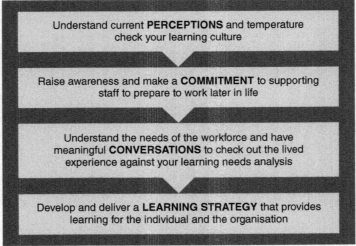

**Figure 8.2**   Valuing older workers (RCN, 2012). (Reproduced with the permission of the Royal College of Nursing)

# Developing a healthy work environment

As previously stated, the NMC (2018a) requires you to be able to work cooperatively with other members of staff, sharing your skills and experience, and respecting their contribution to the efforts of the team. As a manager or leader, part of your role will involve maintaining a healthy work environment. However, this might not be as easy as it sounds. The population of the UK is changing and, along with it, the workforce is becoming more diverse in terms of educational background, roles, professionalisation (e.g. different value systems), ethnicity, gender and age (Hutchinson et al., 2012; Economist Intelligence Unit, 2014).

All of these factors can influence how people act and communicate with each other, for example expectations of behaviour and conformance or differing styles of communication. A nurse leader will need to have an understanding of how these differences can be harnessed in order to build and maintain a healthy workplace (Stanley, 2010).

However, changes in healthcare during the past decade have led many to question whether the organisational culture within many healthcare settings is toxic (i.e. controlling and repressive, where nurses are often afraid to speak out due to a worry about reprisal) rather than facilitative (Cummings and Bennett, 2012; Francis, 2013; Kirkup, 2018). A healthy work environment correlates to job satisfaction which in turn positively influences recruitment and healthier patients (International Council of Nurses, 2007; Cowden et al., 2011; Dawson et al., 2011). Equally, a poor work environment adversely affects health. Employees spiral into burnout, leading to frequent absences and recurrent sickness, and impacting negatively on professional attitudes and behaviours (RCN, 2013). Therefore, the workplace culture has a huge influence on how employees carry out their work and this, in turn, will ultimately affect patient care. There is a growing call for nurse leaders and managers to embrace the core principles of nursing (e.g. caring and compassion), and translate these into the type of nurse management and leadership needed in today's contemporary healthcare settings (Sieloff and Wallace Raph, 2011). Cummings and Bennett (2012: 11) suggest that 'leaders at every level have a responsibility to shape and lead a caring culture'. Indeed, an effective leader needs to be able to deconstruct a work culture if that becomes necessary (Sherwood, 2003). Hewison and Griffiths (2004) agree, arguing that without paying attention to the wider need of transforming a 'sick' organisational culture all of the effort placed in developing future leaders could be wasted.

## AMINA

Amina's first post as a registered nurse was on a 30-bedded rehabilitation ward. She was happy to be joining a well-established team and was looking forward to her new role. The ward appeared well organised and well resourced, providing care for older patients recovering from surgery or falls at home. The ward manager was a forthright individual who held the belief that healthcare providers sometimes 'had to be cruel to be kind' in a bid to ensure that the rehabilitation process (particularly the remobilisation of patients) facilitated patients' return home as quickly as possible. However, Amina soon began to realise that all was not how it first appeared. Long-serving healthcare assistants were

*(Continued)*

(Continued)

often seen to apply the 'mantra' of the ward manager inflexibly and sometimes a little too literally when attempting to encourage patient mobilisation, using behaviour and language that Amina felt lacked compassion and which she perceived to be bullying. Protests from patients were either ignored and often resulted in staff labelling them 'uncooperative' or 'lazy'. Amina raised her concerns with a few of her peers who were more experienced. Some agreed with the approach favoured by the ward manager, others appeared a little more uncomfortable but admitted to having done nothing about it due to a fear of retaliation if they 'stepped out of line'. Amina quickly established that anyone who had challenged this approach was quickly put in their place by key staff (labelled as 'soft' or 'unhelpful') or had simply left. Amina subsequently found it difficult to exert her authority as a registered nurse or establish herself as a 'team leader', even when the ward manager was not on duty.

- Do you consider the culture of the ward above to be toxic or facilitative? Give your reasons.
- What are the key influencing factors?

According to the International Council for Nurses (2007) positive practice environments are characterised by the following:

- Occupational health, safety and wellness policies that address workplace hazards, discrimination, physical and psychological violence, and issues pertaining to personal security;
- Fair, manageable workloads and job demands;
- An organisational climate reflective of effective management and leadership practices, good peer support, worker participation in decision making and shared values;
- Work schedules and workloads that permit a healthy work–life balance;
- Equal opportunity and treatment;
- Opportunities for professional development and career advancement;
- Professional identity, autonomy and control over practice;
- Job security, decent pay and benefits;
- Safe staffing levels;
- Support, supervision and mentorship;
- Open communication and transparency;
- Recognition programmes;
- Access to adequate equipment, supplies and support staff.

### ACTIVITY 8.7

Take a look at the RCN's resource *Healthy Workforce Toolkit for an Agency Workforce* (RCN, 2016) which is available to download from the Royal College of Nursing website. Although this document relates primarily to the use of agency nurses in the workplace, many of the key considerations outlined here could be applicable in any setting.

Is there anything more that you or leaders in your current workplace could do to make sure that the workplace is a healthy one?

# Managing difficult situations

Managing the delivery of health and social care in the UK involves collaborating with a variety of complex organisations and professionals within a diverse workforce. Nowadays, healthcare staff are constantly under pressure to improve services, often when resources are stretched. In certain circumstances this can result in a communication breakdown or poor provision of care, which leads to frustration, particularly when this involves patients and relatives who may be anxious and upset, distressed or angry. Therefore, it is somewhat inevitable that you will encounter difficult situations at some stage in your career.

Conflict is defined as 'a serious disagreement or argument'; 'a state of mind in which a person experiences a clash of opposing feelings or needs'; 'a serious incompatibility between two or more opinions, principles, or interests' (*Oxford English Dictionary*, 2018), and can potentially arise in any situation but particularly where changes have taken place due to restructuring, team working is poor, or there are differing management styles, individual personalities or behaviours. However, although dealing with 'difficult' people or situations can be very uncomfortable and stressful, if ignored or handled inadequately conflict can have a negative impact on individuals, organisations and patient care, resulting in poor job satisfaction, sickness and poor staff retention (Brinkert, 2010). Yet conflict is not always unhealthy. A degree of conflict can sometimes increase understanding and problem solving, leading to higher levels of creativity, and can enhance team motivation if handled appropriately (Almost, 2006). To be able to do this effectively you will need to have an appreciation of all of the contributing factors and an understanding of ways in which conflict can be resolved successfully.

Sources of conflict can be intrapersonal (e.g. a poor work–life balance or role conflict), interpersonal (e.g. a personality clash or differences in beliefs, values, objectives and priorities) or organisational (e.g. competing for resources). Perhaps, not surprisingly, a common source of interpersonal conflict involves other nurse colleagues (Duddle and Boughton, 2007; Leiter et al., 2010), often resulting in incivility, verbal abuse or bullying. Other sources of interpersonal conflict include other healthcare professionals (e.g. nurse–doctor conflict) and patients or their families – usually as a result of poor communication or perceived shortcomings in provision of care (Brinkert, 2010).

## ACTIVITY 8.8

- Identify and list the potential sources of conflict within your current workplace. What are the aggravating or mitigating factors?
- Use the Thomas and Kilman (1977) conflict mode instrument available via the supporting resources website to help identify how you would normally respond to conflict situations. Your score will help to reveal the repertoire of conflict handling skills that you currently use and also help you identify areas for development and to reflect upon how you might improve your skills.

In stressful circumstances each of us will adopt certain strategies or styles in an attempt to manage the situation (Almost et al., 2010). Furthermore, there are recognised gender differences in the way men and women handle conflict. Women commonly use avoidance or accommodating tactics (Duddle and Boughton, 2007) whereas men tend to use power (Almost, 2006).

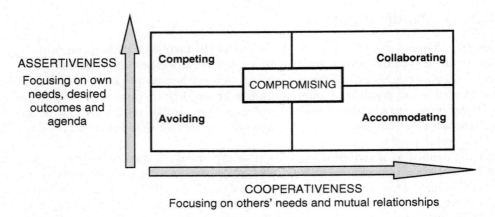

**Figure 8.3**   Thomas–Kilman conflict modes (1977)

Thomas and Kilman (1977) suggest that there are five common approaches to managing conflict (Figure 8.3):

1. Avoiding (e.g. ignoring or withdrawing from the situation);
2. Competing (e.g. dominating as a way of controlling a situation, using whatever power is at your disposal to achieve your goal);
3. Compromising (e.g. respecting and accepting the needs of others, which involves seeking common ground to find a mutually acceptable solution that partially satisfies both parties);
4. Accommodating (e.g. neglecting your own concerns to satisfy the other person, i.e. yielding to another person's point of view);
5. Collaborating (e.g. working with the other person to find some solution that fully satisfies both parties – this involves a full exploration of underlying concerns from all points of view in order to understand the needs of others to find a creative solution).

As with other leadership and management styles no one approach is applicable in every situation. However, Friedman et al. (2000) claim that people who use accommodating, compromising and collaborating styles tend to experience lower levels of conflict and stress. Northouse (2012) also suggests that problem-solving skills (i.e. being able to identify problems and potential solutions and developing effective strategies to deal with conflict) are very useful. At the very least, taking time to actively identify, explore and discuss differences in a non-threatening environment should help to resolve some difficult situations and reduce workplace stress.

In order to be able to do this effectively many would argue that you need to be able to understand your own emotions and those of others, and then apply this knowledge and understanding when choosing strategies to deal with difficult situations as they arise. The five integrated domains of emotional intelligence asserted by Goleman et al. (2013) have already been highlighted earlier in this and previous chapters. However, Huber (2010: 4) interprets these further in relation to the concept of team working as the following:

- Self-awareness (e.g. an ability to read your own emotional state and be aware of your own mood and how this might affect relationships);
- Self-management (e.g. the ability to take corrective action so as not to transfer your own negative moods on to staff relationships);
- Social awareness (e.g. intuitive skill of empathy and expressiveness: being sensitive and aware of the emotions and moods of others);
- Relationship management (e.g. using effective communication with others to disarm conflict and an ability to develop the emotional maturity of other team members).

Make a list of the qualities, skills and abilities that you think may be important when dealing effectively with conflict.

- What measures could be taken to help minimise the sources of conflict in your workplace?

Being open-minded and listening carefully and empathetically to someone else's point of view, concerns and anxieties will help you to demonstrate fairness, respect and emotional maturity. Well-developed communication skills should also assist you to negotiate and collaborate with others in order to attempt to resolve issues and disputes.

## Dealing with unacceptable behaviour

Unacceptable behaviour is defined by the RCN (2017d: 5) as:

> behaviour directed towards a person that in any way attempts to belittle, threaten, intimidate, including verbal, written and physical abuse, and harassment.

Perhaps surprisingly, workplace bullying and discrimination does exist in health and social care settings and can be a major contributing factor to unhealthy and toxic environments (Johnson, 2009; Care Quality Commission, 2014). Bullying has been identified as a factor that not only affects patient outcomes but also increases occupational stress, decreases job satisfaction and adversely affects staff retention (Carter et al., 2013). Bullying can manifest itself physically (e.g. hitting or pushing), verbally (e.g. name calling or arguing) or psychologically (e.g. being ignored, excluded or undermined). Discrimination occurs when an employer, supervisor or co-worker treats another employee unfairly based on religion, age, ethnicity, gender, sexual orientation, disability, skin colour, nationality or race. Bullying can be very unpleasant and in serious cases may be dealt with legally (e.g. Health and Safety at Work Act 1974 [www.legislation.gov.uk/ukpga/1974/37] and Protection from Harassment Act 1977 [www.legislation.gov.uk/ukpga/1997/40/contents]). Discrimination is also unlawful (Equality Act 2010 [www.legislation.gov.uk/ukpga/2010/15/contents]). It is also worth noting that bullying and discrimination can occur within or outside the normal working environment (e.g. staff social gatherings and away days).

Dealing with discriminatory or negative behaviour – whether you are personally on the receiving end or not – can obviously be very challenging. However, Bennett and Sawatzky (2013) argue that individuals with greater emotional intelligence (EI) are more able not only to recognise early signs of negative behaviour but also to deal with it more effectively. The aim is to achieve a workplace culture in which everyone treats each other with dignity and respect and where action is taken to help minimise sources of conflict, bullying or discrimination, including:

- Setting out and clearly verbalising behavioural expectations to other members of staff: linking these expectations of local policies (e.g. bullying and maintaining dignity in the workplace);
- Identifying the risks and warning signs (e.g. levels of staff sickness, staff absence or staff turn-over);
- Improving reporting mechanisms by facilitating a supportive, non-blame and responsive culture to encourage 'victims' to come forward;
- Treating complaints seriously, enforcing expectations where necessary by reiterating these in line with identified policies and clearly outlining these to all parties.

The challenge for any leader or manager will be to deal with conflict in a way that does not add to the stress of the situation within the workplace. It is worth remembering that there are other sources of help that individuals can turn to if necessary (e.g. your mentor/practice supervisor, line manager, university staff or the Royal College of Nursing or other trade union representative).

---

### ACTIVITY 8.9

The RCN provide a useful guide on bullying and harassment. Access a copy of the guide from the following website: www.rcn.org.uk/professional-development/publications/pub-004968.

    After reading this, take a moment to consider the actions you would take if you were to experience or witness unacceptable behaviour in the workplace.

---

## Managing risk and patient safety

Earlier in this chapter we explored the notion that the work environment is influenced not least by the quality of leadership provided within the placement and organisation. Equally, effective leadership plays a pivotal role in maintaining patient safety by creating and maintaining safe working environments and practices (Squires et al., 2010). Critical incidents commonly occur as a result of poor organisational systems or conditions, for example a failure to follow good practice, poor communication, poor record keeping or as the result of equipment failure (Berwick, 2013). As a qualified nurse, ensuring that you have sufficient knowledge and critical understanding of the input and resources needed to manage risk effectively will be crucial to help maintain patient, public and staff safety. Risk can be predictable or unpredictable, environmental (e.g. linked to levels of cleanliness, light, temperature and/or adequacy of space) or human related (e.g. working practices or impaired functioning). Unsafe staffing levels or inappropriate skill mix within teams can also put patients and staff at risk, impacting on the quality of care provision (Francis, 2013; Andrews and Butler, 2014; National Quality Board, 2016).

At this stage, it is important to recognise the difference between 'risk aversion' and 'risk management'. Risk aversion in healthcare relates to an unwillingness to take risks or wanting to avoid risks as much as possible, derived from a belief that risks should be eliminated entirely. Risk-averse behaviour can be driven by a fear of litigation or a reluctance to depart from policy. As you can imagine, risk aversion can often stifle innovation and creativity. The term 'risk management', on the other hand, focuses on understanding and analysing risks, and then taking the appropriate action to avoid or minimise their impact.

Risk assessments comprise a careful examination of what, in your work, could cause harm to people, so that you can decide whether you have taken enough precautions or should do more to prevent harm.

---

### 🗨 ACTIVITY 8.10

Reflecting upon your experience so far:

- Closely examine your current workplace or placement area. Make a list of the common risks and adverse incidents that can occur within this setting.
- Consider the role that you, your colleagues and patients/service users have in creating and maintaining safe working environments.

---

Common incidents in healthcare settings (Health and Safety Executive or HSE, 2017) are outlined below:

- Slips, trips and falls;
- Lifting and handling injuries;
- Physical assault/workplace violence;
- Exposure to materials or substances at work (e.g. soaps, disinfecting agents or latex);
- Spillages and/or chemical injuries;
- Needle-stick injuries;
- Equipment failure;
- Procedural failure (e.g. resulting in the development of pressure ulcers, incorrect surgery, and drug errors or hospital-acquired infections).

It is important to remember also, the potential for psychosocial risks for staff that are associated with poor health, for example work-related stress, lack of influence, discrimination, time and work pressures, working long and irregular hours (HSE, 2017) and the potential impact on patient care as a result of unsafe staffing levels (RCN, 2017b).

The term 'risk management' refers to the process of identifying, assessing/evaluating and reporting risks in order to maintain the safety of patients, relatives and staff, as well as improve the quality of patient care. Risk management is about practising safely and ensuring that the occurrence of harmful or adverse events is reduced by anticipating and preventing potential problems,

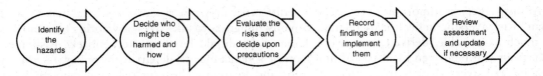

**Figure 8.4**  The HSE's (2014) five-step process to risk assessment

learning from incidents, near misses, patient complaints and litigation, and by introducing systems to help clinical staff reflect on and develop their practice. Figure 8.4 demonstrates the process of risk assessment using the five-step process of the HSE (2014).

To practise safely and manage risk effectively, nurses need to ensure that risk assessment and management strategies are both utilised and applied, not just to the clinical areas they are working in but also to current work practices.

Critical incident reporting is a system that was introduced with the aim of improving patient safety. By thorough investigation of an 'incident', the intention is for practitioners to learn from the event and put additional measures or solutions in place to ensure that the situation is improved. However, fear of reprisals and sometimes a lack of understanding of how these should be reported can sometimes deter individuals from reporting incidents. Nevertheless, all nurses have a statutory duty to report concerns when they believe there is a potential danger to patients. You have a legal responsibility to ensure that no one is harmed as a result of an act or omission on your part. Indeed, it is important to remember that you can still be pursued for compensation as an individual, even if what you are doing is part of your contractual duties and can be prosecuted for criminal damage or negligence. *The Code* demands that you make the care and safety of your patients your main concern (NMC, 2018b: 6) and that you 'share information to identify and reduce risk' (NMC, 2018b: 10) and 'act immediately to put right the situation if someone has suffered actual harm for any reason' (NMC, 2018b: 13). This will involve documenting any concerns carefully as soon as possible, making sure that records are clearly signed, dated and timed, and asking for additional help where necessary (e.g. from more senior staff and/or risk managers). Therefore familiarising yourself with local/national risk management policies and the role/functions of numerous patient safety agencies (outlined in Table 8.7), as well as required reporting systems, is essential to ensure that appropriate action is taken.

## Critical incident analysis

When incidents occur, it is important to ensure that lessons are learned to prevent the same incident occurring again or elsewhere. A root cause analysis framework can be helpful when trying to identify exactly what has happened and, more importantly, why. Getting to the root of the problem and understanding why something has happened will help to ensure that the real cause of the incident will be uncovered rather than just the details of the incident itself. You should then be able to focus on identifying and implementing solutions to improve the situation and ensure that the risk of it happening again is minimal. The NHS Institute for Innovation and Improvement (https://improvement.nhs.uk/resources) provides an array of tools and templates that can be used to assist this process. The 'five whys' approach used in the example below is one of the simplest approaches because it is considered one of the easiest to learn and apply.

**Table 8.7**   Examples of risk management agencies across the UK

| NHS Commissioning Board Special Health Authority | Lead and contribute to improved, safe patient care by *informing*, *supporting* and *influencing* organisations and people working in the health sector. Aim to identify and reduce risks to patients receiving NHS care and lead on national initiatives to improve patient safety |
| --- | --- |
| NHS Improvement | Oversee Foundation Trusts and NHS Trusts, as well as independent providers that provide NHS-funded care. NHS Improvement is the operational name for an organisation that, in 2016, brought together the following organisations:<br>Monitor<br>NHS Trust Development Authority<br>Patient safety (including the National Reporting and Learning System) |
| NHS Resolution (**formerly** the NHS Litigation Authority) | NHS Resolution combines the three operating arms of NHSLA, the National Clinical Assessment Service and the Family Health Services Appeal Unit to assist the NHS to resolve litigation concerns fairly, as well as share lessons learnt to improve clinical practice and preserve resources for patient care |
| Care Quality Commission (CQC) | Statutory independent regulator of health and social care in England responsible for registering and monitoring services and regulating care provided by healthcare providers |
| Medicines and Healthcare products Regulatory Agency (MHRA) | Regulates a wide range of materials from medicines and medical devices to blood and therapeutic products/services that are derived from tissue engineering |
| Health and Safety Executive | Enforces health and safety law in industrial workplaces |
| Regulation and Quality Improvement Authority (RQIA) | An independent body responsible for monitoring and inspecting the availability and quality of health and social care services in Northern Ireland, and encouraging improvements in the quality of those services |

 Root cause analysis using the five 'whys' approach

Step 1: Write down the details of the specific problem. This helps you formalise the problem and describe it accurately. It will also help the team focus on the same problem.

Step 2: Brainstorm to ask why the problem occurs and then write the answer down.

Step 3: If this answer doesn't identify the source of the problem, ask 'why?' again and write that answer down.

Step 4: Loop back to Step 3 until the team agrees that they have identified the problem's root cause. Again, this may take fewer or more than five 'whys?'.

## SABRINA

Practice nurse Sabrina is covering for a colleague who is ill. A busy nurse-led travel vaccination clinic is taking place, and several waiting patients have already complained due to the delays in their appointments as a result of staff shortages. As Sabrina is a little unfamiliar with the clinic processes – and in order to try to save time – a receptionist has offered to assist with the necessary paperwork (e.g. completing forms and checklists before sending the patients through to the treatment room). Sabrina rapidly calls the first patient into the treatment room and quickly checks the paperwork before administering the required injections. However, immediately after doing so she quickly realises that she has given the patient the wrong set of injections. The paperwork she looked at belonged to a different patient and had been mixed up in the process.

Using the 'five whys' approach outlined above consider the following:

- What is the probable cause of the accident/incident?
- What are the underlying causes – if any?
- What immediate action should be taken?
- How could the incident have been prevented?
- Are there any other issues that need to be considered or addressed?

It is clear that several factors contributed to the incident above, for example staff shortages, escalating waiting times leading to patient complaints, unfamiliar processes, poor delegation and/or a lack of acknowledgement on Sabrina's part of her limitations. Obviously the most immediate action would be ensure that the patient had not come to any harm as a result of the mistake. It is also clear that measures could have been taken to prevent this (e.g. informing patients of staff shortages, rearranging appointments, ensuring the availability of appropriately experienced staff or even cancelling the clinic if necessary). Staff education, training and support are also issues that should be considered.

- What opportunities are provided in your placement area to offer staff the chance to critically reflect on such incidents?

# Managing team performance

Earlier in this chapter, we explored some of the leadership approaches that aim to enhance team performance. In your role as a leader you will be responsible for supporting junior staff to fulfil their own professional obligations. According to the Advisory, Conciliation and Arbitration Service (ACAS, 2014), performance management is a continuous process by which managers and employees work together to plan, monitor and review work objectives, with the aim of improving their overall contribution to the organisation, including:

- Agreeing SMART (specific, measurable, achievable, relevant and time-bound) objectives, competencies and development needs;
- Reviewing individual performance against agreed objectives;

- Giving appropriate feedback;
- Agreeing a personal development plan;
- Helping staff to achieve objectives through coaching and providing access to training or other development opportunities.

---

### ACTIVITY 8.11

Access the ACAS website (www.acas.org.uk) and download the booklet *How to Manage Performance*. Consider how this guidance currently relates to performance management activities in your own workplace.

How could you use this guidance in the future to assist you in facilitating the development of others within your team?

---

Occasionally you will need to address concerns about the underperformance or behaviour of members of your team. However, fear and mistrust could lead to staff keeping quiet and not reporting their concerns. Therefore, as a nurse leader one of your key aims should be to build an effective organisational culture in which there is trust and accountability among members of your team, fostering a culture of openness and transparency in order to build an atmosphere in which all staff are encouraged to identify and report unsafe conditions within a 'non-blame' culture (Francis, 2015).

All organisations should have internal mechanisms for investigating and dealing effectively with patient complaints or concerns (e.g. robust policies and procedures). Healthcare professionals also have a duty to report any concerns they may have about the quality of care in their organisation or indeed any other organisation with which they have contact (NMC, 2017b). Raising and escalating concerns or 'whistleblowing' defines the act of bringing an important issue to the attention of someone in authority (RCN, 2017c). Normally, in the first instance, this would involve informing senior staff or clinical leaders. If unresolved, additional external mechanisms, e.g. reporting concerns to the Care Quality Commission, may also be implemented although if this is necessary it is advisable to follow your organisation's published whistleblowing procedures (National Quality Board, 2013). In all instances where practice or procedures are brought into question, clear, comprehensive and unambiguous records will be crucial in determining what has happened. Good record keeping, as well as being a duty of professional practice, will also protect staff.

---

The RCN's *Principles of Nursing Practice* (RCN, 2010) and the NMC's Code (NMC, 2018b) set out what patients, colleagues, families and carers can expect from nurses:

- What factors could contribute to situations where nurses might fail to meet such expectations?
- Are you confident about the quality of care that you and your colleagues deliver?
- If so, what evidence do you have that this is the case?
- If not, what can you do about it?

Berwick (2013: 10) provides a useful summary of the leadership behaviours that are thought to reduce risk and make healthcare provision safer:

- Abandoning blame as a tool;
- Constantly and consistently asserting the primacy of safely meeting patients' and carers' needs;
- Expecting and insisting on transparency, welcoming warnings of problems;
- Recognising that the most valuable information is about risks and things that have gone wrong;
- Hearing the patient voice, at every level;
- Seeking out and listening to colleagues and staff;
- Expecting and achieving cooperation, without exception;
- Giving help to learn, master and apply modern improvement methods;
- Using data accurately, even where uncomfortable, to support healthcare and continual improvement;
- Leading by example, through commitment, encouragement, compassion and a learning approach;
- Maintaining a clear, mature and open dialogue about risk;
- Infusing pride and joy in work;
- Helping develop the leadership potential in others by providing support and work experiences to enable them to improve their own leadership capability;
- Recognising that some problems require technical action but that others are complex and may require many innovative solutions involving all who have a stake in the problem.

## Chapter summary

There is evidence to suggest that effective leadership is positively associated with improved patient outcomes (Wong et al., 2013). Therefore, the need for strong and effective nurse leadership throughout the whole organisation has never been greater. However, leadership and management activities are complex and multifaceted, with many differing theories advocating essential skills, desirable attributes and approaches. It appears that the most effective leaders and managers are those who recognise the importance and impact of emotional intelligence and resilience in developing valuable relationships with others, and who are able to apply well-developed team leadership skills to ensure the delivery of safe and effective practice by every member of the team.

## Useful websites

Healthcare Improvement Scotland: www.healthcareimprovementscotland.org.
Improving Quality Together NHS Wales: www.iqt.wales.nhs.uk/home.
The Regulation and Quality Improvement Authority (Northern Ireland): www.rqia.org.uk.
NHS Improvement: https://improvement.nhs.uk.
ACAS: www.acas.org.uk.
Care Quality Commission: www.cqc.org.uk.

## Further reading

1000 Lives Improvement (2014) *The Quality Improvement Guide: The Improving Quality Together Edition.* Cardiff: 1000 Lives Improvement.
Department of Health, Social Services and Public Safety (2011) *Quality 2020: A Ten-year Strategy to Protect and Improve Quality in Health and Social Care in Northern Ireland.* Belfast: DHSSPS.

National Institute for Health and Care Excellence (2017) *Healthy Workplaces: Improving Employee Mental Health and Wellbeing*. London: NICE. Available at: www.nice.org.uk/guidance/qs147 (last accessed 7 April 2018).

NHS Leadership Academy (2018) Leadership Academy Programmes. Available at: www.leadership academy.nhs.uk/programmes last accessed 22 March 2018).

NHS Quality Improvement Scotland (NHS QIS) (2005) *Standards for Clinical Governance and Risk Management*. Available at: www.healthcareimprovementscotland.org/previous_resources/standards/cgrm_ standards.aspx (last accessed 8 April 2018).

NHS Wales Governance e-manual. Available at: www.wales.nhs.uk/governance-emanual/risk-management.

Whitmore, J. (2017) *Coaching for Performance. The Principles and Practice of Coaching and Leadership*, 5th edn. Boston, MA: Brearley Publishing.

# References

ACAS (2014) *How to Manage Performance*. Available at: www.acas.org.uk/media/pdf/s/n/How-to-manage-performance-advisory-booklet.pdf (last accessed 9 April 2018).

Adair, J. (2009) *Effective Leadership: How to be a Successful Leader*. London: Pan Macmillan.

Almost, J. (2006) 'Conflict within nursing work environments: concept analysis', *Journal of Advanced Nursing*, 53(4): 444–53.

Almost, J., Doran, D.M., McGillis Hall, L.M. and Spence Laschinger, H.K. (2010) 'Antecedents and consequences of intra-group conflict among nurses', *Journal of Nursing Management*, 18: 981–92.

American Psychological Association (2018) *The Road to Resilience*. Available at: www.apa.org/helpcenter/road-resilience.aspx (last accessed 31 January 2018).

Andrews, A. and Butler, M. (2014) *Trusted to Care. An Independent Review of the Princess of Wales Hospital and Neath Port Talbot Hospital at Abertawe Bro Morgannwg University Health Boards (Executive Summary)*. Available at: http://gov.wales/topics/health/publications/health/reports/care (last accessed 8 April 2018).

Barr, J. and Dowding, L. (2012) *Leadership in Healthcare*, 2nd edn. London: Sage.

Bass, B.M. (1990) *Bass and Stodgill's Handbook of Leadership: Theory, Research and Managerial Application*, 3rd edn. New York: Free Press.

Bennett, K. and Sawatzky, J.V. (2013) 'Building emotional intelligence: a strategy for emerging nurse leaders to reduce workplace bullying', *Nursing Administration Quarterly*, 37(2): 144–51.

Berwick, D. (2013) *A Promise to Learn: A Commitment to Act. Improving the Safety of Patients in England*. London: HMSO.

Blanchard, K., Zigarmi, D. and Nelson, R. (1993) 'Situational leadership after 25 years: a retrospective', *Journal of Leadership Studies*, 1(1): 22–36.

Brinkert, R. (2010) 'A literature review of conflict communication causes, costs, benefits and interventions in nursing', *Journal of Nursing Management*, 18: 145–56.

Care Quality Commission (2013) *Supporting Information and Guidance: Supporting Effective Clinical Supervision*. London: CQC.

Care Quality Commission (2014) *Bart's NHS Trust Quality Report*. London: CQC.

Care Quality Commission (2017) *The State of Healthcare and Adult Social Care in England*. London: CQC.

Carsten, M.K., Uhl-Bien, M., West, B.J., Patera, J.L. and McGregor, R. (2010) 'Exploring social constructions of followership: a qualitative study', *The Leadership Quarterly*, 21: 543–62.

Carter, M., Thompson, N., Crampton, P., Morrow, G., Burford, B., Gray, C. and Illing, J. (2013) 'Workplace bullying in the UK NHS: a questionnaire and interview study on prevalence, impact and barriers to reporting', *BMJ Open*, 3(6): 1–12.

Chaleff, I. (2009) *The Courageous Follower: Standing up to and for Our Leaders*. San Francisco, CA: Berrett-Koehler.

Ciulla, J.B. (2003) *The Ethics of Leadership*. Belmont, CA: Wadsworth/Thompson Learning.

Cowden, T., Cummings, G. and Profetto-McGrath, J. (2011) 'Leadership practices and staff nurses intent to stay: a systematic review', *Journal of Nursing Management*, 19: 461–77.

Cummings, J. and Bennett, V. (2012) *Compassion in Practice: Nursing, Midwifery and Care Staff: Our Strategy*. Leeds: NHS Commissioning Board.

Cutliffe, J.R., Sloan, G. and Bashaw, M. (2018) 'A systematic review of clinical supervision evaluation studies in nursing', *International Journal of Mental Health Nursing*, 27(1): 1–19.

Dawson, J.F., West, M.A., Admasachew, L. and Topakas, A. (2011) *NHS Staff Management and Health Service Quality: Results from the NHS Staff Survey and Related Data*. London: Department of Health.

Dimond, B. (2015) *Legal Aspects of Nursing*, 7th edn. Harlow: Pearson Education Ltd.

Duddle, M. and Boughton, M. (2007) 'Intra-professional relations in nursing', *Journal of Advanced Nursing*, 59(1): 29–37.

Economist Intelligence Unit (2014) *Is 75 the New 65? Rising to the Challenge of an Aging Workforce*. Available at: www.eiu.com (last accessed 22 March 2018).

Fayol, F. (1916) *General and Industrial Management*. London: Pitman.

Fiedler, F.E. (1967) A *Theory of Leadership Effectiveness*. New York: McGraw-Hill.

Francis, R. (2013) *Report of the Mid Staffordshire NHS Foundation Trust Public Inquiry Executive Summary*. Available at: http://webarchive.nationalarchives.gov.uk/20150407084003 or www.midstaffspublicinquiry.com/report (last accessed 22 March 2018).

Francis, R. (2015) *Freedom to Speak Up. An Independent Review into Creating an Open and Honest Reporting Culture in the NHS*. Available at: www.gov.uk/government/publications/sir-robert-francis-freedom-to-speak-up-review (last accessed 9 April 2018).

French, J.P.R., Jr and Raven, B. (1960) 'The bases of social power'. In D. Cartwright and A. Zander (eds), *Group Dynamics*. New York: Harper & Row, pp. 607–23.

Friedman, R.A., Tidd, S.T., Currall, S.C. and Tsai, J.C. (2000) 'What goes around comes around: the impact of personal conflict style on work conflict and stress', *International Journal of Conflict Management*, 11: 32–55.

Goleman, D., Boyatzis, R. and McKee, A. (2013) *Primal Leadership. Unleashing the Power of Emotional Intelligence*. Boston, MA: Harvard Business Review Press.

Goss, S. (2015) *Systems Leadership: A View from the Bridge*. London: Office for Public Management.

Greenleaf, R.K. (1977) *Servant Leadership: A Journey into the Nature of Legitimate Power and Greatness*. New York: Paulist.

Hardacre, J., Cragg, R., Shapiro, J., Spurgeon, P. and Flanagan, H. (2011) *What's Leadership Got to Do with It?* London: The Health Foundation.

Hasson, F., McKenna, H.P. and Keeney, S. (2013) 'Delegating and supervising unregistered professionals: the student nurse experience', *Nurse Education Today*, 33(3): 229–35.

Health and Safety Executive (2014) *Five Steps to Risk Assessment*. Belfast: HSE.

Health and Safety Executive (2017) *Health and Safety Statistics for the Public Services Sector in Great Britain 2017*. Available at: www.hse.gov.uk/sTATIsTICs/index.htm (last accessed 8 April 2018).

Hersey, P. and Blanchard, K.H. (1988) *Management of Organizational Behavior*, 5th edn. Upper Saddle River, NJ: Prentice Hall.

Hewison, A. and Griffiths, M. (2004) 'Leadership development in healthcare: a word of caution', *Journal of Health Organisation and Management*, 18(6): 464–73.

Huber, D.L. (2010) *Leadership and Nursing Care Management*, 4th edn. Missouri, IL: Elsevier.

Hutchinson, D., Brown, J. and Longworth, K. (2012) 'Attracting and maintaining the Y Generation in nursing: a literature review', *Journal of Nursing Management*, 20(4): 444–50.

International Council of Nurses (2007) 'Positive practice environments: Quality workplaces = quality patient care'. In *Information and Action Tool Kit*. Geneva: ICN.

Johnson, S.L. (2009) 'International perspectives on workplace bullying among nurses: a review', *International Nursing Review*, 56: 34–40.

King's Fund, The (2011) *The Future of Leadership and Management in the NHS: No More Heroes*. London: The King's Fund.

King's Fund, The (2012) *Leadership and Engagement for Improvement in the NHS*. London: The King's Fund.

King's Fund, The (2014) *Culture and Leadership in the NHS*: The King's Fund 2014 Survey, May 2014. Available at: www.kingsfund.org.uk/sites/files/kf/field/field_publication_file/survey-culture-leadership-nhs-may2014.pdf.

Kirkup, B. (2015) *The Report of the Morecambe Bay Investigation*. Available at: www.gov.uk/government/publications (last accessed 21 March 2018).

Kirkup, B. (2018) *Report of the Liverpool Community Health Independent Review*. Available at: https://improvement.nhs.uk/news-alerts/independent-review-liverpool-community-health-nhs-trust-published (last accessed 21 March 2018).

Kouzes, J. and Posner, B. (2017) *The Leadership Challenge*, 6th edn. Hoboken, NJ: Wiley.

Leiter, M.P., Price, S.L. and Spence Lashinger, H.K. (2010) 'Generational differences in distress, attitudes and incivility among nurses', *Journal of Nursing Management*, 18: 970–80.

Lucas, B. and Buckley, T. (2009) 'Leadership for quality improvement: what does it really take?', *International Journal of Leadership in Public Services*, 5(1): 37–46.

Marquis, B.L. and Huston, C.J. (2006) *Leadership Roles and Management Functions in Nursing: Theory and Application*, 5th edn. Philadelphia, PA: Lippincott.

Mayo, E. (1949) *Hawthorne and the Western Electrical Company: The Social Problems of an Industrial Civilisation*. London: Routledge & Kegan Paul.

McGregor, D. (1960) *The Human Side of Enterprise*. New York: McGraw-Hill.

McKee, L., Charles, K., Dixon-Woods, M., Willars, J. and Martin, G. (2013) '"New" and distributed leadership in quality and safety in health care, or "old" and hierarchical? An interview study with strategic stakeholders', *Journal of Health Services Research & Policy*, 18(Suppl 2): 11–19.

National Leadership and Innovations Agency for Healthcare (2010) *All Wales Guidelines for Delegation*. Llanharan: NLIAH. Available at: www.wales.nhs.uk/sitesplus/861/document/181978 (last accessed 8 April 2018).

National Quality Board (2013) *Quality in the New Health System: Maintaining and Improving Quality (Final Report)*. Available at: https://assets.publishing.service.gov.uk/government/uploads/system/uploads/attachment_data/file/213304/Final-NQB-report-v4-160113.pdf (last accessed 8 October 2018).

National Quality Board (2016) *Supporting NHS Providers to Deliver the Right Staff, with the Right Skills, in the Right Place, at the Right Time*. Available at: www.england.nhs.uk/publication/national-quality-board-guidance-on-safe-staffing (last accessed 8 April 2018).

NHS England (2014) *Five Year Forward Review*. Available at www.england.nhs.uk/wpcontent/uploads/2014/10/5yfv-web.pdf (last accessed 22 March 2018).

NHS Improvement (2016) *Creating a Culture of Compassionate and Inclusive Leadership*. Available at https://improvement.nhs.uk/resources/culture-leadership (last accessed 21 March 2018).

NHS Leadership Academy (2013) *Healthcare Leadership Model*. Available at: www.leadershipacademy.nhs.uk/resources/healthcare-leadership-model (last accessed 22 March 2018).

NHS Management Executive (1993) *A Vision for the Future. The Nursing, Midwifery and Health Visiting Contribution to Health and Health Care*. London: NHS Management Executive.

Northouse, P.G. (2012) *Introduction to Leadership Concepts and Practice*, 2nd edn. London: Sage.

Nursing and Midwifery Council (2017a) *Revalidation*. London: NMC.

Nursing and Midwifery Council (2017b) *Raising Concerns: Guidance for Nurses and Midwives*. London: NMC.

Nursing and Midwifery Council (2018a) *Future Nurse: Standards of Proficiency for Registered Nurses*. London: NMC.

Nursing and Midwifery Council (2018b) *The Code: Professional Standards of Practice Behaviour for Nurses and Midwives*. London: NMC.

Nursing and Midwifery Council (2018c) *Delegation and Accountability: Supplementary Information to the NMC Code*. London: NMC.

*Oxford English Dictionary* (2018) 'Conflict', Oxford: Oxford University Press. Available at https://en.oxforddictionaries.com/definition/conflict.

Rose, L. (2015) *Better Leadership for Tomorrow: NHS Leadership Review*. Available at: www.gov.uk/government/uploads/system/uploads/attachment_data/file/445738/Lord_Rose_NHS_Report_acc.pdf (last accessed 22 March 2018).

Rowland, D. (2017) *Still Moving: How to Lead Mindful Change*. Chichester: Wiley & Sons.

Royal College of Nursing (2009) *Breaking Down Barriers, Driving Up Standards: The Role of the Ward Sister and Charge Nurse*. London: RCN.

Royal College of Nursing (2010) *The Principles of Nursing Practice*. Available at: www.rcn.org.uk/development/practice/principles (last accessed 9 April 2018).

Royal College of Nursing (2012) *Valuing Older Workers*. London: RCN.

Royal College of Nursing (2013) *Beyond Breaking Point*. London: RCN.

Royal College of Nursing (2016) *Healthy Workforce Toolkit for an Agency Workforce*. London: RCN.

Royal College of Nursing (2017a) *Accountability and Delegation*. London: RCN.

Royal College of Nursing (2017b) *Safe and Effective Staffing: Nursing Against the Odds*. London: RCN.

Royal College of Nursing (2017c) *Delegating Record Keeping and Countersigning Records*. London: RCN.

Royal College of Nursing (2017d) *Managing Unacceptable Behaviour. Guidelines for Accredited Representatives and Relevant RCN Staff*. London: RCN.

Senge, P.M. (1990) *The Fifth Discipline: The Art and Practice of the Learning Organization*. London: Random House/Doubleday.

Sherwood, G. (2003) 'Leadership for a healthy work environment: caring for the human spirit', *Nurse Leader*, Sept/Oct: 36–40.

Sieloff, C.L. and Wallace Raph, S. (2011) 'Nursing theory and management (editorial)', *Journal of Nursing Management*, 19: 979–80.

Snowden, D.A., Leggat, S.G. and Taylor, N.F. (2017) 'Does clinical supervision of healthcare professionals improve effectiveness of care and patient experience? A systematic review', *BMC Health Services Research*, 17: 786.

Squires, M., Tourangeau, A., Spence Laschinger, H.K. and Doran, D. (2010) 'The link between leadership and safety outcomes in hospital', *Journal of Nursing Management*, 18: 914–25.

Stanley, D. (2010) 'Multigenerational workforce issues and their implications for leadership in nursing', *Journal of Nursing Management*, 18(7): 846–52.

Stein, S.J. (2017) *The EQ Leader*. Hoboken, NJ: Wiley.

Thomas, K.W. and Kilman, R.H. (1977) 'Developing a forced-choice measure of conflict behaviour: the "mode" instrument', *Educational and Psychological Measurement*, 37: 309–25.

Tuffin, R. (2016) 'Implications of complexity theory for clinical practice and healthcare organization', *BJA Education*, 16(10): 349–52.

West, M. and Chowla, R. (2017) 'Compassionate leadership for compassionate health care', In P. Gilbert (ed.), *Compassion: Concepts, Research and Applications*. New York: Routledge, pp. 237–57.

West, M. and Lyubovnikova, J. (2012) 'Real teams or pseudo teams? The changing landscape needs a better map', *Industrial and Organizational Psychology: Perspectives on Science and Practice*, 5(1): 25–8.

West, M.A., Borrill, C.S., Dawson, J.F., Brodbeck, F., Shapiro, D.A. and Haward, B. (2003) 'Leadership clarity and team innovation in healthcare', *Leadership Quarterly*, 14: 393–410.

West, M.A., Eckert, R., Steward, K. and Pasmore, B. (2014) *Developing Collective Leadership for Healthcare*. London: The King's Fund.

West, M., Armit, K., Loewenthal, L., Eckert, R., West, T. and Lee, A. (2015) *Leadership and Leadership Development in Healthcare: The Evidence Base*. London: Faculty of Medical Leadership and Management.

West, M., Eckert, R., Collins, B. and Chowla, R. (2017) *Caring to Change*. London: The King's Fund.

Wong, C.A. and Cummings, G.G. (2007) 'The relationship between nursing leadership and patient outcomes: a systematic review', *Journal of Nursing Management*, 15(5): 508–21.

Wong, C.A., Cummings, G.A. and Ducharme, L. (2013) 'The relationship between nursing leadership and patient outcomes: a systematic review update', *Journal of Nursing Management*, 21: 709–24.

# DEVELOPING PRACTICE AND MANAGING CHANGE

## DIANNE BURNS

---

### CHAPTER OBJECTIVES

- Appraise the concept of quality, focusing on quality assurance frameworks and methods of monitoring, and improving the quality of care and service provision;
- Outline current legal, ethical and professional drivers for change/service improvement;
- Critically discuss the role of change agents in developing and leading teams to effective change;
- Identify effective strategies for managing change and consider their application to healthcare practice;
- Critically discuss barriers to service improvement implementation and appraise potential solutions to overcome them.

---

One of the biggest challenges for leaders of healthcare today is how to achieve more for less. Not only do healthcare practitioners have to care for more patients/service users (many of whom are highly dependent with complex care needs), but we are also called on to provide high(er)-quality care and improve patient satisfaction while maintaining and enhancing patient safety.

In order for us to be able to deliver safe and effective person-centred healthcare in a timely, cost-effective and efficient manner, we need to continually monitor and improve the way we work. However it sometimes seems that healthcare provision in the UK is constantly changing and this can be unsettling for everyone. Yet change is an integral part of service improvement and being able to live with and manage change is an essential skill. Moreover, as a nurse you have a professional responsibility to make a positive contribution towards shaping a healthcare environment that promotes excellent care and patient satisfaction (NMC, 2018a).

## Related NMC proficiencies for registered nurses

The overarching requirement of the Nursing and Midwifery Council (NMC) is that all nurses must be able to contribute effectively to continuous monitoring and quality improvement processes in order to be able to improve health outcomes for patients (NMC, 2018b).

### To achieve entry to the nursing register you must be able to

- Identify the implications of current health policy and future policy changes for nursing and other professions, and understand the impact of policy changes on the delivery and coordination of care;
- Understand how health legislation and current health and social care policies can be used to influence organisational change;
- Demonstrate an understanding of the principles of health economics and their relevance to resource allocation in health and social care organisations and other agencies;
- Demonstrate an understanding of how to monitor and evaluate the quality and effectiveness of care (including patient experience) and how this can be used to bring about continuous service improvement;
- Demonstrate an understanding of the principles of improvement methodologies, participate in all stages of audit activity and identify appropriate quality improvement strategies;
- Work with people, their families, carers and colleagues, to develop effective improvement strategies for quality and safety, sharing feedback and learning from positive outcomes and experiences, mistakes, and adverse outcomes and experiences;
- Demonstrate an understanding of the mechanisms involved in influencing policy development and change, including the importance of exercising political awareness and skills to maximise the influence and effect of registered nursing on quality of care, patient safety and cost effectiveness;
- Demonstrate an understanding of the processes involved in developing a basic business case for additional care funding, by applying knowledge of finance, resources and safe staffing levels.

(Adapted from NMC, 2018b)

## Drivers for change

In Chapter 8, we focused on the leader's role in leading and managing teams. We also explored the importance of improving patient safety and reducing/managing risk, which are of course important drivers for change. Here, we will begin to explore the nurse's role in managing quality, developing practice and leading change.

It is imperative that healthcare systems across the UK can deliver high-quality patient care. Good quality care is defined by the National Quality Board (2013: 4) as 'care that is effective, safe and provides as positive an experience as possible'. In light of failures highlighted by Francis (2013) and others (Andrews and Butler, 2014; Kirkup, 2015, 2018), monitoring and improving the quality of care we deliver to our patients have never been higher on the political or professional agenda. However, it is also a complex and demanding task. Having a working knowledge of the relevant frameworks, policies, tools and techniques, alongside an ability to enable and facilitate others, is central to leading improvement in the NHS, particularly when dealing with more complex issues (Hardacre et al., 2011). In order to sustain high-quality care, nurses (and their co-workers) will need to maintain and enhance patient safety while also taking action to improve efficiency by managing available resources effectively (NHS England, 2016).

**Clinical governance** is a term used to define the framework though which NHS organisations are accountable for continuously improving the quality of care and services (Department of Health or DH, 1998). The three components of clinical governance that you will no doubt be involved in are clinical effectiveness, patient safety and patient experience (Figure 9.1).

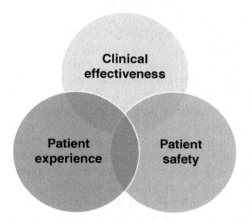

**Figure 9.1**   Clinical governance

This encompasses the whole range of quality improvement activities falling within the three main strands: *clinical effectiveness, patient safety* and *patient experience* (National Quality Board, 2013). As a qualified nurse you will be accountable for the standard of nursing care, dignity and wellbeing of your patients, so you will have a vital role to play in putting these into practice (NMC, 2018a). You will also have the responsibility of promoting awareness of essential standards of quality and safety, monitoring the standard of care delivered and taking action where necessary in the interests of patients. This will involve ensuring that the workplace culture is one in which quality improvement activities flourish and where frontline staff can grasp opportunities to make a positive contribution not only by enhancing their own professional development but also by engaging collaboratively with service users to improve and enhance care delivery.

Good quality care is care that is delivered according to the best evidence of what is clinically effective in improving an individual's health outcomes. Having clear, robust systems and structures in place can help us to identify and report on the quality of patient care. For example, in England, the NHS Outcomes Framework (DH, 2012a), the Public Health Outcomes Framework (DH, 2012b) and the Adult Social Care Outcomes Framework (DH, 2013) set out indicators for measuring outcomes within health and social care systems in an effort to ensure continuous improvement in the quality of NHS services across all care providers. Similar strategies have been implemented in Scotland, Northern Ireland and Wales (NHS Scotland, 2010; Department of Health, Social Services and Public Safety or DHSSPS, 2011; NHS Wales, 2013, 2014).

## Measuring quality

It is more than 30 years ago since the concept of quality improvement in healthcare settings was introduced by Donabedian (2005), among others, who suggested that by observing *structure* (the setting in which care is delivered, e.g. nurse:patient ratio, staffing levels), *focus* (the process or means by which the end point is achieved, e.g. patient care pathways) and *outcomes* (end point, e.g. readmission rates, number of reported falls or hospital-acquired infection rates) we can measure the quality of healthcare. More recently the introduction of agreed standards of care has allowed us to measure the care we deliver against a set standard (e.g. benchmarking). As a bare minimum, current requirements dictate that we should meet essential standards for quality and safety set out by the Care Quality Commission (2018). We should also be aiming to meet standards set by the National Institute for Health and Care Excellence (NICE), for example care pathways (http://pathways.nice.org.uk) and National Service Frameworks (e.g. http://nhs.uk/nhsengland/NSF and www.wales.nhs.uk/sites3/), which focus on the care of patients with a particular condition and set out what high-quality care looks like for a particular patient group.

Regular participation in activities that continuously measure and monitor the quality of care delivered in your current workplace is essential. To do this effectively requires the use of robust systems and processes designed to monitor performance. Examples include:

- *Quality indicators* (QIs), also referred to as *clinical quality indicators* (CQIs), are reliable and valid measures, which can be used to assess health processes and outcomes (Maintz, 2003);
- *Clinical audit*: a cyclical staged process that seeks to improve patient care and outcomes through a systematic review of care measured against explicit criteria (e.g. quality indicators), a course of action taken to improve services and followed by continued monitoring to sustain improvement;
- *Clinical benchmarking*: a systematic process in which current practice and care are compared, and amended to attain best practice and care (DH, 2010); it involves sharing evidence of best practice with colleagues and peers;
- *Patient-reported outcome measures* (PROMs) can be used to evaluate the effectiveness of current service provision, recognise deficits and assist in the development of new evidence-based services.

In order to be successful, healthcare professionals need to fully understand the importance and value of collecting data because the success of such strategies is almost entirely dependent on the values and behaviours of staff working within the system. For example, some nurses may be somewhat sceptical about the benefits of time-consuming 'number crunching', and do not always understand the importance of data collection and how information can be used to benefit patient care. As you continue to read on, you will hopefully begin to see how these data can be used in the drive for service improvement.

## ACTIVITY 9.1

To help improve your own knowledge and understanding of ways in which we can measure performance, the Healthcare Quality Improvement Partnership (HQIP) have published some useful guidance documents:

HQIP (2016) *Documenting Local Clinical Audit: A Guide to Reporting and Recording*. London: HQIP.

HQIP (2016) *Best Practice in Clinical Audit*. London: HQIP.

HQIP (2017) *Guide to Managing Ethical Issues in Quality Improvement or Clinical Audit Projects*. London: HQIP.

## Clinical effectiveness

Quality care is 'care which is delivered according to the best evidence as to what is clinically effective in improving an individual's health outcomes' (National Quality Board, 2013: 13).

The provision of good quality patient care is of great interest to providers and purchasers of care alike. In recent years, the emphasis for care providers has focused on evidence-based practice. Indeed the NMC's *Code* (NMC, 2018a) demands that you deliver care based on the best available evidence. This requires you to keep your knowledge and skills up to date, ensuring that you have a good understanding of the current evidence base and an ability to apply this to your day-to-day practice. In addition, purchasers are keen to ensure that healthcare provision is cost-effective and provides value for money. However, concerns about the quality of care within some healthcare settings have continued to attract national publicity and often focus on the failure of organisations to provide services that deliver high standards of care. For example, in 2011–12 the Care Quality Commission (CQC) reported that only 85% of NHS hospitals met the required standard of ensuring that patients had access to the right food, drink and help that they needed (CQC, 2012).

Clinical effectiveness is about improving patient care and experience by critically reviewing what you/your team do by considering the following:

- What should be happening? (identifying evidence of best practice);
- What is happening? (reviewing current practice);
- How can we do it better? (comparing your practice with good practice and implementing change);
- Evaluating change (using clinical audit and other measures, i.e. PROMs, to demonstrate improvement).

- Consider how you might begin to improve patient care and experience in your current practice setting? What would you need to know? What types of data might you need to collect and why? How might you do this?

## Patient experience

Quality care is care that looks to give the individual as positive an experience of receiving and recovering from illness as possible, including being treated according to what that individual wants or needs with compassion, dignity and respect (National Quality Board, 2013: 13). Patients and service users are being encouraged to take more control of their own care (DHSSPS, 2011; NHS England, 2014; Scottish Government, 2017) and they have an important part to play in determining how services are designed, implemented and evaluated (King's Fund, 2014). By collaborating closely with patients and service users and responding appropriately to their feedback, nurses can deliver more appropriate care and ensure that any concerns raised are dealt with quickly and appropriately (Coulter, 2012). This will usually involve collecting and using information provided by patients/service users and carers (e.g. patient satisfaction surveys or focus groups) in order to deliver the kind of services they want. Whatever approach is used, the key aim is to find out what they really think about the services we provide and provide supporting evidence of this. Ultimately it is very rewarding when you receive compliments from patients about their care. However, unfortunately from time to time complaints will also feature and when they arise it is important to ensure that they are not ignored.

Think of some examples currently used in your practice setting to elicit patient feedback:

- How effective are these methods?
- How is the feedback used?

Luxford et al. (2011) suggest that the following factors are critical in assuring the quality of patients' experience of care:

- Strong and committed senior leadership;
- Communication of the strategic vision;
- Engagement of patients and families;
- A sustained focus on employee satisfaction;
- Regular measurement and feedback reporting;
- Adequate resourcing for care delivery design;
- Building staff capacity to support patient-centred care;
- Accountability and an incentives culture – strongly supportive of change and learning.

## Resource management

Although patient safety and quality care are obvious drivers for change, so too is the need to be able to manage resources effectively. As resources are essentially limited, we now have to make choices about how they are to be used. Resource management is about getting the best value for money and reducing 'unwarranted variations' by addressing overuse, misuse and underuse of treatment (NHS England, 2016). As a nurse, it is important to be able to provide the best quality care in the most efficient and effective way possible. We need to be able to balance available budgets and eliminate waste while improving the quality of the services we provide. All areas of expenditure will need to be carefully monitored and scrutinised. This is a huge challenge at a time where current severe funding restraint is accompanied by major reorganisations of health- and social cares services alongside calls for improvements in care quality (Francis, 2013; NHS England, 2013, 2016). Nevertheless, it is possible. For example Alderwick et al. (2015) highlight significant savings that have already been made by the use of generic medicines and targeted efforts to reduce the length of inpatient stays, driven in part by improved cooperation between clinicians and managers, redesigning patient pathways to maximise good healthcare outcomes, improved data collection/information and 'frontline' support from clinicians in practice.

**Lean thinking** is a philosophy that has been used widely in manufacturing industries, but has been applied more recently in healthcare settings (D'Andreamatteo et al., 2015). It is essentially about simplifying processes, identifying which parts of a process add value to patient care, enabling care to flow more effectively and eliminating waste. The Lean framework incorporates six areas of consideration when seeking to manage available resources more effectively: overproduction; inventory; waiting; transportation; staff movement; and unnecessary processing. Some argue that a Lean approach is being used effectively to manage safety and improve productivity (Amnis Healthcare, 2011) whereas others suggest that there is conflicting evidence of the outcomes of Lean thinking when applied in healthcare settings (Andersen et al., 2014).

> ## 🗨? ACTIVITY 9.2
>
> Closely observing the care that is delivered to patients within a chosen healthcare setting:
>
> 1. Record the care processes (from a patient perspective) that are encountered throughout the day (e.g. waiting times, provision of patient information, contact with other healthcare professionals, investigations and procedures performed).
> 2. Identify where possible savings could be made while maintaining or improving patient safety and service provision.
> 3. What information or evidence might you need to collect to support your claims?

In response to the activity above, you may have witnessed (or been involved in) practices that include undertaking an activity 'just in case' (*overproduction*) – for example unnecessary duplication of diagnostic tests, ordering excess material because the supply is unreliable (*inventory*), or using complex equipment to undertake simple tasks – for example opening a sterile dressing pack to get access to gauze swabs (*overprocessing* or *unnecessary processing*). You may have seen patients *waiting* in queues at the GP surgery, *waiting* for tests or having treatment delayed due to the fact that vital equipment is not ready or missing. You may also be familiar with issues related to the *transportation* of patients or material that is wasteful or ways in which staff movement in the workplace seems inefficient (e.g. layout and organisation of the workplace or poor access to end of life care in the community resulting in admission to hospital). You could also have witnessed misuse or poor use of services, for example poor concordance with prescribed medication or preventable patient complications (e.g. venous thromboembolism, falls, medication errors).

Many of the current targets and organisational aims require us to make changes to patient services in order to improve the quality of care or patient safety (e.g. intervening earlier to avoid the development of possible complications), making more effective use of financial resources by improving stock rotation, or ordering processes or perhaps improving management systems to ensure that you can make better use of human resources and available staff (e.g. reducing sickness and absence, developing staff by providing education and training, motivating staff to be innovative).

## Change management theory

Change is not a single action; it is a challenge to experience, as well as to plan and manage. It requires a variety of resources – both human and material. Although many argue that it needs to involve a *well-planned, stepwise process* (proactive approach), including a combination of interventions, linked to specific needs and obstacles to change (Lewin, 1951; Bullock and Batten, 1985; Grol, 1997; Grol and Grimshaw, 2003), others support the view that change can also be *unplanned* (emergent/reactive) or ad hoc – particularly in rapidly changing environments or when triggered by organisational crisis – and that change will always contain complex emergent elements (Olson and Eoyang, 2001), especially in large-scale projects. Approaches can also be *top-down* (from management downwards) or *bottom-up* (generated by frontline staff upwards). Pearson et al.

(2008) suggest that both can be successful in disseminating nursing interventions depending on the requirements and circumstances.

Although there are many change management theories, one popular theory is that of Lewin (1951). Within this model (Figure 9.2), the *unfreezing* stage is aimed at destabilising the forces that maintain the status quo. Actions of the change agent or leader are focused on gathering data and evidence to support the change, generating an air of discontent among those involved, decreasing the strength of old values, attitudes and behaviours and making others aware of the need for change. Once the need for change has been recognised, goals and objectives can be agreed, planned and implemented. The *change* stage requires the leader to identify areas of support and resistance, developing strategies to support those involved or affected by the proposed change, in addition to dealing with resistance effectively. *Refreezing* is aimed at stabilising the change, sustaining efforts to ensure that the new ways of working are incorporated into practice on a long-term basis.

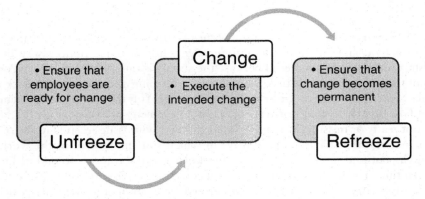

**Figure 9.2** Lewin's model of change (1951)

However, change management and service improvement are complex and demanding processes that will often require consideration of a number of factors (e.g. availability of technology, workforce availability and skill, service user expectations and experience, managing and reducing risk, competition, government policy and economics). It is worth remembering that seeking to change or improve services will always have an impact on someone. Having a critical understanding of the key issues, influencing factors and potential barriers is crucial if you are going to succeed in managing change and improving services within healthcare settings. The Health Foundation (2015) suggests that the key barriers to improvement in the NHS relate to the *initiative* itself (e.g. insufficient evidence base or usability of interventions), the *skills and attitude of individuals* (e.g. resistance, lack of knowledge and skills, role demarcation), *organisational context* (e.g. lack of leadership and management, culture and stability, lack of funding or time) or are system wide (e.g. incentives and funding, NHS culture, lack of stability and partnership working).

Indeed, it would be relatively easy if, once a need for change has been identified, everyone involved readily accepted this and supported the development. However, it is never that simple – not everyone will be willing or interested. Changing entrenched clinical styles can be a difficult and lengthy process. Defensive reactions from colleagues, lack of awareness, incentives or training, time pressures or a fear of losing power can all act as barriers (Coulter, 2012). The organisational culture, changes in roles and responsibilities, and policy shifts can also affect the outcome of improvement work.

According to Silber (1993), the degree of resistance for each individual will often depend upon four factors:

1. Their flexibility to change;
2. Their evaluation of the immediate situation;
3. Their anticipated consequences of the change;
4. Their perception of what they have to lose and/or gain.

Potential barriers include organisational politics and conflict, which sometimes cannot be easily identified or resolved. Therefore, in order to progress with a change idea, all the driving and restraining forces need to be identified (Lewin, 1951). Lewin' force field analysis framework (Figure 9.3) can be a useful tool to assist in the identification of the drivers and restrainers or change within planning and implementation phases.

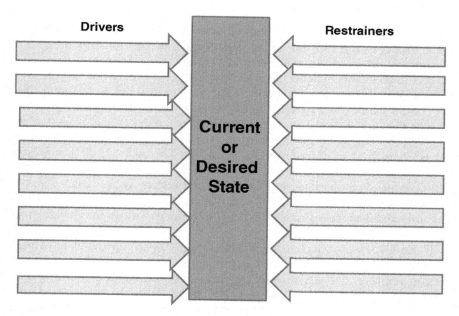

**Figure 9.3**    Force field analysis (Lewin, 1951)

Various types of forces that you will need to consider include:

- Available resources/funding/costs;
- Current targets;
- Current and past practices;
- The vested interests of stakeholders;
- The attitudes of stakeholders and those who will be affected by the proposed change;
- Regulations, policies and procedures (e.g. DH initiatives or local trust policies);
- The organisational structures/traditions and/or culture;
- Relationships;
- Personal and/or group needs;

- The values of both the organisation and individuals;
- Opportunities;
- Productivity.

---

**? ACTIVITY 9.3**

Identify the potential barriers to change in your own workplace and consider how you might overcome these.

TIP: the National Institute for Health and Clinical Excellence (NICE, 2007) have produced a useful guide that aims to help healthcare practitioners change their practice in line with clinical guidance.

---

By (2005) provides a useful critical review of organisational change management exploring the differences in approaches, but concludes that there is still a lack of underpinning evidence to suggest the best approach in any given situation and suggests that more robust research is needed to evaluate organisational change management frameworks. This is particularly vital when considering change involving healthcare organisations. Traditional approaches, for example those suggested by Lewin (1951) and Bullock and Batten (1985), are now viewed as simplistic and, although some would argue that they are still relevant today, emergent approaches (e.g. Kanter et al., 1992 and Kotter, 1996), acknowledging the complexity of working with individuals within multifaceted organisations is considered more appropriate. Grol and Grimshaw (2003) suggest that certain strategies are more effective in increasing the adoption rate of the change process (Grol and Grimshaw, 2003) depending on the desired outcomes (Grimshaw et al., 2012).

Grol's (1997) five-stage implementation process for changing clinical practice takes into account the need to identify and deal with obstacles in order to be able to move the change process forward (Figure 9.4).

Alternatively, Kotter's eight-step change model (Kotter, 2014) comprises eight overlapping accelerators that are proposed to assist those leading transformational change. He argues that, although strategy, structure, culture and systems are important, nothing matters more than changing the behaviour of people by dealing with their feelings. The model is therefore based on how people experience the change process. Updated from previous work (Kotter, 1996; Kotter and Cohen, 2002), Kotter proposes a dual operating system – the hierarchy to take care of business and the network to react quickly to change and opportunities – suggesting that the two operating systems work side by side and are both essential for success.

## Leading and managing change to improve patient services

Lockitt (2004) provides a useful overview of five broad strategies for affecting change, claiming that each has its advantages, disadvantages and potential effects (Table 9.1).

Porter-O'Grady (2003) argues that leader or manager behaviour is the single most important factor in how people accept change. The most successful change agents are people who possess the essential knowledge, skills and attributes for effective leadership and management of service improvement teams. Kouzes and Posner (2017) maintain that having a leadership or management

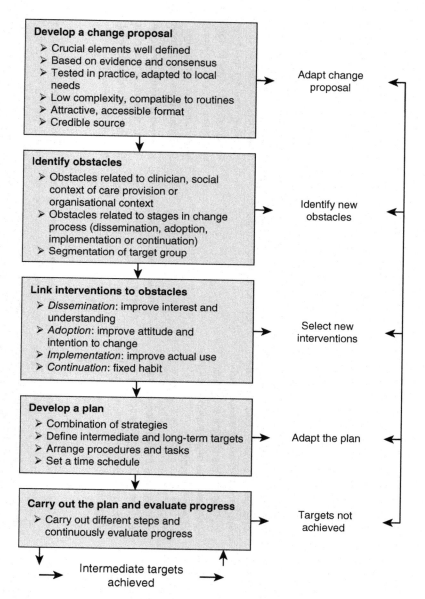

**Figure 9.4**   Grol's (1997) five-stage implementation process

style that generates a shared purpose across all stakeholders is the most effective strategy to ensure success. They identify the following five leadership behaviours that contribute to a leader's ability to engage and empower others, some of which are considered crucial when attempting to affect change within the NHS and other healthcare settings.

*Modelling the way* involves identifying and clarifying shared values (e.g. the application of evidence-based practice and the provision of an excellent standard of patient care) and then setting an example for others to follow. To be able to do this effectively requires an ability to identify new

**Table 9.1** Strategies for affecting change

| Strategy | Advantages | Disadvantages | Potential effects |
|---|---|---|---|
| *Directive*: change is usually imposed by managers with little or no consultation with others (i.e. those affected) | Can be implemented quickly | Fails to take into consideration the views and feelings of those involved in or affected by the change | May lead to valuable information or ideas being missed. May cause resentment from staff and those affected |
| *Expert*: management of change is seen as a problem-solving process that needs to be resolved by an 'expert'. Change is normally led by specialist project team or manager | The 'experts' play a major role in finding the solution and often the solution can be implemented quickly because a small number of 'experts' are involved | Those affected may have different views from those of the 'experts' and may not appreciate the solution being imposed or the outcomes of the changes made | |
| *Negotiating*: recognises the willingness to negotiate and bargain in order to affect change | Those affected by the change have an opportunity to have a say in what changes are made, how they are implemented and the expected outcomes, therefore feeling more involved and more supportive of the changes made | Negotiating effectively takes time and the outcomes cannot be predicted | Adjustments and concessions may be required in order to implement change, so the final changes may not meet the total expectation of the change agent. Relatively slow to implement. More complex to manage. Requires more resources/costs |
| *Educative*: involves changing people's values and beliefs in order for them to fully support the proposed change using a mixture of activities including persuasion, education, training and selection, and led by in-house experts | Encourages the development of a shared set of organisational values that individuals are willing and able to support | Takes longer to implement change | Involves a mixture of activities including persuasion, education, training and selection and is led by in-house experts |
| *Participative*: involves all those affected by anticipated changes. Driven less by managers and more by groups or individuals within an organisation | All views are taken into account before change is made. Any changes made are more likely to be supported due to the involvement of all those affected. The commitment of individuals and groups within the organisation will increase because those individuals and groups feel ownership over the changes being implemented | Can be time-consuming and costly due to the number of meetings needed, etc. Outcomes cannot be accurately predicted | The organisation and individuals also have the opportunity to learn from this experience and will know more about the organisation and how it functions, thus increasing their skills, knowledge and effectiveness to the organisation |

opportunities, and the confidence to be able to speak up, to share fresh ideas and to demonstrate commitment to supporting others in making the change by creating opportunities (e.g. setting interim goals to achieve small wins while working towards larger objectives using pilot studies or small trials).

*Inspiring a shared vision* involves creating a shared picture of how things might be better with the change imposed. The leader needs to be able to inspire others by making the 'shared vision' appeal to a wider audience. Carefully exploring the interests and aspirations of others, listening to their views and finding a common ground to ensure that the 'vision' is shaped, shared and agreed by team members will help everyone involved to develop a strong sense of ownership. The ability to build coalitions of support and counter resistance to change is considered crucial to success (King's Fund, 2012) and the healthcare leader will play a key role in enabling others in the system to contribute their views, expertise and ideas.

*Challenging the process* change often involves taking carefully considered risks so it is important for a leader to be able to develop a supportive climate/culture (Larson and LaFasto, 1989), in which trying out new approaches is considered normal and safe experimentation is encouraged (e.g. using an example from practice where a change when implemented did not work out). Mistakes and failures – while disappointing – are a key component of success because learning from these helps individuals to progress.

*Enabling others to act*: Rogers (2003) suggested that a common process occurs as people adopt a new idea. He identified five categories of adopters of an innovation: innovators (eager and adventurous), early adopters (respected opinion leaders), early majority (may deliberate for some time), late majority (sceptical and cautious) and laggards (traditionalists who prefer to do things as they have always done) – all of whom will have an impact on success. It is clear that a variety of approaches may be needed to engage with all those involved as implementing the 'vision' will require collaboration over an extended period. Regularly reviewing and recognising the contribution of other members of your team as you go – encouraging, empowering and sometimes challenging those involved – can help to develop confidence and competence and in turn generate an overall climate of trust. However, this will often require tolerance and empathy, showing sensitivity to the needs of others to make everyone feel included (Northouse, 2012).

*Encouraging the heart*: successfully managing change in healthcare organisations often involves a lot of hard work and dedication. People can frequently lose heart, particularly if there are no quick wins. Recognition of your own achievements and those of your colleagues (however small) helps to keep optimism and determination alive. Giving praise to others also shows that their support and commitment have been noticed and appreciated. This can involve something as simple as passing an encouraging comment or something a little more 'showy', such as public praise in team meetings, celebration events or 'telling the story'.

Bate et al. (2004) consider the act of connecting and engaging with others as crucial in order to effect change in healthcare settings. Their arguments (based on *social movement theory*) are leading a new way of thinking that has helped to develop a number of wide-ranging initiatives aimed at speeding up the diffusion and adoption of innovation across the country, in the hope of improving and sustaining patient outcomes.

# Service improvement models and frameworks

Improving the quality of nursing care and services involves 'the combined and unceasing efforts of everyone to make the changes that will lead to better patient outcomes (**health**), better system performance (**care**) and better professional development (**learning**)' (Batalden and Davidoff, 2007: 2) (Figure 9.5).

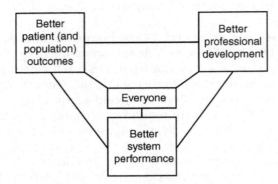

**Figure 9.5**   Illustrative tools and methods in improvement (reproduced from Batalden and Davidoff, 2007, with the permission of the BMJ Publishing Group)

There are a vast array of service improvement frameworks and tools available to support healthcare practitioners in their quest to improve patient services. One approach is the 'six-stage framework for service improvement' (Figure 9.6) (NHS Institute for Innovation and Improvement, 2013), which appears to draw on some of the change management strategies and models we reviewed earlier.

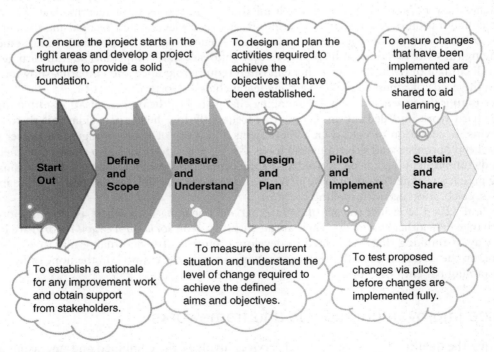

**Figure 9.6**   Six-stage framework for service improvement

Although the six stage framework encourages us to focus on six defined areas, some elements are considered critical to success at all stages (e.g. stakeholder engagement and involvement, risk and issues management and sustainability) of a service improvement project (NHS Institute for Innovation and Improvement, 2010). Above all, although the reasons for change in healthcare settings are numerous, the main focus should be on improving services for patients (directly or indirectly). This will often include the effective introduction of new policies and guidelines (in line with an emerging evidence base), or the consideration of the safe introduction of new technology and equipment, changes to the workforce/team or the need for effective resource management. Patient safety, care quality and the need to manage resources effectively are all key drivers for change that may be required in response to new government policies or legislation, professional guidance (top-down approach) or as a result of practitioners at ground level recognising the need to influence or change local policies, procedures and practice (bottom-up approach). Whatever the circumstances, being able to 'think differently' about care delivery options is considered a crucial skill for future healthcare leaders (Bevan, 2013).

As identified in the six step approach above, the first step towards service improvement is to identify what needs improving. To gain support for a project, it is useful to align the proposal to overall organisational aims, clearly illustrating short-term and long-term benefits.

What are the quality/service improvement drivers in your workplace?
    Tip: find out about existing targets and/or service and organisational aims.

Service or quality improvement projects can vary from local small-scale schemes to the complete redesign of an organisation (Figure 9.7). As a nurse you will be in an ideal position to identify opportunities to make a positive difference to patient care or the working environment, getting involved in service improvement initiatives or even taking the lead on change management projects. The task at this stage is to provide a strong rationale for change which is underpinned by supporting evidence that can be used to help create an impetus for movement, creating a vision for why and how things could be different.

| LOCAL – SMALL SCALE: | MEDIUM SCALE: | LARGE ORGANISATIONAL SCALE: |
|---|---|---|
| e.g. Protected patient meal or rest times | e.g. The Productive Ward Programme (NHS Institute for Innovation and Improvement) | e.g. Health and Social Care Bill and Reconfiguration of the NHS |

**Figure 9.7** Levels of change

## Stakeholder engagement

In order to manage change effectively, there is a need to involve others at every stage (e.g. team members, managers, multidisciplinary staff, service users, family/friends/carers and students). Very early in the life of a project, it is critical to identify all of the organisations and people who may have an impact on the project. It is useful to remember that a 'stakeholder' is any person or organisation that is actively involved in a project, or whose interests may be affected positively or negatively. Once an area for improvement has been identified, it will need to be really clear to others what it is that needs to be improved (e.g. situation, structure, process, treatment pathways, roles, behaviours) and why. We can then effectively share this 'vision' with others by appealing to their values, beliefs, hopes and dreams in an attempt to come together to form a 'shared vision'. The identification of key stakeholders and their potential influence or resistance are somewhat crucial in helping to determine their fears and concerns as well as identifying potential difficulties. In order to be able to overcome resistance you will not only have to create interest in the proposed project but also have to be prepared to face up to and either win over the sceptics or amend the 'vision' in response to their views.

Can you identify all of the potential stakeholders who might influence a service improvement project in your current placement area?
How might you engage with *all* of these?

It is important to recognise that not all stakeholders will be found within your immediate colleagues. Stakeholders can be internal or external to the organisation. Depending on the proposed change this could include service users and carers, team members or other professional groups and employees, suppliers, communities, and representatives from the private or voluntary sector, professional associations and government regulatory agencies. Once identified, it is worth considering each stakeholder's importance and impact on the project. Stakeholder engagement involves understanding the needs of all the different groups or individuals who may be interested or affected by your proposed change and building relationships with them. It also helps to define which stakeholders will be involved while considering a communication strategy that aims to obtain 'buy-in' from all. Table 9.2 provides an overview of the different engagement approaches that can be employed depending on the needs and interests of each individual, group or organisation.

**Table 9.2** Stakeholder engagement approaches

| Engagement approach | Description |
| --- | --- |
| Partnership | Shared accountability and responsibility |
| Participation | Part of the team engaged in delivering tasks or responsibility for a particular area/activity. Two-way engagement within limits of responsibility |
| Consultation | Involved, but not responsible and not necessarily able to influence outside of consultation boundaries. Limited two-way engagement: organisation asks questions, stakeholders answer |
| Push communications | One-way engagement: organisation may broadcast information to all stakeholders or target particular stakeholder groups using various channels, e.g. email, letter, webcasts, podcasts, videos, leaflets |
| Pull communications | One-way engagement: information is made available, and stakeholders choose whether to engage with it, e.g. web pages or construction hoardings |

Reproduced with the permission of stakeholdermap.com

A clear statement of the need for change and what that will mean is essential for rallying support and commitment from stakeholders. Indeed, you may need to create more than one message if stakeholder priorities are different. Dixon-Woods et al. (2012) suggest that it is important to convince people there is a problem that is relevant to them (securing emotional engagement) and this can be achieved by using powerful patient stories and voices.

## Patient and public involvement

Patients, service users, carers and the public can offer valuable first-hand experience of inefficiencies and areas for improvement. There is now a growing recognition of the need to involve patients and the public in service improvement processes. Service user involvement refers to the process by which people who are using or have used a service become involved in the planning, development and delivery of that service. Levels of involvement can vary, ranging from consultation (where they are asked their views but have limited influence on decision making), participation (where their views are sought and have a direct impact on decisions made), partnership working (contributing as equals – sharing decisions and responsibility) to full control (controlling the decision-making process).

Consider the role that service users and carers have in service development. What would you consider to be meaningful engagement? Are there any potential barriers to patient and public involvement (PPI)? How might these be overcome?

Beresford (2013) suggests that to achieve effective and meaningful involvement with people (particularly those whose voices are seldom heard, e.g. those with communication problems, black and ethnic minority groups, travellers, those in residential care or homeless individuals), means exploring, evaluating and monitoring new and creative ways of engaging with and involving them. He goes on to say that some of the common barriers include:

- Devaluing service users: not valuing or listening to what they say;
- Tokenism: asking for their involvement but not taking it seriously, making it an unproductive experience;
- Stigma: the stigma associated with service user identity (e.g. alcohol, drug abuse or ex-offenders), discouraging them from associating themselves with it and getting involved on that basis;
- Low levels of confidence and self-esteem: leaving service users feeling that they don't have much to contribute or are worried about whether they will be able to do it;
- Language and culture: the frequent reliance on jargon and other exclusionary arrangements for involvement, puts off many service users who are not confident in or used to such situations;
- Inadequate information about involvement: this is made worse by the frequent lack of appropriate and accessible information about getting involved, discouraging many from taking the first steps to getting involved.

To overcome these issues, Beresford (2013) recommends reaching out directly to service users, communities and community leaders, ensuring that they are able to gain access to the decision-making structures and collective working opportunities, and providing support and practical help to build their skills and confidence so that they can participate effectively.

[?]          **ACTIVITY 9.4**

Access and read the following articles/documents:

- The King's Fund (2012) *Leadership and Engagement for Improvement in the NHS. Together We Can*. London: The King's Fund.
- Ocloo, J. and Matthews, R. (2016) *From Tokenism to Empowerment: Progressing Patient and Public Involvement in Healthcare Improvement*. Available at: http://qualitysafety.bmj.com/content/qhc/early/2016/03/18/bmjqs-2015-004839.full.pdf.

Now access the Patient Association's website (www.patients-association.org.uk) and consider if there are better ways in which we as nurses could engage with patients and the public.

Capturing all of the information generated from engagement activities should help to ensure that the current situation is understood and will provide a focus for the improvement, assisting in the setting of measurable targets (NHS Institute for Innovation and Improvement, 2010). It is important to have measurable quality outcomes (a change is not necessarily an improvement!), so thought must be given right at the start about how the outcomes might be measured, depending on the aims and objectives. It is helpful to remember that there may already be data available that can initially be used as a baseline to set new targets.

At this stage however, Dixon-Woods et al. (2012) caution against setting overambitious goals that can alienate people, so it is important to try to set and agree realistic targets with the aim to include all stakeholders, in order to counteract perceived lack of ownership and subsequent disengagement. Agreeing goals that are aligned with those of the organisation(s) also helps to ensure that individuals don't feel pulled in too many directions. When attempting to make improvements you should try to ensure that your goals are SMART (Blanchard and Johnson, 1982):

- **Specific**: focused, specific objectives are much easier to manage and execute;
- **Measurable**: you must be able to measure the extent to which your objective has been achieved;
- **Attainable**: goals within reach but challenging enough to motivate;
- **Relevant**: goals aligned to professional or organisational goals;
- **Timely**: goals have target dates that monitor and maintain progression.

Once the goals have been clarified and agreed, activities need to be planned and implemented. At this stage it is really important that all of those involved and affected fully understand the demands of the process. This may require provision of detailed explanations and ongoing support to ensure everyone involved has a clear understanding of the future and agreed action plan (Dixon-Woods et al., 2012). Setting individual and team goals and targets based on the agreed objectives should help to keep the focus. Giving timely constructive feedback should also help to maintain and perhaps improve motivation.

### ACTIVITY 9.5

Identify one area of practice where you think implementing a change (however small) could help improve patient safety, the patient experience or quality of care provision, or perhaps save valuable resources.

Make a list of the skills and attributes you think could be helpful when attempting to implement change within a healthcare setting and explain how and why they would be useful.

What strategies might you use and why? Think about how you might present ideas in a way that the current situation is understood and you can obtain support from relevant stakeholders.

The plan–do–study–act (PDSA) cycle (Langley et al., 2009) is advocated for use by the NHS Institute for Innovation and Improvement when attempting to test new change ideas on a small scale, by temporarily trialling a change and assessing the impact – for example trying out a new way to make appointments for one consultant or clinic or trying out a new patient information sheet with a selected group of patients before introducing the change to all clinics or patient groups. The cyclical process (Figure 9.8) provides an opportunity to allow assessments to be made of whether or not the intervention is successful very early on in a project, thereby allowing adjustments where necessary as the project moves forward.

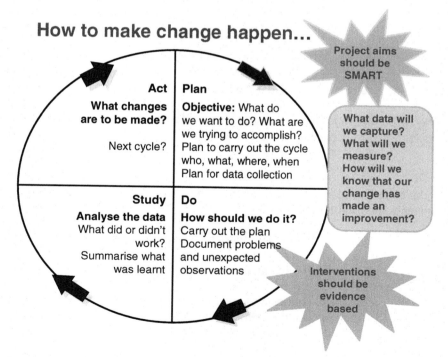

**Figure 9.8**  Plan–do–study–act cycle

However, Taylor et al. (2013) report variations in the way PDSA has been implemented in healthcare settings, suggesting that the process is not being used optimally. In addition, Reed and Card (2016) argue that in some cases (particularly where organisational and cultural changes are required) there is a need for an extensive repertoire of skills and knowledge to be able to use it well.

When evaluating the impact of a change or service improvement, we are seeking to assess how well (or not!) we have managed to achieve all of our aims and objectives. Solberg et al. (1997) suggest there are three characteristics of performance measures; measuring for *improvement*, *accountability* and *research*. However, unlike research measurements taken where the aim is to extend the available knowledge by means of a systematically defensible process of enquiry, measures for improvement may have a lower threshold than that of research (i.e. 'good enough'). It is often better to have just a few good measures, rather than a range of hard-to-collect details. Accountability measurements often relate to whether services meet a defined standard.

Sustaining improvement whereby innovations are embedded into everyday practice is not always easy. Berwick (2003) suggests that only a third of all innovations are successfully adopted and integrated into practice. Indeed, sustainability is vulnerable when improvement efforts are seen as one-off or time-limited projects or when they rely on certain individuals to ensure compliance or success (Dixon-Woods et al., 2012). Greenhalgh et al. (2005) suggest that the spread of innovation can be passive (e.g. unplanned and informal diffusion) or active (e.g. by means of a planned and coordinated approach). The NHS Institute for Innovation and Improvement (2010) sustainability model was designed to help address this problem, proposing a strategy to measure the likelihood of sustaining improvement in practice and suggesting actions to take to ensure that this is increased where possible. Its use can also lead to useful discussions about the improvement process.

---

### ?  ACTIVITY 9.6

Thinking back to the area of practice you identified in Activity 9.5, how would you evaluate your project effectively?

Access the NHS Institute for Innovation and Improvement (2010) sustainability model. Consider what you would do to ensure the success of your project.

---

According to the NHS Institute for Innovation and Improvement (2010), factors that are likely to improve the chances of sustainability include:

- Where there are benefits beyond helping patients (e.g. making a difference to working lives, reducing waste, duplication or costs);
- Where benefits to patients, staff and the organisation are visible, are believed by staff and can be described clearly;
- Where changed processes will continue to meet the need of the organisations and can be maintained when an individual or group of people who initiated it are no longer there;
- When data is easily available to monitor progress or assess improvement and where there are systems to communicate this in the organisation;
- When staff play a part in the implementation of changes to processes and where the training and development of staff are provided to help sustain these changes;

- When staff ideas are taken on board and they are then given the opportunity to test these ideas and their belief that this is a better way of doing things;
- When credible and respected senior and clinical leaders are seen as promoting and investing their own time in changes;
- When the changes being made are seen as an important contribution to the overall organisational aims;
- When staff, facilities, equipment, and policies and procedures are adequate to sustain new processes.

## CASE SCENARIO

You are a registered nurse currently leading a nursing team. Over the last 12 months, the team have found it difficult to maintain the provision of good quality patient care. More recently, two registered nurse members of your team have left, having managed to secure jobs elsewhere, and despite attempts to recruit replacements their positions remain vacant. Although acknowledging the need to replace your registered nurse colleagues as soon as possible, you think there may also be an opportunity to introduce a wider skill mix into the team by recruiting nursing associates, and have been asked to produce a business case to support this plan. How would you go about this?

## Developing a business case

When developing your business case, it could be argued that the process would be similar to that outlined in the six-stage framework mentioned earlier. You would need to carry out a fair amount of research into the key issues and to consider and analyse all possible options. A good business case will explain the key issues clearly and also identify potential solutions, before going on to explain how the proposal would aim to address this. Central to your proposal, of course, should be the current and overall potential impact on patient safety, the quality of patient care provision and the patient experience. You would need to include the benefits, costs, likely timescale and the risks associated with both taking action and/or doing nothing. For example, you would point out the need to ensure sufficient capacity and capability while also making best use of available resources. Finally, you would need to make recommendations for which option you think is best. You may be able to include convincing measures of impact outcomes and success criteria from similar projects that have been implemented elsewhere, perhaps demonstrating the value and benefits your proposal will bring. Relating your proposal back to the organisational strategy or vision is always useful to demonstrate how important it is; convincing the commissioner/funding body that the solution you have proposed is the right one is absolutely key.

## Political influencing

As an adult nurse, you should be aware of the influence of UK government healthcare policies on our day-to-day practice. Undeniably, political decisions impact on every aspect of nursing at every level. Yet, it may be of no surprise to learn that many nurses appear disinterested in the political processes, despite the need more than ever before to stand together in order to be able to ensure the best possible care for patients. Speaking up and speaking out on behalf of our patients and the profession is a vital role if we wish to influence the future of UK healthcare services. Political activity consists of having the knowledge, skills, ability and will to engage and influence politicians. To do so effectively requires knowledge of current healthcare or nursing issues, laws and current health policies, in addition to all of the leadership and influencing skills highlighted in this and previous chapters.

Boswell et al. (2005) highlight that barriers to political activism are heavy workloads, feelings of powerlessness, time constraints, gender issues and a lack of understanding of the political process.

 **ACTIVITY 9.7**

Do you know how UK government works?

Find out about how you can lobby your elected political representative. Irrespective of whether this person is an MP (UK Parliament), MSP (Scottish Parliament), a member of the national Assembly for Wales (AM) or a member of the Northern Ireland Assembly, the principles of lobbying and engagement are the same.

Would you know the most effective way to get your key message across? Think about ways in which you can strengthen your case and arguments by using powerful patient stories to illustrate key issues.

## Chapter summary

The numerous current demands placed on us as nurses sometimes challenge our ability to maintain – let alone improve – patient care. However, nurses in particular will remain the first line of defence in the safeguarding of quality care and patient protection underpinning the use of recognised change management and quality improvement tools and techniques to improve care within their own sphere of influence. Dixon-Woods et al. (2012) suggest that being an effective leader or change agent involves a delicate combination of the ability to set out a clear vision while also being sensitive and aware of the needs of others. By acknowledging the complexity of change management we should recognise there is no prescribed linear order to the change process. Instead frameworks encourage leaders of change to consider and focus on a number of key interacting factors, ensuring that all the components are aligned for sustained success.

Whichever model or framework you choose to use, understanding the nature of the change or improvement you wish to make and the context in which you are working is important in determining your chosen approach. Having a clear understanding of the people, processes and organisational culture that will be affected by your change is considered crucial to success. Burnes (1996: 13) believes that 'successful change is less dependent on detailed plans and projections than on reaching an understanding of the complexity of the issues concerned and identifying the range of available options'. Whilst this seems a most sensible approach to take, research demonstrates that such factors are often overlooked, ignored or underestimated by those wishing to implement change (Kotter, 1996; Fernandez and Rainey, 2006). It is vital to also remember that any changes to services should always take into account the needs of patients and clients first and foremost. Targets require constant monitoring and revising if necessary to remain valid and meaningful.

Therefore evaluation is an essential part of this process, whether or not the change has achieved the desired outcome. Finally, within service improvement or change management initiatives the most effective leadership styles are those that seek to include others, offer clear explanations and apply gentle persuasion most effectively (Dixon-Woods et al., 2012).

## Useful websites

NICE Guidance on Service Improvement Processes: www.nice.org.uk/about/what-we-do/into-practice/audit-and-service-improvement.
NICE Quality Standards and indicators: www.nice.org.uk/standards-and-indicators.
Information on Quality Improvement in Wales: www.iqi.wales.nhs.uk/home.
Safety and Quality Standards Northern Ireland: www.health-ni.gov.uk/topics/safety-and-quality-standards/safety-and-quality-standards-service-frameworks.
NHS Improvement Resources: https://improvement.nhs.uk/resources.
Healthcare Quality Improvement Partnership: www.hqip.org.uk.
NHS Improvement Tools and Resources: https://improvement.nhs.uk/resources/quality-service-improvement-and-redesign-qsir-tools.
NHS RightCare: www.england.nhs.uk/rightcare.

## Further reading

Health Foundation (2013) *Quality Improvement Made Simple*. London: The Health Foundation.
Healthcare Quality Improvement Partnership (2015) *A Guide to Quality Improvement Methods*. London: HQIP.
King's Fund, The (2016) *Improving Quality in the English NHS. A Strategy for Action*. London: The King's Fund.
NHS Scotland Quality Improvement Hub (2014) *The Spread and Sustainability of Quality Improvement in Healthcare*. Edinburgh: Healthcare Improvement Scotland.
NHS Wales (2014) *The Quality Improvement Guide*. Cardiff: NHS Wales.
Scottish Government (2010) *The Healthcare Quality Strategy for Scotland*. Available at: www.gov.scot/Resource/Doc/311667/0098354.pdf (last accessed 23 April 2018).

## References

Alderwick, H., Robertson, R., Appleby, J., Dunn, P. and Maguire, D. (2015) *Better Value in the NHS. The Role of Changes in Clinical Practice*. London: The King's Fund.
Amnis Healthcare (2011) *Safe and Effective Service Improvement. Delivering the Safety and Productivity Agenda in Healthcare Using a LEAN Approach*. San Diego, CA: Amnis Healthcare: Available at: www.choiceforum.org/docs/ses.pdf (last accessed 19 April 2018).
Andersen, H., Røvik, K.A. and Ingebrigtsen, T. (2014) 'Lean thinking in hospitals: is there a cure for the absence of evidence? A systematic review of reviews', *BMJ Open*, 4: e003873. doi:10.1136/bmjopen-2013-003873.
Andrews, A. and Butler, M. (2014) *Trusted to Care. An Independent Review of the Princess of Wales Hospital and Neath Port Talbot Hospital at Abertawe Bro Morgannwg University Health Boards* (Executive Summary). Available at: http://gov.wales/topics/health/publications/health/reports/care (last accessed 8 April 2018).
Batalden, P.B. and Davidoff, F. (2007) 'What is "quality improvement" and how can it transform healthcare?', *Quality and Safety in Healthcare*, 16: 2–3.
Bate, P., Bevan, H. and Robert, G. (2004) *Towards a Million Change Agents: A Review of the Social Movements Literature: Implications for Large Scale Change in the NHS*. London: NHS Modernisation Agency.

Beresford, P. (2013) *Beyond the Usual Suspects*. London: Shaping our lives. Available at: www.shapingourlives.org.uk/documents/BTUSFINDINGS.pdf (last accessed 21 April 2018).

Berwick, D.M. (2003) 'Disseminating innovations in healthcare', *JAMA*, 289(15): 1969–75.

Bevan, H. (2013) *What Can Civil Rights Leaders Teach us about Strategy for Transformation?* Available at: www.hsj.co.uk/opinion/blogs/the-nhs-change-agent/the-nhs-change-agent/5003114.bloglead (last accessed 2 September 2013).

Blanchard, K. and Johnson, S. (1982) *The One Minute Manager*. New York: William Morrow.

Boswell, C., Cannon, S. and Miller, J. (2005) 'Nurses' political involvement: responsibility versus privilege', *Journal of Professional Nursing*, 21(1): 5–8.

Bullock, R.J. and Batten, D. (1985) '"It's just a phase we're going through": a review and synthesis of OD phase analysis', *Group and Organization Studies*, 10: 383–412.

Burnes, B. (1996) 'No such thing as . . . a "one best way" to manage organizational change', *Management Decision*, 34(10): 11–18.

By, R.T. (2005) 'Organisational change management: a critical review', *Journal of Change Management*, 5(4): 369–80.

Care Quality Commission (2012) *The State of Healthcare and Adult Social Care in England*. London: CQC.

Care Quality Commission (2018) *Essential Standards for Quality and Safety*. London: CQC. Available at: www.cqc.org.uk/what-we-do/how-we-do-our-job/fundamental-standards (last accessed 16 April 2018).

Coulter, A. (2012) *Leadership for Patient Engagement*. Available at: www.kingsfund.org.uk/leadershipreview (last accessed 8 October 2018).

D'Andreamatteo, A., Ianni, L., Lega, F. and Sargiacomo, M. (2015) 'Lean in healthcare: A comprehensive review', *Health Policy*, 119: 1197–209.

Department of Health (1998) *A First Class Service Quality in the New NHS*. London: DH. Available at: http://webarchive.nationalarchives.gov.uk (last accessed 8 October 2018).

Department of Health (2010) *Essence of Care*. London: DH.

Department of Health (2012a) *The NHS Outcomes Framework 2013–14*. London: DH.

Department of Health (2012b) *The Public Health Outcomes Framework for England, 2013–2016*. London: DH.

Department of Health (2013) *Adult Social Care Outcomes Framework*. London: DH.

Department of Health, Social Services and Public Safety (2011) *Quality 2020: A Ten Year Strategy to Protect and Improve Quality in Health and Social Care in Northern Ireland*. Belfast: DHSSPS.

Dixon-Woods, M., McNichol, S. and Martin, G. (2012) 'Ten challenges in improving quality in healthcare: lessons from the Healthcare Foundation's programme evaluations and relevant literature', *BMJ Quality & Safety*, 21: 876–84.

Donabedian, A. (2005) 'Evaluating the quality of medical care 1966', *The Milbank Quarterly*, 83(4): 691–729.

Fernandez, R. and Rainey, H.G. (2006) 'Managing successful organisational change in the public sector', *Public Administration Review*, March/April: 168–76.

Francis, R. (2013) *Report of the Mid Staffordshire NHS Foundation Trust Public Inquiry Executive Summary*. Available at: http://webarchive.nationalarchives.gov.uk/20150407084003/http://www.midstaffspublicinquiry.com/report (last accessed 22 March 2018).

Greenhalgh, T., Robert, G., Bate, P., Macfarlane, F. and Kyriakidou, O. (2005) *Diffusion of Innovations in Health Service Organisations: A Systematic Literature Review*. Oxford: Blackwell Publishing.

Grimshaw, J.M., Eccles, M.P., Lavis, J.N., Hill, S.J. and Squires, J.E. (2012) 'Knowledge translation of research findings', *Implementation Science*, 7: 50

Grol, R. (1997) 'Beliefs and evidence in changing clinical practice', *British Medical Journal*, 315: 418–25.

Grol, R. and Grimshaw, J. (2003) 'From best evidence to best practice: effective implementation of change in patients' care', *The Lancet*, 362(9391): 1225–30.

Hardacre, J., Cragg, R., Shapiro, J., Spurgeon, P. and Flanagan, H. (2011) *What's Leadership Got to Do With It?* London: The Health Foundation.

Health Foundation (2015) *What's Getting in the Way? Barriers to Improvement in the NHS*. London: The Health Foundation.

Kanter, R.M., Stein, B.A. and Jick, T.D. (1992) *The Challenge of Organizational Change*. New York: The Free Press.

King's Fund, The (2012) *Leadership and Engagement for Improvement in the NHS. Together We Can*. London: The King's Fund.

King's Fund, The (2014) *People in Control of Their Own Health and Care. The State of Involvement*. London: The King's Fund.

Kirkup, B. (2015) *The Report of the Morecambe Bay Investigation*. Available at: www.gov.uk/government/publications (last accessed 21 March 2018).

Kirkup, B. (2018) *Report of the Liverpool Community Health Independent Review*. Available at: https://improvement.nhs.uk/news-alerts/independent-review-liverpool-community-health-nhs-trust-published (last accessed 21 March 2018).

Kotter, J.P. (1996) *Leading Change*. Boston, MA: Harvard Business School Press.

Kotter, J.P. (2014) *Accelerate: Building Strategic Agility for a Faster-Moving World*. Boston, MA: Harvard Business Review Press.

Kotter, J.P. and Cohen, D.S. (2002) *The Heart of Change: Real-life Stories of How People Change Their Organisations*. Boston, MA: Harvard Business School Press.

Kouzes, J. and Posner, B. (2017) *The Leadership Challenge*, 6th edn. Hoboken, NJ: Wiley.

Langley, G.L., Nolan, K.M., Nolan, T.W., Norman, C.L. and Provost, L.P. (2009) *The Improvement Guide: A Practical Approach to Enhancing Organizational Performance*, 2nd edn. San Francisco, CA: Jossey-Bass.

Larson, C.E. and LaFasto, F.M.J. (1989) *Teamwork: What Must Go Right, What Can Go Wrong*. London: Sage.

Lewin, K. (1951) *Field Theory in Social Science*. New York: Harper & Row.

Lockitt, W. (2004) *Change Management*. Available at: www.scribd.com/doc/50615816/CHANGE-MANAGEMENT (last accessed 8 October 2018).

Luxford, K., Safran, D.B. and Delbanco, T. (2011) 'Promoting patient-centered care: a qualitative study of facilitators and barriers in healthcare organizations with a reputation for improving the patient experience', *International Journal for Quality in Healthcare*, 23(5): 510–15.

Maintz, J. (2003) 'Defining and classifying clinical indicators for quality improvement', *International Journal for Quality in Healthcare*, 15(6): 523–30.

National Institute for Health and Care Excellence (2007) *How to Change Practice*. London: NICE.

National Quality Board (2013) *Quality in the New Health System: Maintaining and Improving Quality* (Final Report). Available at: www.gov.uk/government/publications/quality-in-the-new-health-system-maintaining-and-improving-quality-from-april-2013 (last accessed 5 October 2018).

NHS England (2013) *Review into the Quality of Care and Treatment Provided by 14 Hospital Trusts in England*: Overview report. Available at: www.nhs.uk/NHSEngland/bruce-keogh-review/Documents/outcomes/keogh-review-final-report.pdf (last accessed 19 April 2018).

NHS England (2014) *Five Year Forward View*. London: NHS England.

NHS England (2016) *Leading Change Adding Value. A Framework for Nursing, Midwifery and Care Staff*. London: NHS England.

NHS Institute for Innovation and Improvement (2010) *The Handbook of Quality and Service Improvement Tools*. Coventry: NHS Institute for Innovation and Improvement.

NHS Institute for Innovation and Improvement (2013) *Six-stage Framework for Service Improvement*. Available at: www.institute.nhs.uk/quality_and_service_improvement_tools/quality_and_service_improvement_tools/ (last accessed 23 April 2018).

NHS Scotland (2010) *The Healthcare Quality Strategy for NHS Scotland*. Edinburgh: The Scottish Government.

NHS Wales (2013) *Safe Care, Compassionate Care. A National Governance Framework to Enable High Quality Care in NHS Wales*. Cardiff: NHS Wales.

NHS Wales (2014) *The Quality Improvement Guide*. Cardiff: NHS Wales.

Northouse, P.G. (2012) *Introduction to Leadership Concepts and Practice*, 2nd edn. London: Sage.

Nursing and Midwifery Council (2018a) *The Code: Professional Standards of Practice Behaviour for Nurses and Midwives*. London: NMC.

Nursing and Midwifery Council (2018b) *Future Nurse: Standards of Proficiency for Registered Nurses.* London: NMC.

Olson, E.E. and Eoyang, G.H. (2001) *Facilitating Organizational Change: Lessons from Complexity Science.* San Francisco, CA: Jossey-Bass/Pfeiffer.

Pearson, M.L., Upenieks, V.V., Yee, T. and Needleman, J. (2008) 'Spreading nursing unit innovation in large hospital systems', *Journal of Nursing Administration*, 38(3): 146–52.

Porter-O'Grady, T. (2003) 'A different age for leadership, part 1', *Journal of Nursing Administration*, 33(10): 105–10.

Reed, J.E. and Card, A.J. (2016) 'The problem with plan–do–study–act cycles', *BMJ Quality & Safety*, published online 12 January 2016. Available at: doi:10.1136/bmjqs-2015-005076 (last accessed 25 April 2018).

Rogers, E.M. (2003) *Diffusion of Innovations.* New York: Free Press.

Scottish Government (2017) *Health and Social Care Standards. My Support, My Life.* Edinburgh: Scottish Government.

Silber, M.B. (1993) 'The "Cs" in excellence: choice and change', *Nursing Management*, 24(9): 60–2.

Solberg, L., Mosser, G. and McDonald, S. (1997) 'The three faces of performance measurement: improvement, accountability and research', *Joint Commission Journal on Quality Improvement*, 23(3): 135–47.

Taylor, M.J., McNicholas, C., Nicolay, C., Darzi, A., Bell, D. and Reed, J.E. (2013) 'Systematic review of the application of the plan–do–study–act method to improve quality in healthcare', *BMJ Quality & Safety*, 23: 290–8. Available at: http://dx.doi.org/10.1136/ bmjqs-2013-002703 (last accessed 25 April 2018).

# PART 2

# CARING FOR ADULTS IN A VARIETY OF SETTINGS

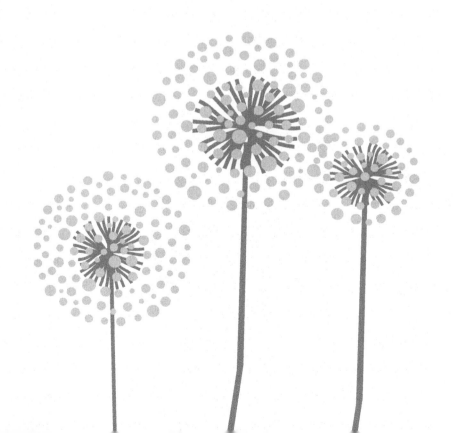

# SUPPORTING AND PROMOTING HEALTH

## HELEN DAVIDSON, KAREN ILEY AND SUSAN RAMSDALE (WITH JANICE CHRISTIE, JULIE GRAILEY AND CAROL MCGLONE)

---

**CHAPTER OBJECTIVES**

- Introduce the principles and practice of epidemiology;
- Consider the range of opportunities available to promote health to a variety of individuals, families and patient groups within any contemporary healthcare setting;
- Outline required health promotion skills for registered nurses.

---

At this point you might be thinking that 'health promotion' is exclusively the domain of practice nurses, school nurses and health visitors. However, although health promotion is indeed a significant aspect of the community practitioner role (Baisch, 2009), there is now an expectation that all nurses will work to promote health whenever the opportunity arises, irrespective of the practice setting (Nursing and Midwifery Council [NMC], 2018a, 2018b). Health promotion interventions may be carried out with individuals, families or communities (National Institute for Health and Care Excellence [NICE], 2007a, 2008a, 2014). Indeed, it is important to remember that individuals at all stages of life can benefit from health promotion (Salva et al., 2009; Rosenberg and Yates, 2014; NICE, 2015; Public Health England [PHE], 2016a).

The range of public health issues affecting populations on both a national and a global level is vast (World Health Organization [WHO], 2002; PHE, 2013, 2014), though this chapter will focus specifically on modifiable lifestyle behaviours/risk factors – particularly in relation to cardiovascular disease (CVD), obesity, sexual health and mental health – because these have significant implications for the health and wellbeing of the adult population across the UK (Health Protection Agency, 2009; Myint et al., 2011).

# Related NMC proficiencies for registered nurses

Adult nurses play a key role in improving and maintaining the mental, physical and behavioural health and wellbeing of individuals, families, communities and populations. They support and enable people at all stages of life and across all care settings to make informed choices about how to prevent ill health and manage health challenges in order to maximise their quality of life and improve health. They also engage in activities aimed at preventing or protecting against disease and ill health, public health, community development, global health agendas and the reduction of health inequalities (NMC, 2018b).

## To achieve entry to the nursing register you must be able to

- Understand the importance of early years' interventions and the impact of adverse life experiences on lifestyle choices and mental and physical wellbeing;
- Understand and explain the contribution of social influences, health literacy, individual circumstances, behaviours and lifestyle choices to mental and physical health outcomes in people, families and communities;
- Demonstrate knowledge of epidemiology, demography, genomics, and the wider determinants of health, illness and wellbeing at all stages of life and apply this to an understanding of patterns of health and illness and health outcomes;
- Understand the aims and principles of health promotion and health improvement and be able to apply these when caring for individuals, families, communities and populations;
- Understand and explain the principles, practice and evidence base for health screening when engaging with individuals, families and populations, in order to promote and improve mental and physical health outcomes;
- Understand and apply the principles of pathogenesis and immunology, and the evidence base for immunisation, vaccination and herd immunity when engaging with individuals, families and populations to promote health and avoid ill health;
- Identify and use every appropriate opportunity to discuss with people the impact of lifestyle choices including smoking, substance use, alcohol, sexual behaviours, diet and exercise on mental, physical, cognitive and behavioural health and wellbeing;
- Critically appraise and apply information about health outcomes when supporting people and families to manage their healthcare needs and make health choices;
- Explain and demonstrate the use of up-to-date approaches to behaviour change to enable individuals, families and populations to use their strengths and expertise, and make informed choices when managing their own health and making lifestyle adjustments.

(Adapted from NMC, 2018b)

## Background

Historically, health concerns have focused on infections and accidents (Rosen, 1993). Although these are still a concern today, the recognition that lifestyle is a major cause of morbidity and mortality (Upton and Thirlaway, 2010) has led to a growing emphasis on a number of UK public health strategies (Department of Health [DH], 2012a; Department of Health, Social Services and Public Safety [DHSSPS], 2014; PHE, 2014) and the role of the nurse in the implementation of these (Royal College of Nursing [RCN], 2012, 2016; DH, 2012a; PHE, 2014).

The evolution of public health has demonstrated that there are a range of factors that influence the health of a population. For health promotion interventions to be carried out effectively, you will need to understand the basic underlying principles (e.g. population health and epidemiology). Epidemiology studies the distribution of health events in particular populations (Last, 1988) and as such can be applied to the control of such events (Mulhall, 1996). These concepts will be discussed and clarified in more detail throughout the chapter. At this point, it is perhaps useful to explore the way public health has evolved over the years.

---

 **THE FOUR STAGES OF PUBLIC HEALTH**

1. *Sanitary reform 1848–1870s*: focused on: environmental issues and change.

   During this time, Dr John Snow used the principles of epidemiology to identify the link between an outbreak of cholera and the use of the Broad Street water pump in London. This is a useful example of a population-based approach to health events because the water pump was disabled by having its handle removed – thereby effectively ending the outbreak (Gunn and Masellis, 2008).

2. *Sanitary science 1870–1930s*: focused on personal preventative measures.

   Interestingly, the lifetime of Florence Nightingale spanned both stages (sanitary reform and sanitary science) and the principles of these stages are evident in the many accounts of her work (Bostridge, 2009).

3. *Therapeutic era 1930s to late 1970s*: focused on therapeutic interventions.

   This stage saw a real increase in emphasis on hospital services and pharmaceutical approaches to medicine and health, although not all were in agreement that this would be the panacea for all health issues (McKeown, 1976).

4. *New public health, the 1980s to the present day*: focuses on medical/social/environmental aspects, personal preventative measures and therapeutic intervention.

---

In 1974, Lalonde highlighted the preventable aspects of ill health. This was presented via a framework called the 'Health Field Concept', which organised the various influences on health into four key areas: human biology, the environment, lifestyle and healthcare organisation. This concept can still be applied to modern-day public health policy and practice. For example, the effective promotion of 'healthy eating' would consider all of these four areas (DH, 2012a, 2012b; PHE, 2016b) (Figure 10.1).

## Health inequalities

To consider why there is a need for good public health it is necessary to look at the variations between the health and life experiences for different individuals and groups in society. Inequalities in health and premature death have been evident since the pioneering work of Edwin Farr in 1842, who noted the difference in the life expectancy of people living in the wealthiest and poorest parts

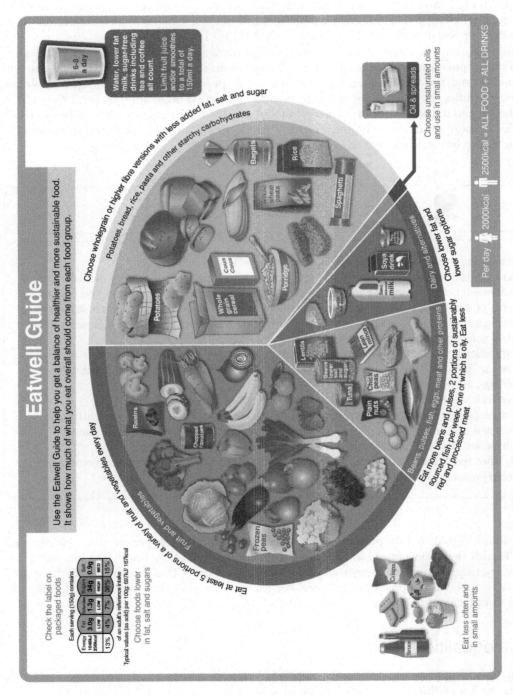

**Figure 10.1** The eatwell guide (Public Health England in association with the Welsh government, Food Standards Scotland and the Food Standards Agency in Northern Ireland)

of London. More recently, the Black Report (Townsend et al., 1992), Acheson (1998) Report and Marmot Review (Marmot, 2010) have continued to show that social factors such as wealth and environment have an impact on health. Other factors also contribute to inequalities in health including age, gender, ethnicity, sexuality and disability, and contemporary evidence continues to demonstrate this relationship. For example, the poorest 10% of the population will have the lowest life expectancy and healthy life expectancy those of the wealthiest 10% (Office for National Statistics, 2018b).

Marmot (2010) suggests that adverse socioeconomic circumstances accumulate over the life course. He proposes that health disadvantage begins at conception and continues through life for the poorest, resulting in early and avoidable mortality. Therefore an understanding of the relationship between health and social factors is crucial for adult nurses so they can support patients in a sensitive manner, appreciating the difficulties faced by poorer families.

In contemporary public health practice, the broad concept of health promotion is underpinned by principles of 'equity', 'participation' and 'empowerment' (WHO, 1986; Davies and Macdowall, 2006). Although it is likely that you will come across these terms as you read around the general nursing literature, we should consider these again within the context of health promotion practice:

*Equity*: it is important to consider this principle when thinking about the many determinants of health. For example, a population may share a similar level of access to healthcare services but have an unequal level of income or education. Broadly speaking, this can have a negative impact on health. Life expectancy can be (among other things) determined by the level of deprivation or affluence in a particular area (Marmot, 2010). In response to this, a number of health promotion initiatives aim to address 'inequalities in health' such as the provision of cookery lessons and food vouchers for low-income young families (DH, 2012b). Nevertheless, the issue of health inequalities continues to be important for modern Britain (Marmot, 2010).

*Participation*: the involvement of service users is a significant feature of contemporary UK healthcare policy (for example, DH, 2010; DHSSPS, 2014) and the views of patients, carers and communities are both desired and valued (Griffiths et al., 2012). As adult nurses it can be easy to overlook the significance of family, friends and the wider community when working with individual patients. Yet in many instances these 'hold the key' to achieving real results in health promotion (Koshy et al., 2010). A good example of this is the 'peer support' schemes available to breastfeeding mothers, where the main source of infant feeding support is another mother from the local community rather than the community nurse (Thomson et al., 2011). Nevertheless, the community nurse would still play a role here by referring mothers on to the peer support service and continuing to liaise with the local community.

*Empowerment*: within health promotion practice 'empowerment' is mainly about ensuring the service user has the resources, support and information required to make decisions about their own health and lifestyle (DH, 2010). For example, many community nurses work with patients who express a desire to stop smoking but do not feel confident in taking control of their smoking behaviour. The nurse might then work with the patient to help them identify the 'stage of change' they are at (Prochaska and DiClemente, 1986) in order to guide the motivational interviewing process (Karatay et al., 2010). In addition, the community nurse could perhaps prescribe a tailored regimen of nicotine replacement therapy, signpost the service user to additional smoking cessation services (DH, 2012a) and offer regular emotional support. Here, the community nurse can empower service users to reduce or stop their smoking at their own pace and on their own terms.

Registered nurses need to be aware of the resources that individuals, families and communities have access to when assessing their health needs and planning interventions. There is a wealth of evidence to show that social factors influence people's health. Current evidence shows that the richest fifth of the population has 12 times more wealth than the poorest fifth in the UK (ONS, 2016b). This has an impact on the choices people can make to keep healthy and presents challenges to us as nurses. For example, if we are promoting healthy eating we should consider the individual or family budget, cultural issues, and the quality of their food storage and preparation facilities. In addition, we need to think about the accessibility, availability and affordability of healthy food because this can vary from place to place. Understanding the various determinants of health will help us anticipate and plan for targeted health promotion activity.

Dahlgren and Whitehead (1991) offer a useful visual representation of the various determinants of health (Figure 10.2). Here they demonstrate that health is not solely dependent on healthcare services. Their work reflects the 'Health Field Concept' as presented by Lalonde (1974), i.e. health is also affected by individuals themselves and their social and material resources, which are in turn influenced by healthcare policy (Naidoo and Wills, 2009). It is therefore clear that the nurse's role in health promotion is wide and far-reaching, and in many instances requires committed, joined-up working with other agencies (Green and Tones, 2010).

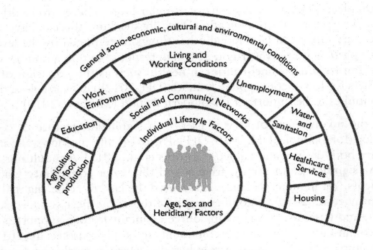

**Figure 10.2**   Influences on health (Dahlgren and Whitehead, 1991)

When thinking about the type of health promotion activity we might use, we need to consider whether the level of prevention we are aiming for is 'primary', 'secondary' or 'tertiary' (Loveday and Linsley, 2011). This is an important concept in health promotion theory because it helps both nurse and service user have realistic expectations of the planned intervention.

## Levels of prevention

- Primary: to prevent the disease developing at all (the likely focus is population wide);
- Secondary: to prevent the disease from progressing (the likely focus is those at risk but not unwell);
- Tertiary: to prevent the consequences of the disease.

Consider the different scenarios below. Make a note of whether you think the level of prevention offered is primary, secondary or tertiary:

- The diabetes nurse specialist advises a 22-year-old woman with type 1 diabetes mellitus on her diet, insulin regimens and glucose monitoring.
- A 78-year-old man is given his annual influenza vaccination by the practice nurse.
- A 37-year-old woman is offered annual mammograms after being identified as carrying the *BRCA1* gene.

Was deciding on the level of prevention clear and straightforward or were some of the scenarios more difficult to appraise?

(Note: do not worry if you found this activity challenging – in clinical practice cases can be more or less complex depending on factors such as age, gender, lifestyle and any other illnesses or 'co-morbidities' a patient may have.)

Deciding whether an intervention is primary, secondary or tertiary is not as easy as it looks. For example, in areas such as cancer care, the distinctions are less clear (Silberstein and Parsons, 2010). Also, although a combination of approaches may have a significant effect on some disease outcomes there are other conditions, such as some musculoskeletal disorders where there is a particular emphasis on primary prevention (Rozenfeld et al., 2010).

'Prevention is better than cure'.

*(Desiderius Erasmus)*

As we consider primary prevention in public health, it is important to include the significant role of immunisation (vaccination) programmes. The prevention of communicable disease by mass inoculation can be extremely effective (Hamami et al., 2017). Indeed, in terms of public health practice, only the provision of clean water performs better (Plotkin et al., 2017). This is particularly the case when a 'critical mass' of the target population is immunised, thus achieving 'herd immunity' (Fine et al., 2011) (Figure 10.3). Although 'disease-specific herd immunity thresholds' can vary (Betsch et al., 2017), the WHO-recommended target for immunisation uptake is 95% for most programmes (Andre et al., 2008). When a sufficient proportion of the 'herd' has been immunised, this affords some protection for the remaining non-immunised population, due to the rate of transmission being slowed or stopped (Vynnycky and White, 2010). This additional benefit of 'herd immunity' is of notable value to those who are immunocompromised (Cesaro et al., 2014). The growing issue of antimicrobial resistance may pose an additional risk to immunocompromised individuals (DH, 2013a) because they may contract an infection without having effective medication as a treatment option (Dumford, 2016).

The impact of 'herd immunity' on the population demonstrates the need for a high uptake of immunisation programmes across the UK. Nevertheless, although it is desirable to aim for as high an uptake as possible, there are a number of factors that can affect participation (Vynnycky and White, 2010). As adult nurses it is important that we are mindful of these, because it will help us to carry out effective, targeted health promotion. For example, health beliefs in relation to the vaccination (and the disease it aims to prevent) can have a significant effect on uptake (Funk and Klepac, 2015). In addition, potential recipients may be allergic to some part of the vaccine (Chung, 2013), and those with a compromised

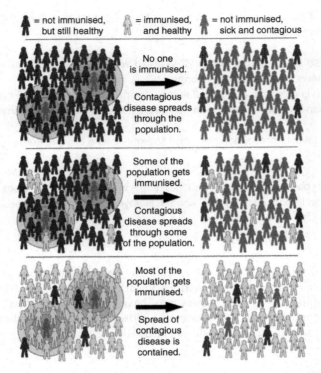

**Figure 10.3** Herd immunity (from National Institute of Allergy and Infectious Diseases)

immune system due to existing morbidity and/or medical treatment would be unable to receive vacci-nations (Andre et al., 2008). Due consideration should also be given to the efficacy of the vaccine (Plotkin et al., 2017), which can vary according to the disease and population even when uptake is high (Fine et al., 2011). For example, the influenza vaccine does not protect against every strain of the virus (Public Health England, 2017a). Conversely, for another disease the specificity of the vaccination may be high (Delves et al., 2017), but some individuals may not produce the desired immune response upon receiving the vaccination, for a variety of reasons (Plotkin et al., 2017).

## ACTIVITY 10.1

- Have a look at the data available on adults' immunisation uptake across the UK: https://gov.uk>statistics. Are there any notable differences in uptake?
- Note down anything you observe in relation to these differences, for example is uptake very different in one part of the UK compared to another? What do you think may have contributed to these differences?
- How could you as an adult nurse positively influence immunisation uptake in your future practice?

# Behaviour change for health

Thus far we have established that the level of 'prevention' can vary depending on the patient's individual risk factors and current diagnosis. However, this is not the only consideration in health promotion practice. Adult nurses can have an impact on the health of individuals, families and communities within a range of settings (NICE, 2007b, 2008a, 2014), while also influencing health policy at a local and national level (Naidoo and Wills, 2009). Here health promotion models are particularly useful, because they identify the different levels of change:

- Individual behaviour change;
- Community development and action;
- Communication strategies;
- Organisational change;
- Public policy change.

For example, the health belief model (Becker, 1974; Rosenstock, 1974) draws on health psychology and focuses on individual belief systems in relation to lifestyle choices. An understanding of health psychology is a key part of effective health promotion because it can provide the practitioner with a range of tools to use. Some of these models are outlined in Table 10.1. Although these models differ, they all share the view that the individual's level of 'self-efficacy' or 'perceived control' may have an impact on the lifestyle decision he or she makes.

**Table 10.1**  An overview of models used in health psychology – and their application to health promotion

| Nature of model/ approach | Author(s) | Key features |
| --- | --- | --- |
| Health belief model | Rosenstock (1974); Becker (1974) | Acknowledge the influence of demographics, social class, gender, age, internal and external cues |
| | | Perceived susceptibility and severity of the negative health outcome plays a key role |
| | | The perceived benefits and barriers to the behaviour change are also important |
| | | Specific 'cues to action'/perception of threat can contribute to a behaviour change |
| | | Levels of self-efficacy inform decision to change |
| Transtheoretical model | Prochaska and DiClemente (1986) | Suggest that change follows 'sequential' stages |
| | | Describe 'processes' which people typically use to facilitate change |
| | | Change can be predicted by consideration of the 'decisional balance' |
| | | Self-efficacy is described as the person's confidence in their ability to make changes |

*(Continued)*

**Table 10.1**   (Continued)

| Nature of model/ approach | Author(s) | Key features |
| --- | --- | --- |
| | | This model has been applied to a variety of unhealthy behaviours (for example, smoking, alcohol consumption, exercise, diet, drug abuse) with evidence to suggest that health promotion programmes that are designed or tailored around each of the stages above are more effective (Noar et al., 2007) |
| Theory of planned behaviour | Ajzen (1991) | An extension of the theory of reasoned action (Ajzen and Fishbein, 1980) |
| | | Used to study cognitive determinants of health behaviours |
| | | Behaviour is determined by the strength of intention and the level of control a person perceives they have |
| | | Acknowledges the role of 'subjective norms' in influencing behaviour choices, e.g. perceived social pressure to perform or not perform a behaviour (Ajzen, 1991) |
| 'Mode of intervention' and 'Focus of intervention' criteria used to generate four models of health promotion activity | Beattie (1991) | *Focus* of intervention may be *individual* or *collective* |
| | | *Mode* of intervention may be *authoritative* (top-down and expert-led) or *negotiated* (bottom-up, individual) |
| | | Health promotion practice identified as: |
| | | Health persuasion (authoritative, individual); Legislative action (authoritative, collective); Personal counselling (negotiated, individual); Community development (negotiated, collective) |
| Three overlapping spheres of activity: health education, prevention and health protection | Tannahill (1990) | Health education: communication to enhance wellbeing and prevent ill-health through influencing knowledge and attitudes |
| | | Prevention: reducing or avoiding the risk of disease and ill health primarily through medical intervention |
| | | Health protection: safeguarding population health through legislative, fiscal or social measures |
| Five approaches to health promotion activity | Ewles and Simnett (2003) | Medical approach: treatment, for example drugs |
| | | Behavioural approach: providing advice and guidance |
| | | Educational approach: specific information and/or training provided |
| | | Empowerment approach: life skills approach, for example assertiveness and communication |
| | | Social change approach: appraisal of services available, lobbying, campaigning |

This table represents some of the health promotion models available. Further reading in relation to each specific model or approach is recommended.

- As an adult nurse, think about how you could influence the patient's level of self-efficacy.
- How does this link to the practice of empowerment?

Due to the varied nature of the nurse's role in health promotion, it can sometimes be difficult to decide which approach to take when working with patients. Fortunately, a number of health promotion models have been created in order to make sense of and simplify the complexity of health promotion (Davies and Macdowall, 2006). Nurses can use these models to help select the most relevant type of health promotion activity and decide whether the intervention is individually or collectively focused. We will look at some of the most commonly used models a little later in the chapter.

The potential scope of health promotion activity is vast and goes beyond working with the individual. Therefore, in addition to models that focus on the individual, there are also 'collective' models such as community development theory (Fawcett et al., 1995) which acknowledge the importance of harnessing the resources within a community.

At this point you may be thinking about the sheer number of theoretical models you could refer to – at times seem a little overwhelming. Table 10.1 above summarises the main features of the most well-known models. These models specifically focus on an area of health promotion and tend to acknowledge both individual and community approaches to public health interventions. 'Health promotion' models are particularly useful because they incorporate the many determinants of health with a combined approach to health promotion (Nutbeam and Harris, 2010).

Although there are only a selection of models here, you will see that there are a number of approaches to health promotion practice with a varied emphasis on each component.

- Consider which of these models appear particularly applicable to your own nursing practice. Why is this so?
- Try to identify three strengths and limitations for each model.

The above activity helps to illustrate that the scope of our practice as adult nurses goes beyond our immediate setting, with the potential for involvement in broader activity such as national campaigns and lobbying parliament (Naidoo and Wills, 2009).

## Health needs assessment

Before any health promotion activity is carried out, we should carry out an effective assessment of health needs – in terms of the individual, family and community – because as highlighted in previous chapters assessment is an important element of the nursing process (Kozier, 2008).

- What is a community health needs assessment?
- What knowledge and information would you need to be able to carry this out effectively?

A community health needs assessment is a process that systematically reviews the health of a population, informing on priorities and the allocation of resources (Cavanagh and Chadwick, 2005). Effective health promotion requires a thorough knowledge of the health issues in any given community (Naidoo and Wills, 2009). Although this is particularly relevant to the work of community practitioners (Rowe et al., 2001), knowledge of an individual's local community is important for all nurses because this also informs effective assessment and discharge planning (Timby, 2012).

## The five stages of a community health needs assessment

1. Planning and beginning the process;
2. Identifying the health priorities;
3. Assessing a priority for action;
4. Action planning for change;
5. Moving on/project review.

(Adapted from Cavanagh and Chadwick, 2005: 20)

It is helpful to refer to Bradshaw's (1972) taxonomy of need when assessing the health of a community:

- *Normative*: an agreed standard that is laid down by an expert professional body, i.e. as defined by professionals;
- *Felt*: as perceived by individuals (a subjective view of need);
- *Expressed*: demanded or felt need turned into action;
- *Comparative*: exists when two groups of people with the same condition receive an unequal provision of services (i.e. the variation between different population groups).

A good community assessment includes standard measurements such as epidemiological data and the views of service users.

Think back over the last few months about any assessment (individual, family or community) that you have encountered and consider the following:

- Was this assessment based on normative needs?
- Were 'other' needs discovered ('expressed', 'felt')?
- What do you think are the challenges in discovering 'expressed' and 'felt' needs?

Health needs assessment is not always straightforward, yet it is a key aspect of service planning (Green and Tones, 2010). We have to make sure that the appropriate modes of assessment are used and that the people involved know about the significant health issues in a community and can make changes happen (DH, 2010).

There are three main perspectives:

1. The epidemiological perspective;
2. The health economist's perspective, e.g. is the health promotion intervention 'clinically effective' and 'cost effective'?;
3. The sociological perspective, e.g. the health issue is considered from a sociological perspective, including a consideration of health inequalities.

Epidemiological data helps us identify the main health issues in a particular area (Mulhall, 1996) and includes morbidity and mortality rates, census data and deprivation scores (Naidoo and Wills, 2009).

*Mortality rates*: the rates of death within a defined population over a defined timeframe.

*Morbidity rates*: the 'incidence' and 'prevalence' of a particular disease, condition or event within a defined population.

*Census data* can demonstrate the social and economic differences between populations. Sources include the Office of National Statistics (ONS) data.

The *Index of Multiple Deprivation* (IMD) measures various indicators to obtain a score of relative deprivation (e.g. affluence).

## What is the difference between 'incidence' and 'prevalence'?

As a nurse you will come across these terms very frequently and at times it will seem that they are used almost interchangeably. There is, however, a notable difference between the two, with implications for your role as an adult nurse. 'Incidence' refers to the number of new cases of a particular disease, condition or event in a particular population (usually within the previous year). 'Prevalence' refers to the total number of cases in a particular population (at a set point or period in time), some of which may have been diagnosed for a number of years.

- What can incidence rates tell us about our health promotion practice?

There are a range of factors to consider when assessing community health needs and as adult nurses it is reassuring for us to know that this information may be obtained from a range of sources. Nevertheless, although population health is a regional, national and global concern (WHO, 2002), the role of the nurse in everyday practice is also significant. For example, a five-minute conversation with a patient before their discharge can help signpost them towards resources of which they would otherwise be unaware. A useful example of this is sexual health screening services for the over-55 age group (DH, 2013b). Alternatively, depending on the setting, adult nurses can form longer-term relationships with patients and can implement more focused health promotion strategies. This could involve the facilitation of a 'patient support' group with diabetic patients (Gillett et al., 2010), the delivery of a cardiac rehabilitation programme within the community (Taylor et al., 2010) or motivational interviewing as part of a smoking cessation package (Karatay et al., 2010). The approach to health promotion can vary depending on the patient, setting and resources available. In this respect, health promotion can either be 'planned', e.g. as part of a wider public health initiative (RCN, 2012), or 'opportunistic', e.g. delivered as the need arises (RCN, 2016). The role of the nurse in 'making every contact count' (NHS Future Forum, 2012) is an essential element of the national health promotion strategy (Percival, 2014).

- What are the potential health needs (and any challenges to health promotion) of your workplace/ placement setting or geographical area?
- How might these be addressed?
- What are the challenges and what steps could be taken to overcome these?
- What opportunities do you have to incorporate health promotion within your everyday nursing practice?

## Policy and health promotion

In general, a policy is a statement about a goal in healthcare and a plan for achieving that goal (Earle et al., 2007). For example, to prevent a flu epidemic in older people, a policy relating to inoculating that population is developed and implemented. A White Paper is an official government report that sets out the government's policy on a matter that is presented to parliament. Acts, on the other hand, are laws, for example the Clean Air Act 1956 (see www.legislation.gov.uk/ukpga/Eliz2/4-5/52/ enacted), the Smoking (Northern Ireland) Order (see www.legislation.gov.uk/nisi/2006/2957/contents) or the Tobacco and Primary Medical Services (Scotland) Act (see www.legislation.gov.uk/ asp/2010/3/contents). These are usually preceded by a White Paper (Masterson, 2011).

 **London's Great Smog 1952 and the Clean Air Act 1956**

London's Great Smog in 1952 occurred between 5 and 9 December 1952 (Davis and Bates, 2002). This resulted in 12,000 immediate deaths and a further 6000 subsequent deaths (Bell et al., 2004). Despite these shocking figures, the government was initially reluctant to act. Nevertheless, in 1956 the Clean Air Act banned emissions of black smoke (Naidoo and Wills, 2009). The impact of the Clean Air Act on many private households influenced the debate about public health, individual choice and the scope of government intervention.

You may come across this 'nanny state' debate today – 'individual autonomy' versus the 'needs of a population' continues to be a tension in health promotion practice.

Can you think of any examples of this?

In addition to the tension described above, there are a number of different challenges to the implementation of health promotion policy. Laws and policies are often insufficient as 'stand-alone' agents to completely change health behaviour, although they can play an important role.

For example, despite the Health Act 2006 and subsequent smoking ban, people across the UK continue to smoke (ONS, 2017a). Nevertheless, the overall prevalence of smoking has reduced since

2010 (ONS, 2017b). This demonstrates the need for us to look closely at the data available because an overall 'prevalence rate' may not provide an accurate account of adult smoking (or quit rates) in the UK. Although the overall prevalence of smoking has reduced (ONS, 2017b), this is most notable in the 18- to 24-year age group (ONS, 2017a). As the quit rates are higher in the older age groups (ONS, 2017a), this would suggest that younger adults are not starting to smoke, whereas older adults are more likely to have smoked in the past and then attempted to stop. This of course has implications for targeted health promotion, because we would need to ascertain the health promotion approach required. Similarly, we would be mindful that smoking can be more prevalent in different parts of the UK (ONS, 2017b) and in groups with lower socioeconomic status (ONS, 2017a).

Psychological theory suggests that people have to want to stop smoking (Prochaska and DiClemente, 1986) and hence there will be a group of people who do not want to stop smoking for a range of reasons (Buck and Frosini, 2012). An important consideration in a smoking cessation policy is therefore how this group of people are accessed and targeted.

Each government launches their main 'flagship' health policy, which sets out their long-term vision for the NHS. The fact that 'Public Health' was the first priority to be mentioned in *Five Year Forward View* (DH, 2014a) demonstrates the government's recognition of population health as a concern for all. Moving on from this, Public Health England has, as a subsection of the British government, also set out its strategy for protecting and improving the nation's health (PHE, 2016c).

- Reflect upon your current abilities within health promotion; do you think you have any areas for improvement?
- Have a closer look and review your answers to the previous opportunities for health promotion reflective activity and ask yourself 'How does my practice incorporate the recommendations of public health policy?'

In addition to the government policies that address a range of health issues, there are also those that address specific issues, or lifestyle factors, such as alcohol use and smoking (DH, 2011a, 2011b; Scottish Government, 2008, 2009, 2013a, 2018; Department of Health and Social Care, 2015; Cabinet Office, DHSC, HM Treasury and Prime Minister's Office, 2016).

## Lifestyle and public health

It is interesting that four lifestyle factors are associated with nearly half of the overall 'illness burden' in the UK and the developed world (Newton, 2015): excessive alcohol use, drug misuse, smoking, poor diet (including low consumption of fruit and vegetables) and low levels of physical activity. These factors often occur together (NHS Information Centre, 2012) and there is a growing interest in the reasons for this (Buck and Frosini, 2012), much like the coexistence of different illnesses in patients with long-term conditions and 'co-morbidities' (DH, 2014b). As the 'clustering' of unhealthy behaviours can have a compound effect on patients' health outcomes (Spring et al., 2012; Meader et al., 2016), these can also have implications for the approach to health promotion practice and the nurse's role (RCN, 2012).

As adult nurses we come across a range of health issues (both acute and long term) that can be influenced in part by lifestyle choices (ONS, 2011). A clear and well-known example of this is the link between smoking, lung cancer (Doll and Hill, 1950) and chronic obstructive pulmonary disease (Fletcher and Peto, 1977). Similarly, alcohol, diet, drug use and physical activity can all play a significant role in health outcomes for adults across the lifespan (Fuller, 2011). As these lifestyle behaviours often occur together (Littleton et al., 2007) this can often have a compound effect on the health of an individual (Buck and Frosini, 2012).

Alcohol intake is a recognised aspect of the British culture and lifestyle (HM Government, 2012), and in 2017 across the UK an estimated 29.2 million adults drank alcohol (ONS, 2018a). Despite this, the first national strategy for England was only published in 2003 (Prime Minister's Strategy Unit, 2003). There have been updates since then (Home Office and DH, 2007; HM Government, 2012) replicated in similar policies across the UK (Scottish Government, 2009; DHSSPS, 2011). Excess alcohol intake has been linked to a range of public health and social issues (WHO, 2014), with an increased incidence of crime (Chaplin et al., 2011) and hospital admissions when binge drinking has occurred (HM Government, 2012). At first glance we could assume that binge drinking is only a small part of our national lifestyle, yet half of the total alcohol consumption in the UK is attributed to binge drinking (HM Government, 2012).

A number of strategies have been put forward to address this issue. A notable recent policy change is that which has been implemented in Scotland, a 'Minimum Unit Pricing' strategy to reduce alcohol consumption (Scottish Government, 2018). Similarly, strategies to address the use of drugs have also been publicised (DH, 2007; Scottish Government, 2008).

- What does this mean for us as adult nurses?

We have to remember that our role is to promote health when working with individuals, groups and communities (NMC, 2018a), while also remaining non-judgemental of individual lifestyle choices (Jarvis et al., 2005).

## ⟦?⟧ ACTIVITY 10.2

Find out more about motivational interviewing. You can access some of the following websites or articles or books suggested below:

1. Wagner, C. and Ingersol, K.S. (2012) *Motivational Interviewing in Groups*. London: Guilford.
2. Miller, W.R. and Rollnick, S. (2012) *Motivational Interviewing: Helping People Change*. London: Guilford.
3. Copello, A., Velleman, R. and Templeton, L. (2005) 'Family interventions in the treatment of alcohol and drug problems', *Drug and Alcohol Review*, 24: 369–85.

Make a list of the key elements you consider important and then reflect upon how these might influence your work with:

- Individuals;
- Families;
- Groups.

Would your approach differ depending on the lifestyle behaviour being addressed?

Despite the need to consider the coexistence of unhealthy behaviours, it does not mean that we should immediately reject any intervention that focuses on just one behaviour (for example, smoking). Indeed, it may be that coexisting unhealthy behaviours do need to be addressed 'one at a time', because success in one lifestyle change may empower and motivate an individual to make other changes (Paiva et al., 2012).

We have already acknowledged the value in looking at health issues and lifestyle behaviours, both in clusters and on an individual basis. We will now focus on four specific areas – obesity, cardiovascular disease/coronary heart disease (CVD/CHD), sexual health and mental health – in more detail. These areas are all affected by at least one of the four lifestyle behaviours, as outlined by the WHO (2002), and as such can be effectively targeted for health promotion intervention (Table 10.2).

**Table 10.2**   Lifestyle problems in the UK

| Health issue | Scale of the problem | Associated lifestyle behaviours – examples |
|---|---|---|
| Obesity | Adult morbid obesity has tripled since 1993. Prevalence has increased from 15% in 1993 to 27% in 2015 (HSIC, 2014) | Low level of physical activity<br>Poor diet |
| Cardiovascular disease/coronary heart disease (CVD/CHD) | One of the leading causes of death in the England (ONS, 2016a) and across the UK | Poor diet, smoking, low levels of physical activity |
| Sexual health | Rates of infectious syphilis highest since the 1950s<br><br>Nearly 50% of pregnancies are unplanned (DH, 2013b) | Excessive alcohol use increases likelihood of risk-taking behaviour (Corte and Sommers, 2005) |
| Mental health | Suicide is the most common cause of death in men aged 20–49 years in England and Wales (ONS, 2016a)<br><br>16.6% of adults in England drinking to hazardous levels (Drummond et al., 2016)<br><br>3.1% show signs of drug dependence (Roberts et al., 2016) | |

# Obesity

Although obesity is an increasing problem, we must also consider safety, comfort, dignity and respect with regard to the nursing care of this group. Obesity can have a range of consequences on both physical and mental health (Cabinet Office, DHSC, HM Treasury and Prime Minister's Office, 2016; PHE, 2016b) and, as such, it is never too late to start or continue any intervention for addressing obesity.

## LUCY AND PAUL

Lucy is a 27-year-old woman with a BMI (body mass index) of 35. (Note that BMI is [weight in kg]/[height in m]$^2$.) She is married to Paul, 31, who has a BMI of 21. Both Lucy and Paul are smokers. Lucy works as a receptionist but has recently had a long period of absence due to back pain. Paul is a long-distance lorry driver who works erratic hours. Lucy attends an asthma clinic appointment with the practice nurse, and asks for advice about healthy weight loss. She discloses that she and Paul would like to start a family.

- What are Lucy's main health needs?
- What are the key influencing factors?
- What would be your approach to promoting Lucy's health in this scenario?
- Can you always rely on the BMI as an accurate indicator of obesity?

There are a range of factors that contribute to obesity (e.g. poor diet, physical inactivity and /or alcohol intake – NICE, 2013a, 2013b; Shelton and Knott, 2014). The impact of obesity can have consequences, for both an individual and the wider family (Flodgren et al., 2010). This is evident within this scenario, because there could be a potential impact on fertility (Pasquali et al., 2007) in addition to an increased risk of heart disease (Yusuf et al., 2001, 2004) and diabetes (Daousi et al., 2006). The good news, how-ever, is that there are a number of health promotion strategies to use in cases such as this. For example, as an adult nurse the work you do with Lucy and Paul could be on an individual, family or community basis (Naidoo and Wills, 2009) and target a range of lifestyle issues. For example, motivational inter-viewing could be implemented as part of an individual smoking cessation programme (Karatay et al., 2010), with the additional benefit of Lucy and Paul supporting each other. In turn, this would facilitate an improvement in the ability to exercise (DH, 2011a) in which case a referral to a community diet and exercise programme (NICE, 2008b; DHSSPS, 2012) would be beneficial.

However, care must be taken when evaluating the success of certain initiatives because any data gathered must be a valid measure of their impact (Flodgren et al., 2010). For example, you may have already come across the difficulty with BMI as a 'universal' measurement, e.g. some individuals with a 'high' BMI may simply have a higher muscle mass (Shah and Braverman, 2012) and/or be from a different ethnic group (NICE, 2013b) as opposed to being 'obese'. In such instances additional meas-urements such as 'waist:height ratio' should also be considered (NICE, 2013b), as well as a broader, holistic assessment of the individual (Roper et al., 2000).

## Cardiovascular disease/coronary heart disease

CVD is an umbrella term that includes disease involving the heart and/or blood vessels (Mendis et al., 2011). In 2016, 152,465 people died as a result of CVD (ONS, 2017b). Nevertheless, the overall mor-tality for CVD has been declining, although death rates are falling more slowly in younger age groups (ONS, 2017b). Mortality from CHD in England is highest in the north-west region (ONS, 2017b).

- What are the lifestyle risk factors associated with the development of CVD?

A knowledge of both risk and protective factors can help a nurse to deliver targeted and effective health promotion.

## JEAN

You are due to assess a 60-year-old woman, Jean, who has been referred to you as part of a community rehabilitation programme. She is overweight and has type 2 diabetes. She has a strong family history of CVD and suffered a myocardial infarction two weeks ago. Jean is retired, and lives with her retired husband Andy. They have one son, Martin, who lives in Australia. Jean and Andy each smoke 20 cigarettes a day.

- What assessment tools would you use to ascertain Jean's health needs?
- What health promotion initiatives could be accessed that may benefit Jean?

Jean's case scenario demonstrates the multifactorial nature of CVD (WHO, 2002; Tolstrup et al., 2014) and the implications of this for health promotion practice. The importance of a case-specific assessment is apparent here, because it would appear that the evidence for home and centre-based cardiac rehabilitation services demonstrates a broadly equal level of effectiveness (Taylor et al., 2010). Therefore, further exploration of factors such as personal preference and convenience would enable the nurse to implement an appropriate health promotion initiative (Naidoo and Wills, 2009).

# Sexual health

Sexual health needs vary according to factors such as age, gender, sexuality and ethnicity. Some individuals are particularly at risk of poor sexual health. However, although individuals' needs may vary, there are certain core needs that are common to everyone (DH, 2013b: 4). Although there is a growing awareness of sexual health within the UK, there are a number of ongoing issues in England. For example, there has been a small but steady increase in diagnosis of infection with *Chlamydia* in women over the age of 65 since 2012 (PHE, 2017b).

## RICHARD AND DAVID

Richard and his partner David have both attended the sexual health clinic as part of the local screening services for MSM (men who have sex with men). Both Richard and David attend the clinic for their results and state that they are happy to obtain their results together. When you access the records you see that David has tested positive for *Chlamydia* but Richard hasn't.

- What are the wider issues involved here?
- How could you overcome these challenges to health promotion?
- What nursing skills would be required in this scenario?

*(Continued)*

(Continued)

Now consider the many factors that may affect or inform sexual health. This may include religious beliefs, social norms, drug and alcohol use, and issues of vulnerability, coercion and abuse.

- What strategies could you employ as an adult nurse to address these factors as part of your nursing assessment?

## Promoting mental health

About one in four people in the UK suffers from mental health problems each year, with many going untreated. Mental illness is estimated to account for almost a quarter of the total burden of disease (Parkin and Powell, 2017).

- Mental health – as opposed to mental illness – has many benefits including healthier lifestyles, better physical health, improved recovery from illness, and better employment prospects and income (Friedli, 2009). But what is 'mental health'?

Concepts of mental health include subjective wellbeing, perceived self-efficacy, autonomy, competence, intergenerational dependence and recognition of the ability to realise one's intellectual and emotional potential. It has also been defined as a state of wellbeing whereby individuals recognise their abilities, can cope with the normal stresses of life, work productively and fruitfully, and make a contribution to their communities. Mental health is about enhancing competencies of individuals and communities and enabling them to achieve their self-determined goals. Mental health should be a concern for all of us, rather than only for those who have a mental disorder (WHO, 2003: 7).

However, mental health is more than a lack of mental illness (WHO, 2003). Keyes (2009) prefers to view mental health at one end of a continuum with mental illness at the other end (Figure 10.4). People may move along this continuum at different times in their lives. Friedli (2009) argues that mental illness should be understood less in terms of individual pathology and more in terms of the response to adversity.

Mental health ————————————————————— Mental illness

**Figure 10.4**  Mental health continuum

In recent years the government has sought to raise the profile of mental healthcare, treatment and services achieving parity of esteem between mental and physical health. The government strategy for mental health, *No Health Without Mental Health* (DH, 2011c) makes explicit its objective to give equal priority to mental and physical health. *Closing the Gap: Priorities for Essential Change in Mental Health* (DH, 2014c) supports the longer-term aims of the mental health strategy but also seeks to speed up the pace of change, identifying 25 areas where changes can be made within a shorter timescale. Central to this is the aim of gathering more information about mental health and illness, the needs of clients and the services that are available. One of the aims of enhanced information is to establish waiting time limits for mental health services in order to match the existing standards for access to services for physical health problems (DH, 2014c). Improving access to mental health services by 2020, NHS England (2016) and the DH (2014c) set out to ensure that mental and physical health services are given equal priority in terms of waiting times and service quality. This is against the background of concerns raised about waiting times for the treatment of anxiety and depression.

Another aim is to tackle inequalities in access to mental health services (for example, in relation to black and minority ethnic communities and older people) particularly concerning access to psychological therapies which have been found to help many people manage long-term mental health problems (DH, 2014c). Psychological therapies are often referred to as 'talking therapies' (e.g. cognitive-behavioural therapy and counselling). The *Five Year Forward View for Mental Health* (NHS England, 2016) makes recommendations for improvements in outcomes in mental health in three broad areas:

1. Achieving parity of esteem between mental and physical health for children, young people, adults and older people;
2. Wider action relating to mental health in areas such as housing, employment and social inclusion;
3. Tackling inequalities, including higher incidence of mental health problems among people living in poverty, those who are unemployed, those who face discrimination, and people from certain black and minority ethnic groups whose first experience of mental healthcare is often when they are detained under the Mental Health Act 2007 (see www.legislation.gov.uk/ukpga/2007/12/pdfs/ukpga_20070012_en.pdf), often with police involvement.

## Culture and mental health

The issue of mental health, illness and ethnicity is a complex and controversial one. The term 'minority ethnic group' encompasses many different groups with different experiences and beliefs about mental health and illness. For example, there is a long history of higher admission rates to psychiatric hospitals for black men than those for the majority white population (Balarajan and Soni Raleigh, 1993; Smaje, 1995). In 2011, the Care Quality Commission reported that 23% of people receiving inpatient care in mental health units in England and Wales were from ethnic minority groups with admissions for people from black Caribbean, black African and mixed white/black groups at least two times higher than average. Afro-Caribbean people are also more likely to be subject to compulsory treatment under the Mental Health Act than the majority UK population (DH, 2011c) with over four times the rate of detention for black or black British groups over those of the white group (NHS Digital, 2017). The boundary between mental health and mental illness is related to the question of normality, which is culturally relative (Sashidharan and Commander, 1998; Fernando, 2002). Mental health and illness are socially constructed, in terms of both the person suffering from the 'abnormality' and the person making any judgement on 'abnormality' (Helman, 2000), suggesting that cultural misunderstanding may contribute to some misdiagnosis. Helman notes that, as well as having a higher rate of mental illness than the majority population in their adopted countries, immigrants also have higher rates of mental illness than the populations of their countries of origin. This suggests that mental health problems among immigrants may be associated with experiences in host countries. The government acknowledges that progress in tackling inequalities for minority ethnic groups has been disappointing (DH, 2011c; Salway et al., 2016). The role of social disadvantage also cannot be ignored. One study (Thomas et al., 1993) found that second-generation (UK-born) Afro-Caribbean people had nine times the rate of schizophrenia of the white indigenous population. They explained that this could be because of their greater socioeconomic disadvantage (i.e. poor inner-city housing and higher rates of unemployment) rather than psychiatric misdiagnosis. Socioeconomic disadvantage is known to be correlated with schizophrenia (Thomas et al., 1993).

---

### ACTIVITY 10.3

Find out more about culture and mental health by accessing the Department of Health (2010) report *Race Equality Action Plan: A Five-Year Review* and the Scottish Government's (2016) *Race Equality Framework for Scotland 2016–2030*.

---

## Labelling and stigma

People with mental health problems often suffer from labelling and social stigma (WHO, 2013). Stigma has connotations of shame and deviations from normal. The process of stigmatising involves making adverse social judgements about a person or a group. People who are stigmatised often experience rejection and exclusion and may be treated as outcasts (Scambler, 2009), so it is not surprising perhaps that current policy aims to raise awareness of mental health and illness and to promote positive views on mental health.

## Maladaptive coping strategies

Stressful circumstances can be damaging to health. Ongoing adverse social and psychological circumstances (e.g. low pay and difficulties in supporting a family, paying a mortgage or rent, difficult working conditions and/or social isolation) can cause long-term stress, which in turn can have a detrimental effect on physical and mental health (Marmot, 2010). In such situations some people might turn to health-damaging behaviours as a way of dealing with their problems. Misuse of drugs and alcohol can then lead to addiction. The Centre for Social Justice (2013) reports the following statistics:

- 1.6 million adults (1 in 20) are dependent on alcohol;
- 380,000 people (1 in 100) are addicted to heroin or crack cocaine;
- 335,000 children (1 in 37) live with a parent who is addicted to drugs;
- 1 in 7 children under the age of one lives with a substance-abusing parent.

Drug and alcohol abuse has significant effects on individuals, families and communities (WHO, 2003; Centre for Social Justice, 2013). Such abuse can lead to child poverty, family breakdown, welfare dependency and severe personal debt as well as crime (Centre for Social Justice, 2013). For example, the WHO (2003) demonstrates how excessive alcohol consumption can result in more money being spent on alcohol, which in turn can lead to financial problems and less money being available to spend on food. Living conditions can deteriorate, the individual and family may experience social stigma and the health of the entire family may be affected as a consequence of the stigma and poor nutrition. The impact of drug and alcohol abuse is felt particularly in Britain's most deprived communities (Centre for Social Justice, 2013). Drinking alcohol at dangerous levels is increasing and alcohol-related hospital admissions and deaths are rising (Centre for Social Justice, 2013). Furthermore, coping strategies such as smoking are linked to physical health problems (WHO, 2003). Poor mental health can also cause and be the result of being homeless. The rate of mental health problems is higher among the homeless population than the general population and one report found that homeless people were twice as likely to have mental health problems and the rate of psychosis was much higher than in the general population (Rees, 2009). A later report (Sanders and Brianna, 2015) also found that two-thirds of homeless people cited drug or alcohol use as a reason for becoming homeless, and those who used drugs were seven times more likely to be homeless. The Unhealthy State of Homelessness report (Homeless Link, 2014) found that most of the homeless population did not have regular access to health services, resulting in heavy use of acute services, for both physical and mental health. Their data showed that the number of A&E visits per homeless person were four times higher than for the general public.

What health promotion activities are targeted towards homeless individuals in your area?

## Suicide prevention

The *Preventing Suicide in England* strategy (DH, 2012c) seeks to identify those deemed at high risk of suicide and provide tailored approaches to reducing risk. It also aims to increase research in this area and work with media sources towards sensitive reporting to minimise stigma and harm.

### PAUL

Paul, a 24-year-old man, is brought into A&E having self-harmed. He is accompanied by his partner who claims that he is suicidal.

- As a nurse working in the A&E department, what could you do?

Suicide is everyone's business and not just the realm of specialist mental health nurses. Although specialist mental health nurses are expected to use evidence-based models of suicide prevention, intervention and harm reduction to reduce risk, adult nurses also have their part to play. For example, Scotland's suicide prevention strategy (Scottish Government, 2013b) has a broad approach, promoting emotional resilience and wellbeing initiatives across schools and the wider public, tackling issues related to discrimination, stigma and poverty. There has also been work to improve the knowledge and understanding of suicide among all frontline NHS staff, with more than 50% completing at least one of the suicide prevention courses: STORM,

ASIST, safeTALK of SMHSA. Between 2009 and 2012 there has been an 18% reduction in the overall suicide rate across Scotland. Northern Ireland is planning a similar approach (DHSSPS, 2016).

---

### ACTIVITY 10.4

Access the Health and Social Care Alliance Scotland Suicide Prevention Strategy Report (2018) at www.samaritans.org/sites/default/files/kcfinder/files/SPR%20final%20WEB.pdf and identify the key issues faced by those at risk of suicide.

You can find out more about the STORM, ASIST and safeTALK programmes by accessing the websites below:

https://mentalhealthpartnerships.com/project/storm-skills-training

www.gov.scot/Publications/2008/05/21112543/4

www.chooselife.net/Training/safetalk.aspx

Consider how you could respond sensitively and effectively to patients at risk of suicide.

---

## Health promotion in prisons

Watson et al. (2009) identified the tension that exists between the correctional aspects of being in prison (such as separation from society and confinement) and healthcare issues that may arise in prison. It is estimated that 80% of prisoners in England and Wales smoke and are allowed to do so in their cells (Ginn, 2013). Other health issues relate to poor mental health, substance misuse and communicable diseases (Heidari et al., 2014). As a nurse working within a prison setting, you may come across several challenges. Nevertheless, Exworthy et al. (2012) suggested that the principle of 'equivalence of care' is not wholly applicable, because prisons are not equivalent to the outside, civilian community in some areas. This is evident in the primary care provision in prisons and, interestingly, the number of consultations within a prison setting is much higher than the community equivalents (Exworthy et al., 2012). Also long-term conditions such as respiratory and ischaemic heart disease are very common, especially in older prisoners (Condon et al., 2007). This is unsurprising given that the relationship between poor health and social circumstance is well documented. There is therefore an opportunity to implement more involved health promotion strategies in such settings.

## Travelling communities

Members of travelling communities are more likely to suffer from poor health and also have a lower life expectancy (Lhussier et al., 2015). A number of health concerns include poor infant and child health, maternal mortality, and high rates of depression, anxiety and suicide (McFadden et al., 2016). Engaging with travelling communities presents a number of challenges, including cultural beliefs as well as poor access to services (Lhussier et al., 2015). Van Cleemput et al. (2007) highlights the specific cultural beliefs that inform many travellers' health behaviours, including clear rules about what is 'pure' and 'impure' and a notable 'fear of death'. The beliefs about 'pure' and 'impure' extends to the uptake of vaccinations, whereas the 'fear of death' means that a general anaesthetic might be avoided, because it might be considered a 'little death' (Van Cleemput et al., 2007). Accessing services can also be difficult because of a mobile lifestyle or discrimination by staff (McFadden et al., 2016). This can be further compounded by higher levels of illiteracy and mistrust of healthcare professionals (Lhussier et al., 2015). Having no fixed address often means not being registered with a GP, resulting in limited access to services, which is further complicated by primary healthcare staff who are reluctant to visit traveller sites or camps (McFadden et al., 2016).

## Promoting the health of mothers and babies

The health of a mother during pregnancy is vital to the health of the unborn baby. The foundations of adult health are laid before birth and during early childhood (Wilkinson and Marmot, 2003). Unfavourable circumstances during pregnancy, for example poor nutrition, stress, smoking, the misuse of drugs and alcohol, can affect the developing baby and set the scene for poor health in later life (Wilkinson and Marmot, 2003), so ensuring a good start means supporting mothers and young children (Wilkinson and Marmot, 2003). Most families are receptive to help and advice during this period because most parents will want their children to have the best possible start in life. Therefore, healthcare professionals are in a prime position to make use of this opportunity to provide support to families and give advice about a healthy lifestyle during pregnancy (PHE, 2016d).

## Nutrition in pregnancy

A healthy diet is key during pregnancy in order to meet the needs of both the mother and developing fetus (Shepherd, 2008). Epidemiological research led by Barker (cited in Wadsworth, 1996) concluded that maternal under-nutrition during fetal life or immediately after birth can have lasting consequences on the child and may extend into adulthood. The general advice for nutrition during pregnancy is to find a balance of eating a wide variety of foods, appropriate weight gain and physical exercise (Shepherd, 2008). As an adult nurse you should familiarise yourself with the advice that is offered to expectant mothers concerning their diets.

### ACTIVITY 10.5

Locate *The Pregnancy Book* (DH, 2017) at www.publichealth.hscni.net/publications by placing the term 'The Pregnancy Book' in the website's search engine.

Read the section 'Your health in pregnancy – advice on nutrition'. You should ensure that you are able to pass on this advice to expectant mothers if required.

## Smoking cessation in pregnancy

In pregnancy, the adverse effects of smoking include the risk of miscarriage, a premature birth, a low birth weight, stillbirth and sudden infant death (Wisborg et al., 2000; Anderson et al., 2005; Duaso and Duncan, 2012; Percival, 2013). Furthermore, mothers who are exposed to environmental smoke – including second-hand smoke – are more likely to give birth to babies with low birth weights (Duaso and Duncan, 2012). Children who are exposed to passive smoking are at an increased risk of developing pneumonia, bronchitis and asthma. Guidelines on quitting smoking in pregnancy and after childbirth (NICE, 2010) state that anyone planning a pregnancy, or who is already pregnant or has an infant under 12 months, should receive smoking cessation support. Therefore, healthcare professionals should assess expectant mothers' exposure to cigarette smoke, inform them of the dangers of smoking, ask smokers if they would like to stop smoking and refer them to NHS Stop Smoking Services appropriately.

## Vulnerable families

Women who experience stress during pregnancy may give birth to babies of low birth weight and as they grow up these children may have emotional and behavioural problems (Wilkinson, 2005). Thus, alongside the mainstream services for pregnant women and young children are some initiatives that focus on more vulnerable families. Women living in complex social situations (e.g. those at risk from substance abuse, recent migrants with language barriers, and victims or potential victims of domestic abuse) often avoid antenatal care and so there is a need to reach out to such women. Many healthcare trusts have specialist midwives with a responsibility to target and support vulnerable women. The Healthy Start programme is a UK-wide government scheme to improve the health of low-income pregnant women and families on benefits and tax credits. The programme provides vouchers for healthy food, for example milk, fresh or frozen fruit and vegetables. Another initiative that aims to help vulnerable, young, first-time mothers across the UK is the Family Nurse Partnership Programme (FNP) (DH, 2012d). This programme aims to improve pregnancy outcomes, improve child health and development, and improve parents' economic self-sufficiency. All first-time mothers aged 19 and under at conception are eligible and participation in the programme is voluntary. Healthcare professionals use theory and expertise to engage in behaviour change methods to foster the adoption of healthier lifestyles by the families.

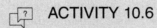

## ACTIVITY 10.6

Find out about the services available in your area that aim to assist pregnant women and support vulnerable families.

## Vaccinations for pregnant women

The pertussis (whooping cough) vaccine is recommended for all pregnant women from 16 weeks' gestation (ideally around 20 weeks after the anomaly scan). This was commenced in 2012 in response to the increase in morbidity and mortality rates of newborn infants contracting pertussis before the normal vaccination age of around 8 weeks (PHE, 2016d). The influenza vaccine is now offered to all pregnant women and can be given at any stage of pregnancy. This was introduced in 2012 after the Confidential Enquiry into Maternal Deaths 2009–2012 which reported that 36 women died during pregnancy from flu-related problems (Hinton, 2014). Both vaccines are safe for pregnant women and the unborn child, providing immunity to the fetus and protecting the newborn for the first two months of life.

# Postnatal care and transition to the community

Before being discharged from hospital, mothers will receive a postnatal examination by a midwife. This examination includes an assessment of the mother's emotional state and her physical wellbeing (Kinge and Gregory, 2011). All newborn babies are examined within 72 hours of birth by a competent practitioner. New mothers are offered advice on contraception and are advised to make an appointment for a postnatal check-up with their GP in six weeks' time for themselves and their babies. A health visitor will also visit the mother and baby at home between 10 and 14 days after the birth, and will advise where and how often to take the baby for regular assessments.

The period of six to eight weeks after childbirth is referred to as the puerperium and it is a time of enormous adjustment (Kinge and Gregory, 2011). NICE (2013c) has developed a quality standard (QS37) for postnatal care, outlining the care and support that every woman should receive during the postnatal period. This care should be individualised to meet the needs of the mother and baby (including partners and family as appropriate). The midwife will normally visit the family at home following discharge from hospital until 10–14 days postnatal. However, this care and support can be extended beyond the 6- to 8-week period if necessary. The health visitor will visit from day 10 postnatal. NICE (2013c) recommends the provision of postnatal education programmes delivered by a multidisciplinary team, which provides advice, information and support for new mothers and their families (Kinge and Gregory, 2011).

## Physical health

Women who have just given birth should be provided with information about how to look for signs that they are becoming ill. For example, if they have flu-like symptoms they should report this immediately to their midwife or GP (NICE, 2013c). Other symptoms such as persistent headache and aches and pains should not be ignored. Maternal sepsis has been a leading cause of maternal death (Knight et al., 2016). It can affect women during pregnancy and in the first few weeks after birth. Women and their families need to remain aware of early warning signs:

- High temperature (>38.3°C);
- Very low temperature (<36°C);
- Chills and shivering;
- Fast heartbeat;
- Fast breathing, breathlessness;
- Headache;
- Severe abdominal pain;
- Extreme sleepiness (Hinton, 2014: 3).

If any of these symptoms appear that urgent, medical advice should be sought. This can be via a GP or the local hospital.

## Perinatal mental health

Perinatal mental health problems are those that occur during pregnancy or in the first year after the birth of a child, affect up to 20% of women and cover a wide range of conditions. If left untreated, they can have significant and long-lasting effects not only on the woman but also on her children's emotional, social and cognitive development. The NICE clinical guidelines (NICE, 2013c) require that at a pregnant woman's first contact with services, healthcare professionals should ask questions about past and present severe mental illness, previous treatment by mental health professionals and family history of perinatal mental illness. The aim here is early detection and treatment. It is important to be aware of the mental health problems that can arise in the postnatal period and to be able to differentiate 'baby blues' (e.g. irritability, anxiety and tearfulness three to four days after childbirth, stopping by the time the baby is about ten days old), postnatal depression (e.g. a depressive disorder that can affect women in the months after childbirth, Robertson, 2010) and postpartum (or puerperal) psychosis (e.g. a severe episode of mental illness representing a psychiatric emergency, with a sudden onset during the days or weeks after childbirth (Royal College of Psychiatrists, 2014).

### ACTIVITY 10.7

Access the patient information leaflet: *Postpartum Psychosis: Severe Mental Illness after Childbirth* (Royal College of Psychiatrists, 2014). Available at: www.rcpsych.ac.uk/healthadvice/problemsand disorders/postpartumpsychosis.aspx.
    Consider how useful this leaflet might be when educating new mothers about postnatal mental health.

## Breastfeeding

Breast milk supplies all the nutrients a baby needs for around the first six months of life (NHS, 2010). Policies on breastfeeding across the UK promote feeding babies solely on breast milk for the first six months of life, after which time it is suggested that breastfeeding can continue as long as the mother and baby wish while gradually introducing a more varied diet (NICE, 2008b). Breastfeeding contributes to the health of both mother and baby. It has been found that babies who are not breastfed are more likely to acquire infections such as gastroenteritis and respiratory problems during their first year of life (NICE, 2008b). Women who are disadvantaged are less likely to breastfeed than their better-off counterparts.

### ACTIVITY 10.8

Read about the Baby Friendly Initiative at www.unicef.org.uk/babyfriendly/what-is-baby-friendly.
    Read the following document: NHS (2010) *Off to the Best Start: Important Information about Feeding Your Baby.* Available at www.unicef.org.uk/babyfriendly/wp-content/uploads/sites/2/2010/11/Off_to_the_Best_Start_Leaflet_4_Pages-2017_.pdf.

## Promoting the health of children and young people

As a registered nurse you may encounter children or young people while working in an accident and emergency department, in primary care, in any adult care ward or indeed in your personal day-to-day life. The United Nations' convention on the Rights of the Child (UN, 1989; ratified by the UK in 1991) defines a child as anyone under the age of 18. The General Medical Council (GMC) defines 'young people' as 'older or experienced children who could make important decisions for themselves' (GMC, 2018). Currently 18.9% of the UK population is aged under 15 years though this may decrease to about 17.7% by 2046 as the current population ages (ONS, 2017c). None the less, children and young people are any country's future and each of the four countries (England, Scotland, Wales and Northern Ireland) that make up the UK has a Commissioner for Children and Young People. These Commissioners work independently to uphold children's rights under the UN convention, and represent the views of children and young people to policy makers and other stakeholders with a view to improving the lives of all children, particularly the most vulnerable.

## ? ACTIVITY 10.9

There are 54 Articles contained within the UN Convention.

Access this online and identify those articles that are most readily applicable to nursing practice.

The UN's Convention stresses that the family (as the natural place for nurturing children) should be afforded the necessary protection and assistance to fulfil its responsibilities (UN, 1989). The ONS defines a family as 'married, civil partnered or cohabiting couple with or without children, or a lone parent, with a least one child, who live at the same address' (ONS, 2018b: 2). Families come in all 'shapes and sizes' including co-habiting, lone parent, same sex and reconstituted forms. Families may be 'nuclear' in form, consisting of adults and dependent children. Extended families include a wider network of kin, for example including grandparents, aunts, uncles and cousins.

All types of families are important for meeting children's and young people's psychological and physical needs, providing support and finances for shelter, food, health, development and protection, and socialisation (enabling children to learn about identity, roles, values and culture) (Friedman et al., 2003). Ideals about family life and child rearing may vary according to the family structure, cultural beliefs and values. It is important to develop cultural competency so that care for families is neither too intrusive nor so lax that it results in children's needs being overlooked (Akilapa and Simkiss, 2012). Despite the importance of families to children's wellbeing, families living in difficult circumstances, such as domestic violence/intimate partner violence, drug or alcohol dependency, can negatively impact on children's lives (WHO and International Society for Prevention of Child Abuse and Neglect [ISPCAN], 2006).

## ? ACTIVITY 10.10

If you have access to Open Athens you may wish to undertake cultural competence training: www. e-lfh.org.uk/programmes/cultural-competence.

Think point: Reflect on your own upbringing. What type of help and support did you need as you grew up?

## Universal services

Current UK policies aim to ensure that all children and young people have the best start in life (HSC Public Health Agency, 2011; Welsh Government, 2013; PHE, 2016d; Scottish Government, 2017).

Universal services are those that are provided to everyone. Every child and young person in the UK is offered a range of universal health, education and welfare support. A child or young person can have needs for additional education, health or social care support (i.e. resulting from learning difficulties, disabilities or abuse) and require a comprehensive assessment in order to ensure that additional targeted services are provided to meet their needs. Families may also need additional support when their child is ill or has additional needs. Thomas and Price (2012) explored the experiences of some mothers caring for children with complex needs. They identified that parents felt physically burdened and isolated, and experienced emotional turmoil, yet they valued additional support services.

The Healthy Child Programme offers universal services from pregnancy to 19 years (DH, 2009a, 2009b) and is part of 'giving every child the best start in life' initiative (PHE, 2016d). The programme offers children, young people and their families health promotion (such as immunisations, or advice and support about physical or emotional wellbeing), health and developmental reviews, and screening (e.g. the UK newborn screening programme for various disorders).

Universal health and development reviews are a key feature of the Healthy Child Programme (PHE, 2016d). These reviews are carried out by healthcare professionals (often, health visitors) who have skills in assessing child development, and an understanding of the factors that influence family health and wellbeing. One of the aims of the review is to support keeping children and the family healthy (for example, with regard to oral health, nutrition or safety), and also detecting any potential health issues early so that appropriate support can be offered to the child and the family (early intervention). The Healthy Child Programme 0–5 years offers the following health and development reviews:

- Prenatal: at 28 weeks of pregnancy;
- Within 14 days of birth;
- The baby's 6- to 8-week examination;
- At 9–12 months old;
- Between 2 and 2½ years old.

## Keeping children healthy

UK policy documents emphasise the importance of good child health, for example through encouraging families to have their children immunised and by encouraging healthy lifestyles.

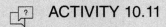 **ACTIVITY 10.11**

What vaccinations are children given in the UK and what diseases do they prevent?
Follow this link to find out: www.nhs.uk/conditions/vaccinations/childhood-vaccines-timeline.

Childhood obesity is a national concern because approximately a third of children are overweight or obese and this can negatively impact on their health as children and adults (Gov.uk, 2017). As part of 'making every contact count' we should ask parents about their family's diet and physical activity – encouraging parents to find out more information on healthy living or letting them know about weight loss services, as appropriate (Health Education England, 2018). We can also educate children and their parents to understand what child-size portions are (Marteau et al., 2015) and encourage 60 minutes of daily moderate-to-vigorous physical activity for children (Gov.uk, 2017).

## ACTIVITY 10.12

Get familiar with NHS choices. What advice does the website offer for parents with overweight children? Check out: www.nhs.uk/Livewell/childhealth6-15/Pages/child-health-measurement-programme-very-overweight-advice.aspx.

## The importance of play

A key component in 'giving every child a good start in life' is preparing children to be ready to learn and to be ready for school (PHE, 2016d). Play is important for children because it is a pleasurable activity and assists with the development of peer friendships, learning about social dynamics and the rules of engagement (Lester and Russell, 2010). Lester and Russell suggest that without play, a child's development may be compromised. Article 31 of the Rights of a Child (UN, 1989: 10) recognises the right of the child to 'rest and leisure, to engage in play and recreational activities appropriate to the age of the child and to participate freely in cultural life and the arts'. Lester and Russell (2010: ix) argue that play contributes to health, wellbeing and resilience through promoting:

- Pleasure and enjoyment;
- Emotional management;
- Stress regulation;
- Attachment;
- Learning and creativity.

Protective factors in early childhood, such as secure attachment, consistent parenting, appropriate play and learning opportunities, contribute to children's emotional wellbeing and chances of reaching their potential (Fearn and Howard, 2012). During play children create imaginary worlds and through play children can develop a range of adaptive capacities and strategies to help them cope or adapt with abuse, conflict, displacement and/or poverty (Lester and Russell, 2010). Fearn and Howard (2012) found that play can provide a healing experience for children affected by war and conflict and that play encourages the growth of resilience.

## Early education

A child's intellectual, social and behavioural development is also enhanced by pre-school education; pre-school provision particularly enhances children's attainments at school when they are from challenging social environments (Sylva et al., 2004). The UK offers universal free entitlement to early education and child care for some pre-school children (with between-country differences in provision) (Gov.uk, 2018). This education helps the transition to school (Department for Education, 2011).

## Safeguarding children

Safeguarding is any action taken to promote the wellbeing of children or young people and to protect them from harm (National Society for the Prevention of Cruelty to Children [NSPCC], 2018). All nurses have a responsibility to raise a concern with an appropriate person for anyone who is vulnerable, at risk and needing protection (NMC, 2018a). There are clear guidelines in the UK about how to raise a safeguarding concern about a child. The first government Act to prevent cruelty to children was passed in 1889, but UK policies were strengthened after the death of Victoria Climbié. The Laming Report (DH, 2003) identified poor communication, interprofessional working and team work as being among the factors that contributed to the failure of professional services to protect Victoria. This report influenced the establishment of local children's Trusts, consisting of multidisciplinary teams of health, education and social service professionals. Other policy developments included the Children Act 2004 (www.legislation.gov.uk/ukpga/2004/31/contents) which defined the duties of agencies working with children to promote health and wellbeing, as well as protecting children from harm (Powell, 2013).

In spite of these policy changes, there have been subsequent high-profile and shocking cases of child abuse and neglect. Below, we encourage you to consider the case of Daniel Pelka, a very sad case which resulted in his death at the hands of his mother and her male partner. Daniel's case was extensively covered in the media and in a Serious Case Review (Coventry Safeguarding Children Board, 2013).

A Serious Case Review (SCR) is commissioned to determine what can be learned from a case about the way in which local professionals and organisations worked individually and together to safeguard children.

### DANIEL PELKA

Daniel was aged 4 years and 8 months at the time of his death. He had one older and one younger sibling. His family had migrated to the UK from Poland in 2005. Daniel was born in the UK in 2007. His family life was chaotic – his mother had relationships with three different partners whilst in the UK. All of these relationships involved high alcohol consumption and abuse. The family was known to the police, who were called to the home on many occasions, including 27 reported incidents of domestic abuse. In 2011 Daniel was taken to A&E with a spiral fracture to his arm. As the fracture had occurred on the previous day (the mother and stepfather had delayed taking Daniel to hospital), and with the knowledge that this type of fracture is associated with non-accidental injury, the hospital referred the case to the police. Although a social worker carried out an assessment, professionals accepted the mother's account of what led to the fracture and no continuing need for intervention was identified.

In September 2011 Daniel started school and over the ensuing months his attendance was poor. He grew thinner, was constantly hungry, stopped growing and went to school with bruises. His teachers reported seeing facial injuries, black eyes and bruises on his neck and head. Daniel was found scavenging in bins at school for food, but when school staff spoke to his mother about his hunger she told them he had an eating disorder that caused him to feel constantly hungry. She also told them that they should not give him any food.

It is reported that Daniel spoke little English, had few friends, often played in isolation and sometimes displayed ritualistic behaviours. He did, however, have a strong bond with his older sibling. When teachers asked him how he got his injuries, he looked down at the ground and did not answer.

Daniel's mother and stepfather were both sentenced to life imprisonment when he died of a subdural haematoma after a severe blow to the head in March 2012. The trial and SCR revealed that, for at least six months before his death, Daniel had been starved, assaulted, neglected and abused. Daniel was frequently locked in a 'box room' without a window, heating or toys – the only 'furniture' in this room was a soiled mattress. Daniel was plunged into cold baths, he was beaten and denied meals. He was force fed salt until he vomited. A postmortem examination found him to be emaciated, grossly malnourished and dehydrated with bruising over his body – a total of 40 injuries. There was evidence of long-standing neglect.

The SCR reported that his mother and stepfather set out to deliberately harm Daniel and deceive professionals. The professionals who had contact with Daniel and his family included teachers, classroom assistants, school nurses, an education welfare officer, a general practitioner, a community paediatrician, social workers and the police. Teachers variously described Daniel as 'losing weight', 'pale', 'ashen' and 'a bag of bones'. There was poor communication between the professionals who met Daniel and professionals' concerns were not well recorded. As in previous cases, there were many missed opportunities to protect Daniel. The SCR claims that no professional tried hard enough to engage with Daniel about his eating habits or home life, and concluded that all professionals need to 'think the unthinkable' and believe and act on what they see and not accept parents' versions of events without challenging.

---

- Having read the case study about Daniel, can you identify any areas where professionals might have identified concerns or 'professional curiosity'?

Apart from Daniel's visible injuries there are several issues that you might have identified. For example, Daniel was not growing well. Growth is an important indicator of a child's health and wellbeing and slow growth during childhood can have psychosocial causes (Wilkinson, 2005). Daniel's apparent isolation or bin scavenging might have also caused you concern. You might have considered his lack of response when asked about his injuries in terms of 'professional curiosity', you might have asked the question 'What eating disorder?' in response to his mother's explanation of Daniel losing weight and being constantly hungry.

Many of the professionals who were in contact with Daniel were concerned about him but they did not act adequately on those concerns and the various professional groups did not communicate with each other. The revised document *Working Together to Safeguard Children: A Guide to Interagency Working to Safeguard and Promote the Welfare of Children* (HM Government, 2015) emphasises that safeguarding children is everyone's responsibility; everyone who comes into contact with children and their families has a role to play. The document stresses that a child's needs remain paramount (first and foremost). Professionals' failures to protect children are often the result of losing sight of the needs of children or placing the interests of adults ahead of those of children (HM Government, 2015). Acknowledging that no single professional can have a full picture of a child's needs and circumstances, the document stresses the need to share information. Lack of sharing information has often resulted in a failure to protect children.

## A registered nurse's role in relation to safeguarding children

HM Government (2015) identifies that safeguarding is everyone's responsibility, everyone should have a child-centred approach and good understanding of the needs and views of children, and all professionals should share information in a timely way and discuss their concerns. This means that no one should assume that someone else will pass on information about a child, and everyone should share information about concerns as soon as possible to ensure early intervention and prevention of any further difficulties for the child. Early and effective communication is key to protecting children and young people. Children are best protected when professionals are clear about what is required of them individually, and how they need to work together (HM Government, 2015: 7).

As a registered nurse, you need to be aware of the factors that might place a child at risk of maltreatment (HM Government, 2015: 13); these are children who:

- Are disabled and has specific additional needs;
- Have special educational needs;
- Are a young carer;
- Are showing signs of engaging in antisocial or criminal behaviour;
- Are in family circumstances presenting challenges for the child, such as substance abuse, adult mental health, domestic violence; and/or
- Are showing early signs of abuse and/or neglect (see the next section).

- Are you aware of the different types of maltreatment? Are you familiar with the procedures for safeguarding the welfare of children in your area?

## Child and young person maltreatment: what is it and what do you need to do?

Child maltreatment can involve physical, emotional or emotional abuse, neglect or exploitation of children or young people (WHO and ISPCAN, 2006). Maltreatment causes significant harm to a child's or young person's current and future health, development and wellbeing; the health and social effects of such abuse can last a lifetime (NICE, 2017).

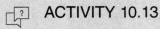 ACTIVITY 10.13

Read the WHO's (2017) document about child maltreatment: at www.who.int/violence_injury_prevention/violence/child/Child_maltreatment_infographic_EN.pdf?ua=1.

- What are some of the different forms of maltreatment?
- How common are these?
- What are the consequences of maltreatment?
- What increases the risk of maltreatment?

It is important that a child's needs are paramount (considered first and foremost) and is child-centred (focused on their needs, concerns and wishes). To protect, safeguard and promote the wellbeing of children and young people effectively, everyone in education, health or social care organisations need to do their part in identifying concerns and promptly sharing information with appropriate, child-safeguarding professionals. This is because no one professional will know everything about a child and the family (HM Government, 2015).

There are some regional and national variations in child safeguarding policies in the UK; it is, therefore, important to be aware of your local policies and also to keep yourself up to date with policy through regular training. There are two important things to know no matter where you work. The first is to be aware of the types of child maltreatment, so that you can be vigilant and recognise signs that may indicate that a child is being maltreated. The second is to know to whom, and how to, communicate any concerns.

## Recognising child maltreatment

Although maltreatment is often classified as neglect, physical, sexual or emotional, it is important to remember that children or young people can experience more than one type of maltreatment.

 **Some types of maltreatment (adapted from WHO and ISPCAN, 2006; HM Government, 2015)**

Neglect happens when there has been a failure to meet a child's basic needs over a period of time (e.g. neglect of a child's health, education, emotional development, food or safety needs);

Physical abuse is the intentional use of physical force (e.g. hitting, beating, kicking, shaking, biting, scalding, pinching, poisoning or suffocating a child);

Emotional or psychological abuse occurs when there is a persistent failure to provide an appropriate environment for mental wellbeing (e.g. by telling a child that they are not loved, or not good enough, by belittling, blaming, threatening, frightening, discriminating, ridiculing, rejecting or showing hostility to a child);

Sexual abuse happens when a child is involved in inappropriate sexual activity (this includes physical contact or non-contact activities such as forcing children to watch sexual images), which the child does not understand and is not developmentally prepared for.

## How can you recognise maltreatment?

NICE have produced two guidelines of what you might see or hear that can suggest maltreatment (NICE calls these 'alerting features'). NICE (2009, 2017) describes these altering features as either 'suspect' or 'consider'. 'Suspect' is an altering feature that should trigger a 'serious level of concern' that maltreatment might be occurring, and 'consider' is where maltreatment may be a possible explanation for a child's injury or presentation.

**ACTIVITY 10.14**

Read the alerting features section of the following NICE guidelines: physical maltreatment (NICE, 2017) and NICE (2009) for alerting features to other forms of maltreatment.
Make a note of what should alert you to consider or suspect maltreatment.

Children and young people may be maltreated by parents or other family members, caregivers, people in authority, strangers, friends or other children (WHO and ISPCAN, 2006). If a child tells you that they are being maltreated, you should listen to them, pay attention and respect what they are saying. Then you should reassure the child that you will 'act to keep them safe' (by enacting your local safeguarding guideline) (HM Government, 2015). It is also important to be alert for 'unsuitable explanations' where a child's or young person's or carer's or parent's account about an injury or presentation is not adequate or plausible, or if explanations are contradictory or inconsistent (NICE, 2017).

## Communicating and recording

You need to become familiar with procedures for safeguarding the welfare of children in your area and know whom to contact to express any concerns you might have. Every NHS trust has a named member of staff who takes the lead on concerns relating to child maltreatment and safeguarding. If you suspect that a child is being maltreated you should report your concerns; if you are a student you may report to your practice supervisor or an experienced colleague. He or she may well refer the matter to the named nurse for safeguarding children who could then make a referral to social services. You must record your concerns clearly – exactly what you observed and heard from whom and when. In addition, record why this is of concern and what you did about your concerns.

The focus of this section has been on maintaining health during childhood so that everyone can have 'the best start in life'. We have considered the importance of assessing every child's needs and how being vigilant and good communication with appropriate professionals can support vulnerable children and young people.

## Promoting the health of adults with learning disabilities

Traditionally services for people with learning disabilities were based around long-stay institutions (Leaning and Adderley, 2016). However, there has been a move away from institutional care for people with learning disabilities towards practices that promote more ordinary lives following the 1971 White Paper, *Better Services for the Mentally Handicapped* (Health Foundation, 2018). This shift continued and there was a move from a medical model to a social model of care (i.e. an approach that considers how disability and dependency are socially constructed). This move stems very much from a government White Paper, *Valuing People* (DH, 2001), which emphasises the rights of people with learning disabilities, particularly in relation to exerting choice and control over their lives. People with learning disabilities may live in a wide range of settings but the majority live in their own home or the family home (Burt, 2015). There are a range of support services available according to the level of ability of the individual. These services may include supported housing provided by social services, the private sector or the voluntary sector.

A learning disability can be mild, moderate or severe, or profound (RCN, 2013). Some people experience profound and multiple learning disabilities which include more than one disability, a significant learning disability and complex healthcare needs (Brown et al., 2010). These individuals need full-time care and support with most aspects of daily life. They may also have physical disabilities.

## Health problems associated with learning disabilities

Public Health England (2016d) estimates that, in 2015, there were around 1,087,100 people with learning disabilities, including 930,400 adults. An increasing number of people with a learning disability live into old age and, as a consequence of co-morbidities, can become frequent users of health services (Brown et al., 2010; Phillips, 2012). Governments from all four countries of the UK promote the provision of mainstream healthcare services for people with learning disabilities, supported by specialist services as appropriate (Gibson, 2009). However, evidence suggests that the needs of people with learning disabilities are often not met sufficiently in general healthcare services (MENCAP, 2007, 2018), resulting in inequalities in healthcare provision (Phillips, 2012; NHS England, 2017). The health problems associated with learning disabilities include the following:

- Circulatory diseases are the main cause of death (PHE, 2016d) for people with learning disability. People with Down's syndrome experience a higher risk of congenital heart problems in addition to problems with sight and hearing (RCN, 2013);
- Respiratory disease is also one of the main causes of death. This may be related to aspiration or gastro-oesophageal reflux, because swallowing problems are more prevalent in people with learning disabilities (RCN, 2013);
- Higher levels of gastrointestinal cancers (RCN, 2013);
- Greater vulnerability to mental health problems (RCN, 2013);
- There is also a higher prevalence of epilepsy, constipation, obesity and dental problems (RCN, 2013).

---

### ACTIVITY 10.15

Review the LeDeR (NHS England, 2017) report and consider the actions you might need to take to ensure that you are able to promote the health of patients with learning disabilities within healthcare settings.

---

## Chapter summary

In this chapter we have considered the registered nurse's role in promoting the health of individuals from the moment of conception. We have explored some of the health needs of individuals, groups and communities and have also identified unifying threads in terms of the needs of disadvantaged people within these groups. It is clear that there are many different issues and needs to consider when promoting health, but perhaps the most important principle to remember, as a registered nurse, is to promote both physical and mental health whenever the opportunity arises – because even five minutes can make a difference (DH, 2012a).

Health promotion is becoming much more prominent than in previous years and all registered nurses are expected to be able to engage in health promotion activities regardless of the practice setting (DH, 2012a; RCN, 2012; NMC, 2018b). As an adult nurse you will need always to refer to the most up-to-date and best available evidence to inform your health promotion activities and be able to appraise the effectiveness of your interventions – with individuals, families and communities (NICE, 2007a, 2007b, 2008a, 2014).

## Useful websites

Public Health Agency, Northern Ireland: www.publichealth.hscni.net.
Department of Health (NI), Health Promotion Website: www.health-ni.gov.uk/topics/public-health-policy-and-advice/health-promotion.
Health Promotion Scotland: www.healthscotland.scot.
Public Health Wales: www.wales.nhs.uk/sitesplus/888/page/59338.
World Health Organization: www.who.int/topics/health_promotion/en.

## Further reading

Boyce, T., Peckham, S., Hann, A. and Trenholm, S. (2010) *A Pro-active Approach. Health Promotion and Ill-health Prevention*. London: The King's Fund.
NHS England (2017) *Next Steps on the NHS Five Year Forward Review*. London: NHS England.

## References

Acheson, D. (1998) *Independent Inquiry into Inequalities in Health Report*. London: The Stationery Office.
Ajzen, D. (1991) 'The theory of planned behaviour', *Organizational Behavior and Human Decision Processes*, 50: 179–211.
Ajzen, D. and Fishbein, M. (1980) *Understanding Attitudes and Predicting Social Behaviour*. Englewood Cliffs, NJ: Prentice Hall.
Akilapa, R. and Simkiss, D. (2012) 'Cultural influences and safeguarding children', *Paediatrics and Child Health*, 22(11): 490–5.
Anderson, M.E., Johnson, D.C. and Batal, H.A. (2005) 'Sudden infant death syndrome and prenatal maternal smoking: rising attributed risk in the back to sleep era', *BMC Medicine*. Available at: www.biomedcentral.com/1741-7015/3/4 (last accessed 19 January 2015).
Andre, F.E., Booy, R., Bock, H.L., Clemens, J., Datta, S.K., John, T.J., Lee, B.W., Lolekha, S., Peltola, H., Ruff, T.A., Santosham, M. and Schmitt, H.J. (2008) 'Vaccination greatly reduces disease, disability, death and inequity worldwide', *Bulletin of the World Health Organization*, 86: 140–6.
Baisch, M.J. (2009) 'Community health: an evolutionary concept analysis', *Journal of Advanced Nursing*, 65: 2464–76.
Balarajan, R. and Soni Raleigh, V. (1993) *Ethnicity and Health: A Guide for the NHS*. London: Department of Health.
Beattie, A. (1991) 'Knowledge and control in health promotion: a test case for social policy and theory'. In J. Gabe, M. Calnan and M. Bury (eds), *The Sociology of the Health Service*. London: Routledge, pp. 162–202.
Becker, M.H. (ed.) (1974) 'The Health Belief Model and personal health behaviour', *Health Education Monographs*, 2: 324–473.

Bell, M.L., Davis, D.L. and Fletcher, T. (2004) 'A retrospective assessment of mortality from the London Smog episode of 1952: the role of influenza and pollution', *Environmental Health Perspectives*, 112 (1): 6–8.

Betsch, C., Bohm, R., Korn, L. and Holtmann, C. (2017) 'On the benefits of explaining herd immunity in vaccine advocacy', *Nature Human Behaviour*, 1(56) doi:10.1038/s41562-017-0056.

Bostridge, M. (2009) *Florence Nightingale: The Woman and Her Legend.* Harmondsworth: Penguin.

Bradshaw, J. (1972) 'A taxonomy of social need', *New Society*, March: 640–3.

Brown, M., MacArthur, J., McKechanie, A., Hayes, M. and Fletcher, J. (2010) 'Equality and access to general healthcare for people with learning disabilities: reality or rhetoric?', *Journal of Research in Nursing*, 15(4): 351–61.

Buck, D. and Frosini, F. (2012) *Clustering of Unhealthy Behaviours Over Time: Implications for Policy and Practice.* London: The King's Fund.

Burt, A. (2015) *Understanding the Needs of People with Learning Disabilities.* Available at: www.gov.uk/government/speeches/understanding-the-needs-of-people-with-learning-disabilities (last accessed 9 May 2018).

Cabinet Office, DHSC, HM Treasury and Prime Minister's Office (2016) *Childhood Obesity: A Plan for Action.* London: HMSO.

Cavanagh, S. and Chadwick, K. (2005) *Summary: Health Needs Assessment at a Glance.* London: Health Development Agency/NICE.

Centre for Social Justice (2013) *No Quick Fix: Exposing the Depth of Britain's Drug and Alcohol Problem.* London: CSJ. Available at: www.centreforsocialjustice.org.uk/library/no-quick-fix-exposing-depth-britains-drug-alcohol-problem (last accessed 20 May 2018).

Cesaro, S., Giacchino, M., Fioreda, F., Barone, A., Battisti, L., Bezzio, S., Frenos, S., De Santis, R., Livadiotti, S., Marinello, S., Zanazzo, A.G. and Caselli, D. (2014) 'Guidelines on vaccinations in paediatric haematology and oncology patients', *Biomedical Research International*, doi:10.1155/2014/707691. PMC 40205020. PMID 24868544.

Chaplin, R., Flatley, J. and Smith, K. (2011) *Crime in England and Wales 2010/11. Home Office Statistical Bulletin 10/11.* London: The Home Office.

Chung, E.H. (2013) 'Vaccine allergies', *Clinical and Experimental Vaccine Research*, 4(3): 50–7.

Condon, L., Gill, H. and Harris, F. (2007) 'A review of prison health and its implications for primary care nursing in England and Wales: the research evidence', *Journal of Clinical Nursing*, 16(7): 1201–9.

Corte, C.M. and Sommers, M.S. (2005) 'Alcohol and risky behaviors', *Annual Review of Nursing Research*, 23: 327–60.

Coventry Safeguarding Children Board (2013) *Serious Case Review: Daniel Pelka.* Available at: https://cscb-new.co.uk/downloads/Serious%20Case%20Reviews%20-%20exec.%20summaries/SCR_Archive/Coventry%20SCR%20-%20Daniel%20Pelka%20(2013).pdf (last accessed 18 August 2018).

Dahlgren, G. and Whitehead, M. (1991) *Policies and Strategies to Promote Social Equity in Health.* Stockholm: Institute for Future Studies.

Daousi, C., Casson, I.F., Gill, G.V., MacFarlane, I.A., Wilding, J.P.H. and Pinkney, J.H. (2006) 'Prevalence of obesity in type 2 diabetes in secondary care: association with cardiovascular risk factors', *Postgraduate Medical Journal*, 82: 280–4.

Davies, M. and Macdowall, W. (2006) *Health Promotion Theory.* Maidenhead: Open University Press.

Davis, D.L. and Bates, D. (2002) 'A look back at the London smog of 1952 and the half century since', *Environmental Health Perspectives*, December.

Delves, P.J., Martin, S.J., Burton, D.R. and Roitt, I.M. (2017) *Roitt's Essential Immunology*, 13th edn. London: Wiley Blackwell.

Department for Education (2011) *Supporting Families in Foundation Years.* Available at: www.gov.uk/government/publications/supporting-families-in-the-foundation-years (last accessed 16 August 2018).

Department of Health (2001) *Valuing People. A New Strategy for Learning Disability for the 21st Century*. London: DH. Available at: https://assets.publishing.service.gov.uk/government/uploads/system/uploads/attachment_data/file/250877/5086.pdf (last accessed 15 May 2018).

Department of Health (2003) *The Victoria Climbié Inquiry: Report of an Inquiry by Lord Laming*. Cm5730. London: DH.

Department of Health (2007) *Drug Misuse and Dependence: UK Guidelines on Clinical Management*. London: HMSO.

Department of Health (2009a) *Healthy Child Programme: Pregnancy and the First Five Years of Life*. London: DH. Available at: www.gov.uk/government/publications/healthy-child-programme-pregnancy-and-the-first-5-years-of-life (last accessed 16 May 2018).

Department of Health (2009b) *Healthy Child Programme: 5–10 Years*. London: DH. Available at: www.gov.uk/government/publications/healthy-child-programme-5-to-19-years-old (last accessed 16 May 2018).

Department of Health (2010) *Equity and Excellence: Liberating the NHS*. London: HMSO.

Department of Health (2011a) *Healthy Lives, Healthy People: A Call to Action on Obesity in England*. London: HMSO.

Department of Health (2011b) *Healthy Lives, Healthy People: A Tobacco Control Plan for England*. London: HMSO.

Department of Health (2011c) *No Health Without Mental Health*. London: HMSO.

Department of Health (2012a) *The Public Health Outcomes Framework for England, 2013–2016*. London: HMSO.

Department of Health (2012b) *Government Response to NHS Future Forum's Second Report*. London: HMSO.

Department of Health (2012c) *Preventing Suicide in England: A Cross Government Outcome Strategy to Save Lives*. London: HMSO.

Department of Health (2012d) *Family Nurse Partnership Programme*. Available at: www.gov.uk/government/publications/family-nurse-partnership-programme-information-leaflet (last accessed 16 May 2018).

Department of Health (2013a) *UK 5 Year Antimicrobial Resistance Strategy 2013–2018*. London: DH.

Department of Health (2013b) *A Framework for Sexual Health Improvement in England*. London: HMSO.

Department of Health (2014a) *Five Year Forward View*. London: HMSO.

Department of Health (2014b) *Better Care for People With 2 or More Long Term Conditions*. London: HMSO.

Department of Health (2014c) *Closing the Gap. Priorities for Essential Change in Mental Health*. London: DH.

Department of Health (2017) *The Pregnancy Book*. London: DH. Available at: www.publichealth.hscni.net/publications/pregnancy-book-0.

Department of Health and Social Care (2015) *Rules about Tobacco, e-cigarettes and Smoking*. London: HMSO. Available at: www.gov.uk (last accessed 13 April 2018).

Department of Health, Social Services and Public Safety (2011) *New Strategic Direction for Alcohol and Drugs (Phase 2) 2011–2016: A Framework for Reducing Alcohol and Drug Related Harm in Northern Ireland*. Belfast: DHSSPS.

Department of Health, Social Services and Public Safety (2012) *A Fitter Future for All: Framework for Preventing and Addressing Overweight and Obesity in Northern Ireland 2012–2022*. Belfast: DHSSPS.

Department of Health, Social Services and Public Safety (2014) *Making Life Better: A Whole System Strategic Framework for Public Health 2013–2023*. Belfast: DHSSPS.

Department of Health, Social Services and Public Safety (2016) *Protect Life 2: A Draft Strategy for Suicide Prevention in the North of Ireland*. Belfast: DHSSPS.

Doll, R. and Hill, A.B. (1950) 'Smoking and carcinoma of the lung: a preliminary report', *British Medical Journal*, 30: 738–47.

Drummond, C., McBride, O., Fear, N. and Fuller, E. (2016) 'Alcohol dependence'. In S. McManus, P. Bebbington, R. Jenkins and T. Brugha (eds), *Mental Health and Wellbeing in England: Adult Psychiatric Morbidity Survey 2014*. Leeds: NHS Digital, Chapter 10.

Duaso, M.J. and Duncan, D. (2012) 'Health impact of smoking and smoking cessation strategies: current evidence', *British Journal of Community Nursing*, 17(8): 356–63.

Dumford, D.M. (2016) 'Antibiotic-resistant infections and treatment challenges in the immunocompromised host', *Infectious Disease Clinics of North America*, 30(2): 465–89.

Earle, S., Lloyd, C.E., Sidell, M. and Spur, S. (2007) *Theory and Research in Promoting Public Health*. London: Sage.

Ewles, L. and Simnett, I. (2003) *Promoting Health*, 5th edn. London: Baillière Tindall.

Exworthy, T., Samele, C., Urquía, N. and Forrester, A. (2012) 'Asserting prisoners' right to health: progressing beyond equivalence', *Psychiatric Services*, 63: 270–5.

Fawcett, S.B., Paine-Andrews, A., Francisco, V.T., Schultz, J.A., Richter, K.P., Lewis, R.K., Williams, E.L., Harris, K.J., Berkley, J.Y., Fisher, J.L. and Lopez, C.M. (1995) 'Using empowerment theory in collaborative partnerships for community health and development', *American Journal of Community Psychology*, 23(5): 677–97.

Fearn, M. and Howard, J. (2012) 'Play as a resource for children facing adversity: an exploration of indicative case studies', *Children and Society*, 26: 456–68.

Fernando, S. (2002) *Mental Health, Race and Culture*, 2nd edn. Basingstoke: Palgrave.

Fine, P., Eames, K. and Heymann, D.L. (2011) '"Herd immunity": a rough guide', *Clinical Infectious Diseases*, 52(7): 911–16.

Fletcher, C. and Peto, R. (1977) 'The natural history of chronic airflow obstruction', *British Medical Journal*, i: 1645–8.

Flodgren, G., Deane, K., Dickinson, H.O., Kirk, S., Alberti, H., Beyer, F.R., Brown, J.G., Penney, T.L., Summerbell, C.D. and Eccles, M.P. (2010) 'Interventions to change the behaviour of health professionals and the organisation of care to promote weight reduction in overweight and obese adults (Review)', *Cochrane Database of Systematic Reviews*, (3): 1–106.

Friedli, L. (2009) *Mental Health, Resilience and Inequalities*. Copenhagen: WHO. Available at: www.euro.who.int/__data/assets/pdf_file/0012/100821/E92227.pdf (last accessed 16 May 2018).

Friedman, M.M., Bowden, V.R. and Jones, E.G. (2003) *Family Nursing, Research, Theory and Practice*, 5th edn. Upper Saddle River, NJ: Prentice Hall.

Fuller, E. (2011) *Smoking, Drinking and Drug use among Young People in England in 2010*. London: Information Centre for Health and Social Care,.

Funk, S. and Klepac, P. (2015) 'Nine challenges in incorporating the dynamics of behavior in infectious disease models', *Epidemics*, 10(15): 21–5.

General Medical Council (2018) *Who are Children and Young People?* [Online]. London: General Medical Council. Available at: www.gmc-uk.org/ethical-guidance/ethical-guidance-for-doctors/protecting-children-and-young-people/definitions-of-children-young-people-and-parents (last accessed 16 May 2018).

Gibson, T. (2009) 'Learning disabilities education in the common foundation programme', *Nursing Standard*, 23(46): 35–9.

Gillett, M., Dallosso, H.M., Dixon, S., Brennan, A., Carey, M.E., Campbell, M.J., Heller, S., Khunti, K., Skinner, T.C. and Davies, M.J. (2010) 'Delivering the diabetes education and self management for ongoing and newly diagnosed (DESMOND) programme for people with newly diagnosed type 2 diabetes', *British Medical Journal*, Aug 20, 341: c4093.

Ginn, S. (2013) 'Promoting health in prison', *British Medical Journal*, 346: 2216f. doi:10.1136/bmj.f2216.

Gov.uk. (2017) *Guidance: Childhood Obesity: A Plan for Action* [online]. Available at: www.gov.uk/government/publications/childhood-obesity-a-plan-for-action/childhood-obesity-a-plan-for-action#fn:2 (last accessed 10 May 2018).

Gov.uk. (2018) *Help Paying for Childcare* [online]. Available at: www.gov.uk/help-with-childcare-costs/free-childcare-and-education-for-2-to-4-year-olds (last accessed 16 May 2018).

Green, J. and Tones, K. (2010) *Health Promotion: Planning and Strategies*, 2nd edn. London: Sage.

Griffiths, J., Speed, S., Horne, M. and Keeley, P. (2012) '"A caring professional attitude": what service users and carers seek in graduate nurses and the challenge for educators', *Nurse Education Today*, 32: 121–7.

Gunn, S.W. and Masellis, M. (2008) *Concepts and Practice of Humanitarian Medicine*. New York: Springer.

Hamami, D., Cameron, R., Pollock, K.G. and Shankland, C. (2017) 'Waning immunity is associated with periodic large outbreaks of mumps: a mathematical modeling study of Scottish data', *Frontiers in Physiology*, 8(233). doi:10.3389/fphys.2017.00233.

Health and Social Care Information Centre (2014) *Statistics on Obesity, Physical Activity and Diet, England 2014*. Available at: www.hscic.gov.uk/catalogue/PUB13648 (last accessed 20 May 2018).

Health Education England (2018) *Making Every Contact Count* [online]. Available at: www.makingevery contactcount.co.uk (last accessed 10 May 2018).

Health Foundation (2018) *The Better Services for the Mentally Handicapped*. Available at: https://navigator. health.org.uk/content/better-services-mentally-handicapped-white-paper-was-published-department-health-june-1971 (last accessed 9 May 2018).

Health Protection Agency (2009) *Sexual Health: Chlamydia Rates Continue to Rise*. Available at: www. statistics.gov.uk (last accessed 20 May 2018).

Heidari, E., Dickinson, C. and Newton, T. (2014) 'An overview of the prison population and the general health status of prisoners', *British Dental Journal*, 217(1): 15–19. doi:10.1038/sj.bdj.2014.548.

Helman, C.G. (2000) *Culture, Health and Illness*, 4th edn. Oxford: Butterworth-Heinemann.

Hinton, L. on behalf of the MBRRACE-UK Lay Summary Writing Group (2014) *Saving Lives, Improving Mothers' Care* – Lay Summary 2014. Report of MBRRACE (Mothers and Babies Reducing Risk through Audits and Confidential Enquiries across the UK). Available at: www.npeu.ox.ac.uk/downloads/files/ mbrrace-uk/reports/Saving%20Lives%20Improving%20Mothers%20Care%20report%202014%20 Lay%20Summary.pdf (last accessed 15 May 2018).

HM Government (2012) *The Government's Alcohol Strategy*. London: HMSO.

HM Government (2015) *Working Together to Safeguard Children, A Guide to Inter-agency Working to Safeguard and Promote the Welfare of Children*. London: HM Government.

Home Office and Department of Health (2007) *Safe, Sensible and Social: The Next Steps in the National Alcohol Strategy*. London: The Home Office.

Homeless Link (2014) *The Unhealthy State of Homelessness*. London: Homeless Link.

HSC Public Health Agency (2011) *Give Every Child the Best Start in Life* [Online]. Available at: www.publichealth. hscni.net/directorate-public-health/health-and-social-wellbeing-improvement/give-every-child-best-start-life (last accessed 10 May 2018).

Jarvis, T.J., Tebbutt, J., Mattick, R.P. and Shand, F. (2005) *Treatment Approaches to Drug and Alcohol Dependence: An Introductory Guide*, 2nd edn. Chichester: Wiley.

Karatay, G., Kublay, G. and Emiroglu, O.N. (2010) 'Effect of motivational interviewing on smoking cessation in pregnant women', *Journal of Advanced Nursing*, 66(6): 1328–37.

Keyes, C.L.M. (2009). *Atlanta: Brief Description of the Mental Health Continuum Short Form (MHC-SF)*. Available at: www.aacu.org/sites/default/files/MHC-SFEnglish.pdf (last accessed 16 August 2018).

Kinge, S. and Gregory, I. (2011) 'Maternity focus: postnatal classes and effective care', *British Journal of Healthcare Assistants*, 5(8): 399–400.

Knight, M., Nair, M., Tuffnell, D., Shakespeare, J., Kenyon, S. and Kurinczuk, J.J. (eds) (2018) *Saving Lives, Improving Mothers' Care*. MBRRACE-UK. Available at: www.npeu.ox.ac.uk/downloads/ files/mbrrace-uk/reports/MBRRACE-UK%20Maternal%20Report%202017%20-%20Web.pdf (last accessed 15 May 2018).

Koshy, P., Mackenzie, M., Tappin, D. and Bauld, L. (2010) 'Smoking cessation during pregnancy: the influence of partners, families and friends on quitters and non-quitters', *Health and Social Care in the Community*, 18(5): 500–10.

Kozier, B. (2008) *Fundamentals of Nursing: Concepts, Process and Practice*. London: Pearson.

Lalonde, M. (1974) *A New Perspective on the Health of Canadians. A working document*. Ottawa: Government of Canada.

Last, J.M. (1988) *A Dictionary of Epidemiology*, 2nd edn. New York: Oxford University Press.

Leaning, B. and Adderley, H. (2016) 'From long-stay hospitals to community care: reconstructing the narratives of people with learning disabilities', *British Journal of Learning Disabilities*, 44(2): 167–71.

Lester, S. and Russell, W. (2010) *Children's right to play: an examination of the importance of play in the lives of children worldwide*, Working paper no. 57. The Hague, The Netherlands: Bernard van Leer Foundation. Available at: www.researchgate.net/publication/263087157_Children's_Right_to_Play_An_Examination_of_the_Importance_of_Play_in_the_Lives_of_Children_Worldwide.

Lhussier, M., Carr, S.M. and Forster, N. (2015) 'A realist synthesis of the evidence on outreach programmes for health improvement of Traveller Communities', *Journal of Public Health*, 38(2): e125–32.

Littleton, J., Barron, S., Prendergast, M. and Nixon, S.J. (2007) 'Smoking kills (alcoholics): shouldn't we do something about it?', *Alcohol and Alcoholism*, 42: 167–73.

Loveday, I. and Linsley, P. (2011) 'Implementing interventions: delivering care to individuals and communities'. In P. Linsley, R. Kane and S. Owen (eds), *Nursing for Public Health: Promotion, Principles and Practice*. Oxford: Oxford University Press, pp. 134–43.

Marmot, M. (2010) *Fair Society, Health Lives. The Marmot Review*. Available at: www.instituteofhealthequity.org/resources-reports/fair-society-healthy-lives-the-marmot-review (last accessed 8 October 2018).

Marteau, T.M., Hollands, G.J., Shemilt, I. and Jebb, S.A. (2015) 'Downsizing: policy options to reduce portion sizes to help tackle obesity', *British Medical Journal*, 351: h5863.

Masterson, A. (2011) 'The importance of nursing to public health: the political and policy context'. In P. Linsley, R. Kane and S. Owen (eds), *Nursing for Public Health: Promotion, Principles and Practice*. Oxford: Oxford University Press, pp. 89–97.

McFadden, A., Atkin, K., Bell, K., Innes, N., Jackson, C., Jones, H., MacGillivary, S. and Siebelt, L. (2016) 'Community engagement to enhance trust between Gypsy/Travellers, and maternity, early years' and child dental health services: protocol for a multi method exploratory study', *International Journal for Equity in Health*, 15: 183.

McKeown, T. (1976) *The Role of Medicine: Dream, Mirage or Nemesis?* London: Nuffield Provincial Hospitals Trust.

Meader, N., King, K., Moe-Byrne, T., Wright, K., Graham, H., Petticrew, M., Power, C., White, M. and Sowden, A.J. (2016) 'A systematic review on the clustering and co-occurrence of multiple risk behaviours', *BMC Public Health*, 16: 657.

MENCAP (2007) *Death by Indifference: Following up the Treat me Right! Report*. London: MENCAP. Available at: www.mencap.org.uk/sites/default/files/2016-06/DBIreport.pdf (last accessed 16 May 2018).

MENCAP (2018) *Health Inequalities*. Available at: www.mencap.org.uk/learning-disability-explained/research-and-statistics/health/health-inequalities (last accessed 9 May 2018).

Mendis, S., Puska, P. and Norrving, B. (2011) *Global Atlas on Cardiovascular Disease Prevention and Control*. Geneva: WHO, 3–18.

Mulhall, A. (1996) *Epidemiology, Nursing and Healthcare: A New Perspective*. Basingstoke: Macmillan.

Myint, P.K., Smith, R.D., Luben, R.N., Surtess, P.G., Wainwright, N.W., Wareham, N.J. and Khaw, K.T. (2011) 'Lifestyle behaviours and quality-adjusted life years in middle and older age', *Age and Ageing*, 40(5): 589–95.

Naidoo, J. and Wills, J. (2009) *Foundations for Health Promotion*, 3rd edn. London: Baillière Tindall/Elsevier.

National Institute for Health and Care Excellence (2007a) *Behaviour Change: The Principles for Effective Interventions NICE Public Health*, Guidance 6. London: NICE.

National Institute for Health and Care Excellence (2007b) *One to One Interventions to Reduce the Transmission of Sexually Transmitted Infections (STIs) Including HIV, and to Reduce the Rate of under 18 Conceptions, Especially Among Vulnerable and At Risk Groups*. London: NICE.

National Institute for Health and Care Excellence (2008a) *Community Engagement*, NICE Public Health Guidance 9. London: NICE.

National Institute for Health and Care Excellence (2008b) *Maternal and Child Nutrition*, NICE Public Health Guidance 11. Last updated 2014 Available at: www.nice.org.uk/guidance/ph11 (last accessed 16 May 2018).

National Institute for Health and Care Excellence (2009) *Child Maltreatment: When to Suspect Maltreatment in under 18s (Clinical guideline CG89; last updated 2017)*. London: NICE.

National Institute for Health and Care Excellence (2010) *Quitting Smoking in Pregnancy and Following Childbirth, NICE Public Health Guidance PH26*. Available at: www.nice.org.uk/guidance/ph26 (last accessed 16 May 2018).

National Institute for Health and Care Excellence (2013a) *Physical Activity: Brief Advice for Adults in Primary Care*, NICE Public Health Guidance 44. London: NICE.

National Institute for Health and Care Excellence (2013b) *Assessing Body Mass Index and Waist Circumference Thresholds for Intervening to Prevent Ill Health and Premature Death Among Adults from Black, Asian and Other Minority Groups in UK*, NICE Public Health Guidance 46. London: NICE.

National Institute for Health and Care Excellence (2013c) *Quality Standard 37. Postnatal Care*. Available at: www.nice.org.uk/guidance/qs37 (last accessed 16 May 2018).

National Institute for Health and Care Excellence (2014) *Behaviour Change: Individual Approaches*, NICE Public Health Guidance 49. London: NICE.

National Institute for Health and Care Excellence (2015) *Dementia, Disability and Frailty in Later Life: Mid-life Approaches to Delay or Prevent Onset*. London: NICE. Available at: www.nice.org.uk/guidance/ng/16.

National Institute for Health and Care Excellence (2017) *Child Abuse and Neglect*. NICE Guideline [NG76]. London: NICE.

National Society for the Prevention of Cruelty to Children (NSPCC) (2018) *Safeguarding Children, What Organisations Need to Do to Protect Children from Harm*. Available at: www.nspcc.org.uk/preventing-abuse/safeguarding (last accessed 10 May 2018).

Newton, J. (2015) 'Changes in Health in England, with analysis by England regions and areas for deprivation, 1990–2013: a systematic analysis for the Global Burden of Disease Study 2013', *The Lancet*, published online, 15 September 2015, http://dx.doi.org/10.1016/S0140-6736 (15) 00195-6 (last accessed 11 May 2018).

NHS (2010) *Off to the Best Start: Important Information about Feeding Your Baby*. Available at: www.unicef.org.uk/babyfriendly/wp-content/uploads/sites/2/2010/11/Off_to_the_Best_Start_Leaflet_4_Pages-2017_.pdf.

NHS Digital (2017) *Mental Health Act Statistics, Annual Figures: 2016–17, Experimental Statistics*. Available at: https://digital.nhs.uk/data-and-information/publications/statistical/mental-health-act-statistics-annual-figures/mental-health-act-statistics-annual-figures-2016-17-experimental-statistics (last accessed 16 May 2018).

NHS England (2016) *Five Year Forward View for Mental Health*. London: NHS England.

NHS England (2017) *The Learning Disabilities Mortality Review (LeDeR Programme) Annual Report*, December 2017. Bristol: Norah Fry Centre for Disability Studies.

NHS Future Forum (2012) *NHS Future Forum Summary Report: Second Phase Overarching Report*. Available at: www.gov.uk/government/publications/nhs-future-forum-recommendations-to-government-second-phase (last accessed 28 March 2018).

NHS Information Centre (2012) *The Health Survey for England*. Available at: https://digital.nhs.uk/data-and-information/publications/statistical/health-survey-for-england (last accessed 8 October 2018).

Noar, S.M., Benac, C.N. and Harris, M.S. (2007) 'Does tailoring matter? Meta-analytic review of tailored print health behavior change interventions', *Psychological Bulletin*, 4: 673–93.

Nursing and Midwifery Council (2018a) *The Code: Professional Standards of Practice and Behaviour for Nurses and Midwives*. London: NMC.

Nursing and Midwifery Council (2018b) *Future Nurse: Standards of Proficiency for Registered Nurses*. London: NMC.

Nutbeam, D. and Harris, E. (2010) *Theory in a Nutshell: A Guide to Health Promotion Theory*. Melbourne: McGraw-Hill.

Office for National Statistics (2011) *Statistics on CHD and CVD in England*. London: ONS.

Office for National Statistics (2016a) *Statistical Bulletin: Avoidable Mortality in England and Wales: 2014*. London: ONS.

Office for National Statistics (2016b) *Statistical Bulletin: Effects of Taxes and Benefits on UK Household Income: Financial Year Ending 2016*. London: ONS.

Office for National Statistics (2017a) *Adult Smoking Habits in the UK: 2016*. London: ONS. Available at: www.ons.gov.uk/peoplepopulationandcommunity/healthandsocialcare/healthandlifeexpectancies/bulletins/adultsmokinghabitsingreatbritain/2016 (last accessed 11 May 2018).

Office for National Statistics (2017b) 'Research and analysis'. In *Major Causes of Death and How They Have Changed*. London: ONC, Chapter 2.

Office for National Statistics (2017c) *Overview of the UK Population: July 2017*. London: ONS. Available at: www.ons.gov.uk/peoplepopulationandcommunity/populationandmigration/populationestimates/articles/overviewoftheukpopulation/july2017 (last accessed 4 May 2018).

Office for National Statistics (2018a) *Adult Drinking Habits in Great Britain: 2017*. London: ONS. Available at: www.ons.gov.uk (last accessed 11 May 2018).

Office for National Statistics (2018b) *Families and Households: 2017*. London: ONS. Available at: file://nask.man.ac.uk/home$/Families%20and%20Households%202017.pdf (last accessed 5 May 2018).

Paiva, A.L., Prochaska, J.O., Yin, H.G., Rossi, J.S., Redding, C.A., Blissmer, B., Robbins, M.L., Velicer, W.F., Lipschitz, J., Amoyal, N., Babbin, S.F., Blaney, C.L., Sillice, M.A., Fernandez, A., McGee, H. and Horiuchi, S. (2012) 'Treated individuals who progress to action or maintenance for one behaviour are more likely to make similar progress on another behaviour: coaction results of a pooled data analysis of three trials', *Preventive Medicine*, 54(5): 331–4.

Parkin, E. and Powell, T. (2017) *Mental Health Policy in England*. London: House of Commons.

Pasquali, R., Patton, L. and Gamberini, A. (2007) '"Obesity and infertility": current opinion in endocrinology', *Diabetes and Obesity*, 14(6): 482–7.

Percival, J. (2013) 'Smoking cessation: reducing harm and improving the health of children', *Journal of Health Visiting*, 1(12): 689–95.

Percival, J. (2014) 'Promoting health: making every contact count', *Nursing Standard*, 28(29): 37–41.

Phillips, L. (2012) 'Improving care for people with learning disabilities in hospital', *Nursing Standard*, 26(23): 42–58.

Plotkin, S., Orenstein, W., Offitt, P. and Edwards, K.M. (2017) *Plotkin's Vaccines*, 7th edn. New York: Elsevier.

Powell, J. (2013) 'Use of the common assessment framework in an acute setting', *Nursing Children and Young People*, 25(5): 24–8.

Prime Minister's Strategy Unit (2003) *Alcohol Misuse: How Much Does It Cost?* London: Prime Minister's Strategy Unit.

Prochaska, J.O. and DiClemente, C.C. (1986) 'Towards a comprehensive model of change'. In W.R. Miller and N. Heather (eds), *Treating Addictive Behaviors: Processes of Change*. New York: Plenum, 3–27.

Public Health England (2013) *Our Priorities for 2013/14*. London: PHE.

Public Health England (2014) *Evidence into Action*. London: PHE.

Public Health England (2016a) *Making a Difference in Dementia: Nursing Vision and Strategy Refreshed*. London: PHE.

Public Health England (2016b) *The Eatwell Guide*. London: PHE.

Public Health England (2016c) *Strategic Plan for the Next Four Years: Better Outcomes by 2020*. London: PHE.

Public Health England (2016d) *Health Matters: Giving Every Child the Best Start in Life* [Online]. Available at: www.gov.uk/government/publications/health-matters-giving-every-child-the-best-start-in-life/health-matters-giving-every-child-the-best-start-in-life#summary (last accessed 10 May 2018).

Public Health England (2017a) *Influenza Vaccine Effectiveness (VE) in Adults and Children in Primary Care in the United Kingdom (UK): Provisional End-of-season Results 2016–17*. Available at: www.gov.uk/government/uploads/system (last accessed 15 April 2018).

Public Health England (2017b) 'Table 2'. In *New STI Diagnoses & Rates by Gender, Sexual Risk & Age Group, 2012–2016*, London: Public Health England, p. 7.

Rees, S. (2009) *Mental Ill Health in the Adult Single Population. A Review of the Literature*. London: Crisis.

Roberts, C., Lepps, H., Strang, J. and Singleton, N. (2016) 'Drug use and dependence'. In S. McManus, P. Bebbington, R. Jenkins and T. Brugha (eds), *Mental Health and Wellbeing in England: Adult Psychiatric Morbidity Survey 2014*. Leeds: NHS Digital, Chapter 11.

Robertson, K. (2010) 'Understanding the needs of women with postnatal depression', *Nursing Standard*, 24(46): 47–55.

Roper, N., Logan, W.W. and Tierney, A.J. (2000) *The Elements of Nursing*. Edinburgh: Churchill Livingstone.

Rosen, G. (1993) *A History of Public Health*. Baltimore, MA: Johns Hopkins University Press.

Rosenberg, J.P. and Yates, P. (2014) 'Health promotion in palliative care: the case for conceptual congruence', *Critical Public Health*, 20(2): 201–10.

Rosenstock, I.M. (1974) 'Historical origins of the health belief model', *Health Education Monographs*, 2: 328–35.

Rowe, A., McClelland, A. and Billingham, K. (2001) *Community Health Needs Assessment: An Introductory Guide for the Family Health Nurse in Europe*. Geneva: World Health Organization.

Royal College of Nursing (2012) *Going Upstream: Nursing's Contribution to Public Health: RCN Guidance for Nurses*. London: RCN.

Royal College of Nursing (2013) *Meeting the Health Needs of People with Learning Disabilities: RCN Guidance for Nursing Staff*. London: RCN. Available at: www.rcn.org.uk/professional-development/publications/pub-003024 (last accessed 16 May 2018).

Royal College of Nursing (2016) *Nurse 4 Public Health: Promote, Prevent and Protect: The Value and Contribution of Nursing to Public Health in the UK: Final Report*. London: RCN.

Royal College of Psychiatrists (2014) *Postpartum Psychosis: Severe Mental Illness after Childbirth*. Available at: www.rcpsych.ac.uk/healthadvice/problemsdisorders/postpartumpsychosis.aspx (last accessed 20 May 2018).

Rozenfeld, V., Ribak, J., Tsamir, J. and Carmeli, E. (2010) 'Prevalence, risk factors and preventive strategies in work-related musculoskeletal disorders among Israeli physical therapists', *Physiotherapy Research International*, 15(3): 176–84.

Salva, A., Andrieu, S., Fernandez, E., Schiffrin, E.J., Moulin, J., Decarli, B., Guigoz, Y. and Vellas, B. (2009) 'Health and nutritional promotion program for patients with dementia (NutriAlz study): design and baseline data', *Journal of Nutrition, Health and Aging*, 13(6): 529–37.

Salway, S., Mir, G., Turner, D., Ellison, G.T.H., Carter, L. and Gerrish, K. (2016) 'Obstacles to "race equality" in the English National Health Service: insights from the healthcare commissioning arena', *Social Science and Medicine*, 152: 102–10.

Sanders, B. and Brianna, B. (2015) *I Was on My Own: Experiences of Loneliness and Isolation amongst Homeless People*. London: Crisis.

Sashidharan, S.P. and Commander, M.J. (1998) 'Mental health'. In S. Rawaf and V. Bahl (eds), *Assessing Health Needs of People from Minority Ethnic Groups*. London: Royal College of Physicians.

Scambler, G. (2009) 'Health-related stigma', *Sociology of Health and Illness*, 31(3): 441–55.

Scottish Government (2008) *The Road to Recovery: A New Approach to Tackling Scotland's Drug Problem*. Edinburgh: The Scottish Government.

Scottish Government (2009) *Changing Scotland's Relationship with Alcohol: A Framework for Action*. Edinburgh: The Scottish Government.

Scottish Government (2013a) *Creating a Tobacco-Free Generation. Tobacco Control Strategy for Scotland*. Edinburgh: The Scottish Government.

Scottish Government (2013b) *Suicide Prevention Strategy*. Available at: www.gov.scot/Publications/2013/12/7616 (last accessed 16 May 2018).

Scottish Government (2016) *Race Equality Framework for Scotland 2016–2030*. Available at: www.gov.scot/Resource/0049/00497601.pdf (last accessed 16 August 2018).

Scottish Government (2017) *Our Children have the Best Start in Life and are Ready to Succeed* [online]. Available at: www.gov.scot/About/Performance/scotPerforms/outcome/children (last accessed 10 May 2018).

Scottish Government (2018) *Minimum Unit Pricing*. Scotland: The Scottish Government. Available at: www.minimumunitpricing.scot (last accessed 11 May 2018).

Shah, N.R. and Braverman, E.R. (2012) 'Measuring adiposity in patients: the utility of body mass index (BMI), percent body fat, and leptin', *PLoS ONE*, 7(4): e33308.

Shelton, S.J. and Knott, C.S. (2014) 'Association between alcohol calorie intake and overweight and obesity in English adults', *American Journal of Public Health*, 104(4): 629–31.

Shepherd, A.A. (2008) 'Nutrition through the life-span. Part 1: preconception, pregnancy and infancy', *British Journal of Nursing*, 17(20): 1261–7.

Silberstein, J.L. and Parsons, J.K. (2010) 'Prostate cancer prevention: concepts and clinical recommendations', *Prostate Cancer and Prostatic Disease*, 13(4): 300–6.

Smaje, C. (1995) *Health, 'Race' and Ethnicity: Making Sense of the Evidence*. London: King's Fund Institute.

Spring, B., Moller, A.C. and Coons, M.J. (2012) 'Multiple health behaviours: overview and implications', *Journal of Public Health*, 34(Suppl i): i3–10.

Sylva, K., Melhuish, E., Sammons, P., Siraj-Blatchford, I. and Taggart, B. (2004) 'Effective provision of pre-school education (EPPE)', Project, Research Online, University of Woolongong. Available at: http://ro.uow.edu.au/cgi/viewcontent.cgi?article=3155&context=sspapers (last accessed 16 August 2018).

Tannahill, A. (1990) In R.S. Downie, C. Fyfe and A. Tannahill (eds), *Health Promotion: Models and Values*. Oxford: Oxford University Press.

Taylor, R.S., Dalal, H., Moxham, T. and Zawada, A. (2010) 'Home-based versus centre-based cardiac rehabilitation', *Cochrane Database of Systematic Reviews*, (1): CD007130. doi:10.1002/14651858. CD007130.pub2.

Thomas, C.S., Stone, K., Osborn, M., Thoma, P.F. and Fisher, M. (1993) 'Psychiatric morbidity and compulsory admission among UK-born Europeans, Afro-Caribbeans and Asians in Central Manchester', *British Journal of Psychiatry*, 163: 91–9.

Thomas, S. and Price, M. (2012) 'Respite care in seven families with children with complex care needs', *Nursing Children and Young People*, 24(8): 24–7.

Thomson, G., Crossland, N. and Dykes, F. (2011) 'Giving me hope: women's reflections on a breastfeeding support service', *Maternal and Child Nutrition*, 8: 340–53.

Timby, B.K. (2012) *Fundamental Nursing Skills and Concept*, 10th edn. Philadelphia, PA: Lippincott, Williams & Wilkins.

Tolstrup, J.S., Hvidtfeldt, U.A., Flachs, E.M., Spiegelman, D., Heitmann, B.L., Balter, K., Goldbourt, U., Hallmans, G., Knekt, P., Liu, S., Pereira, M., Stevens, J., Virtamo, J. and Feskanich, D. (2014) 'Smoking and risk of coronary heart disease in younger, middle-aged, and older adults', *American Journal of Public Health*, 104(1): 96–102.

Townsend, P., Davidson, N. and Whitehead, M. (eds) (1992) *Inequalities in Health: The Black Report: The Health Divide*. London: Penguin Books.

UN (1989) *Convention on the Rights of the Child*. Available at: www.ohchr.org/EN/ProfessionalInterest/Pages/CRC.aspx (last accessed 16 May 2018).

Upton, D. and Thirlaway, K. (2010) *Promoting Healthy Behaviour: A Practical Guide for Nursing and Healthcare Professionals*. London: Pearson Education.

Van Cleemput, P., Parry, G., Thomas, K., Peters, J. and Cooper, C. (2007) 'Health-related beliefs and experiences of Gypsies and Travellers: a qualitative study', *Journal of Epidemiology and Community Health*, 61(3): 205–10.

Vynnycky, E. and White, R.G. (2010) *An Introduction to Infectious Disease Modelling*. Oxford: Oxford University Press.

Wadsworth, M. (1996) 'Family and education as determinants of health'. In D. Blane, E. Brunner and R. Wilkinson (eds), *Health and Social Organisation: Towards a Health Policy for the 21st Century*. London: Routledge, Chapter 9.

Watson, R., Stimpson, A. and Hostick, C. (2009) 'Prison health care: a review of the literature', *International Journal of Nursing Studies*, 41(2): 119–28.

Welsh Government (2013) *Building a Brighter Future: Early Years and Childcare Plan* [online]. Available at: http://dera.ioe.ac.uk/18045/1/130716-building-brighter-future-en.pdf (last accessed 16 May 2018).

Wilkinson, R.G. (2005) *The Impact of Inequality: How to Make Sick Societies Healthier*. London: Routledge.

Wilkinson, R. and Marmot, M. (2003) *The Solid Facts*, 2nd edn. Copenhagen: WHO. Available at: www.euro.who.int/document/e81384.pdf (last accessed 16 May 2018).

Wisborg, K., Kesmodel, U., Henriksen, T.B., Olsen, S.F. and Secher, N.J. (2000) 'A prospective study of smoking during pregnancy and SIDS', *Archives of Disease in Childhood*, 83: 203–6.

World Health Organization (1986) *Ottawa Charter for Health Promotion: An International Conference on Health Promotion*. Geneva: WHO.

World Health Organization (2002) *The World Health Report 2002: Reducing Risks, Promoting Healthy Life*. Geneva: WHO.

World Health Organization (2003) *Investing in Mental Health*. Geneva: WHO. Available at: www.who.int/mental_health/media/investing_mnh.pdf (last accessed 16 May 2018).

World Health Organization (2013) *Mental Health Action Plan, 2013–2020*. Geneva: WHO.

World Health Organization (2014) *Global Report on Alcohol and Health 2014*. Geneva: WHO.

World Health Organization (2017) *Child Maltreatment*. WHO/NMH/NV1/18.6. Geneva: WHO.

World Health Organization and International Society for Prevention of Child Abuse and Neglect (2006) *Preventing Child Maltreatment: A Guide to Taking Action and Generating Evidence*. Geneva: WHO, ISPCAN.

Yusuf, S., Reddy, S., Ounpuu, S. and Anand, S. (2001) 'Global burden of cardiovascular diseases, part 1: general considerations, the epidemiological transition, risk factors, and impact of urbanization', *Circulation*, 104: 2746–53.

Yusuf, S., Hawken, S., Ounpuu, S., Dans, T., Avezum, A., Lanas, F., McQueen, M., Budaj, A., Pais, P., Varigos, J. and Lisheng, L. (2004) 'Effect of potentially modifiable risk factors associated with myocardial infarction in 52 countries (the INTERHEART study): case-control study', *The Lancet*, 364(9438): 937–52.

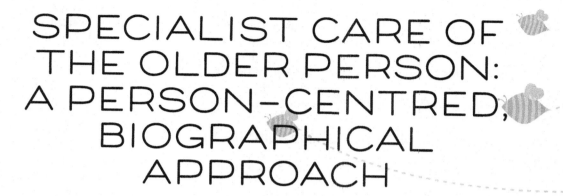

# SPECIALIST CARE OF THE OLDER PERSON: A PERSON-CENTRED, BIOGRAPHICAL APPROACH

## EMMA STANMORE AND CHRISTINE BROWN WILSON

---

### CHAPTER OBJECTIVES

- Outline the specialist needs and challenges around planning and delivering high-quality care to pre-frail and frail older people, and supporting their carers in a variety of settings;
- Consider the principles of anti-discriminatory practice through examining myths and stereotypes that may detrimentally influence the care of older people, including those with dementia;
- Explain the importance of preventative care and health promotion for older people, including those with dementia with particular reference to physical activity and falls prevention;
- Explore the principles of independence, empowerment and choice for the delivery of care, and the role of technology in supporting these principles;
- Identify how dignity and compassion might be promoted for older people in everyday practice;
- Evaluate the role of the nurse in establishing the needs and preferences of older people and their carers through the use of person-centred and biographical care planning.

---

This chapter considers the knowledge, skills and attitudes required by nurses for the optimum care of the older person and how we as nurses might promote individualised, person-centred care in everyday practice. We explore how the principles of health promotion (with particular reference to physical activity and falls prevention) can be applied to promote independence and improve the quality of life for older people. We address other important topics such as dignity in care, empowerment and choice in relation to the care of older people, including people with dementia or 'frailty'. We also consider the role of carers and how we might support the carers of older people, including those with dementia. A key aim is for readers to question current perceptions of older people, using examples of myths and stereotypes that can often influence how ageing is viewed and valued in our society. The chapter promotes an understanding of the principles of anti-discriminatory practice with reference to age and considers how this is applied in practice. Most importantly, we also demonstrate the importance of using biography throughout the assessment process, appreciating the experience, skills and wisdom of older people to both enrich our nursing practice and enhance person-centred care.

## Related NMC proficiencies for registered nurses

The overarching NMC requirements are that all registered nurses should be able to

manage the complex nursing and integrated care needs of people at any stage of their lives; supporting and enabling them to make informed choices about how to manage health challenges in order to maximise their quality of life and improve health outcomes. Working in partnership with people, nurses need to be able to use information obtained during assessments (taking into account their circumstances, characteristics, wishes and preferences) to identify the priorities and requirements for person-centred and evidence based nursing interventions. They should also assess risks to safety or experience and take appropriate action to manage those, putting the best interests, needs and preferences of people first . . . across a range of organisations and settings.

(Nursing and Midwifery Council [NMC], 2018)

 **To achieve entry to the nursing register you must be able to**

- Understand the principles and processes involved in supporting people and families with a range of care needs in order to maintain optimal independence and avoid unnecessary interventions and disruptions to their lives;
- Take into account knowledge of body systems and homoeostasis, human anatomy and physiology, biology, pharmacology, social, physical, behavioural and cognitive health conditions, medication usage and treatments when undertaking full and accurate person-centred nursing assessments;
- Demonstrate the ability to accurately process all information gathered during the assessment process (including an understanding of co-morbidities and the need to meet people's complex nursing and social care needs) to individualise nursing care, developing and applying person-centred evidence-based plans for nursing interventions with agreed goals;
- Demonstrate the ability to work in partnership with people, families and carers (encouraging shared decision making) to continuously monitor, evaluate and reassess the effectiveness of all agreed nursing care plans and care, readjusting agreed goals, documenting progress and decisions made in order to support individuals, their families and carers to manage their own care when appropriate;

- Effectively assess a person's capacity to make decisions about their own care and to give or with-hold consent, and understand and apply the principles and processes for making reasonable adjustments and best interest decisions where people do not have capacity;
- Recognise and assess people at risk of harm and the situations that may put them at risk, using a range of contemporary assessment and improvement tools, and ensuring that prompt action is taken to safeguard those who are vulnerable;
- Demonstrate knowledge of when and how to refer people safely to other professionals or services for clinical intervention or support.

(Adapted from NMC, 2018)

## Background

It is a cause for celebration that people in the UK are living longer and, on the whole, healthier lives than ever before (Government Office for Science, 2016). This reflects our advancement in areas such as healthcare technologies, pharmacology, education, better living conditions and reduced child-hood mortality. For the first time in history we have more people over the age of 60 than those under the age of 18 (Office for National Statistics [ONS], 2017) with the 'oldest old' (over the age of 85) being the fastest growing demographic. It is for this very reason that all adult nurses need to be educated in the specialism of care of older people to ensure that their individual needs are met.

It would be logical to think that, as older people are the core users of the NHS, this would lead to more expertise within this field of care in nursing and healthcare. However, this does not appear to be the case, with recent reports repeatedly highlighting a picture of poor or variable care for older people (Cornwell, 2012; Royal College of Physicians [RCP], 2012; Francis, 2013; Humphries et al., 2016). The Mid Staffordshire enquiry highlighted the need for the delivery of compassionate care for older people. This public enquiry and other similar reports (Andrews and Butler, 2014) revealed a negative culture of disengagement, low morale, tolerance of poor care and long-term understaffing which led to high mortality rates, undignified care, and excessive levels of patient and staff complaints that had been previously unaddressed by those in authority. Since then, issues of quality of care for older people have more than ever been in the public eye (Age UK, 2017).

The positive side of these perturbing reports is that they have led to an unparalleled opportunity to transform services for older people, in which nurses have a key role. As older people account for the majority of patients, all adult nurses should be educated in this specialism, including the aware-ness and skills in working with patients who are cognitively impaired (such as those with dementia) or frail. One of the key recommendations in the Francis Report (2013) is that the specialist require-ments of caring for older people should be recognised by the introduction of a new status of a registered older person's nurse. There have been a number of other government actions to help put the care of older people at the centre of healthcare, which include an improved publicly available ratings system for the inspection of healthcare organisations with a greater emphasis on compas-sionate care. There has been a governmental drive to promote more research and improved standards for the care of older people with dementia (Department of Health [DH], 2016). Similarly, following the recognition that mild frailty or pre-frailty is potentially reversible, the e-frailty index tool has been implemented to highlight those at risk with a view to preventing frailty progression (National Institute for Health and Care Excellence [NICE], 2016). Tailored education and support are to be offered for nursing staff to promote the values of compassion, dignity and respect, and there is to be a reduction in unnecessary bureaucracy through streamlining inspections, information sharing and the improved use of technology among frontline staff, to give more time to and emphasis on caring.

There has also been a governmental push to recruit people into the care workforce who demonstrate a desire and ability to care for others (DH, 2013; Government Office for Science, 2016). Therefore, as a result of these policies, we may see some important leadership changes in the care of older people, with a greater recognition of the skills required for competent and compassionate care, and nurses need to seize these opportunities to make a difference.

Identify the key nursing skills required to care effectively for older people to overcome the shortcomings of the public enquiries mentioned above.

- When providing care to an older adult, how could you ensure that you are able to develop your clinical skills outlined in annexes A and B of the NMC (2018) proficiency framework?
- How might you demonstrate these skills in everyday practice?
- Provide one or two examples where you might implement these skills.

## Myths and stereotypes of older people

Before discussing the challenges of caring for the growing population of older people further, it is important to recognise the value and importance of older people as individuals with beneficial societal roles and influences. Ageing should not signify decline and disease. Many older adults continue to perform at exceptionally high levels and learn new skills, as well as coping with major life changes such as retirement and bereavement. With age comes a wealth of experience, wisdom and skills that are a rich resource for all generations. At present, these skills do not seem to be fully realised by society at large, although since 2011 older people can, if they wish, continue working past the age of 65. A 2015 Eurobarometer report found that people in the UK are the second most likely in Europe to see ageism as a problem, with those in the 50–64 and 65–74 age groups most likely to be worried that employers will show preference to those in their 20s (Age UK, 2011; European Commission, 2015; Government Office for Science, 2016). However, we know that older people can be as productive as younger generations and we need to discard any stereotypes about what we think it means to be 'old' (Bowers et al., 2013). Older people should not be seen as a homogeneous group with burdensome needs, but as diverse individuals with the ability to contribute to society and the same right to dignified, personalised care as any other generation.

Myths can be described as stories propagated within a society and were often a means of educating people in the values and morals of society. In the global society in which we currently live, myths now emerge from advertising through a range of media. In terms of ageing, myths portray old age either as a sign of decline and increasing decrepitude or as a heroic point in life, where older adults overcome adverse effects of ageing to do things that would be expected of younger members of society such as running marathons. Neither of these views are particularly helpful for older people because they do not recognise the individual nature of ageing or the context in which people live their later years (Minkler, 1996). These views have been perpetuated by early sociological research, resulting in the disengagement and activity theories and, more latterly, the theory of successful ageing (for a discussion on these theories, please see Bond et al., 2007).

We stereotype people by placing them in a group with others whom we believe all have similar traits and so will behave in similar ways, and this is often used as a mechanism to mentally organise workload. In addition, by stereotyping people in this way, we risk seeing them as 'different' and so can justify treating them differently. For older people, this may mean treating them with less dignity than other groups of people in our care. The language we use often refers to the stereotypes to which we subscribe (Fiske et al., 2002; Oliver, 2013). For example, referring to older people as 'the elderly' suggests we believe that all older people have limited capacity for development because they are in a period of decline. This may be used to justify nursing older people in bed for longer periods, because they already have limited mobility and limited capacity to recover. However, when we consider the personal nature of ageing we cannot assume that all older people approach their ageing in the same way (Bond et al., 2007). Therefore, we might conclude that myths and stereotypes of ageing in our society may have an adverse impact on older people when they present to healthcare environments. For example, nurses in busy environments may unknowingly use stereotypes to make quick decisions when faced by an increasing workload. Students have recounted how staff nurses see older people being admitted to wards and make assumptions based on these stereotypes, such as the expectation that an older person will suffer from incontinence or that they have dementia (Brown Wilson, 2013). These decisions may have an adverse impact on the care of older people, because nurses are often the gatekeepers for referrals to other healthcare professionals/services.

Consider two older people you know or have cared for who are similar ages.

- What influences their approach to their ageing?
- Are there similarities and differences?
- What do you attribute these to?
- What do you think this means for your care of the older person?

No one will be immune from societal stereotypes but an awareness of when myths or stereotypes are being used to make judgements about the older person and their care is the first step in minimising the potential harm they may cause. In addition, adopting an approach to care that focuses on the person and enables the practitioner to see the condition in context to the person will also lessen the impact negative stereotypes may have. As nurses, we must challenge the stereotype of ageing as a period of decline, and support older people to maintain and enhance their quality of life by improving their health in ways that are meaningful to them.

## The opportunities and challenges of caring for older people

Older people are the main users of health services in both hospitals and the community, and this trend is likely to continue. With increasing age the risk of living with one or more long-term medical conditions increases, and hospitals are struggling to cope with fewer beds and increasing numbers of emergency admissions, largely due to the increase in older patients (RCP, 2012). The Office for Budget Responsibility (2015) projects total public spending to increase by nearly 5% of

GDP between 2019–20 and 2064–65 – equivalent to £79 billion in today's terms, mainly due to the ageing population. The growing number of older people will bring new challenges to those nurses responsible for the care of older people, as well as new opportunities to ensure high-quality care is experienced and maintained for older people and their carers.

Traditionally, care of the older person has been seen as a less attractive career pathway compared with other nursing specialisms, but in reality it is a rewarding, challenging field of nursing that is ripe for further development and innovation. There are opportunities for nurses to pioneer and transform services designed to support older people to live longer in their own homes using assistive technologies, and to deliver better preventative care or specialist inpatient care that incorporates their needs and preferences. Social media, ubiquitous computing and digital health technologies such as mobile health apps are proving to be of great value to healthcare. Patients and doctors are increasingly using social media such as Twitter and Facebook to post medical problems and seek help finding diagnoses, and apps are commonly used to provide information about conditions and support self-management of care. Telehealth (also known as telecare or remote patient monitoring) is currently expanding due to its potential to enable more older people to receive care under the supervision of a healthcare team, reducing costly home visits and improving quality of care as well as preventing accidents and crises. Findings from a large, 'Whole System Demonstrator' trial in the UK found that telehealth is associated with lower mortality and emergency admission rates (Steventon et al., 2013). There are also growing numbers of 'smart homes' with embedded health devices such as movement and fall sensors, programmes to manage complex medication regimens, and microprocessors in appliances, furniture and clothing that collect health-monitoring data.

Despite these technological advances which aim to enable people to remain active at home age for longer, benefits achieved to date still require further research (Greenhalgh et al., 2012). The process of developing and implementing telehealth technologies requires coordination and commitment between numerous professions and organisations. However, nurses are in a key position to support, implement and evaluate new technologies to ensure that they are introduced using best evidence, with joined-up service provision and, most importantly, what older people want.

- Consider an older person that you know: what technology do they use in everyday life? How might this or similar technology be used to enhance their health or maintain their independence as they age?

The care of older people can be emotionally demanding and requires qualities such as compassion, empathy and patience, alongside specialist gerontological education to ensure that nurses are equipped to meet the complex care needs using a person-centred approach. Caring for older people requires an understanding of the physiological changes that take place as we age, with in-depth knowledge of long-term conditions such as diabetes, depression, arthritis, cardiovascular disease, respiratory conditions and dementia, to name but a few (see Arking, 2006, for more information about the biology of ageing and Goodwin et al., 2010, to learn more about the long-term conditions affecting older people).

We know that older people, given the right help and support, would prefer to live in their familiar homes and communities for as long as possible. However, Smith et al. (2011) argue that much of the current undergraduate nurse education programme is focused on acute hospital care for patients with single organ or infectious diseases, whereas many older people have complex care needs and multiple co-morbidities and predominantly use primary care services as well as hospitals. Indeed, the current model of acute care is geared to treatment and cure, and is not well suited to older patients living with complex needs. There is also the consideration of the complexities of polypharmacy, and the interaction between multiple medications and their side effects, the need to give preventative care to enable older people to stay independent and disease free. As a registered nurse you will need to develop your knowledge and understanding of these issues in order to be able to support those with complex, often interrelated co-morbidities, the frail 'oldest old' and the growing number of people with dementia in an already over-stretched health service. This may require you to undertake additional gerontological courses in the future to gain the skills required for the care of older people.

Developing the specialised skills and knowledge to care for older people and a positive attitude to ageing at the individual as well as the organisational level should drive a sustainable improvement in service provision and improve dignity in care for older people.

## Maintaining dignity for the older person

Dignity in care refers to the care and support in any setting that promotes and maintains a person's self-respect whatever their circumstances, health, age or any other such difference. The Social Care Institute for Excellence (2013) defines dignity as a state, quality or manner worthy of esteem or respect, and (by extension) self-respect. Although dignity may be difficult to define, it is clear to an older person when they have not received dignified care, and this can result in feelings of embarrassment and humiliation. From the perspective of the older person in hospital, it can be the small actions, such as finding out their usual routines, needs and preferences rather than conforming to standardised hospital routines, that can make an older person feel like a valued individual. Being thoughtful, polite and caring not only enriches the care that is delivered, but can also reduce the person's anxiety and increase their confidence. For example, simply reading an excerpt from a book that is of interest to a patient who is blind shows that you are trying to do what really matters to the patient and applying this to your practice.

Nordenfelt and Edgar (2005) describe four ways of understanding dignity (Figure 11.1): dignity we earn by our actions (Dignity of Merit) and for whom we are in society (Dignity of Identity), dignity we feel within ourselves (Dignity of Moral Status) and dignity we deserve because we are human (Menschenwürde). These are interrelated concepts with Dignity of Merit and Dignity of Identity conferred on us by others. If people treat us with dignity because they feel our position in society warrants this, then this will support our own sense of worth, leading to self-respect. Each of these notions is underpinned by the respect we should show to all people because they are human beings. However, if this respect is not shown, then our sense of dignity becomes eroded, which then impacts adversely on our self-respect (Nordenfelt and Edgar, 2005).

This conceptual definition of dignity was part of a wider European study conducted by Bayer et al. (2005) that examined how older people themselves experienced dignity. They reported that older people gave examples of how their dignity was compromised when their views were not respected by healthcare professionals, they were not addressed directly or their opinion was not asked. Such actions implied a lack of respect. A report for Help the Aged (Levenson, 2007) also identified a number of principles of how dignity might be enhanced (Box 11.1). These included the importance of staff respecting older people and ensuring that facilities were well maintained and clean. Autonomy was a key issue and included supporting older people to maintain independence

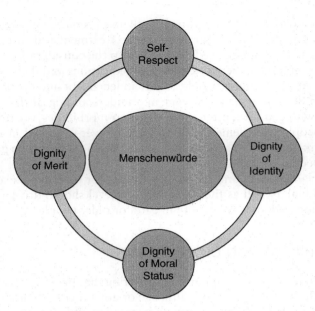

**Figure 11.1**   Four ways of understanding dignity (Nordenfelt and Edgar, 2005)

wherever possible, ascertaining people's wishes to be involved in their care and then involving them in the decision-making process (Magee et al., 2008). Overall, maintaining dignity is about treating people as people, not as objects. This demonstrates respect for the person and builds trust between the professional and the person receiving care.

## BOX 11.1 (LEVENSON, 2007)

- Dignity in care is inseparable from the wider context of dignity as a whole;
- Dignity is about treating people as individual persons;
- Dignity is not just about physical care;
- Dignity thrives in the context of equal power relationships;
- Dignity must be actively promoted;
- Dignity is more than the sum of its parts.

When older people are admitted to hospital, the dignity of the person can be undermined while they are unwell because their key focus is recovering (Jacelon, 2003; Goodrich, 2011). However, as they transition from the acute phase of their illness they become more aware of such assaults on their dignity. Jacelon (2003), in her observational study, found that many older people attempted to address this by interacting with staff and developing reciprocal relationships. One interpretation of this study might be that healthcare professionals become so focused on one approach to care that they don't always realise the impact their actions have on a person's dignity. If we return to the four notions of Dignity (see Figure 11.1), we might understand such actions as an effort by the older person to enhance their dignity of moral status (because they were trying to help staff) because the dignity conferred by others has not been forthcoming.

Furthermore, people with dementia are more likely to suffer assaults on their dignity because they may not be able to communicate in a way that is understandable to busy healthcare professionals. This is often compounded by them being in a unfamiliar environment and having their usual routines disrupted. Moreover, many people with dementia may be admitted to a healthcare environment with an underlying medical problem such as an infection, that is not recognised due to the overlying symptoms of dementia, which then results in poor consequences for the person (All-Party Parliamentary Group on Dementia, 2011).

## MRS CROSS

Consider the needs of Mrs Cross, a 70-year-old woman with impaired hearing and poor eyesight, who has been admitted to hospital for treatment due to viral pneumonia.

Think of the practical ways in which nursing and hospital staff could work to maintain the dignity of Mrs Cross.

Consider simple methods such as keeping the person informed and being polite, for example: How would you communicate effectively, considering the needs and preferences of the person? What would you need to consider to assist the person effectively with her personal hygiene needs? What may be the difficulties that you may face in a busy acute hospital? Write down your thoughts and reflections. There are some websites listed at the end of this chapter that contain useful information when considering dignity and the care of older people.

## Compassion, choice and empowerment in healthcare

Previous chapters have highlighted the value of compassion, patient choice and empowerment in healthcare provision. However, we feel this is important enough to reiterate it again here in relation to caring for the older person.

According to Cummings (DH, 2012: 13), compassion in nursing care is defined as 'how care is given through relationships based on empathy, respect and dignity – it can also be described as intelligent kindness, and is central to how people perceive their care'. Compassionate and effective care for the older person requires nurses to be able to respond in an ever-changing environment and place the care of the older person and their individual needs at the forefront. We also need to focus on the things that matter to older patients and their families and not just their medical care.

The Care Quality Commission (CQC) regularly inspects hospitals, care homes and primary care centres in Scotland, England and Wales to ensure that services are effective, safe and compassionate. In Northern Ireland, the Regulation and Quality Improvement Authority has a similar remit for their province. All regulatory authorities across the UK publish their findings from these inspections, and encourage services to make improvements where shortfalls in care are identified. In terms of the care of the older person, the CQC in England and Wales has made recommendations to a number of NHS services including the recruitment of specialist care nurses for the older person, more consultant geriatricians, increasing staffing levels and the introduction of the compassionate care training programme for all staff working with older people.

However, it is often difficult from these reports to identify what is meant by terms such as 'caring' and 'compassion'. If we examine these in more detail, we see examples of nurses telling older people to use the incontinence aid rather than being taken to the toilet (Abrahams, 2011). Similarly, research reports comparable issues such as nurses or carers making the assumption that an older person is not hungry rather than finding out the underlying reason why they are not eating (Tadd et al., 2011). These reports describe everyday occurrences observed in busy ward environments that imply a lack of dignity. This is another term that is considered integral to modern-day healthcare but may be difficult for nurses to see how it applies to their everyday care, allowing practices such as described above to creep into the workplace culture. Such practices may occur when we fail to consider the impact of our approach to care when we care for older people.

 Consider how you might improve your practice in each of the 6Cs in your workplace and how any improvements that you introduce could be measured to demonstrate change.

The measurement of compassion may be difficult because compassion is not always visible. Think about novel ideas such as collecting patient case studies where compassion was demonstrated or introducing short patient feedback forms in your work setting, which could be used to recognise good examples of care or areas that need further improvements.

The responsibility for improving the quality of older people's care needs to taken at the individual level as well as by nurses in leadership positions. As nurses lead by best example, the culture and environment of undervaluing older people can be changed to one of empowerment of older people and putting their perspective first. Many older patients are reliant on support from family carers, and it's generally these carers who raise concerns and complaints about the quality of care, as acknowledged in the Francis Report (Francis, 2013).

Nurses need to be proactive in involving older people in their care decisions from the onset: giving explanations, managing expectations, and involving families in decision making and discharge planning. In a study on the views of older people in the choice of care for intermediate care services (this could involve care at home, a short admission to a care home or an intermediate care unit), there appeared to be mixed views from the patients on whether they received choice about their care and also about how much they wanted to be involved in the decisions about this (Stanmore, 2011). A study by Pickard and Glendinning (2002) recommends that older carers should receive real choice about the extent of their involvement in care giving and that healthcare professionals should anticipate the needs of older carers and provide a more proactive service when offering help. The implementation of this advice would ensure that older carers would feel more supported and valued.

In a systematic review of the literature, carers' needs are described in two key areas: meeting the needs of the person receiving care and meeting their own needs (McCabe et al., 2016). Although professionals may recognise and support carers in how to provide care and meet the needs of the person receiving care, it is rare that they also consider the needs of the carers themselves. For example, the health of carers demonstrated that they are more likely to experience worse physical and mental health than those without caregiving duties living in the community (Pinquart and Sorensen, 2003).

Depression, in particular, is associated with the amount of caregiving per week, alongside the care recipients' physical impairment in the absence of dementia, with stronger associations found for spouses than for adult children (Pinquart and Sorensen, 2003). However, those caring for a person with dementia are more likely to experience poorer physical and mental health than other carers (Pinquart and Sorensen, 2004), with care recipient behaviour more likely to result in greater caregiver burden and depression for this group (Pinquart and Sorensen, 2003). Differences also exist between groups of carers, with spouses experiencing worse physical and mental health than adult children (Pinquart and Sorensen, 2011).

However, there are also benefits or 'uplifts' experienced by carers in the caregiving relationship which may result in subjective wellbeing, including positive affect, life satisfaction and perceived quality of life (Pinquart and Sorensen, 2004). When considering the impact of uplifts on subjective wellbeing, Pinquart and Sorensen (2004) undertook a meta-analytical study and found that depression was more directly correlated with caregiver burden than uplifts, which contributes directly to subjective wellbeing. This demonstrates that the subjective wellbeing of carers may be encouraged by enabling carers with time to continue activities that contribute to their subjective wellbeing or ensuring that they are still experiencing the 'uplifts' of caregiving rather than reducing their burden. For example, positive pre-caregiving relationships have been associated with better outcomes, suggesting that interventions that take into account the context of family relationships may support improved outcomes for the caregiving and the person receiving the care (Quinn et al., 2012).

In the UK, the Care Act 2014 (see www.legislation.gov.uk/ukpga/2014/23/contents/enacted) provides family carers with the same recognition in their need for support as the person they are caring for (Department of Health and Social Care, 2016). The carer assessment might be undertaken by a social worker or another trained professional such as a registered nurse (district/community or psychiatric) and may occur together with the assessment of the person receiving care. The assessment covers caring responsibilities, housing, work, study, leisure opportunities, relationships and social activities, as well as the goals of the caregiver (Carers UK, 2016). This may result in services such as support with meals, help around the home, replacement care or gym membership, depending on the outcome of the assessment (Department of Health and Social Care, 2016). However, looking at the literature, we can see the importance of understanding that different carers have different needs. For example, spousal carers may benefit from respite care to reduce burden whereas adult children may benefit from interventions that strengthen their relationship with the person receiving care (Pinquart and Sorensen, 2011). Adult children might also have caring responsibilities for young children alongside their responsibilities for an ageing parent, suggesting they will have different needs to adult children with no additional caregiving responsibilities (Schumacher et al., 2012). In addition, the more recent phenomenon of adult children staying at home for longer delays the transition to adulthood, further compounding stressors for those caring for ageing parents as well (Mitchell et al., 2015).

As nurses supporting carers, we also need to understand the impact of the conditions experienced by care recipients on the needs of carers. Dementia is one such condition that creates additional issues for carers due to the nature of the condition. It is estimated that 850,000 people are living with dementia in the UK alone, a figure expected to rise to over a million by 2025, which represents a rise of 35% (Prince et al., 2014). One in 14 people over the age of 65 has dementia in the UK (Prince et al., 2014) and it is projected that one in three people born in 2015 will develop dementia in their lifetime (Lewis, 2015). This means that 34% of the UK population are affected by dementia in their family, with 700,000 people involved in caregiving (Alzheimer's Research UK, 2015a). Of these, 60–70% are women with 20% having to drop from full-time to part-time work due to caregiving responsibilities (Alzheimer's Research UK, 2015b). Over a third of carers provide over 100 hours per week in caregiving and 30% of caregivers had been providing care for a person with dementia for over five years (SACE, 2017). Of dementia caregivers 15% say that they are not in paid work due to caregiving commitments (SACE, 2017). The nature of dementia being a progressive loss of the person's identity alongside their cognitive and physical abilities creates additional stressors for these carers, and subsequently impacts on the life decisions of other members of the family. In this way, the caregiving trajectory in dementia has been liked to a 'career' due to the transition points of diagnosis, behavioural changes, institutionalisation and bereavement (Gaugler et al., 2005). Understanding this caregiving 'career' is vital for nurses and other healthcare professionals in supporting dementia carers. For example, the nature of dementia alters the dynamics of family relationships and so may impact on the caregiver's social support as well as their wellbeing. There is limited literature that considers the wider family dynamics, although these altered relationships may impact on the level of support received and, subsequently, the caregiving trajectory (Ablitt et al., 2009).

Some older people, including carers, may not initially appear to be particularly interested in being involved in the choice and decision making for their care. There is still an attitude of 'whatever the doctor thinks is best', rather than voicing their own preferences or opinions, which reflects the medical model of healthcare. This involves paternalism, whereby the doctors tell patients what they need and patients submissively accept it. In addition, not all older patients are in a fit state to make decisions when they are acutely ill. It is at this point that we need to ensure involvement of the family carer, who will know the older person's wishes or have an idea of what they might want if they are unable to be involved in the decision-making process. Recognising and valuing the knowledge that families/carers bring is the first step to working in partnership. Working in partnership with carers involves working with mutual respect and trust, developing communication with carers, where their contribution is valued, transparency of decision making involves the caregiver and encourages patients and their families to participate in healthcare decisions and management (Gaugler et al., 2014). This is not simply having people and their families in the same room but enabling them to feel comfortable enough to participate in the decision-making process. To achieve this, healthcare professionals and family carers need to demonstrate respect for each other's input, with families feeling able to ask questions and to be fully informed, and not be afraid of disagreeing or offering their own goals for treatment and care (Gaugler et al., 2014).

We must beware of engaging in substitute decision making because we believe the older person or the person with dementia is unable to engage in the decision-making process. We must endeavour to provide opportunities for involvement and where necessary facilitate supported decision making, ensuring that information is provided at times when the person is alert and not medicated, the environment is conducive and the information is provided in accessible language. If people wish to opt out of the decision-making process, then they will be able to make this known, but it is also important to support people in identifying an advocate until they wish to be involved in the decision-making process. Person-centred care does not stop at assessment and should be incorporated throughout the patient's care. Patients are entitled to be involved in their healthcare decisions and involvement of patients should be embedded in the structures of all aspects of NHS healthcare (DH, 2001).

# Biographical approach to care

So how can we ensure that older people receive the person-centred care that they deserve? It is by valuing the older person for whom they are, understanding what is important and ensuring that significant routines are maintained in their care that we deliver person-centred care. We start this by developing an understanding of the biography of the older person which supports us in valuing them as a person first and then considers their needs as a patient or client in this context (Box 11.2).

---

## BOX 11.2 BIOGRAPHICAL APPROACH TO CARE PLANNING

- Encourage client to talk about how they approach their life;
- Develop rapport by talking about everyday events and people during care routines;
- Use personal belongings and photos as triggers for discussion;
- Recognise unique assets and characteristics of each person and build on these when care planning;
- Build on lifelong interests to offer clients opportunities to experience new things and interests in context to their care.

---

We may think we do this, but as busy healthcare professionals we often focus on the condition the person presents with first, with the needs of the older person a secondary consideration. It is when focusing on the condition rather than the person becomes established practice that we begin to see examples of poor care, as described by the Ombudsman (Abrahams, 2011) and other enquiries (e.g. Francis, 2013). These reports talk about established practice which results in care that lacks compassion and dignity, and often provides examples of older people and/or people with dementia. As nurses are often in the frontline of patient care, it is their care that comes under scrutiny, with reports talking about nurses not having time to care or losing their compassion.

## Promoting person-centred care with older people and those with dementia

Person-centred care has been identified as a way of improving the care of older people (McCormack and McCance, 2006) and those with dementia (Brooker, 2004).

Dementia is not one condition but a syndrome characterised by decline of mental and physical abilities, including recent memory, problem solving, language, visuospatial skills and orientation (Alzheimer's Society, 2017). There are many types of dementia, the most common being Alzheimer's disease, accounting for two-thirds of people living with dementia. Vascular dementia is the second most common cause with dementia with Lewy bodies being the third most common (Alzheimer's Society, 2014). Although most people affected by dementia are aged over 65, approximately 42,000 people under this age are also affected by early onset dementia in the UK (Prince et al., 2014). However, 72% of people living with dementia will have co-morbid conditions (Dowrick and Southern, 2014), with those aged over 65 likely to have four co-morbid conditions when compared with people aged over 65 without dementia (Poblador-Plou et al., 2014). (For further details of the aetiology of dementia, see SCIE resources at the end of this chapter.)

Older lesbian, gay, bisexual, transgender and intersex (LGBTI) people have greater challenges in accessing healthcare where heterosexuality is considered the norm (Crameri et al., 2015).

Treating LGBTI older people as the 'same' as other older people does not acknowledge the history of the lives they have lived, usually experiencing discrimination, stigma and potential imprisonment or forced 'cures' (Crameri et al., 2015). This collective experience contributes to a culture of shared values, beliefs and behaviours, which is distinct from the shared experience of the heterosexual population. This perspective supports us in recognising that older LGBTI people have additional needs and requires us to provide a culturally safe environment in the delivery of services. LGBTI older people's fear about discrimination may result in delay in accessing services with greater dependency and strain on intimate partners, particularly when one partner has dementia (Barrett et al., 2015). In speaking with LGBTI couples, some of whom had dementia, and service providers, it is evident that older people do not change their sexuality or gender recognition following dementia (Barrett et al., 2015). LGBTI people will require additional support to maintain their support structures with their intimate partners and 'family of choice', to prevent social isolation and depression when entering services. Indeed, it can be the attitudes of service providers and families of origin that can be more damaging to a person's identity than the dementia itself (Barrett et al., 2015). Developing culturally safe services requires engagement with LGBTI people in planning of services, organisational leadership, staff education and inclusive service literature where LGBTI people are visible (Crameri et al., 2015).

Not all older people will have dementia, but the risk of some dementias, such as Alzheimer's disease, increase with age. This suggests that increased longevity may also increase the number of people diagnosed with a dementia. Person-centred care, as developed by Tom Kitwood (1997), aimed to focus the attention of professionals on to the person rather than the condition. Kitwood believed that considering the emotional needs of the person alongside their physical needs would enhance the care of people with dementia. Dawn Brooker developed these principles into the VIPS model (valuing the person with dementia, providing individualised care, recognising the perspective of the person with dementia and examining the social environment in which the person is located – Røsvik et al., 2011). Recognising that the patient is a person first is now considered a guiding principle across all models of healthcare. For example, the Institute of Medicine's (2001) definition of patient-centred care includes respecting needs, values and preferences, as well as providing for emotional and physical support. However, many of these models lack specific guidance as to how these models might be put into practice (Dewing, 2004), with Goodrich and Cornwell (2008) finding that few healthcare professionals in the UK could describe what was meant by patient-centred care.

---

### ⁇ ACTIVITY 11.1

Draw a timeline of your life and consider how some of the events that have been significant in your life have shaped how you approach your life today.

- Consider an older person you know in your personal life. How have events in their life shaped how they make decisions about their health?

- For this older person, what are the significant routines in their life that might be interfered with if they required health and social care support?
- How might you as a concerned relative try to influence their care?

Person-centred care is an approach that nurses should use with all older people, and is characterised by understanding the biography of the person and seeing beyond the immediate context of illness (McCormack and McCance, 2006). A systematic review of patient experience in acute hospitals suggests that older people and their families want staff to recognise who they are and what is important to them, to involve them in decision making and to support them in maintaining links with their community while in hospital (Bridges et al., 2010). This is of particular importance for older LGBTI people who may not have traditional social support networks as reflected in the heterosexual population. Intimate partners and wider friendships in the LGBTI community are often the only environments where LGBTI people feel safe to be themselves, with such networks becoming 'families of choice' (Barrett et al., 2015). However, it is also important not to treat all LGBTI people as the same, particularly people of trans or non-binary experience who may require additional support for personal care and grooming (Ansara, 2015).

Brown Wilson (2013) develops the use of biography to consider what is significant in a person's life, including day-to-day routines that give the older person's life meaning, or, for the person with dementia, provides an understandable structure to their day. Nurses often develop insights into this biographical information through the daily contact they have with patients in providing care, such as giving out medication, bathing, dressing and supporting people at meal times. This information may not be shared as routine because it might not be considered relevant to the nursing care of this person (Brown Wilson, 2013). The challenge for nurses at this point is how to document information such as this so it becomes part of accepted practice for the older person, and not dependent on one nurse being on duty for that older person.

Sexuality and intimacy are another important aspect of ageing and one often neglected both in the literature and in practice, which suggests that older people are not seen as sexual beings (Simpson et al., 2017a). As nurses, we might feel very uncomfortable in speaking about these issues but older people speak about their needs to engage in ongoing intimate and sexual relationships (Simpson et al., 2017b). Indeed, the highest incidence of sexually transmitted infections are now in the over-60 age group (Lee, 2016), suggesting an important role for nurses in speaking to older people about their sexual health. This work suggests that we need to move away from the perspective that sexuality is only about providing choice in what an older person wishes to wear or how they express their gender. However, this element of care is of particular importance for transgender and intersex people who do not necessarily conform to the binary gender of male or female (Ansara, 2015). Also maintaining connection with LGBTI networks and safe spaces for the continuation of intimate relationships are aspects of care important to LGBTI people as they age and enter services (Barrett et al., 2015). However, the need to maintain intimate and sexual relationships is largely ignored in the design of care systems (Simpson et al., 2017a) with staff identifying the structural barriers in addressing such needs (Simpson et al., 2017b). A first step in addressing the sexuality and intimacy needs of older people might be finding out what important relationships they have and developing trusting relationships, enabling older people to feel comfortable in speaking about these issues.

## Implementing person-centred care

So far we have suggested a number of ways in which the principles of person-centred care can be implemented as a mechanism by which to promote dignity when working with and/or caring for older people. However, it is recognised that the environment in which care is delivered and organised also has an impact on the implementation of approaches such as person-centred care (McCormack and McCance, 2010; Brown Wilson, 2013).

McCormack and McCance (2010) identify the care environment as a key feature of their model of person-centred nursing, suggesting that a range of factors such as organisational systems, physical environment, skill mix and staff relationships, needs to be taken into consideration. Each of these factors will make a contribution or act as a barrier to the implementation of person-centred care. Often person-centred care may be considered something additional because some of these factors may require additional work and sometimes be beyond the control of ward-based staff. Brown Wilson (2009) offers a number of factors based on smaller organisations that may be of value in supporting ward-based staff and students in implementing a person-centred approach by integrating the following into current practice:

- Leadership;
- Staff motivation;
- Team work;
- A consistent approach to care;
- Continuity of care.

In order to develop person-centred services, nurses need to consider how to use their leadership irrespective of their position in the organisation. Indeed nurses may be working at every level in some organisations and as such have the power to influence person-centred care, whether it be at the bedside or at the executive level (Brown Wilson, 2017). As we have already established in Chapter 8, leadership that is approachable, able to generate trust, supportive of staff in resolving conflict and promotes an exchange of information to support staff in their decision making is more likely to develop positive relationships in the workplace (Anderson et al., 2003). Brown Wilson (2009) suggests that this style of leadership can also come from those delivering day-to-day care in ways such as role modelling good practice.

To get to know a person and then to implement significant changes to their care plan requires the continuity of staff who will adopt a person-centred approach. Initially, sharing biographical knowledge may be dependent on developing relationships with specific members of staff, but, once this information has been disseminated, continuity can be promoted even when the same nursing staff are on duty through a consistent approach to care. This is possible even when staffing levels and skill mix may be suboptimal.

The personal philosophy of staff, their beliefs and values are integral to a person-centred approach (McCormack and McCance, 2006; Brown Wilson and Davies, 2009). This has been represented in Figure 11.2, as staff motivation with a 'do unto others' philosophy is more likely to create a focus on the person. This means that the staff consider what the older person considers important in their care and seeks to implement care in this way. In her work, Brown Wilson (2009) found that a critical mass of staff working with the same philosophy was more likely to result in a focus on the person. Therefore, this implies that developing a culture in the work environment where the older person is listened to and their needs are acted on is more likely to deliver a person-centred approach to care.

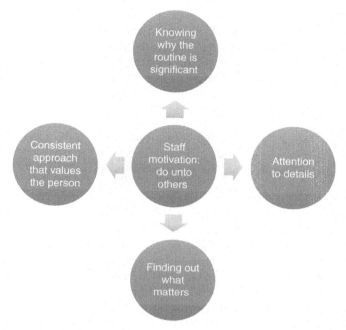

**Figure 11.2**   Brown Wilson's (2013) person-centred approach

Older people and families often seek to make a direct contribution to, or influence their care through the development of relationships with staff (Jacelon, 2003; Brown Wilson, 2009). Adopting a biographical approach to care planning is one way of recognising and valuing this contribution. This may highlight reasons behind different behaviours, supporting staff in making sense of these given their workload.

## MR SMITH

Mr Smith's pain had been attributed to his age and he was currently being treated for depression as he appeared withdrawn. On speaking with Mr Smith, the nurse found that he had always been an active and outgoing man and enjoyed volunteering at the local hospital but was unable to continue this due to the pain in his knees, which restricted his mobility. Finding out what was significant to Mr Smith was then transferred into action by referring to other members of the multidisciplinary team to investigate the cause of the pain. In the meantime, the nurse arranged for transport for Mr Smith to attend a day centre, which he enjoyed.

## Understanding frailty in the older person

One of the key challenges for supporting people as they age is the increasing level of frailty. Frailty is a complex, age-related health state in which people progressively lose their in-built reserves and ability to recover from seemingly minor events or illness (Cowdell et al., 2018). Frailty as a term is often used but remains poorly defined with little consensus on definitions (Rockwood and Koller, 2013). Some have defined frailty as a collection of deficits – the more people have wrong with them, the frailer they are (Mitnitski et al., 2005) – with some researchers suggesting it is a specific syndrome represented by weight loss, exhaustion, low physical activity and slowness (Fried et al., 2004). Despite these different definitions there is increasing recognition that frailty is a physiological syndrome that causes an older person to be more vulnerable to adverse health outcomes (Ferrucci et al., 2004). This is due mainly to a decline in physiological function across multiple systems often caused by co-morbid conditions. This results in the older person's body system having limited ability to respond to internal stressors such as viruses or environmental stressors such as changes in temperature. This approach suggests that frailty is not simply a result of the ageing process and so should not be defined by chronological age, but by how the older person's body responds to different stressors.

Rockwood and colleagues (2006) undertook a large-scale study testing the hypothesis that, at a given age, frailty can be defined in relation to how many deficits an older person has, such as problems with mobility, nutrition, and the ability to undertake activities of daily living. The accumulation of deficits is important because it may tip the balance between an older person being able to live independently in the community or requiring institutional care (Rockwood et al., 1994). A Frailty Index has been developed to summarise a person's health status by counting the number of deficits, which is then used to infer relative frailty of an individual (Mitnitski et al., 2005). This has more recently been further developed and implemented as an electronic frailty index (eFI) in many GP practices throughout the UK (Clegg et al., 2016). Both the work undertaken by Rockwood et al. (2006) and Clegg et al. (2016) suggest that it is the accumulation of these deficits that is important for health outcomes, rather than the individual nature of each deficit. This is important for nurses in healthcare, because we often focus on the nature of the deficit.

It is very tempting to think about frailty as a fixed condition, e.g. once you become frail there is no going back. However, this work should challenge us to consider how older people may be supported to reduce their deficits rather than accepting they are a result of age. Rockwood et al. (1994) consider frailty as a balance (Figure 11.3). For well older people, the scales are tipped towards the side of the assets (medical and social). Increasing frailty then brings the scales into alignment until one additional problem may tip the scales in favour of the deficits. However, the nature of those deficits may be amenable to treatment to enable the balance between asset and deficit to change. For example, if a deficit is related to walking, then simple exercises can improve this deficit.

There is substantial evidence that older people with frailty benefit from assessment and intervention that is whole person centred, multidisciplinary, iterative and case managed – this is also known as the comprehensive geriatric assessment (CGA: Ellis et al., 2011). Physiological function, the reactions of the body to pharmaceutical treatments, and responses to health challenges and injury all change with age. The syndromes frequently presenting in older patients – cognitive impairment, stroke, fragility fractures, falls, syncope and incontinence – are different from those in younger populations.

When using the CGA to assess frailty (Box 11.3) (Jones et al., 2004) the more deficits the older person has, then the greater their risk of poor outcomes. However, when nurses consider these domains, they tend to consider each issue as an isolated problem. Considering issues of nutrition, mobility and continence, for example, as indicators of frailty may promote a more holistic assessment of the person. In any assessment, it is vital that we understand the significance of the presenting issues to the older person themselves. So we need to consider the clinical significance of

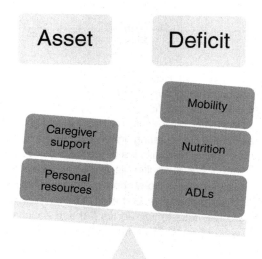

**Figure 11.3**   Interpretation of the 'Frailty Balance' based on Rockwood et al. (1994)

these issues from the person's perspective, i.e. what is most important to that person and what intervention is required to support that person in achieving his or her personal goal. By doing this, we place the older person at the centre of the assessment process and provide an opportunity to learn more about individuals, their current situation and their desires for the future.

### BOX 11.3   ASSESSING FRAILTY USING CGA DOMAINS BASED ON JONES ET AL. (2004)

Cognitive status (no cognitive impairment = no problem; cognitive impairment/no dementia = mild problem; delirium or dementia = severe problem)

Mood and motivation

Communication (vision, hearing, speech)

Mobility, balance (scored at the highest level of independence with aids where used)

Bowel function

Bladder function

IADLs (instrumental activities of daily living) and ADLs (activities of daily living) (rated as no impairment = no problem; IADL impairment = mild problem; ADL impairment = major problem)

Nutrition

Social resources (scored as a problem if there was need for additional help)

Instructions:

For a Frailty Index, score problems in each domain were scored as 0 (no problem), 1 (a minor problem) or 2 (a major problem). For evaluating the contribution of each domain, the mode of the three ratings determined the value for each subject.

## MR JONES

Mr Jones has been admitted to your ward. He is generally a well 88-year-old man but was unable to get out of bed this morning. The community nurses could not find a specific problem with him but were unable to move him from the bed and so he was admitted to hospital. On further assessment, Mr Jones states he is eating regularly but admits he has lost weight over the past three months because his trousers now feel loose. He is eating light meals that can be prepared in a microwave because he has lost interest in cooking. He walks his dog once a day but only walks a short distance. He has a slow walking speed and tends to shuffle his feet when he walks. He is struggling to do his housework and needs help with the garden. He wishes to remain in his own home.

Using the domains of the Comprehensive Geriatric Assessment identify how frail you think Mr Jones is and why. What are the risks for Mr Jones if these deficits are not addressed? What nursing actions do you think would benefit Mr Jones and how would this enable him to retain his independence?

## Health promotion for older people

Caring for older people is not just about treating them during illness. It is also about keeping them well and educating them about how to stay healthy and active for as long as possible. Although it is widely understood that health promotion for older people may encompass activities such as blood pressure control, flu immunisation or smoking cessation, it should be recognised that every contact with an older person may present an opportunity to promote healthy behaviour and lifestyles.

Opportunities for nurses to promote health may be related to screening for the early detection of conditions, identifying whether the older person would benefit from preventative advice or assessment for asymptomatic disease such as hypertension or osteoporosis. Early identification of dementia is also important to ensure that treatment, support and follow-up can be put into place, so that sufferers and their families can receive ongoing care and review. Likewise, recognising through assessment the need for screening for cancers such as breast, prostate and colon (which are increasingly remediable through surgery or chemotherapy) can lead to much improved outcomes when these diseases are identified early on in their natural history. Similarly, being on the lookout for signs of depression, another common condition in older people, can lead to early diagnosis and treatment that can greatly improve the quality of life in older people.

Simple health-promoting measures such as checking when an older person last had his or her vision or hearing ability checked and referring to appropriate services can improve their general health and wellbeing, and assist in maintaining their ability to remain independent. Similarly, establishing whether an older person is experiencing difficulties with urinary incontinence can lead to effective prevention and treatment that also impacts positively on the person's self-esteem. Although urinary incontinence is treatable, fewer than half of patients with urinary incontinence report their symptoms to a physician and suffer in silence (Orrell et al., 2013). This is usually because they are too embarrassed; they consider their problem a normal part of ageing, absorbent devices are readily available, or they have low expectations of treatment or fear surgery. Developing positive, therapeutic relationships with older people may enable them to disclose symptoms that may be a source of embarrassment more readily (Fultz and Herzog, 2000), leading to diagnosis and treatment.

Educating older people to manage chronic conditions such as arthritis or diabetes optimally should also be a key part of nurses' health-promoting role. For instance, reinforcing healthy dietary advice or encouraging physical activity will not only improve the condition but also reduce the likelihood of developing other co-morbid diseases. Diet and lifestyle influences can have a considerable influence on health during the life course (World Health Organization [WHO], 2002). In a study of dietary patterns and lifestyle among individuals aged 70–90 years, adherence to a Mediterranean diet and healthy lifestyle was associated with a more than 50% lower rate of all-cause and cause-specific mortality (Knoops et al., 2004). Similarly, risk factors associated with dementia include the reduction of saturated fat, eating a balanced diet, not smoking, moderate alcohol intake, controlling blood pressure, preventing diabetes, increasing physical and leisure activities, and cognitive stimulation (Barnes and Yaffe, 2011). The prevailing health promotion messages are to modify these lifestyle factors and, although these may not guarantee that a person will not develop dementia, the brain will be in better health with greater cognitive reserves to deal with the condition if it develops.

Health-promoting activities may also encompass the reassessment or review of the patient's medication, considering ongoing needs or their understanding of safe administration and possible side effects. For older people taking four or more medicines (known as polypharmacy), referral to the GP or pharmacist for a medication review has been shown to be very beneficial in reducing medication-related complications. These increase with the number of medications consumed, both prescribed and over the counter. Medication management studies in older people have shown that they are more likely to experience adverse consequences and have lower tolerance of drug side effects, and be at greater risk of inappropriate prescribing, more likely to be uncertain about physician instructions, more likely to have greater difficulties ordering and collecting their medicines, and prone to have difficulties administering their medicines because of cognitive, sensory or physical impairment (Rogers et al., 2014). Therefore, taking the time to assess the patient's needs in managing their medication, teaching about the safe administration and possible side effects could save much distress, reduce hospital admissions and potentially be life saving.

## MRS FIELDS

Mrs Fields, a 78-year-old woman, with coronary heart disease, congestive heart failure and hypertension lives at home with her spouse. She decided to stop taking her diuretics due to continence problems and was admitted to hospital with worsening heart failure. The nursing assessment revealed that a number of general practitioners had visited Mrs Fields and adjusted her medication to improve control of her heart failure. One of the community nurses was also visiting to assess and manage continence problems but neither the doctors nor the nurse was aware of each other's visits.

- In your area of practice, do you think that medication management is considered within the nursing assessment and organisation of care?
- What additional training would you find useful in enabling you to support older people to manage their medicines effectively?

What nursing and health-promoting actions do you think would benefit Mrs Fields? How would these actions enable her to return home safely and manage her medication effectively? What could be done to improve multidisciplinary communication to prevent incidents like this case from occurring again?

# Promoting physical activity in older people

For many older people, an inactive life can lead to poor mental health and feeling dissatisfied, depressed and socially isolated. Participation in meaningful activity is important for maintaining relationships and feelings of purpose, as well as improving physical and mental health (NICE, 2008). Research over the last 25 years has shown that physically active older people experience a better quality of life and less social isolation, and maintain their function and independence compared with those who remain sedentary (Wilmoth and Ferraro, 2013).

Current evidence suggests that nurses should be encouraging older people to remain active and independent rather than disempowering them or overly increasing their reliance on health professionals.

There are a number of important reasons for encouraging physical activity or exercise in older people – it can be health promoting, for instance resistance exercises (those that incorporate strength training) can maintain or improve bone health to prevent osteoporosis. Exercise can also be disease preventing, for example it can lower blood pressure and cholesterol, prevent heart disease and diabetes, and has also been associated with preventing certain types of cancer (Centers for Disease Control and Prevention [CDC], 1996; WHO, 2007; British Heart Foundation, 2010).

There are further myths and stereotypes about older people being unable to remain physically fit and active. Those working in exercise science could inform us that older people are capable of functioning at exceptionally high levels and that decline occurs on an individual basis, dependent on factors such as lifestyle and genetics. We know from research studies that older people, even in their 90s can reverse the effects of ageing through regular muscle-strengthening and balance exercises (Fiatarone et al., 1990). Therefore, it is important for nurses to encourage activity and exercise with older people, whatever their ability, and to assist them to find local facilities or give advice on home-based exercises that will maintain and improve their physical function.

Some of the benefits that can be used to encourage older people to become more active and remain active are listed in Table 11.1. Possibly the most important points listed here are the benefits in maintaining independence and a social network, losing these abilities are some of the biggest

**Table 11.1** Advantages of physical activity and risks associated with sedentary behaviour

| Physically active behaviour | Sedentary behaviour |
|---|---|
| Increases ability to maintain social network | Reduces postural stability |
| Reduces fatigue | Decreases function and independence |
| Improves ability to maintain a stable weight | Decreases quality of life |
| Better quality of life | Increases risk of pressure ulcers |
| Possible improved survival | Significantly decreases bone density and increases risk of osteoporosis |
| Improves bone density and lower risk of osteoporosis | |
| Improves muscle strength and balance | Can negatively affect mental health |
| Quicker reaction time | Increases risk of obesity and associated morbidities (e.g. cardiovascular disease, type 2 diabetes, cancer) |
| Improves proprioception | |
| Improves mental health and cognitive function | |

Based on Chief Medical Officer (2011) and Sherrington et al. (2016).

fears of older people. When talking to patients about staying active and not sitting for longer than an hour they may not be not be highly motivated to do so, but if it is explained that this could be the difference in staying independent at home for longer they may be much more motivated to increase their physical activity.

As a nation we are becoming increasingly sedentary and this is the first generation to need to make a conscious decision to build physical activity into daily lives (Public Health England [PHE], 2016). Societal changes (such as fewer manual jobs, increased car use and automation) have designed physical activity out of our lives, and there have been many recent governmental campaigns aimed at getting people to be more active to target obesity, social isolation and encourage longer working lives (DH, 2009; PHE, 2016). Sedentary behaviour accelerates the loss of performance and sarcopenia (loss of muscle mass), and older people already lose 1–2% of functional ability each year. Just one week of bed rest reduces a person's strength by approximately 20% and spine bone density by 1% (LeBlanc et al., 1987). If you consider how much time older people in care homes spend either sitting down or in bed you can understand their increased risk of fractures and falls. All older adults should minimise the amount of time spent being sedentary (sitting) for extended periods, and nurses can educate and encourage older people to be as active as possible.

The question is how active should older people be? This very much depends on the individual, taking into consideration their current health and how active they already are. In 2011, the first-ever, UK-wide, published guidelines (Chief Medical Officer, 2011) outlined the amount of physical activity older adults (65 years and over) should be doing to benefit their health:

- Older adults who participate in any amount of physical activity gain some health benefits, including maintenance of good physical and cognitive function;
- Some physical activity is better than none, and more physical activity provides greater health benefits;
- Older adults should also undertake physical activity to improve muscle strength on at least two days a week;
- Older adults at risk of falls should incorporate physical activity to improve balance and coordination on at least two days a week.

Research also suggests that there are many barriers (actual and perceived) for older people to overcome to be able to effectively participate in physical activity. For some patients they are just too unwell, and yet others may think that exercise is not good due to their condition. In actual fact their health would greatly benefit if they did increase their physical activity (e.g. patients needing cardiac rehab or patients with rheumatoid arthritis; Stanmore et al., 2013). Some patients try exercise but don't see any immediate observed positive effects – this is because some of the benefits are not immediately obvious and the person may need to become a little fitter before they experience any improvements in health. Other people may not like the social contact in classes or find they get too fatigued or feel pain, whereas others struggle with motivation or feel they have other more important priorities in their life. For some there may be practical difficulties such as getting to an available class. These barriers can be overcome with help and an individualised approach, so when encouraging an older person to exercise involve them in developing a programme and help them to find a class or sport that they can take part in. Remember there is something for everyone. Skelton et al. (2005) demonstrated in their strength and balance training study of older people, that in three months 65–90 year olds were able to rejuvenate 20 years of lost strength.

Exercise should incorporate some kind of aerobic or endurance tasks, some flexibility and resistance exercises, e.g. weight bearing, in particular the lower limb, and some functional task training that is individualised according to the needs and preferences of the person. There is even published research about the benefits of Wii fit, Xbox kinect and other virtual reality gaming systems for exercise which are being found to be beneficial for older people in the home or care home environment (van Diest et al., 2013).

Consider the types of exercise facilities, classes or services suitable for older people in your local community.

- What do you think might be the barriers to the attendance of older people at each of these activities? How might these barriers be overcome, using an individualised approach and considering the person's significant routines?

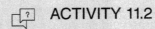 ACTIVITY 11.2

Visit your library or search the internet for facilities local to you that are suitable for older people – remember the importance of finding out what are the older person's interests and the need to tailor this to their preferences. There are also some websites listed at the end of this chapter that contain useful information when considering physical activity and older people.

## Falls prevention for older people

A common myth or stereotype of older people is that falling is often accepted as a natural part of the ageing process. When we look at the research, we find that as many as 40% of falls can be predicted and prevented (Gillespie et al., 2012), but this message needs to reach older people (and some health professionals) who continue to think that falls are inevitable. The National Council on Aging (2013) produced a list of the ten most common misconceptions about falls in older adults such as: 'It won't happen to me', 'It's just a normal part of growing older', 'If I limit my activity, I won't fall', 'As long as I stay at home, I can avoid falling', 'Muscle strength and flexibility can't be regained' and 'Taking medication doesn't increase my risk of falling'. So we can conclude that older people also need re-educating about these misconceptions and we, as nurses, should be reiterating the positive message that with support falls can be prevented.

It is true, however, that falls are common in older people, yet many older people are unaware of their risk of falling. Around one in three people aged over 65, and half of those aged over 80, fall at least once a year and this rate increases with age and in those living in care homes (American Geriatrics Society, British Geriatrics Society, and American Academy of Orthopaedic Surgeons Panel on Falls Prevention [AGS/BGS], 2010). Approximately 10% of falls will result in fractures, and most concerning is that falls resulting in hip fractures commonly lead to death or institutional care within a year. Fear of falling is also an important concern that can restrict social activity and lead to older adults becoming more sedentary and isolated. The risk of falls is exacerbated due to the resulting muscle weakness and balance difficulties. Therefore, it is imperative that nurses raise awareness of the importance of falls risk screening and assessment of older people with other health professionals, older people and their carers/relatives.

We can easily identify those who are most at risk of a fall by asking questions related to the most important risk factors. Fall risk factors for older people can be categorised as biological, behavioural and psychosocial (Figure 11.4). A history of a previous fall is the best predictor of a future fall and any older person who responds positively to this question should receive support on preventing further falls. For some older people, reduced physical activity causes their balance and muscle strength to deteriorate, and their reaction time and gait speed slow, so the ability to remain steady and upright becomes much more challenging. We know that older people are generally more sedentary and this can increase the likelihood of a fall.

Having poor strength and balance, gait problems and fear of falling also increase your fall risk. Some diseases such as Parkinson's disease, stroke, rheumatoid arthritis and dementia also increase the likelihood of falls, as does having poor vision, foot pain and incontinence (WHO, 2007; Stanmore et al., 2013). We know that taking more than four types of medicine and certain types of medicine (antidepressants, diuretics, analgesics and antipsychotic medicines) also increases a person's falls risk. A person's environment can also increase the likelihood of falls, for instance if there were lots of tripping hazards or uneven surfaces in the home (NICE, 2013).

Over the last three decades, researchers have conducted falls prevention trials with older people by modifying either a single risk factor or multiple risk factors. Both strategies have been shown to be effective in reducing the rate of falling. A Cochrane Systematic Review (Gillespie et al., 2012)

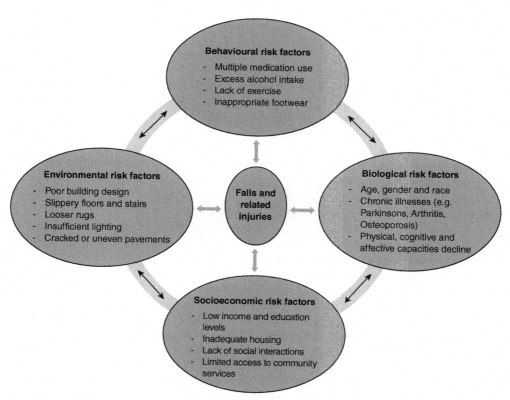

**Figure 11.4**   Fall risk factors (WHO, 2007; NICE, 2013)

assessed the effects of interventions to reduce the incidence of falls in older people living in the community and included 159 clinical trials. They concluded that group and home-based exercise programmes, incorporating balance and strength-training exercises, effectively reduced falls, as did Tai Chi. Overall, these exercise programmes reduced fractures. Home safety interventions were found to be effective, especially in people at higher risk of falling and when carried out by occupational therapists. The reviewers concluded that falls prevention strategies can be cost saving. This evidence could be used by nurses to reduce the risk of falling and improve the quality of life for older people.

A first-line approach for nurses (in the hospital, home and care homes) to identify older individuals at high risk of falls would be to ask if the patient has fallen in the last year and, if so, the frequency, injuries and circumstances of the fall(s). How older people and health professional classify a fall can differ. A stumble or trip where the person is able to respond and recover is not a fall. The following wording is recommended when asking older people about falls, 'In the past month, have you had any fall including a slip or trip in which you lost your balance and landed on the floor or ground or lower level?' (Lamb et al., 2005). A positive history of falls should trigger an in-depth assessment to identify modifiable risk factors that can be dealt with by the health professional (Figure 11.5).

To target those who are at a high risk of falls but who have not yet fallen, a short assessment of the individual's functional and physical ability may be carried out using:

- The FICSIT Four Test Balance Scale (Rossiter-Fornoff et al., 1995);
- The Timed Up and Go Test (Podsiadlo and Richardson, 1991).

The FICSIT Four Test Balance Scale is a short balance test that includes four timed static balance tasks of increasing difficulty, using different positioning of the participants' feet; it has also been extensively tested for validity and reliability (Rossiter-Fornoff et al., 1995). The validated Timed Up and Go Test measures the time it takes for an individual to rise from a chair, walk three metres at a normal pace with their usual assistive device, turn, return to the chair and sit down. A time of 12 or more seconds indicates an increased risk of falling (Podsiadlo and Richardson, 1991). These physical checks have been safely performed on thousands of older people (Robertson et al., 2002) and there are videos available on the internet that can teach health professionals to perform them correctly with older people (see www.cdc.gov/homeandrecreationalsafety/Falls/steadi/videos.html).

Strength and balance exercises are particularly good at reducing the risk of falls, increasing bone health (therefore reducing the risk of fractures) and can have other beneficial properties such as improving mood and social contact. To find out more about trained postural stability instructors or therapists who deliver strength and balance exercises for older people, nurses should contact their local community physiotherapy departments or visit the website of Later Life Training, for a directory of trained staff within local regions (see www.laterlifetraining.co.uk/falls-directory). Tai chi is also known to reduce the risk of falls and is a type of exercise that many older people enjoy due to its relaxing properties; many local leisure centres and libraries can give further details about available classes. In terms of prescribing, the optimum dose and timing of exercise programmes for reducing falls, and the criterion for a minimal effective exercise dose, equate to a twice-weekly programme over 24 weeks (Sherrington et al., 2008). More recent reviews suggest that the higher the dose of exercise and the more challenging to balance the greater the reduction in rate of falls (Sherrington et al., 2016). Referrals to physiotherapists, specialist falls services, occupational therapists, postural stability instructors and GPs (for medication review) could be carried out by nurses to ensure that evidence-based practice is carried out for older people. A home assessment by an occupational therapist or

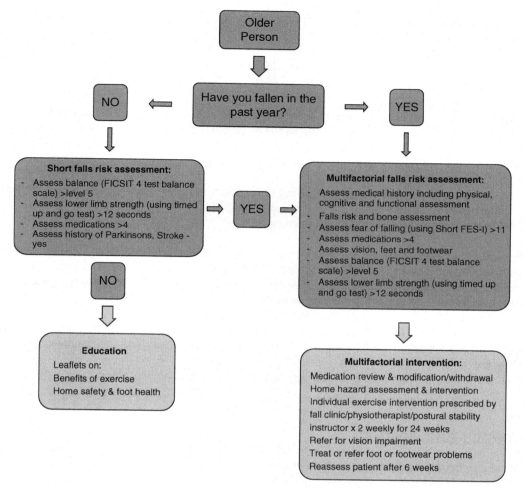

**Figure 11.5** Algorithm of falls risk-screening tool. (Adapted from Nandy et al., 2004; AGS/BGS, 2010; Stanmore, 2013)

community nurse would also be invaluable to highlight any fall hazards that may be present on the person's home environment.

Ensuring that older people receive regular eyesight checks and treatment for visual problems (e.g. cataract surgery) can be helpful in preventing falls, as can wearing well-fitting, anti-slip shoes. As many older people can be taking a number of different types of medicines, it is important that they receive a regular review of their medication (in particular the review of psychotropic medicines) so that they can be modified if necessary.

Fear of falling can negatively affect individuals and their ability to maintain social networks and maintain independence. A simple measure of fear of falling, such as the validated Short Falls Efficacy Scale – International (Kempen et al., 2008) can be undertaken to identify those with low levels of confidence. People who fall recurrently would benefit from a more detailed multi-factorial assessment, and an individual falls prevention programme from a trained clinician or at a falls prevention clinic.

## MRS BIRCH

Mrs Birch is a 79-year-old independent woman who lives at home with her frail husband who has Parkinson's disease. She has been having difficulties sleeping and has recently had a couple of falls during the night, resulting in some minor bruising and a small laceration to her right shin. As a registered nurse, you are requested to visit and assess Mrs Birch.

- How would you conduct a bio-psychosocial assessment with Mrs Birch, thinking about her individual needs and care?
- What is normal for Mrs Birch? What has changed?

*Physical assessment*: past medical history, current health status, co-morbidities; nocturia: detailed falls assessment (see Figure 11.5); medications: prescribed and use of over the counter, type and frequency; sleep duration, quality, difficulties falling asleep/staying asleep/un-refreshing sleep/daytime sleepiness, sleep apnoea; wound assessment.

     *Psychological assessment*: assess mood, anxiety, cognition.

     *Social assessment*: lifestyle; formal and informal support; environment; exercise levels; husband's needs; what is important to Mrs Birch and her husband, their interests, past occupations, hobbies, family, etc.

     How could you ensure a biographical approach is incorporated into the assessment?

## Dementia and delirium

The most important issue for nurses is to understand that the behaviour exhibited by people living with dementia will be dictated by the type of dementia they have and the area of the brain most affected. The deterioration of abilities will also vary from person to person, which further instils the need for individualised, person-centred care (Social Care Institute for Excellence, 2013). As an example, Alzheimer's dementia is characterised by a progressive deterioration of brain function, whereas people with a diagnosis of vascular dementia may experience a stepped decline in function, alongside cognitive symptoms such as apathy, anxiety or depression, and mood swings (Alzheimer's Society, 2014). As with the general population, people with dementia will require hospital treatment for conditions as they age. However, 42% of unplanned admissions for people over 70 will be due to dementia. This demonstrates the complexity of addressing healthcare needs for people with dementia, particularly as 20% of admissions involving people with dementia will be for preventable conditions such as urinary tract infections (National Dementia Intelligence Network, 2015). To further compound the difficulties experienced by people with dementia in hospitals, around 83% of admissions involving people with dementia are via the accident and emergency department (National Dementia Intelligence Network, 2015). The person with dementia will be exposed to the confusing effects of waiting for long periods, moving between departments and/or wards and seeing a number of different people, when they may be used to seeing only one or two people per day. Equally, they may be experiencing pain or feeling ill and, being bombarded with information from multiple sources which may cause stress with the person's behaviour being adversely impacted. This may present challenges for staff in acute and busy environments because people with dementia are not able to communicate in the same way as older people without dementia. Quite often it may be the situation impacting on a person with dementia's behaviour and, if we can create a more appropriate environment, the behaviour may create fewer challenges for staff (Table 11.2).

**Table 11.2**   Common responses to hospital environment for people with dementia

| Psychological | Physical |
| --- | --- |
| Stress | Disturbance in relation to activities of living, |
| Fear | e.g. |
| Agitation and/or aggression | Sleep patterns |
| Vocalisations | Nutrition |
| Wandering or excessive walking | Hydration |
| Searching | Elimination |
| Wanting to go home | Mobility |

Clarke et al. (2003) undertook a pilot investigation into how staff understanding the life history of a person with dementia might improve person-centred care in an acute context. The philosophy of this project emphasised that attitudes, desires and interests of older people are a culmination of life experience, and sought to support staff in viewing later decades as a time of ongoing development and self-determination. By encouraging older people to talk about their life experiences staff can gain a fuller appreciation of people's needs, concerns and aspirations (Clarke et al., 2003). Life story work is being used more widely across dementia care and usually involves the construction of a life storybook (McKeown et al., 2006). However, a practice development project undertaken with staff in a dementia environment suggests that the focused use of biographical information can also promote person-centred practice (Brown Wilson et al., 2013).

It is important that nurses do not make assumptions about the behaviour of people living with dementia, attributing it solely to their dementia; changes in behaviour may also be a result of underlying physical issues such as pain or the onset of infection. For example, a urinary tract infection (UTI) continues to be a reason for older people being admitted to hospital. Using questionnaires to document the cues an older person might exhibit to suggest a change in their condition has been found to be acceptable to both nurses and patients in acute services (Hill, 2012). Infection in older people may result in delirium, which often presents with cognitive confusion and may be misdiagnosed as dementia. The key difference between the two conditions is that the cognitive confusion that presents with delirium is acute in onset and improves with appropriate treatment.

Delirium is a little understood condition that, when experienced by older patients, often results in increased length of stay and poorer outcomes because older people may have less resources to cope with illness and/or ill effects caused by hospitalisation. This situation may be further compounded if nurses subscribe to the myth that all older people are likely to be confused because of their age, rather than a result of underlying and treatable conditions. Delirium is different from dementia because it is acute in onset, often with families telling healthcare staff that their family member is not generally confused. There are a number of risk factors associated with delirium, for example: age, fever, co-morbidities, malnutrition, dehydration and low serum albumin (Siddiqi et al., 2007). There are few effective known interventions, but there is recognition that, after a comprehensive assessment, a multi-factorial approach is required to treat the underlying causes (Siddiqi et al., 2007).

In undertaking a practice development project, one ward found that nurses can identify and treat the early onset of delirium when patients and relatives identify early behavioural or cognitive changes that might go unrecognised by staff (Hill, 2012).

## MR BANKS

Mr Banks has been sent by his GP to the emergency department due to second-degree burns on his right leg from his electric fire. On initial assessment he appears unkempt, is wearing soiled clothes, in a confused state, disorientated to time and place. The doctor requests an urgent care home placement and prescribe pain-killers and non-adhesive, antimicrobial wound care dressings. You are asked to assist the social worker to set up the care home package and to contact the family. On contacting the family you discover that Mr Banks is usually self-caring, but since his wife died 6 weeks ago he has not been coping at home, has not been eating and drinking and has stopped going out bowling with his friends.

What further assessments need to be carried out in order to gain a comprehensive and systematic nursing assessment of Mr Banks' needs? What acute problems or illnesses could have led to his delirium? What nursing actions do you think would benefit Mr Banks and how would these enable him to return home and maintain his independence?

## Chapter summary

Nurses must be aware of the myths and stereotypes of ageing and ensure that these are not influencing key decisions in how they support older people. Subscribing to the myths of ageing or stereotyping older people may precipitate decisions, leading to lack of dignity in care giving. Seeing the person not the condition is essential to ensure that the dignity of older people, including those living with dementia, is maintained.

Person-centred care challenges the nurse to see the person rather than the condition, and is a further mechanism whereby dignity can be enhanced in care giving. Adopting a biographical approach to care planning is a first step in identifying what is important to the older person, and how this might be integrated into their care. For people living with dementia, knowing their usual routines and working to ensure that these are maintained in unfamiliar environments will enable staff to understand their responses.

Healthy lifestyles are as influential as genetic factors in helping older people avoid the decline traditionally associated with ageing. Many chronic diseases can also be prevented by maintaining a healthy and active lifestyle throughout the life course. Nurses are well placed to advise on health promotion factors such as physical activity, healthy diets, smoking cessation, immunisation uptake, and optimum management of chronic diseases to prevent deterioration in health. Regular physical activity has been shown to contribute to both improvements in physical and psychological function, including a reduction in depressive symptoms. It contributes to a healthier independent lifestyle by significantly improving the functional capacity and quality of life for older people.

Older people also need to be aware of the high risk of falls and should be encouraged to undertake strength and balance exercises to try to reduce falls and fall-related fractures and injuries, as well as improve their functioning. Older people with a history of falls should be referred to a fall prevention clinic or a trained therapist for a comprehensive assessment of risk factors and a tailored programme to prevent further falls.

Not all older people are frail, but the risk of frailty increases with age, and sometimes a small loss of function may precipitate a crisis with a risk of poor outcomes. Frailty is a physiological syndrome characterised by multiple deficits in system functioning. Some of the manifestations such as reduced walking speed or gait problems are reversible even at advanced age.

Registered nurses may be the first contact when a patient struggles with memory problems or the one with whom families discuss their concerns when a relative is not coping. They need to be aware of the support available and encourage patients with early signs of dementia to seek a diagnosis, and recognise the impact on the person and family when a diagnosis of dementia is made. Nurses also need to have an understanding of the differences between acute delirium and dementia, and act as advocates for older people to ensure that they receive a comprehensive assessment and person-centred care. The behaviour exhibited by people living with dementia will vary from person to person, so personalised care needs to be given to ensure that individual needs are met.

In summary, there is still much to explore about caring effectively for older people, but we hope that this chapter will encourage adult nurses to use approaches that value the older person and achieve positive changes that will affect us all as we grow old.

## Useful websites

Age UK website for information on health and wellbeing for older people: www.ageuk.org.uk.
British Geriatric Society resources on diagnosis and treatment of delirium: www.bgs.org.uk.
Dignified Revolution: www.dignifiedrevolution.org.uk.
Healthcare Quality Strategies website for more information about the issues of medication and falls: www.hqsi.org/index/providers/Adverse-Drug-Events/Medication-and-Falls.html.
The King's Fund project on dementia: www.kingsfund.org.uk/projects/enhancing-healing-environment/ehe-design-dementia.
Later Life Training website for online support and audio files on specific exercises and training programmes for falls prevention: www.laterlifetraining.co.uk.
Prevention of Falls Network for dissemination website for resources, updates and an online forum for advice and discussion: http://profound.eu.com.
Royal College of Nursing's dignity campaign: www.rcn.org.uk/professional-development/publications/pub-003292.
Royal College of Nursing Dementia Resources: www.rcn.org.uk/development/practice/dementia.
Social Care Institute for Excellence Dementia Resources: www.scie.org.uk/publications/dementia/index.asp.

## Further reading

Arking, R. (2006) *The Biology of Aging: Observations and Principles*, 3rd edn. Oxford: Oxford University Press.
Baillie, L., Gallagher, A. and Wainwright, P. (2008) *Defending Dignity: Challenges and Opportunities*. London: Royal College of Nursing. Available at: www.rcn.org.uk/__data/assets/pdf_file/0011/166655/003257.pdf.

Bridges, J., Flatley, M., Meyer, J. and Brown Wilson, C. (2009) 'Best practice for older people in acute care settings (BPOP): guidance for nurses', *Nursing Standard*, 24, CD.

Brown Wilson, C. (2013) *Caring for Older People: A Shared Approach*. London: Sage.

Elvish, R., Burrow, S., Cawley, R., Harney, K., Pilling, M., Gregory, J. and Keady, J. (2016) '"Getting to know me": the second phase roll-out of a staff training programme for supporting people with dementia in general hospitals', *Dementia: The International Journal of Social Research and Practice*, doi:10.1177/1471301216634926.

McCormack, B. and McCance, T. (2010) *Person Centred Nursing. Theory and Practice*. Oxford: Wiley Blackwell.

National Institute for Health Research (2017) *Comprehensive Care. Older People Living with Frailty in Hospitals*. London: NIHR. Available at: www.dc.nihr.ac.uk/themed-reviews/frailty-in-hospital-research. htm (last accessed 19 August 2018). This review covers four key aspects of caring for older people living with frailty in hospital: assessment; identifying and managing symptoms associated with frailty in hospital; discharge planning; and caring environments.

Reed, J., Clarke, C. and McFarlane, A. (2011) *Nursing Older People: A Textbook for Nurses*. Milton Keynes: Open University Press.

Tolson, D., Booth, J. and Schofield, I. (eds) (2011) *Evidence Informed Nursing with Older People*. Oxford: Blackwell.

# References

Ablitt, A., Jones, G. and Muers, J. (2009) 'Living with dementia: A systematic review of the influence of relationship factors', *Aging and Mental Health*, 13(4): 497–511.

Abrahams, A. (2011) *Care and Compassion? Report of the Health Service Ombudsman on Ten Investigations into NHS Care of Older People*. London: The Stationery Office.

Age UK (2011) *Ageism in Europe: Findings from the European Social Survey*. Available at: www.ageuk. org.uk/Documents/EN-GB/For-professionals/ageism_across_europe_report_interactive.pdf?dtrk=true (last accessed 14 February 2018).

Age UK (2017) *Briefing: Health and Care of Older People in England 2017*. Available at: www.ageuk. org.uk/Documents/EN-GB/For-professionals/Research/The_Health_and_Care_of_Older_People_in_ England_2016.pdf?dtrk=true (last accessed 14 February 2018).

All-Party Parliamentary Group on Dementia (2011) *The £20 Billion Question: An Inquiry into Improving Lives through Cost-effective Dementia Services*. Available at: www.alzheimers.org.uk/site/scripts/ download_info.php?fileID=1207 (last accessed 11 April 2018).

Alzheimer's Research UK (2015a) *Dementia in the Family: The Impact on Carers*. Available at: www. alzheimersresearchuk.org/wp-content/uploads/2015/12/Dementia-in-the-Family-The-impact-on-carers.pdf (last accessed 28 January 2018).

Alzheimer's Research UK (2015b) *Women and Dementia: A Marginalized Majority*. Available at: www. alzheimersresearchuk.org/wp-content/uploads/2015/03/Women-and-Dementia-A-Marginalised-Majority1.pdf (last accessed 28 January 2018).

Alzheimer's Society (2014) *Vascular Dementia*. Factsheet 402LP. Available at: www.alzheimers.org.uk/ download/downloads/id/2427/factsheet_what_is_vascular_dementia.pdf (last accessed 28 January 2018).

Alzheimer's Society (2017) *What is Dementia?* Factsheet 400LP. Available at: www.alzheimers.org.uk/ download/downloads/id/3416/what_is_dementia.pdf (last accessed 28 January 2018).

American Geriatrics Society, British Geriatrics Society, and American Academy of Orthopaedic Surgeons Panel on Falls Prevention (AGS/BGS) (2010) 'Clinical practice guideline: prevention of falls in older persons', *Journal of the American Geriatric Society*. Available at: www.bgs.org.uk/fallsresources-307/ subjectreference/fallsandbones/bgsagsfalls2010 (last accessed 11 April 2018).

Anderson, R.A., Issel, L.M. and McDaniel, Jr, R.R. (2003) 'Nursing homes as complex adaptive systems: relationship between management practice and resident outcomes', *Nursing Research*, 52(1): 12–21.

Andrews, A. and Butler, M. (2014) *Trusted to Care. An Independent Review of the Princess of Wales Hospital and Neath Port Talbot Hospital at Abertawe Bro Morgannwg University Health Boards* (Executive Summary). Available at: http://gov.wales/topics/health/publications/health/reports/care (last accessed 8 April 2018).

Ansara, Y.G. (2015) 'Challenging cisgenderism in the ageing and aged care sector: meeting the needs of older people of trans and/or non-binary experience', *Australasian Journal on Ageing*, 34(Suppl 2): 14–18.

Arking, R. (2006) *The Biology of Aging: Observations and Principles*. New York: Oxford University Press.

Barnes, D.E. and Yaffe, K. (2011) 'The projected effect of risk factor reduction on Alzheimer's disease prevalence', *Lancet Neurology*, 10(9): 819–28.

Barrett, C., Crameri, P., Lambourne, S., Latham, J.R. and Whyte, C. (2015) 'Understanding the experiences and needs of lesbian, gay, bisexual and trans Australians living with dementia, and their partners', *Australasian Journal on Ageing*, 34(Suppl 2): 34–8.

Bayer, T., Tadd, W. and Krajcik, S.(2005) 'Dignity: the voice of older people', *Quality in Ageing*, 6(1): 22–9.

Bond, J., Peace, S.M., Dittmann-Kohli, F. and Westerhof, G. (2007) *Ageing in Society: European Perspectives on Gerontology*. London: Sage.

Bowers, H., Lockwood, S., Eley, A., Catley, A., Runnicles, D., Mordey, M., Barker, S., Thomas, N., Jones, C. and Dalziel, S. (2013) *Widening Choices for Older People with High Support Needs*. York: Joseph Rowntree Foundation.

Bridges, J., Flatley, M. and Meyer, J. (2010) 'Older people's and relatives' experiences in acute care settings: systematic review and synthesis of qualitative studies', *International Journal of Nursing Studies*, 47: 89–107.

British Heart Foundation (2010) *A Toolkit for the Design, Implementation and Evaluation of Exercise Referral Schemes*. Loughborough: BHF National Centre, Loughborough University.

Brooker, D. (2004) 'What is person centred care in dementia?', *Reviews in Clinical Gerontology*, 13: 215–22.

Brown Wilson, C. (2009) 'Developing community in care homes through a relationship-centred approach', *Health and Social Care in the Community*, 17(2): 177–86.

Brown Wilson, C. (2013) *Caring for Older People: A Shared Approach*. London: Sage.

Brown Wilson, C. (2017) *Caring for People with Dementia: A Shared Approach*. London: Sage.

Brown Wilson, C. and Davies, S. (2009) 'Using relationships in care homes to develop relationship centred care: the contribution of staff', *Journal of Clinical Nursing*, 18: 1746–55.

Brown Wilson, C., Swarbrick, C., Pilling, M. and Keady, J. (2013) 'The senses in practice: enhancing the quality of care for residents with dementia in care homes', *Journal of Advanced Nursing*, 69(1): 77–90.

Carers UK (2016) *Factsheet e-1029 Assessments: Getting the Help you Need*. Available at: www.carersuk.org/help-and-advice/practical-support/getting-care-and-support/carers-assessment (last accessed 11 April 2018).

Centers for Disease Control and Prevention (1996) *Physical Activity and Health: A Report of the Surgeon General Executive*. Summary. Atlanta, GA: US Department of Health and Human Services.

Chief Medical Officer (2011) *Public Health Guidelines on Physical Activity for Older Adults*. London: DH.

Clarke, A., Hanson, E.J. and Ross, H. (2003) 'Seeing the person behind the patient: enhancing the care of older people using a biographical approach', *Journal of Clinical Nursing*, 12: 697.

Clegg, A., Bates, C., Young, J., Ryan, R., Nichols, L., Teale, E.A., Mohammed, M.A., Parry, J. and Marshall, T. (2016) 'Development and validation of an electronic frailty index using routine primary care electronic health record data', *Age and Ageing*, 45(3): 353–60.

Cornwell, J. (2012) 'The care of frail older people with complex needs: time for a revolution'. The Sir Roger Bannister Health Summit, The King's Fund, Leeds Castle.

Cowdell, F., Kelly, F., Board, M., Gilmore, C. and Stanmore, E. (2018) 'What is the contribution of nurses and allied health professionals to the care of the frail older person? A narrative review of empirical literature', *Age and Ageing*, in press.

Crameri, P., Barrett, C., Latham, J.R. and Whyte, C. (2015) 'It is more than sex and clothes: culturally safe services for older lesbian, gay, bisexual, transgender and intersex people', *Australasian Journal on Ageing*, 34(Suppl 2): 21–5.

Department of Health (2001) *Involving Patients and the Public in Healthcare: A Discussion Document.* London: DH.

Department of Health (2009) *Be Active, Be Healthy. A Plan for Getting the Nation Moving.* London: DH.

Department of Health (2012) *Compassion in Practice: Nursing, Midwifery and Care Staff, Our Vision and Strategy.* London: DH.

Department of Health (2013) *Patients First and Foremost: The Initial Government Response to the Report of The Mid Staffordshire NHS Foundation Trust Public Inquiry.* London: DH.

Department of Health (2016) *Making a Difference in Dementia: Nursing Vision and Strategy.* London: DH.

Department of Health and Social Care (2016) Care Act 2014. Part 1 Fact sheets. Available at: www.gov.uk/government/publications/care-act-2014-part-1-factsheets/care-act-factsheets#factsheet-8-the-law-for-carers (last accessed 11 April 2018).

Dewing, J. (2004) 'Concerns relating to the application of frameworks to promote person-centredness in nursing older people', *International Journal of Older People Nursing*, 13(3a): 39–44.

Dowrick, A. and Southern, A (2014) *Dementia 2014: Opportunity for Change.* London: Alzheimer's Society. Available at: www.alzheimers.org.uk/download/downloads/id/2317/dementia_2014_opportunity_for_change.pdf (last accessed 11 April 2018).

Ellis, G., Whitehead, M.A., O'Neill, D., Langhorne, P. and Robinson, D. (2011) 'Comprehensive geriatric assessment for older adults admitted to hospital', *Cochrane Database of Systematic Reviews*, 7: CD006211. doi:10.1002/14651858.CD006211.pub2.

European Commission (2015) *Eurobarometer on Discrimination 2015: General Perceptions, Opinions on Policy Measures and Awareness of Rights.* Available at: http://ec.europa.eu/justice/fundamental-rights/files/factsheet_eurobarometer_fundamental_rights_2015.pdf (last accessed 14 February 2018).

Ferrucci, L., Guralnik, J.M., Studenski, S., Fried, L.P. and Cutler, G.B. for Interventions on Frailty Working Group (2004) 'Designing randomized, controlled trials aimed at preventing or delaying functional decline and disability in frail, older persons: a consensus report', *Journal of the American Geriatric Society*, 52: 625–34.

Fiatarone, M.A., Marks, E.C., Ryan, D.T., Meredith, C.N., Lewis, A., Lipsitz, M.D. and Evans, W.J. (1990) 'High-intensity strength training in nonagenarians', *Journal of the American Medical Association*, 263(22): 3029–34.

Fiske, S.T., Cuddy, A.J., Glick, P.C. and Xu, J. (2002) 'A model of (often mixed) stereotype content: competence and warmth respectively follow from perceived status and competition', *Journal of Personality and Social Psychology*, 82(6): 878–902.

Francis, R. (2013) *Report of the Mid Staffordshire NHS Foundation Trust Public Enquiry.* London: HMSO.

Fried, L.P., Ferrucci, L., Darer, J., Williamson, J.D. and Anderson, G.F. (2004) 'Untangling the concepts of disability, frailty, and comorbidity: implications for improved targeting and care', *Journal of Gerontology A Biology, Science and Medical Science*, 59A: M255–63.

Fultz, N.H.A. and Herzog, A.R. (2000) 'Prevalence of urinary incontinence in middle-aged and older women: a survey-based methodological experiment', *Journal of Aging and Health*, 12: 459–69.

Gaugler, J.E., Kane, R.L., Kane, R.A. and Newcomer, R. (2005) 'The longitudinal effects of early behavior problems in the dementia caregiving career', *Psychology and Aging*, 20(1): 100–16.

Gaugler, J.E., Potter, T. and Pruinelli, L. (2014) 'Partnering with caregivers', *Geriatric Psychiatry, Clinics in Geriatric Medicine*, 30(3): 493–515.

Gillespie, L.D., Robertson, M.C., Gillespie, W.J., Sherrington, C., Gates, S., Clemson, L.M. and Lamb, S.E. (2012) 'Interventions for preventing falls in older people living in the community', *Cochrane Database of Systematic Reviews*, 9: CD007146. doi:10.1002/14651858.CD007146.pub3.

Goodrich, J. (2011) *The Point of Care Programme. Consultation on Improving Dignity in Care Submission from The King's Fund to the Partnership on Dignity in Care* (AGE UK, NHS Confederation and Local Government Group). London: The King's Fund.

Goodrich, J. and Cornwell, J. (2008) *Seeing the Person in the Patient: The Point of Care Review Paper.* London: The King's Fund.

Goodwin, N., Curry, N., Naylor, C., Ross, S. and Duldig, W. (2010) *Managing People with Long-term Conditions: An Inquiry into the Quality of General Practice in England*. London: The King's Fund. Available at: www.kingsfund.org.uk/document.rm?id=8757 (last accessed 11 April 2018).

Government Office for Science (2016) *Future of an Ageing Population*. London: Government Office for Science.

Greenhalgh, T., Procter, R., Wherton, J., Sugarhood, P. and Shaw, S. (2012) 'The organising vision for telehealth and telecare: discourse analysis', *BMJ Open*, 2: 4.

Hill, K. (2012) *Critical to Care: Improving the Care to the Acutely Ill and Deteriorating Patient*. Foundation of Nursing Studies Project Report. Available at: http://fons.org/library/report-details.aspx?nstid=18132 (last accessed 11 April 2018).

Humphries, R., Thorlby, R., Holder, H., Hall, P. and Charles, A. (2016) *Social Care for Older People: Home Truths*. London: The King's Fund and the Nuffield Trust. Available at: www.kingsfund.org.uk/sites/default/files/field/field_publication_file/Social_care_older_people_Kings_Fund_Sep_2016.pdf (last accessed 14 February 2018).

Institute of Medicine (IOM) (2001) *Crossing the Quality Chasm: A New Health System for the 21st Century*. Washington, DC: National Academy Press.

Jacelon, C. (2003) 'The dignity of elders in acute care hospital', *Qualitative Health Research*, 13(4): 543–56.

Jones, D., Song, X. and Rockwood, K. (2004) 'Operationalizing a frailty index from a standardized comprehensive geriatric assessment', *Journal of the American Geriatric Society*, 52: 1929–33.

Kempen, G.I., Yardley, L., van Haastregt, J.C., Zijlstra, G.A., Beyer, N., Hauer, K. and Todd, C. (2008) 'The Short FES-I: A shortened version of the falls efficacy scale-international to assess fear of falling', *Age and Ageing*, 37(1): 44–50.

Kitwood, T. (1997) *Dementia Reconsidered: The Person Comes First*. Milton Keynes: Open University Press.

Knoops, K.T., de Groot, L.C., Kromhout, D., Perrin, A.E., Moreiras-Varela, O., Menotti, A. and van Staveren, W.A. (2004) 'Mediterranean diet, lifestyle factors, and 10-year mortality in elderly European men and women: the HALE project', *Journal of the American Medical Association*, 292(12): 1433–9.

Lamb, S.E., Jorstad-Stein, E.C., Hauer, K. and Becker, C. (2005) 'Development of a common outcome data set for fall injury prevention trials: the prevention of falls network Europe consensus', *Journal of the American Geriatric Society*, 53: 1618–22.

LeBlanc, A., Schneider, V., Krebs, J., Evans, H., Jhingran, S. and Johnson, P. (1987) 'Spinal bone mineral after 5 weeks of bed rest', *Calcified Tissue International*, 41: 259–61.

Lee, D. (2016) 'Sexual health'. In M. Moore (ed.), *Annual Report of the Chief Medical Officer, 2015. On the State of the Public's Health Baby Boomers: Fit for the Future*, pp. 137–56. Available at: https://assets.publishing.service.gov.uk/government/uploads/system/uploads/attachment_data/file/654806/CMO_baby_boomers_annual_report_2015.pdf (last accessed 23 August 2018).

Levenson, R. (2007) *The Challenge of Dignity in Care. Upholding the Rights of the Individual*. London: Help the Aged.

Lewis, F. (2015) *Estimation of Future Cases of Dementia from Those Born in 2015: Consultation Report for Alzheimer's Research UK*. Office of Health Economics Consulting. Available at: www.ohe.org/publications/estimation-future-cases-dementia-those-born-2015 (last accessed 10 February 2018).

Magee, H., Parsons, S. and Askham, J. (2008) *Measuring Dignity in Care for Older People. A Research Report for Help the Aged*. London: Help the Aged.

McCabe, M., You, E. and Tatangelo, G. (2016) 'Hearing their voice: a systematic review of dementia family caregivers' needs', *Gerontologist*, 56(5): e70–88. doi:10.1093/geront/gnw078.

McCormack, B. and McCance, T. (2006) 'Development of a framework for person centred nursing', *Journal of Advanced Nursing*, 56(5): 472–9.

McCormack, B. and McCance, T. (2010) *Person Centred Nursing. Theory and Practice*. Oxford: Wiley Blackwell.

McKeown, J., Clarke, A. and Repper, J. (2006) 'Life story work in health and social care: systematic literature review', *Journal of Advanced Nursing*, 55(2): 237–47.

Minkler, M. (1996) 'Critical perspectives on ageing: new challenges for gerontology', *Ageing and Society*, 16: 467–87.

Mitchell, W., Brooks, J. and Glendinning, C. (2015) 'Carers' roles in personal budgets: tensions and dilemmas in front line practice', *British Journal of Social Work*, 45(5): 1433–50.

Mitnitski, A., Song, X., Skoog, I., Broe, G.A., Cox, J., Grunfeld, E. and Rockwood, K. (2005) 'Relative fitness and frailty of elderly men and women in developed countries and their relationship with mortality', *Journal of the American Geriatric Society*, 53: 2184–9.

Nandy, S., Parsons, S., Cryer, C., Underwood, M., Rashbrook, E., Carter, Y., Eldridge, S., Close, J., Skelton, D., Taylor, S. and Feder, G. on behalf of the falls prevention pilot steering group (2004) 'Development and preliminary examination of the predictive validity of the falls risk assessment tool (FRAT) for use in primary care', *Journal Public Health*, 26(2): 138–43.

National Council on Aging (2013) *Debunking the Myths of Older Adult Falls*. Available at: www.ncoa.org (last accessed on 19 August 2014).

National Dementia Intelligence Network (2015) *Reasons Why People with Dementia are Admitted to a General Hospital in an Emergency*. Public Health England. Available at: http://webarchive.nationalarchives.gov.uk/20170302124526/http://www.yhpho.org.uk/default.aspx?RID=207311 (last accessed 28 January 2018).

National Institute for Health and Care Excellence (2008) *Mental Wellbeing and Older People*, NICE Public Health Guidance 16. Available at: www.nice.org.uk/guidance/ph16 (last accessed 14 February 2018).

National Institute for Health and Care Excellence (2013) *Falls: Assessment and Prevention of Falls in Older People*: NICE Public Health Guidance CG161. Available at: www.nice.org.uk/guidance/CG161 (last accessed 14 February 2018).

National Institute for Health and Care Excellence (2016) *Multimorbidity: Clinical Assessment* and *Multimorbidity: Clinical Assessment and Management*. NICE guideline. Available at: www.nice.org.uk/guidance/ng56 (last accessed 14 February18).

Nordenfelt, L. and Edgar, A. (2005) 'The four notions of dignity', *Quality in Ageing* 6(1): 17–21.

Nursing and Midwifery Council (2018) *Future Nurse: Standards of Proficiency for Registered Nurses*. London: NMC.

Office for Budget Responsibility (2015) *Fiscal Sustainability Report June 2015*. Available at: http://budgetresponsibility.org.uk/fsr/fiscalsustainability-report-june-2015 (last accessed 14 April 2018).

Office for National Statistics (2017) *Estimates of the Very Old (including Centenarians): 2002 to 2016*. Available at: www.ons.gov.uk/peoplepopulationandcommunity/birthsdeathsandmarriages/ageing/bulletins/estimatesoftheveryoldincludingcentenarians/2002to2016 (last accessed 11 April 2018).

Oliver, D. (2013) *We Must End Ageism and Age Discrimination in Health and Social Care*. London: The King's Fund. Available at: www.kingsfund.org.uk/blog/2013/05/we-must-end-ageism-and-age-discrimination-health-and-social-care (last accessed 14 February 2018).

Orrell, A., McKee, K., Dahlberg, L., Gilhooly, M. and Parker, S. (2013) 'Improving continence services for older people from the service-providers' perspective: a qualitative interview study', *BMJ Open*, 3: 7.

Pickard, S. and Glendinning, C. (2002). 'Caring for a relative with dementia: the perceptions of carers and CPNs', *Quality in Ageing*, 2: 3–11.

Pinquart, M. and Sorensen, S. (2003) 'Predictors of caregiver burden and depressive mood: a meta-analysis', *Journal of Gerontology, Psychological Sciences*, 58: 112–28.

Pinquart, M. and Sorensen, S. (2004) 'Associations of caregivers' stressors and uplifts with subjective well-being and depressive mood: a meta-analytic comparison', *Aging & Mental Health*, 8(5): 438–49.

Pinquart, M. and Sorensen, S. (2011) 'Spouses, adult children, and children-in-law as carers of older adults: a meta-analytic comparison', *Psychology of Aging*, 26(1): 1–14.

Poblador-Plou, B., Calderón-Larrañaga, A., Marta-Moreno, J., Hancco-Saavedra, J., Sicras-Mainar, A., Soljak, M. and Prados-Torres, A. (2014) 'Comorbidity of dementia: a cross-sectional study of primary care older patients', *BMC Psychiatry*, 14: 84.

Podsiadlo, D.A. and Richardson, S. (1991) 'The timed up and go: a test of functional mobility for frail elder persons', *Journal of the American Geriatrics Society*, 39: 142–8.

Prince, M., Knapp, M., Guerchet, M., McCrone, P., Prina, M., Comas-Herrera, A., Wittenberg, R., Adelaja, B., Hu, B., King, D., Rehill, A. and Salimkumar, D. (2014) *Dementia UK – Overview*, 2nd edn. London: Alzheimer's Society.

Public Health England (2016) *Guidance Health Matters: Getting Every Adult Active Every Day*. Available at: www.gov.uk/government/publications/health-matters-getting-every-adult-active-every-day/health-matters-getting-every-adult-active-every-day (last accessed 15 February 2018).

Quinn, C., Clare, L., McGuinness, T. and Woods, R. (2012) 'The impact of relationships, motivations, and meanings on dementia caregiving outcomes', *International Psychogeriatrics*, 24(11): 1816–26.

Robertson, M.C., Campbell, A.J., Gardner, M.M. and Devlin, N. (2002) 'Meta-analysis of the four trials', *Journal of the American Geriatric Society*, 50: 905–11.

Rockwood, K. and Koller, K. (2013) 'Frailty in older adults: implications for end-of-life care', *Cleveland Clinic Journal of Medicine*, 80(3): 168–74.

Rockwood, K., Fox, R., Stolee, P., Robertson, B. and Beattie, L. (1994) 'Frailty in elderly people: an evolving concept', *Canadian Medical Association Journal*, 150(4): 489–95.

Rockwood, K., Mitnitski, A., Song, X., Steen, B. and Skoog, I. (2006) 'Long-term risks of death and institutionalization of elderly people in relation to deficit accumulation at age 70', *Journal of the American Geriatric Society*, 54(6): 975–9.

Rogers, S., Martin, G. and Rai, G. (2014) 'Medicines management support to older people: understanding the context of systems failure', *BMJ Open*, 4: 7.

Røsvik, J.J., Kirkevold, M., Engedal, K., Brooker, D. and Kirkevold, Ø. (2011) 'A model for using the VIPS framework for person-centred care for persons with dementia in nursing homes: a qualitative evaluative study', *International Journal of Older People Nursing*, 6: 227–36.

Rossiter-Fornoff, J.E., Wolf, S.L., Wolfson, L.I. and Buchner, D.M., FICSIT Group (1995) 'A cross-sectional validation study of the FCSIT common database static balance measures', *Journal of Gerontology: Medical Sciences*, 50A: M291–7.

Royal College of Physicians (2012) *Hospitals on the Edge*. London: RCP.

SACE (2017) *Personal Social Services Survey of Adult Carers in England, 2016–17*. London: NHS Digital. Available at: https://digital.nhs.uk/catalogue/PUB30045 (last accessed 28 January 2018).

Schumacher, L., MacNeill, R., Mobily, K., Teague, M. and Butcher, H. (2012) 'The leisure journey for sandwich generation caregivers', *Therapeutic Recreation Journal*, 46(1): 42–59.

Sherrington, C., Whitney, J.C., Lord, S.R., Herbert, R.D., Cumming, R.G. and Close, J.C. (2008) 'Effective exercise for the prevention of falls: a systematic review and meta-analysis', *Journal of the American Geriatrics Society*, 56: 2234–43. doi:10.1111/j.1532-5415.2008.02014.x.

Sherrington, C., Michaleff, Z.A., Fairhall, N., Paul, S.S., Tiedemann, A., Whitney, J., Cumming, R.G., Herbert, R.D., Close, J.C.T. and Lord, S.R. (2016) 'Exercise to prevent falls in older adults: an updated systematic review and meta-analysis', *British Journal of Sports Medicine*, 51(24): 1750–8.

Siddiqi, N., Stockdale, R., Britton, A.M. and Holmes, J. (2007) 'Interventions for preventing delirium in hospitalised patients', *Cochrane Database of Systematic Reviews*, 2: CD005563. doi:10.1002/14651858. CD005563.pub2.

Simpson, P., Horne, M., Brown, L.J.E., Brown Wilson, C., Dickinson, T. and Torkington, K. (2017a) 'Old(er) care home residents and sexual/intimate citizenship', *Ageing and Society*, 37: 243–65.

Simpson, P., Brown Wilson, C., Horne, M., Brown, L.E.J. and Dickinson, T. (2017b) '"We've had our sex life way back": older care home residents, sexuality and intimacy', *Ageing and Society*, 37(2): 243–65.

Skelton, D.A., Dinan, S.M., Campbell, M.G. and Rutherford, O.M. (2005) 'Tailored group exercise (Falls Management Exercise – FaME) reduces falls in community-dwelling older frequent fallers (an RCT)', *Age and Ageing*, 34: 636–9.

Smith, M.E., Dunphy, L.M. and Mainous, R.O. (2011) 'Innovative nursing educational curriculum for the 21st century'. In National Research Council (ed.), *The Future of Nursing: Leading Change, Advancing Health*. Washington, DC: The National Academies Press.

Social Care Institute for Excellence (2013) *Dignity*. Available at: www.scie.org.uk/publications/guides/guide15/index.asp (last accessed 11 April 2018).

Stanmore, E.K. (2011) 'Choice, appropriateness and adequacy of care for older people: utilising patients and professionals views to identify future service improvements', *International Journal of Person-Centered Medicine*, 1(3): 522–6.

Stanmore, E.K. (2013) 'The importance of falls assessment in patients with rheumatoid arthritis', *Journal of Health Visiting*, 1(2): 5.

Stanmore, E.K., Oldham, J., Skelton, D.A., O'Neill, T., Piling, M., Campbell, A.J. and Todd, C. (2013) 'Fall incidence and outcomes of falls in a prospective study of adults with rheumatoid arthritis', *Arthritis Care and Research*, 65(5): 737–44.

Steventon, A., Bardsley, M., Billings, J., Dixon, J., Doll, H., Beynon, M., Hirani, S., Cartwright, M., Rixon, L., Knapp, M., Henderson, C., Rogers, S., Hendy, J., Fitzpatrick, R. and Newman, S. (2013) 'Effect of telecare on use of health and social care services: findings from the Whole Systems Demonstrator cluster randomised trial', *Age and Ageing*, 42(4): 501–8.

Tadd, W., Hillman, A., Calnan, S., Calnan, M., Bayer, T. and Read, S. (2011) *Dignity in Practice: An Exploration of the Care of Older Adults in Acute NHS Trusts*. Service Delivery and Organisation Programme. Available at: www.sdo.nihr.ac.uk/files/project/SDO_FR_08-1819-218_V01.pdf.

van Diest, M., Lamoth, C.J., Stegenga, J., Verkerke, G.J. and Postema, K. (2013) 'Exergaming for balance training of elderly: state of the art and future developments', *Journal of Neuroengineering and Rehabilitation*, 10: 101.

Wilmoth, J.M. and Ferraro, K.F. (eds) (2013) *Gerontology Perspectives and Issues*. New York: Springer Publishing Co.

World Health Organization (2002) *Keep Fit for Life: Meeting the Nutritional Needs of Older Persons*. Geneva: WHO.

World Health Organization (2007) *WHO Global Report on Falls Prevention in Older Age*. Geneva: WHO.

# CARING FOR ADULTS WITH LONG–TERM CONDITIONS

## JUDITH ORMROD AND DIANNE BURNS

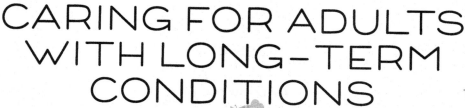

---

### CHAPTER OBJECTIVES

- Identify the common problems encountered by individuals living with a long-term condition;
- Recognise the adult nurse's role in supporting individuals (and their carers) living with long-term conditions in the UK;
- Identify treatment and care pathways that provide the evidence base used to underpin your practice;
- Identify relevant government policies that aim to support self-management, personalised care planning, and working in partnership with patients and carers;
- Demonstrate how the concepts of *patient empowerment*, *shared decision making* and *concordance* can be used to inform the adult nurse's role in partnership working.

---

## Introduction

This chapter aims to offer an introduction to the role of the registered adult nurse in supporting individuals who are living with a chronic illness or a long-term condition (LTC). Chronic illness is defined by the Department of Health (DH, 2005) as a long-term health condition that cannot at present be cured, but can be controlled by medication and other therapies.

Reading and completing the activities in Chapter 10 you will be aware of the nurse's public health role, the importance of identifying and reducing recognised risk factors, and educating patients and their families to help them stay healthy, thereby preventing or minimising (as far as possible) the impact on health of many LTCs. This chapter will help you to build on this knowledge, requiring you to draw on it when considering the role of the registered nurse in supporting patients suffering from a variety of LTCs.

Although it is beyond the remit of this chapter to include every single LTC you might encounter during your pre-registration programme, we intend to focus on some common conditions, because it could be argued that many of the associated issues/problems encountered by patients are shared across a wide spectrum of conditions.

## Related NMC proficiencies for registered nurses

The overarching requirements of the Nursing and Midwifery Council (NMC) are that all registered nurses must be able to provide nursing care that is person centred, safe and compassionate. They should support and enable people at all stages of life and in all care settings to make informed choices about how to manage health challenges in order to maximise their quality of life and improve health outcomes. They need to prioritise the needs of people when assessing and reviewing their mental, physical, cognitive, behavioural, social and spiritual need, and use the information obtained during assessments to identify the priorities and requirements for person-centred and evidence-based nursing interventions and support. They should work in partnership with people to develop person-centred care plans that take into account their circumstances, characteristics and preferences, supporting people of all ages in a range of care settings. They also need to work in partnership with people, families and carers to evaluate whether care is effective and the goals of care have been met in line with their wishes, preferences and desired outcomes; coordinating and managing the complex nursing and integrated care needs of people at any stage of their lives, across a range of organisations and settings (NMC, 2018a).

 **To achieve entry to the nursing register you must be able to**

- Understand and recognise the complexities of providing mental, cognitive, behavioural and physical care services across a wide range of integrated care settings and the need to respond to the challenges of providing safe, effective and person-centred care for people who have co-morbidities and complex care needs;
- Demonstrate the ability to process accurately all information gathered during the assessment process (including an understanding of co-morbidities and the need to meet people's complex nursing and social care needs) to individualise nursing care, developing and applying person-centred, evidence-based plans for nursing interventions with agreed goals;
- Demonstrate the ability to work in partnership with people, families and carers (encouraging shared decision making) to monitor, evaluate and reassess continuously the effectiveness of all agreed nursing care plans and care, readjusting agreed goals, documenting progress and decisions made in order to support individuals, their families and carers to maintain optimal independence and manage their own care when appropriate;
- Facilitate equitable access to healthcare for people who are vulnerable or have a disability and demonstrate the ability to advocate on their behalf when required; make necessary reasonable adjustments to the assessment, planning and delivery of their care;
- Use up-to-date approaches to behaviour change to support and enable people to make informed choices when managing their own health, and making lifestyle adjustments in order to have satisfying and fulfilling lives within the limitations caused by reduced capability, ill health and disability;

- Understand and apply the principles of partnership, collaboration and interagency working across all relevant sectors;
- Understand the principles and processes involved in planning and facilitating the safe discharge and transition of people across caseloads, settings and services, and demonstrate the ability to coordinate and undertake the processes and procedures involved in routine planning and management of safe discharge home or transfer of people between care settings.

(Adapted from NMC, 2018a)

## Background

The incidence of chronic illness across the UK currently presents a significant cost burden for the economy and the healthcare system. In England approximately 15 million people (one in three of the population) are living with a LTC (Health Education England, 2017). Similarly in Wales it is estimated that one in three of all adults have at least one LTC whereas in Scotland and Northern Ireland these figures rise to 40% and 42%, respectively (Gray and Leyland, 2013). Moreover, it is expected that these figures will rise further in the future (Department of Health Northern Ireland, 2012; Scottish Government, 2017) as a result of an increasingly ageing population, increasing obesity levels, low levels of physical activity, the effects of tobacco/alcohol consumption, and improving treatments and interventions that allow individuals to survive previously fatal events (Figure 12.1).

Snell et al. (2011) suggest that by 2030, the number of older people with personal care needs (e.g. washing and dressing) is expected to rise from 2.5 million to 4.1 million (an increase of 61%). Furthermore, the burden of living with an LTC affects the most disadvantaged in society. It is estimated that those belonging to social class V have a 60% higher prevalence of LTCs and a 60% higher severity, as we have already highlighted in Chapter 10. There also appears to be clear links between LTCs, lifestyle factors, deprivation and wider determinants of health (World Health

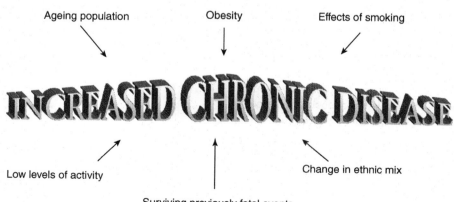

**Figure 12.1** Causes of increased chronic disease

Organization [WHO], 2011). These lifestyle risk factors include tobacco use, high cholesterol (hypercholesterolaemia), high blood pressure (hypertension), obesity/poor diet, alcohol abuse, exposure to certain infectious diseases and physical inactivity. Other factors such as socioeconomic status, social isolation, access to adequate education and health literacy, together with an environmental disadvantage, should also be taken into account. Those living with an LTC may experience disadvantage in opportunities in education, employment and income (Salway et al., 2007; Bajorek et al., 2016). They are also more likely to experience psychological problems, particularly stress and depression. Experiencing stress over a long period of time is detrimental to immunity and may increase the likelihood of an increased disease burden and prolonged recovery (Keller et al., 2000). Therefore, when providing ongoing support to patients with LTCs it is important for you to be able to recognise the associated multi-factorial causes and also the opportunities available to help your patients/clients to minimise or alleviate such risks.

## Long-term conditions

### Chronic neurological conditions

The Alzheimer's Society (Prince et al., 2014) report that there are over 850,000 people living with dementia in the UK today and this is predicted to increase rapidly over the next 30 years. In 2016 dementia/Alzheimer's disease was the leading cause of death across the UK, accounting for 12% of all deaths. Furthermore, although the disease mainly affects people over the age of 65, approximately 42,000 are people with young-onset dementia. Other examples of long-term neurological conditions include epilepsy, multiple sclerosis, Parkinson's disease, traumatic brain injury and chronic fatigue syndrome/myalgic encephalomyelitis (CFS/ME).

---

### ⬚? ACTIVITY 12.1

Find out more about how common neurological conditions currently affect people in the UK.

- Alzheimer's Society: www.alzheimers.org.uk or www.alzheimersresearchuk.org/about-dementia/facts-stats;
- Epilepsy Society: www.epilepsysociety.org.uk;
- Multiple Sclerosis Society: www.mssociety.org.uk;
- Parkinson's UK: www.parkinsons.org.uk;
- Traumatic Brain Injury: www.headway.org.uk;
- ME Association: www.meassociation.org.uk;
- Action for ME: www.actionforme.org.uk.

Make a list of the potential problems encountered by patients suffering from a neurological LTC (remember to include physical/motor, sensory, cognitive, communication, psychosocial and emotional effects).

# Heart and circulatory disease

Cardiovascular disease (CVD) is an umbrella term that describes all diseases of the heart and circulation. Although CVD is preventable and the incidence is falling across the UK, it remains a leading cause of illness and death (Table 12.1) (British Heart Foundation, 2018), particularly in Scotland (e.g. approximately 8000 deaths per year) where there is a high prevalence of associated risk factors such as smoking, poor diet and physical inactivity (Information Services Division Scotland, 2017). Furthermore, it is estimated that 2.7 million UK residents are living with the condition and, although most are men, women over the age of 50 have a similar chance of developing the condition. In addition, half a million people across the UK are currently living with heart failure (British Heart Foundation, 2018).

Hypertension (high blood pressure) affects more than one in four adults in England and is the third biggest risk factor for premature death and disability (Public Health England [PHE], 2016a) and one of the most preventable causes of premature illness and death across the UK (National Institute for Health and Care Excellence [NICE], 2011). It is a common condition, affecting at least 50% of adults over the age of 60, and is a major risk factor for stroke, heart disease, heart failure, chronic kidney disease and cognitive decline. Although the exact cause is unknown, several factors are thought to play a part, including obesity, smoking, insufficient exercise, stress, high salt intake, alcohol consumption and genetic predisposition. There is evidence to indicate that lowering blood pressure reduces the risk of long-term ill health (Ettehad et al., 2016).

**Table 12.1**   Deaths from cardiovascular disease (CVD) and numbers living with CVD

|  | No. of CVD deaths, 2016 | No. of CVD deaths at age <75, 2016 | Estimated no. of people living with CVD, 2016 |
|---|---|---|---|
| England (2016–17) | 124,615 | 33,812 | 5.9 million |
| Scotland (2015–16) | 15,131 | 4644 | 685,000 |
| Wales (2016–17) | 8655 | 2495 | 375,000 |
| Northern Ireland (2016–17) | 3629 | 1070 | 225,000 |
| UK | 152,465 | 42,311 | 7 million+ |

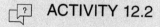 ACTIVITY 12.2

Access and read the resources identified below:

1. Department of Health (2000) *The National Service Framework for Coronary Heart Disease.* London: DH.
2. NHS Wales (2009) *The Cardiac Disease National Service Framework for Wales.* Cardiff: NHS Wales.

*(Continued)*

(Continued)

3. NICE (2011) *Hypertension in Adults: Diagnosis and Management.* Available at: www.nice.org.uk/guidance/cg127.
4. Scottish Intercollegiate Guidelines Network (SIGN) (2016) *Management of Chronic Heart Failure.* Edinburgh: SIGN.

Using the resources above and relating to CHD/CVD, hypertension and heart failure (HF):

- Identify the contributing lifestyle factors;
- Outline the development of each condition and list the common symptoms;
- List the treatment options/aims for each condition;
- List the short- and long-term complications of each of the above.

Access the following article: Hopp, F.P., Thornton, N. and Martin, L. (2010) 'The lived experience of heart failure at the end of life: a systematic literature review', *Health Society and Work*, 35(2): 109–17, and make a note of the key issues faced by patients.

## Cancer

Cancer can develop at any age but it is most commonly diagnosed in older people aged 75 years and above. There are more than 360,000 new cancer cases in the UK every year and the risk of developing cancer in people born after 1960 is 1 in 50 (Cancer Research UK, 2015). Smittenaar et al. (2016) suggest that, although overall cancer mortality seems to be decreasing, the incidence of thyroid, liver, oral and anal cancer appears to be on the increase. In addition, breast, prostate, lung and bowel cancers together accounted for over half (53%) of all new cancer cases in the UK (Cancer Research UK, 2015).

### ACTIVITY 12.3

Go to the Cancer Research UK website (www.cancerresearchuk.org) and identify the potential contributing factors to the incidence of cancer in the UK, the presenting symptoms and the treatment options for all common UK cancers.

Go to the National Institute for Health and Care Excellence (NICE) website (www.nice.org.uk) and review guidelines and NICE pathways for breast, prostrate, lung, liver and bowel cancers.

Go to the National Cancer Patient Experience Survey website (www.ncpes.co.uk/reports) and access the latest report of patient experiences of cancer services and care provision.

Access the Macmillan Routes from Diagnosis report at www.macmillan.org.uk. Make a note of the key issues faced by patients who have survived cancer.

## Respiratory disease

It is estimated 64 million people worldwide are living with chronic obstructive pulmonary disease (COPD) (WHO, 2015). Within the UK it is thought that over 3 million people are living with the disease, but only 900,000 have been diagnosed. In addition, asthma affects over 5.4 million people in the UK and causes the death of around 1200 people every year (Asthma UK, 2016). It is a commonly occurring LTC that often commences in childhood.

### ACTIVITY 12.4

Go to the NICE website (www.nice.org.uk) and review the current COPD guidelines.
   Access British Thoracic Society and Scottish Intercollegiate Guidelines Network (SIGN) (2016) *British Guidelines on the Management of Asthma*. Edinburgh and London: BTS & SIGN.

Using the above documents as supporting evidence:

- Outline the main differences between asthma and COPD.
- What lifestyle and/or environmental factors contribute to the onset of asthma/COPD?
- Make a list of the symptoms of asthma and COPD.
- Identify the short- and long-term complications of poorly controlled asthma/COPD.

   Now go to the British Lung Foundation website and review some of the patient video stories (www.blf.org.uk/support-for-you/copd/stories-and-videos). Make a note of the issues faced by people living with COPD.

## Diabetes

In the UK approximately 3.6 million people are living with diabetes (which is an estimated 9% of the population). The Diabetes Prevalence Model (PHE, 2016b) suggests that an estimated 940,000 individuals are unaware that they have the condition. There are two main types: type 1 and type 2 and the risks of developing type 2 diabetes mellitus include being overweight, although family history, ethnicity and age also increase risk. There are almost 4.6 million people with diabetes living in the UK. By 2025 it is estimated that this number will rise to over 5 million (Diabetes UK, 2017).

### ACTIVITY 12.5

Access the following resources:

1. Diabetes UK (2016) *State of the Nation 2016. Time to Take Control of Diabetes*. Separate reports available for England, Wales, Scotland and Northern Ireland. Available at: www.diabetes.org.uk/professionals/position-statements-reports/statistics/state-of-the-nation-2016-time-to-take-control-of-diabetes.
2. SIGN (2010, updated 2017) *Management of Diabetes. A National Clinical Guideline*. Edinburgh: SIGN.

*(Continued)*

(Continued)

Go to the NICE website (www.nice.org.uk) and review the latest guidelines for the diagnosis and management of type 1 and type 2 diabetes.

- Identify the factors that contribute to the onset of type 1 and type 2 diabetes;
- Outline the main symptoms of undiagnosed or poorly controlled diabetes;
- Summarise the main treatment aims and make a list of the short- and long-term complications of type 1 and type 2 diabetes mellitus;
- Review the nutritional guidance published by Diabetes UK and consider how you could use this to provide information, education and support for patients with diabetes. (Diabetes UK (2018) *Evidence Based Nutrition Guidelines for the Prevention and Management of Diabetes.* Available at: https://diabetes-resources-production.s3.eu-west-1.amazonaws.com/resources-s3/2018-03/1373_ Nutrition%20guidelines_0.pdf.)

## Chronic liver disease

Liver disease is now the fourth most common cause of death in the UK in people under the age of 75. Indeed PHE and Rightcare (2017) suggest that the rate of people dying early from liver disease in some parts of England is almost eight times higher than other parts. Over the last ten years there has been a fivefold increase in the development of cirrhosis in 35–55 year olds and deaths from liver disease appear to be rising steadily (National End of Lifecare Intelligence Network, 2012). Liver disease is almost entirely preventable, with the major risk factors – alcohol, obesity, and hepatitis B and C – accounting for up to 90% of cases (PHE and Rightcare, 2017).

### ⎙ ACTIVITY 12.6

Access the following websites and documents to find out more about caring for patients with liver disease:
    British Liver Trust website: www.britishlivertrust.org.uk.
    Royal College of General Practitioners' Liver Disease Toolkit. Available at: www.rcgp.org.uk/liverdisease.
    Royal College of Nursing (2015) *Caring for People with Liver Disease: A Competency Framework for Nursing*, revised edn. Available at: www.rcn.org.uk/professional-development/publications/pub-004983 (last accessed 29 April 2018).
    Go to the NICE website (www.nice.org.uk) and review the latest guidelines for the diagnosis and management of liver disease.

## Chronic kidney disease

Chronic kidney disease (CKD) is a term used to describe abnormal kidney function and/or structure. It is common, frequently unrecognised and often exists together with other conditions (for example, CVD and diabetes). According to Kidney Research UK (2017), it is estimated that there are 60,000 premature deaths each year from CKD, and in the UK 64,000 people are being treated for kidney failure. Furthermore, a National Confidential Enquiry into Patient Outcome and Death (NCEPOD) in 2009 found that only 50% of the patients who died from acute kidney disease had received 'good' care before their deaths.

---

### ACTIVITY 12.7

Access and review the following journal articles:

Roshni, P.R. and Mathew, M. (2016) 'Risk factors associated with chronic kidney disease: an overview', *International Journal of Sciences Review and Research*, 40(2): 255–7.

- Make a list of the risk factors associated with the development of CKD.

Clarke, A.L., Yates, T., Smith, A.C. and Chilcot, J. (2016) 'Patients' perceptions of chronic kidney disease and their association with psychosocial and clinical outcomes: a narrative review', *Clinical Kidney Journal*, 9(3), 494–502.

Outline the associated health burdens and complications of CKD

Go to the NICE website (www.nice.org.uk) and review the latest guidelines for the diagnosis and management of chronic kidney disease.

---

## Chronic musculoskeletal conditions

The term 'musculoskeletal' describes conditions that affect the joints, muscles and bones. Although the prevalence of musculoskeletal (MSK) conditions tends to increase with age, they can affect any age group and account for 40% of all disabilities across the UK. Conditions include those caused by an abnormal inflammatory process (e.g. rheumatoid arthritis and ankylosing spondylitis), general 'wear and tear' (e.g. osteoarthritis), and bone disease (osteoporosis). Fibromyalgia is a common condition characterised by widespread muscle and joint pain and stiffness. According to Arthritis Research UK (2018), there are estimated to be around 8.75 million people over the age of 44 in the UK with osteoarthritis, 9.11 million with back pain and 2.8 million affected by fibromyalgia.

---

### ACTIVITY 12.8

Go to the Arthritis Research UK website and download the following article: Ryan, S., Lillie, K. and Adams, J. (2013) *The Absent Professional*. London: Arthritis UK. Available at: www.arthritisresearchuk.org/health-professionals-and-students/the-absent-health-professional.aspx.

- Make notes on the report's key findings;
- Now think about what adult nurses could do to help.

## Mental health issues

Around one in four people in the UK suffers from mental health problems each year, with many going untreated. Mental illness is estimated to account for almost a quarter of the total burden of disease, yet NHS spending on mental health services has only accounted for 13% of its budget (Parkin and Powell, 2017). Moreover, people living with long-term depression are also at risk of developing co-morbidities (HM Government/Department of Health, 2011).

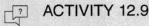 **ACTIVITY 12.9**

Access the following websites to gain a better understanding of how long-term mental health conditions impact on the lives of people and the care they receive:

www.centreformentalhealth.org.uk/a-day-in-the-life

www.centreformentalhealth.org.uk/long-term-conditions

www.centreformentalhealth.org.uk/collaborative-care

www.centreformentalhealth.org.uk/bridging-the-gap

 At this point it would also be worth accessing annexes A and B of the NMC *Proficiency Framework* (NMC, 2018a) and identifying all of the clinical skills required of registered nurses.

- Within a supportive care environment, how could you ensure that you are able to develop your clinical skills to meet the required competencies outlined?

As a registered nurse, it is important that you continue to update your knowledge and understanding, making sure that the care you deliver is based on the best available evidence (2018b: 9). Having undertaken all of the activities in this chapter thus far, you should have a good level of knowledge and understanding of the common LTCs that affect individuals living in the UK, and the lifestyle factors that often contribute to the onset of some of these conditions. This knowledge and understanding will prove crucial when we focus upon the role of the nurse in supporting patients later in this chapter.

## Living with a long-term condition: the patient experience

Most people have to learn to live with rather than die from a chronic illness. Therefore, we need to consider the psychosocial impact that living with an LTC can have on individuals and their families.

 - What percentage of the patients whom you have met have been living with either one or more LTCs?

**ACTIVITY 12.10**

Using the notes you have made when undertaking the previous activities, consider the potential impact that an LTC has on job prospects, lifestyle, and relationships with family or significant others, as well as the physical, psychological and behavioural aspects of life. This is a good opportunity to explore some of these issues with your patients too (although you will need to do this sensitively).

Make a list of as many impact factors you can think of (including those that you identified earlier). Points you might want to consider include the following:

- If your patients/clients were admitted to hospital, what factors led to their admission (e.g. a link to hospital or community care provision)?
- Are there any contributing factors that may have led to other admissions?
- If a patient/client was based in a community setting, what care was required and how often was the intervention undertaken?

Try also to consider how the LTC may have affected either their ability to work or their choice of job if working. Also consider how an LTC can affect lifestyle, hobbies, holidays taken, family and social interaction.

Over the years researchers have sought to describe patients' lived experiences of living with chronic illness (Crumbie and Lawrence, 2002; Barnett, 2005; Salway et al., 2007; Clancy et al., 2009; Lempp et al., 2009; Hopp et al., 2010) and, although many of these studies focus on a specific disease or condition, there are a number of frequently occurring issues and symptoms that appear to be present no matter what the diagnosis or condition may be. Most commonly, these include:

- Symptoms (e.g. tiredness/fatigue, increasing disability, anxiety or depression);
- Perceived loss (e.g. in terms of independence and social activity linked to increasing disability affecting daily activities, occupation, confidence, self-worth/value, intimacy, role within family, control and individuality);
- Feelings (e.g. fear, frustration, blame, denial, and sometimes anger).

## Associated mental health issues

As previously stated, those living with an LTC are two to three times more likely to experience mental ill health such as anxiety and depression than those in the general population. Biessels et al. (2006) report that individuals with CVD and diabetes are also at increased risk of developing mild cognitive impairment, vascular dementia and Alzheimer's disease. Furthermore, the relationship between mental and physical health is a complex one. Prince et al. (2007) have suggested that a combination of environmental, psychological, biological and behavioural factors is involved. A number of studies highlight how depression can exacerbate the distress, pain, sleeplessness and fatigue experienced by many people living with an LTC. Ultimately it appears that those living with two or more LTCs are much more likely to have depression than a healthy person.

Many would argue that this aspect of care is often overlooked, and that patients suffering from chronic medical conditions and co-occurring depression or anxiety are often never diagnosed or treated for their psychiatric conditions (Melek and Norris, 2008). The impact of this can be a reduced quality of life, poorer self-care and adverse health behaviours, as well as poorer health outcomes and overall prognosis (Naylor et al., 2012) (Figure 12.2). Mental health problems can also negatively impact on a person's ability to self-manage their condition (HM Government/DH, 2011). Salway et al. (2007) suggest that positively adapting to chronic illness requires both mental adjustments and the ability to gain control by developing coping strategies, and that patients may need additional support from adult nurses and other external sources in order to positively adapt to their changed health status.

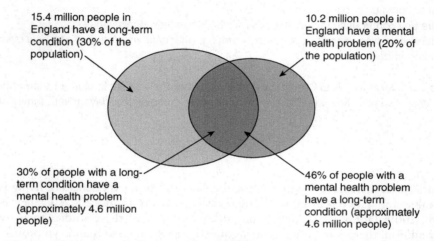

15.4 million people in England have a long-term condition (30% of the population)

10.2 million people in England have a mental health problem (20% of the population)

30% of people with a long-term condition have a mental health problem (approximately 4.6 million people)

46% of people with a mental health problem have a long-term condition (approximately 4.6 million people)

**Figure 12.2**   The overlap between long-term conditions and mental health problems (Naylor et al., 2012)

## Fatigue

Fatigue is commonly experienced by people suffering from a variety of chronic illnesses. The concept of fatigue was initially used in the sixteenth century to describe a tedious duty, although nowadays fatigue is regarded as feeling tired for 'no reason'. Barsevick et al. (2010) have described it as being subjective, a feeling unrelated to being tired after exercise and being relieved after rest. It may be regarded as exhaustive, unpredictable in its course and affecting cognitive ability. Fatigue is often described as multidimensional and disabling, affecting the quality of life of those living with it. Negative emotions such as anxiety, numbness and vulnerability may also be experienced, and are likely to have an impact on social relationships and family life, often leading to withdrawal and social isolation. In a recent qualitative meta-analysis, Whitehead et al. (2016) suggest that many patients feel that others (including healthcare professionals) do not always understand the overwhelming nature of their symptoms. Indeed, Wilson et al. (2006) suggest that gaining an understanding of how each individual conceptualises their own unique experience would be a good starting point for nurses, allowing them to tailor interventions that would best suit their patients rather than merely suggesting strategies for successful living.

## Chronic insomnia

Chronic insomnia is defined as a difficulty initiating and/or maintaining sleep, early waking and sleep that is non-restorative, together with daytime fatigue and poor concentration lasting over six months (Matin and Benca, 2012). Chronic insomnia is often found in individuals suffering from chronic illness (Lempp et al., 2009). However, according to Kay-Stacey (2016) it may be difficult to determine the cause because predisposing conditions, precipitating circumstances and perpetuating factors may be included. Examples include:

- A person who has an anxious personality trait may predispose to sleep problems, resulting in hyperarousal;
- A precipitating event (maybe a decline in health);
- A stressful event;
- Insomnia that is maintained by perpetuating factors, such as having a nap during the day or having an extended lie-in;
- Use of prescribed medications, alcohol or other stimulants (e.g. caffeine);
- Pain.

## Social isolation and loneliness

Loneliness is a complex concept and a variety of definitions exist, although those with poor health report experiencing loneliness more often (ONS, 2018). Loneliness is associated with an increased mortality risk of 26% (Holt-Lunstad et al., 2015). Predisposing factors include partnership status, ethnicity, gender, disability, physical and mental health issues, access to technology, the internet and social media, being a carer and having a limited income that restricts opportunities (ONS, 2018). It appears crucial for nurses to be able to identify those who are lonely, although this may be problematic due to the degree of stigma attached to the concept. There is obviously a need for nurses to facilitate discussion once a rapport has been established with an individual living with a chronic condition. Individuals who have experienced major losses (for example, being widowed or having a chronic health condition) are at risk of loneliness. An early indicator is the difference in everyday activities, although the need to assess for low mood is also important because changes in everyday activities are one indicator of depression.

# Management of long-term conditions

In 2000, the Department of Health established a strategy focusing on a number of chronic diseases through the implementation of a series of National Service Frameworks (NSFs). The various NSFs outline both the actions that need to be taken to reduce the incidence of specific diseases and the treatment and care that should be provided for patients. The NSF for Long Term Conditions (DH, 2005) highlights the importance of a 'person-centred' approach to care provision, and sets out the way in which all healthcare professionals are expected to support patients to live as independently as possible by:

- Giving people choice, through services planned and delivered around their individual needs;
- Coordinating partnership working between health and social services and other local agencies.

Underpinned by a Health and Social Care Framework (DH, 2007) (Figure 12.3), the NSF for LTCs stresses the need for patients to have access to the relevant information necessary to be able to make an informed choice about their treatment.

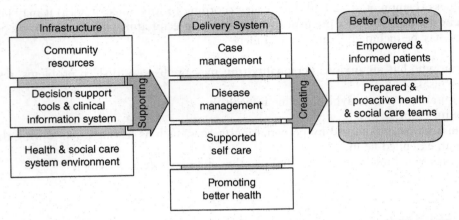

**Figure 12.3**   The NHS and social care long-term conditions model. (*Source:* Department of Health, 2005; © Crown copyright)

## Supported self-care

Around 80–90% of all care for people with LTCs is undertaken by patients themselves and/or their families (Entwistle and Cribb, 2013). Self-care is defined by the Department of Health (2009: 4) as:

> people taking responsibility for their own health and well-being. It includes staying fit and healthy, taking action to prevent illness and accidents, using medicines effectively, treating minor ailments appropriately, and seeking professional help when necessary.

Supported self-care requires a healthcare professional to support patients in making decisions that will help them effectively manage their LTC. The Department of Health (2009) suggests that this involves offering patients timely information and support to empower them to take an active role in maintaining their health. Similarly, the Long Term Conditions Alliance Scotland (LTCAS) defines self-management as:

> the successful outcome of the person and all appropriate individuals and services working together to support him or her to deal with the very real implications of living the rest of their life with one or more long term condition.
>
> (Scottish Government, 2009: 2)

The supported self-care approach requires registered nurses to provide information, care and encouragement for patients in order to help them understand and manage their illness themselves, make informed decisions about their care and engage in healthy behaviours. It also includes working to enhance a patient's capacity for self-management, providing support to ensure that they have more control of their conditions and therefore their life. Evidence suggests that supported self-care can result in beneficial health outcomes for people and more appropriate use of health and social care services (DH, 2009). However, self-management also involves the patient coming to terms with and effectively dealing with the consequences of their condition(s). This requires the patient having the confidence and ability to problem solve and make decisions about their care in partnership with healthcare professionals (we will explore this aspect again later in the chapter). Furthermore, there is no one single approach advocated. Corben and Rosen (2005) argue that individuals often have different ways of coping with an LTC and not everyone will want to be actively involved in managing their own condition, although it is necessary to recognise that a patient's willingness to be involved might also fluctuate over time and depending on the circumstances.

Disease management is defined as a system of coordinated, multidisciplinary healthcare interventions for people with LTCs, the aim of which is to ensure that patients are monitored regularly and defined outcomes/indicators are achieved in order to reduce the risk of health deterioration (Dusheiko et al., 2011). Disease management strategies are targeted at those patients at lower risk of admission to hospital and are usually delivered within a community setting (often by GPs, practice nurses, pharmacists and other healthcare workers). For example, nurses working in general practice will aim to improve the health of individual patients with chronic conditions via monitoring (e.g. checking the blood sugar levels of patients with diabetes, the blood pressure of patients with hypertension) and/or providing lifestyle advice for smokers or obese individuals.

## Case management

Hutt et al. (2004: 1) describe case management (Figure 12.4) as 'the process of planning, co-ordinating and reviewing the care of an individual'. The intended focus is aimed at patients who are the most vulnerable, who have highly complex needs or multiple LTCs (multiple morbidity), and are therefore at greater risk of admission to hospital. A case management approach is used to anticipate and coordinate health and social care, with the aim of reducing hospital admissions and/or length of hospital stay, improving care outcomes for patients and enhancing the patient experience. Ross et al. (2011) suggest that case management involves:

- Case finding;
- Assessment;
- Care planning;
- Care coordination (usually undertaken by a case manager in the context of a multidisciplinary team).

There is some evidence to suggest that ongoing and personalised case management can improve care and reduce inpatient and outpatient costs (Roland et al., 2012).

However, case management is not always implemented in a cost-effective way or for the benefit of patients and carers (Ross et al., 2011; Roland et al., 2012). Furthermore, Purdy (2010) argues that other approaches are more beneficial (e.g. patient self-management, continuity of GP care, and the integration of primary/secondary care and health/social care). In particular, those patients who have more than one LTC, as well as older patients, often face an increasingly fragmented and specialised response. You may well have noticed this yourself, especially in terms of patients you may have come across who have experienced multiple admissions to hospital over the last 12 months.

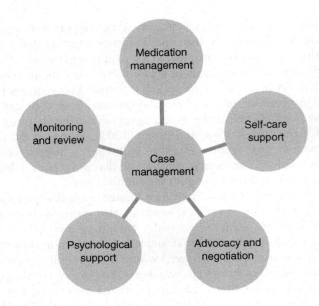

**Figure 12.4**   Case management

Therefore, in contrast to the reactive, disease-focused and clinically driven care of the recent past, integrated care models are now being explored as a means of meeting the challenges of changing disease burdens (Goodwin et al., 2013, 2014). It is proposed that The 'House of Care Model' (Figure 12.5) will help to deliver holistic, patient-centred, preventative and proactive care in England by 'taking as its starting point the active involvement of patients in developing their own care plans through a shared decision-making process with clinicians' (Coulter et al., 2013: 2).

Establishing a collaborative approach with active client/patient involvement is considered crucial. Another key aspect of the model is to ensure that the care planning for individuals and commissioning for local populations are closely linked. The aim is for local services, community resources, social care and healthcare – together with more traditional health services – to work together (Coulter et al., 2013). Furthermore, it is argued that the whole health and social care system should be interdependent.

The aim is for planning, implementation and evaluation of care to be an ongoing process and that the healthcare provider can recognise the personal strengths and the lived experiences of the patient. This requires time, especially for those individuals who may be living with multiple LTCs, for whom longer appointment times are necessary. It is hoped that by using integrated health and social care planning, care is personalised, the patient is an active participant and sufficient support is offered for self-management.

It is also crucial that the health and social care are coordinated and cross team and geographical boundaries, so that care planning moves away from a reactive illness model of care towards a proactive one, which aims to help individuals stay active as long as possible (Foot et al., 2012). The Mandate for NHS England (DH, 2014) and the NHS Constitution (DH, 2013) aim to ensure that everyone who is living with an LTC (either primarily physical or psychological) has their wishes about care respected and an agreed single personalised care plan formulated.

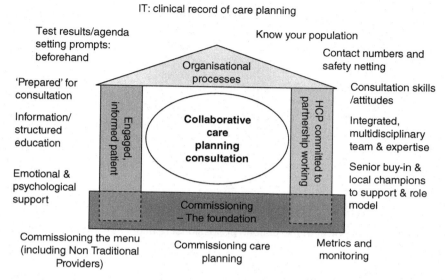

**Figure 12.5**   The 'House of Care Model'

# Patient empowerment and partnership working

People with an LTC are now increasingly working in partnership with health and social care professionals, taking an active role in managing their condition. However, many say that they want to be listened to and be more involved in decisions about their care (McDonald, 2014). They also want access to information to help them make those decisions, and more support in developing the confidence to manage and understand their condition(s), particularly in relation to medications and treatments, and general health advice (DH, 2006; Ipsos MORI, 2011).

Partnership working is a fundamental aspect of the registered nurse's role. Therefore a nurse must be able to develop an inclusive and mutually beneficial relationship with patient/clients and carers in order to improve the quality and experience of care.

In the past a paternalistic/maternalistic relationship (reflecting a medical model of care) often meant that patients were expected to accept a passive role in any healthcare encounter, whereby the doctor/nurse would tell patients what they needed and patients would submissively accept this. Nowadays, however, the power relationship between healthcare professionals and patients should be more equal (Figure 12.6). The concept of patient 'empowerment' has many facets that can differ, depending upon on whether this is applied to a community, organisational or individual context.

However, in this case we refer to it as being suggestive of the nurse handing over or 'giving power' to the patient. It is a process that aims to change the nature and distribution of power in the nurse–patient therapeutic relationship, with the intention of increasing the patient's control over their own health. Patients become active partners in the management of their own condition (e.g. planning care, and deciding on and evaluating treatment options). By acknowledging that the patient is an expert in terms of their own experience and condition, a more equal and facilitative relationship is established.

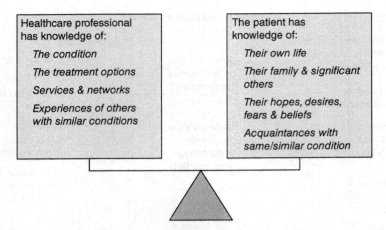

**Figure 12.6**   The balance of power in the patient–professional relationship. (*Source:* Crumbie and Lawrence, 2002)

 Reflecting on the care that you have provided to one of your patients recently, think about what you did and how you did it.

- Was it possible to take every opportunity to empower your patient? If so, how? If not, why not?
- How did this impact on the care provided?

We have established that working in partnership should involve acknowledging and respecting a patient's views, circumstances and preferences for care. Yet research findings suggest that true collaboration or 'power sharing' can be rare and this can act as a barrier to patient participation in care. Examples of 'overt' power and persuasion can still be found (Upton et al., 2011). Barriers to partnership working can include a nurse's (or patient's) lack of confidence or experience, or a perceived lack of time, as well as the attitude of the healthcare professional and/or patient (Millard et al., 2006; Zoffmann and Kirkevold, 2005, 2007; Upton et al., 2011). We also need to ensure that we take account of cultural differences.

## How can we work to empower patients?

Dowling et al. (2011) suggest that in order to be able to empower patients, we ourselves must first feel empowered. We must also be able to communicate effectively and be willing to surrender 'control' to our patients. Conversely, our patients will need to be motivated to change and have the ability to engage in the empowerment process. To make this happen we must see our patients as individuals, make time to listen to their concerns and develop a good understanding of their values and goals. We will also have to ensure that we help them access the information they need in order for them to be able to make appropriate decisions about their care. Perhaps, most importantly, there is a need to regard the person as an individual who is living with a condition but not defined by it.

Zoffmann and Kirkevold (2012) suggest that the use of a guided self-determination (GSD) model can assist healthcare practitioners in helping patients to identify, express and share the unique and unexpected difficulties they face while living with an LTC. Using a life-skills approach, the five-stage process involves:

1. The establishment of an I–you sorted relationship;
2. Self-exploration;
3. Self-understanding;
4. Action;
5. Feedback from action.

Zoffmann and Kirkevold (2012) argue that use of the model has helped nurses establish meaningful therapeutic relationships with their patients, raise awareness of the 'life versus disease conflicts' faced by both patient and nurse, and, in doing so, has helped to overcome many of the barriers to empowerment.

There are a wide range of initiatives aimed at supporting self-care (Figure 12.7), varying from the provision of information and education to developing technical skills, to proactive strategies aimed at changing behaviour and increasing self-efficacy. All of these approaches are important but there is evidence to suggest that adopting proactive strategies is the most effective (De Silva, 2011).

## Providing health information

The NHS Constitution (DH, 2013) sets out a commitment to offer easily accessible, reliable and relevant information to enable people to participate fully in healthcare decisions and support them in making choices. In Chapter 10 we explored the role of the adult nurse in helping patients to make healthy lifestyle choices, particularly in terms of taking adequate exercise, good nutrition and the avoidance of unhealthy behaviours, such as excessive alcohol consumption and smoking. There is also a clear need to ensure that patients can access the information and support needed in order to gain the knowledge and confidence to communicate effectively with healthcare workers. This could include the provision of written or electronic information, videos/DVDs, online courses, patient-held records or care plans, and the use of web-based technologies such as the internet or e-health initiatives. Evidence suggests that self-management behaviours can be facilitated through the exchange of health information and disease experience (Willis, 2013).

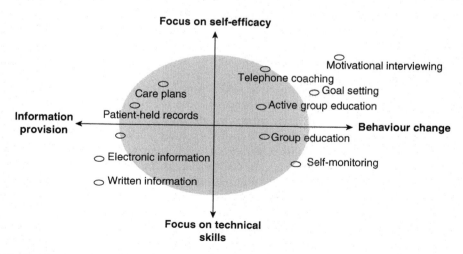

**Figure 12.7** Continuum strategies to support self-management. (De longh et al. (2015), reproduced with permission of the Health Foundation)

## Tools and self-monitoring devices

Tools and self-monitoring devices can help individuals play an integral role in monitoring their LTCs. This can involve the monitoring of physiological measurements (e.g. blood pressure or blood glucose/cholesterol levels) via electronic devices or written self-management plans that help patients to self-medicate and self-refer when appropriate. Moreover the use and impact of tele-healthcare is expanding with evidence of benefits to patients and healthcare professionals (Steel et al., 2011; Zanaboni et al., 2017; Mounessa et al., 2018). The term 'telehealthcare' relates to the real-time monitoring of physiological data (which can include remote professional assistance). Examples include closed circuit TV/video conferencing, the use of email and remote monitoring. Other approaches such as M-health involve the use of mobile apps or personalised systems down-loaded to phones or personal computers, which are used for the personal monitoring of chronic conditions. These systems can communicate with remote call centres, thereby providing data for a professional review.

Make a list of the equipment and tools you have come across that assist your patients to self-care and maintain their independence.

- Do you (and your patients) know how to use these properly?
- Are there any other devices or tools that your patients might be able to access?
- How would they gain access to these?

(Remember that in addition to devices related to health and social care, you should consider the contribution of other aids and adaptations that can be accessed via the voluntary and private sectors.)

The voluntary and community sector also has a key role in terms of providing advice and infor-mation about equipment and tools to help people self-care and maintain their independence. Housing and care services, such as home improvement agencies, will install aids and adapt and repair people's homes to help them live independently (DH, 2009).

## Skills training and support networks

As previously mentioned LTCs appear to affect those with lower socioeconomic status and poorer health literacy disproportionately. Although there is a need for skills training and continuing sup-port to help people engage with healthcare professionals, nurses and other healthcare professionals also need to support the collaborative process and encourage patients into being better-informed active participants. For some individuals referral to a self-help group or a lay-led educational pro-gramme such as the Expert Patient Programme (EPP) may be beneficial. Entwistle and Cribb (2013) suggest that proactive, behaviourally focused, self-management support can have a positive impact on clinical symptoms, attitudes and behaviours, patient quality of life and the use of health-care resources. Self-management programmes such as EPP have been shown to reduce costs and improve health (Sibbald et al., 2010). Reported positive patient outcomes include reductions in depression, anxiety, pain and fatigue, fewer GP visits and increased use of cognitive symptom management techniques, for example goal setting, exercise and relaxation. However, the Mental Health Foundation (2012) has also called for improvements in the access, quality and professional support provided to peer support schemes aimed at addressing the mental health needs of patients with LTCs, an aspect of care that is often overlooked.

What programmes, courses or voluntary groups are available to patients in your area?

- What referral criteria are used?

Consider how you might use this information to help you to support patients with LTCs in your workplace.

## Personalised care planning

Personalised care planning (PCP) is defined by the Department of Health as:

> addressing an individual's full range of needs, taking into account their health, personal, social, economic, educational, mental health, ethnic and cultural background and circumstances. It recognises that there are other issues in addition to medical needs that can affect a person's total health and well-being.

(DH, 2009: 4)

PCP involves helping people with an LTC to identify their desired outcomes and then setting agreed goals, action planning, problem solving, and providing information and access to additional support and treatments where necessary to help them achieve those goals. The process of developing a care plan can help people understand the aims of the care and support they are receiving, as well as any actions they may need to take if their condition worsens (e.g. emergency or crisis planning). The benefits of having a care plan include greater concordance with agreed treatment plans and an increased sense of control for patients.

The PCP journey has three distinct phases:

1. Preparing;
2. Planning;
3. Maintaining.

It is a process that will call on your numerous skills and developing knowledge base.

- What skills do you have that will assist you in supporting patients through this process?
- What new knowledge and skills might you need to access in order to develop and/or review an individual plan?

Developing a personal care plan in partnership with patients and carers will call on all of the skills, attributes, values and behaviours, outlined in previous chapters, that are considered crucial when attempting to build a therapeutic relationship. The process involves discussion, negotiation, shared decision making and review. Care plans (written or otherwise) should include information on the individuals' concerns, their wellbeing needs, actions, goals, information relating to support organisations and any other specific needs they may have.

## MURIEL

Muriel lives with her 76-year-old husband Clive in a ground-floor maisonette in an inner city area. Clive has been living with COPD and type 2 diabetes for over 28 years and had to retire early (at 50) from his job as a joiner due to increased breathlessness and his poorly controlled diabetes. Since that time he has, until recently, enjoyed socialising with his friends, trying to keep his allotment going (he enjoys growing West Indian vegetables and peppers), and has remained the patriarch of his extended family. Muriel has tried to support her husband both physically and emotionally while still taking on some cleaning jobs in the city. Clive admits to being rather stubborn with regard to his dietary control, alcohol intake and occasional cigarette smoking. However, the development of an ulcer on his right leg has led to a prolonged period of physical inactivity, disturbed sleep and increasing social isolation. Clive confides in you that he has been feeling tired, lonely, isolated and depressed, which has resulted in his 'comfort eating'. He is becoming increasingly breathless and tells you that he still occasionally has a secret cigarette in the back garden. His grandchildren visit after school and try to keep him company, but both Muriel and Clive wonder (for different reasons) if he will be able to resume his previous levels of activity. In your role as an adult nurse, you have been asked to provide support for Muriel and Clive.

- How would you assess the bio-psychosocial needs of this family?
- What do you consider to be the main areas of concern?
- What information might Clive and Muriel (and you) need in order to ensure an evidence-based approach to care?
- How could you encourage personalised care planning, working in partnership and self-management?
- Are there any issues connected with Muriel being a carer for Clive as well as working part-time? How may this dual role affect Muriel physically, emotionally and socially?
- Compare your answers by discussing this case scenario with your mentor and/or other colleagues in practice. Is there anything they would do differently?

You will no doubt have identified a number of key issues that need addressing in order to improve Clive's health. However, first and foremost the most important thing to do would be to begin to try to build a therapeutic relationship with Clive and Muriel. To do this, you will need to make time to communicate effectively with them in order to establish their key concerns. Clive exhibits a number of physical illnesses, exacerbating symptoms and unhealthy lifestyle choices. He also reports a deterioration in his mental health and social activity. As nurses, we are often driven by the need to 'make things better' and so there is a temptation to jump right in and begin to plan the care we think is needed to address all of the health issues we have identified. Yet, by listening carefully to Clive and Muriel, you will be able to ascertain their priorities for care. You will then need to consider what valid and reliable assessment tools you might use to assist in this process. For example, how might you assess Clive's sleeping difficulties, fatigue, loneliness and emotional distress?

By assessing and discussing Clive's needs in more depth and providing information about how identified issues could be addressed, you can empower Clive to take an active role in improving his health and any agreed interventions are more likely to be successful. For example:

- Use a holistic approach to assessment to ensure that social and psychological factors are also taken in to account;
- Refer to local/national guidelines and evidence-based care pathways;
- Explore how access to a wider multi-agency team, private or voluntary agencies could help;
- Negotiate and agree a culturally sensitive, person-centred action plan.

Muriel's needs should also be considered. Carers can often feel overlooked and as a nurse you will be responsible for ensuring that she also receives individualised information, advice and support, thereby adopting a family rather than a patient-focused approach.

## The role of carers

A carer as defined by HM Government, is an individual who:

> spends a significant proportion of their life providing unpaid support to family or friends. This could be caring for a relative, partner or friend who is ill, frail, disabled or has mental health or substance misuse problems.

> (HM Government, 2008: 20)

Immediate family members are often seen as a primary resource for managing the impact of long-term ill health across all cultures and groups (Salway et al., 2007), although we should remember that cultural concepts of caring are not universal. In 2011 there were around six million carers across England and Wales (ONS, 2011) and an estimated 788,000 people in Scotland (Scottish Government, 2017). Many of these report a significant negative impact on their own health as a result. According to Carers UK (2017), three in five carers have a long-term health condition themselves, 78% report feeling stressed and many struggle financially having had to give up work to care for family members or friends.

Registered nurses play a vital role in ensuring that the health needs of carers are addressed so that they are able to maintain their own health and wellbeing.

### ACTIVITY 12.11

Access a copy of The Care Act 2014 at: www.legislation.gov.uk/ukpga/2014/23/contents/enacted. What are the responsibilities of local authorities in terms of promoting wellbeing and assessing the needs of individuals and their carers?

- What support services are available to carers in your area (e.g. financial entitlement, respite care/carer breaks and all other forms of support available in the locality)?
- How can you use this knowledge to provide information and support to carers?

# Integrated care

Many patients with an LTC will require support from a range of professionals. As a nurse you will need to be able to work in partnership with other organisations and services (including those in the statutory, voluntary, community and independent sectors) in order to ensure streamlined and integrated care delivery. This may include working across organisational boundaries in the statutory, voluntary, community and independent sectors, demanding effective communication and collaborative multi-agency working skills. Guthrie et al. (2012) argue that current clinical guidelines that focus on single conditions do little to assist healthcare practitioners in supporting people with multiple LTCs and suggest that clinical guidelines are adapted in future to take account of multi-morbidity, emphasising the need to ensure that an individual personalised approach is taken.

Although there is no single definitive model of integrated care, the WHO (2016) provides a useful overview of various models and suggests that, irrespective of the model used, the concept is likely to be shaped by the views and expectations of a number of stakeholders. The expanded chronic care model (Barr et al., 2003) highlights the essential components of care, suggesting that the best outcomes for patients are achieved when these components are integrated, joint professional working is accomplished and a patient-centred approach is adopted – thus moving away from the more traditional 'single disease silo' approach that can sometimes result in duplication or patients 'falling through the gaps' as they attempt to navigate their way through the complex array of health- and social care services, via a series of uncoordinated interactions or patient pathways.

## PATRICK

Patrick, a 79-year-old man, lives with his wife Sadie. They have known each other since childhood and have been together for more than 50 years. Patrick is admitted to hospital after suffering a cerebrovascular accident (CVA). His left side is weakened and he has a catheter *in situ*. He is able to stand and walk for short distances with the aid of a frame. Patrick can understand what is being said to him but he sometimes has difficulty expressing himself as a result of dysphasia caused by the CVA. During his time in hospital he has been diagnosed with type 2 diabetes. Sadie has been recently diagnosed with Parkinson's disease. Patrick is her main carer and they have no children. They live in a house with stairs where the only bathroom and toilet are upstairs. They both want to stay together in their own home.

- What are the overall health and social needs that you would need to consider in order to plan for Patrick's discharge?
- Which other healthcare professionals and organisations would need to be involved?
- How would you reach an agreed plan of care?

The term 'revolving door syndrome' is often used for the readmission of patients to hospital within a few days of their discharge. Although some of these readmissions may be difficult to prevent, often they are a result of poor communication, a fragmented care system or inadequate discharge planning. In 2013 the Royal Voluntary Service (RVS, 2013) found that 150,000 older people had no support on returning home from hospital, and for those who did get some kind of help a fifth didn't receive essential continuing support. Not surprisingly, therefore, 15.3% of those aged over 75 were admitted to hospital again within 28 days of discharge (Health and Social Care Information Centre, 2013).

## Effective discharge planning

Most patients with LTCs will be cared for in a community setting. However, there will be occasions when admission or transfer to and from acute, intermediate or respite care will be required. Individualised discharge planning has been identified as having the potential to reduce a length of stay in hospital and readmission rates (Shepperd et al., 2013). To ensure continuity of care, the Department of Health (2010) has outlined ten key steps involved in the transfer of care process:

1. Start planning for discharge or transfer before or on admission;
2. Identify whether the patient has simple or complex discharge and transfer planning needs, involving the patient and carer in your decision;
3. Develop a clinical management plan for every patient within 24 hours of admission;
4. Coordinate the discharge or transfer of care process through effective leadership and the handover of responsibilities at ward level;
5. Set an expected date of discharge or transfer within 24–48 hours of admission and discuss this with the patient and carer;
6. Review the clinical management plan with the patient each day, take any necessary action, and update progress towards the discharge or transfer date;
7. Involve patients and carers so that they can make informed decisions and choices that will deliver a personalised care pathway and maximise their independence;
8. Plan discharges and transfers to take place over seven days to deliver continuity of care for the patient;
9. Use a discharge checklist 24–48 hours before a transfer;
10. Make decisions to discharge and transfer patients each day.

Planning a patient's discharge or transfer from any care setting is an important part of PCP and will ensure that individuals and their families continue to be supported. As a registered nurse you must be able to liaise effectively with patients, their families and all other agencies involved to achieve a smooth transition of care. Safe and effective discharges/transfers rely on robust decision-making processes and reaching a consensus with patients, families and carers, as well as other members of the multidisciplinary team. Patients with LTCs often have complex needs and as such this process is reliant on therapeutic engagement and a shared philosophy of care where ethical principles are identified as vital to the nursing endeavour, in terms of doing good, avoiding harm, promoting autonomy and affording justice.

## Chapter summary

This chapter has encouraged you to find out more about common LTCs that affect adults across the UK and the evidence-based interventions that aim to help patients manage their conditions. We have explored the impact that many LTCs have on both our patients and their families. We have also examined some of the contemporary approaches aimed at providing help and support to patients, carers and families in our role as registered nurses. The concept of patient-centred, supported self-care, and the importance of integrated care provision in order to deliver good quality effective nursing care have also been highlighted.

## Useful websites

Department of Health: www.gov.uk/government/policies/improving-quality-of-life-for-people-with-long-term-conditions (improving quality of life for people with long term conditions policy page).
Expert Patient Programme: www.nhs.uk/NHSEngland/AboutNHSservices/doctors/Pages/expert-patients-programme.aspx.
Integrated Care and Support Exchange (ICASE): http://lx.iriss.org.uk/content/integrated-care-and-support-exchange-icase (a learning community focused on integrated care and support that helps you to make connections, share information and find answers to key challenges).
National Voices: www.nationalvoices.org.uk/ (a registered charity that stands up for the rights of patients, service users and carers).

## Further reading

Burd, H. and Hallsworth, M. (2016), *Realising the Value, Empowering People: Engaging Communities*. Available at: www.nesta.org.uk/realising-value-programme-reports-tools-and-resources (last accessed 3 May 2018).
Egan, G. (2017) *The Skilled Helper. A Client-centred Approach*. Andover: Cengage Learning EMEA.
Griffin, J. (2010) *The Lonely Society*. London: The Mental Health Foundation. Available at: www.mentalhealth.org.uk/publications/the-lonely-society (last accessed 29 April 2018).
Health Foundation (2014) *Person Centred Care Made Simple*. London: The Health Foundation.
Jopling, K. (2015) *Promising Approaches to Reducing Loneliness and Isolation in Later Life*. London: Age UK. Available at: www.campaigntoendloneoiness.org/wp-content/uploads/promosing-approaches-to-reducing-loneliness-and-isolation-in-later-life.pdf (last accessed 4 April 2018).

## References

Arthritis Research UK (2018) *State of Musculoskeletal Health 2018*. Available at: www.arthritisresearchuk.org/arthritis-information/data-and-statistics/state-of-musculoskeletal-health.aspx (last accessed 29 April 2018).
Asthma UK (2016) *Asthma Facts and Statistics*. Available at: www.asthma.org.uk/about/media/facts-and-statistics (last accessed 29 April 2018).
Bajorek, S., Hind, A. and Bevan, S. (2016) *The Impact of Long Term Conditions on Employment and the Wider UK Economy*. London: The Work Foundation.
Barnett, M. (2005) 'Chronic obstructive pulmonary disease: a phenomenological study of patients' experiences', *Journal of Clinical Nursing*, 14: 805–12.
Barr, V.J., Robinson, S., Marin-Link, B., Underhill, L., Dotts, A., Ravensdale, D. and Salivaras, S. (2003) 'The expanded chronic care model: an integration of concepts and strategies from population health promotion and the chronic care model', *Hospital Quarterly*, 7(1): 73–82.
Barsevick, A.M., Cleelan, C.S., Manning, D.C., O'Mara, A.M., Reeve, B.B., Scott, J.A. and Sloan, J. for AASCPRO (Assessing Symptoms of Cancer Using Patient Reported Outcomes) (2010) 'ASCPRO recommendations for the assessment of fatigue as an outcome in clinical', *Journal of Pain Symptom Management*, 39: 1086–99.

Biessels, G.J., Stackenborg, S., Brunner, E., Brayne, C. and Scheltens, P. (2006) 'Risk of dementia in diabetes mellitus: a systematic review', *Lancet Neurology*, 5(1): 64–7.

British Heart Foundation (2018) *CVD Statistics*. BHF UK Factsheet. Available at: www.bhf.org.uk/research/ heart-statistics/heart-statistics-publications (last accessed 29 April 2018).

Cancer Research UK (2015) *Cancer Statistics for the UK*. Available at: www.cancerresearchuk.org/health-professional/cancer-statistics-for-the-uk (last accessed 29 April 2018).

Carers UK (2017) *State of Caring*. Available at: www.carersuk.org/stateofcaring (last accessed 3 May 2018).

Clancy, K., Hallett, C.E. and Caress, A. (2009) 'The meaning of living with chronic obstructive pulmonary disease', *Journal of Nursing and Healthcare of Chronic Illness*, 1(1): 78–86.

Corben, S. and Rosen, R. (2005) *Self-management for Long-term Conditions: Patients' Perspectives on the Way Ahead*. London: The King's Fund.

Coulter, A., Roberts, S. and Dixson, A. (2013) *Delivering Better Services for People With Long-Term Conditions: Building the House of Care*. London: The King's Fund.

Crumbie, A. and Lawrence, J. (eds) (2002) *Living with a Chronic Condition: A Practitioner's Guide*. London: Elsevier.

de Iongh, A., Fagan, P., Fenner, J. and Kidd, L. (2015) *A Practical Guide to Self-management Support*. London: Health Foundation. Available at: www.health.org.uk/publication/practical-guide-self-management-support.

De Silva, D. (2011) *Helping People Help Themselves*. London: The Health Foundation.

Department of Health (2005) *National Service Framework for Long Term Conditions*. London: DH.

Department of Health (2006) *Our Health, Our Care, Our Say: A New Direction for Community Services*. London: DH.

Department of Health (2007) *The NHS and Social Care Long Term Conditions Model*. Available at: webarchive. nationalarchives.gov.uk/+/.../Healthcare/Longtermconditions/DH_413065(last accessed 3 May 2018).

Department of Health (2009) *Your Health, Your Way: A Guide to Long Term Conditions and Self-care: Information for Healthcare Professionals*. Leeds: DH.

Department of Health (2010) *Ready to Go: Planning the Discharge and the Transfer of Patients from Hospital and Intermediate Care*. Leeds: DH.

Department of Health (2013) *The NHS Constitution*. London: DH.

Department of Health (2014) *The Mandate: A Mandate from the Government to NHS England: April 2014–March 2015*. Available at: www.gov.uk/government/uploads/system/uploads/attachments_data/file/383495/2902896_DoH_Mandate (last accessed 22 February 2015).

Department of Health Northern Ireland (2012) *Living with Long Term Conditions: A Policy Framework*. Belfast: DHNI. Available at: www.health-ni.gov.uk/sites/default/files/publications/dhssps/living-longterm-conditions.pdf (last accessed 19 August 2018).

Diabetes UK (2017) *Diabetes Prevalence 2017*. Available at: www.diabetes.org.uk/professionals/position-statements-reports/statistics/diabetes-prevalence-2017 (last accessed 29 April 2018).

Dowling, M., Murphy, K., Cooney, A. and Casey, D. (2011) 'A concept analysis of empowerment in chronic illness from the perspective of the nurse and the client living with chronic obstructive pulmonary disease', *Journal of Nursing and Healthcare in Chronic Illness*, 3: 476–87.

Dusheiko, M., Gravelle, H., Martin, S., Rice, N. and Smith, P.C. (2011) *Does Better Disease Management in Primary Care Reduce Hospital Costs?* York: University of York, The Centre for Health Economics.

Entwistle, V.A. and Cribb, A. (2013) *Enabling People to Live Well: Fresh Thinking about Collaborative Approaches to Care for People with Long-term Conditions*. London: The Health Foundation.

Ettehad, D., Emdin, C.A., Kiran, A., Anderson, S.G., Callender, T., Emberson, J., Chalmers, J., Rodgers, A. and Rahimi, K. (2016) 'Blood pressure lowering for prevention of cardiovascular disease and death: a systematic review and meta-analysis', *The Lancet*, 387: 957–67.

Foot, C., Goodwin, N. and Sonola, L. (2012) *From Vision to Action: Making Patient-centred Care a Reality*. London: The King's Fund. Available at: www.kingsfund.org.uk/sites/default/files/field/field_publication_file/Richmond-group-from-vision-to-action-april-2012-1.pdf (last accessed 19 August 2018).

Goodwin, N., Sonola, L., Thiel, V. and Kodner, D.L. (2013) *Co-ordinated Care for People with Complex Chronic Conditions: Key Lessons and Markers for Success.* London: The King's Fund.

Goodwin, N., Dixon, A., Anderson, G. and Wodchis, W. (2014) *Providing Integrated Care for Older People with Complex Needs. Lessons from Seven International Case Studies.* London: The King's Fund.

Gray, L. and Leyland, A. (2013) 'Long-term conditions'. In *Scottish Health Survey 2012*, Volume 1, *Main Report.* Edinburgh: Scottish Government Health Directorate.

Guthrie, B., Payne, K., Alderson, P., McMurdo, M.E.T. and Mercer, S.W. (2012) 'Adapting clinical guidelines to take account of multimorbidity', *British Medical Journal*, 345: e6341. doi:10.1136/bmj.e6341.

Health and Social Care Information Centre (2013) *The Quality Outcomes Framework 2012–13.* Available at: https://digital.nhs.uk/data-and-information/data-collections-and-data-sets/data-collections/quality-and-outcomes-framework-qof (last accessed 20 May 2018).

Health Education England (2017) *Facing the Facts, Shaping the Future: A Draft Health and Care Workforce Strategy for England to 2027.* Available at: www.hee.nhs.uk/our-work/workforce-strategy (last accessed 20 August 2018).

HM Government (2008) *Carers at the Heart of 21st-century Families and Communities: 'A Caring System on Your Side. A Life of Your Own'.* London: DH.

HM Government/Department of Health (2011) *No Health Without Mental Health: A Cross Government Mental Health Outcomes Strategy for People of All Ages.* London: DH.

Holt-Lunstad, J., Smith, T.B., Baker, M., Harris, T. and Stephenson, D. ( 2015) 'Loneliness and social isolation as risk factors for mortality: a meta-analytic review', *Perspectives on Psychological Science*, 10(2): 227–37.

Hopp, F.P., Thornton, N. and Martin, L. (2010) 'The lived experience of heart failure at the end of life: a systematic literature review', *Health Society and Work*, 35(2): 109–17.

Hutt, R., Rosen, R. and McCauley, J. (2004) *Case-managing Long-term Conditions: What Impact does it Have in the Treatment of Older People?* London: The King's Fund.

Information Services Division Scotland (2017) *Heart Disease Statistics.* Update: Year ending 31 March 2013. Available at: www.isdscotland.org/Health-Topics/Heart-Disease/Publications/2017-02-21/2017-02-21-Heart-Disease-Report.pdf (last accessed 20 May 2017).

Ipsos MORI (2011) *Long Term Health Conditions 2011: Research Study.* Leeds: Ipsos MORI.

Kay-Stacey, M. (2016) 'Advances in the management of chronic insomnia', *British Medical Journal*, 354: i2123.

Keller, S.E., Schleifer, S.J., Bartiett, J.A., Shiflett, S.C. and Rameshwar, P. (2000) 'Stress, depression, immunity and health'. In K. Goodkin and A.P. Visser (eds), *Psychoneuroimmunology: Stress, Mental Disorders, and Health.* Washington, DC: American Psychiatric Press, pp. 1–25.

Kidney Research UK (2017) *Renal Research. From a Pioneering Past to a Positive Future for Kidney Patients.* London: Kidney Research UK. Available at: www.kidneyresearchuk.org/file/pioneering_past.pdf (last accessed 20 August 2018).

Lempp, K.H., Hatch, S.L., Carville, S.F. and Choy, E.H. (2009) 'Patients' experiences of living with and receiving treatment for fibromyalgia syndrome: a qualitative study', *BMC Musculoskeletal Disorders*, 10(24). doi:10.1186/1471-2474-10-124.

Matin, C. and Benca, R. (2012) 'Chronic insomnia', *The Lancet*, 379: 1129–41.

McDonald, C. (2014) *Patients in Control. Why People with Long Term Conditions Must be Empowered.* London: Institute for Public Policy Research.

Melek, S. and Norris, D. (2008) *Chronic Conditions and Co-morbid Psychological Disorders.* Seattle, WA: Milliman.

Mental Health Foundation (2012) *Developing Peer Support for Long Term Conditions (Final Report).* Edinburgh: Mental Health Foundation.

Millard, L., Hallett, C.E. and Luker, K.A. (2006) 'Nurse–patient interaction and decision-making in care: patient involvement in community nursing', *Journal of Advanced Nursing*, 55(2): 142–50.

Mounessa, J.S., Chapman, J., Braunberger, T., Qin, R., Lipoff, J.B., Dellavalle, R.P. and Dunnick, C.A. (2018) 'A systematic review of satisfaction with teledermatology', *Journal of Telemedicine and Telecare*, 24(4): 263–70.

National Confidential Enquiry into Patient Outcome and Death (NCEPOD) (2009) *Acute Kidney Injury: Adding Insult to Injury*. Available at: www.ncepod.org.uk/2009report1/Downloads/AKI_report.pdf (last accessed 29 April 2018).

National End of Lifecare Intelligence Network (2012) *Deaths from Liver Disease. Implications for End of Life Care in England*. Bristol: National End of Life Care Intelligence Network. Available at: www.endoflifecare-intelligence.org.uk/resources/publications/deaths_from_liver_disease (last accessed 19 August 2018).

National Institute for Health and Care Excellence (2011) *Hypertension: Clinical Management of Primary Hypertension in Adults* [CG127]. Available at: www.nice.org.uk/guidance/cg127/chapter/introduction (last accessed 20 May 2018).

Naylor, C., Parsonage, M., McDaid, D., Knapp, M., Fossey, M. and Galea, A. (2012) *Long-term Conditions and Mental Health: The Cost of Co-morbidities*. London: The King's Fund. Available at: www.kingsfund.org.uk/publications/long-term-conditions-and-mental-health (last accessed 20 May 2018).

Nursing and Midwifery Council (2018a) *Future Nurse: Standards of Proficiency for Registered Nurses*. London: NMC.

Nursing and Midwifery Council (2018b) *The Code*. London: NMC.

Office for National Statistics (2011) *2011 Census: Unpaid Care Snapshot*. London: ONS.

Office for National Statistics (2018) *Loneliness: What Characteristics and Circumstances are Associated with Feeling Lonely?* Available at: www.gov.uk/government/statistics/loneliness-what-characteristics-and-circumstances-are-associated-with-feeling-lonely (last accessed 3 May 2018).

Parkin, E. and Powell, T. (2017) 'Mental health policy in England', Mental Health Briefing Paper, Number CBP 07547, 23 August. Available at: researchbriefings.files.parliament.uk/documents/CBP-7547/CBP-7547.pdf (last accessed 19 August 2018).

Prince, M., Patel, V., Saxena, S., Maj, M., Maselko, J., Philips, M.R. and Rahman, A. (2007) 'No health without mental health', *The Lancet*, 370(9590): 859–77.

Prince, M., Knapp, M., Guerchet, M., McCrone, P., Prina, M., Comas-Herrera, A., Whittenburg, R., Adelaja, B., Hu, B., King, D., Rehill, A. and Salimkumar, D. (2014), *Dementia UK*, 2nd edn. London: Alzheimer's Society.

Public Health England (2016a) *Hypertension Prevalence Estimates in England: Estimated from the Health Survey for England*. London: PHE.

Public Health England (2016b) *Technical Document for Diabetes Prevalence Model for England*. Available at: www.gov.uk/government/uploads/system/uploads/attachment_data/file/612307/Diabetesprevalencemodeltechnicaldocument.pdf (last accessed 4 April 2018).

Public Health England and Rightcare (2017) *The Second Atlas of Variation in Risk Factors and Healthcare for Liver Disease in England*. September 2017. Available at: http://tools.england.nhs.uk/images/LiverAtlas17/atlas.html (last accessed 29 April 2018).

Purdy, S. (2010) *Avoiding Hospital Admissions: What Does the Research Evidence Say?* London: The King's Fund.

Roland, M., Lewis, L., Steventson, A., Abel, G., Adams, J., Bardsley, M., Brerton, L., Chitnis, X., Conklin, A., Staetsky, L., Tunkel, S. and Ling, T. (2012) 'Case management for at-risk elderly patients in the English integrated care pilots: observational study of staff and patient experience and secondary care utilisation', *International Journal of Integrated Care*, 12: e130. Available at: https://zdoc.site/queue/delivering-better-services-for-people-with-long-term-the.kin.html (last accessed 20 May 2018).

Ross, S., Curry, N. and Goodwin, N. (2011) *Case Management: What it is and How it Can Best be Implemented*. London: The King's Fund. Available at: www.kingsfund.org.uk/sites/default/files/Case-Management-paper-The-Kings-Fund-Paper-November-2011_0.pdf (last accessed 20 May 2018).

Royal Voluntary Service (2013) *Avoiding Unhappy Returns: Radical Reductions in Readmissions Achieved with Volunteers*. Cardiff: RVS. Available at: www.royalvoluntaryservice.org.uk/Uploads/Documents/Get%20involved/avoiding_unhappy_returns.pdf (last accessed 20 May 2018).

Salway, S., Platt, L., Chowbey, P., Harriss, K. and Bayliss, E. (2007) *Long Term Ill Health, Poverty and Ethnicity*. York: Joseph Rowntree Foundation.

Scottish Government (2009) *Improving the Health and Wellbeing of People with Long Term Conditions in Scotland*. Available at: www.gov.scot/Resource/Doc/294270/0090939.pdf (last accessed 3 May 2018).

Scottish Government (2017) *Scottish Carers*. Available at: www.gov.scot/Topics/Health/Support-Social-Care/Unpaid-Carers (last accessed 3 May 2018).

Shepperd, S., Lannin, N.A., Clemson, L.M., McCluskey, A., Cameron, I.D. and Barras, S.L. (2013) 'Discharge planning from hospital to home', *Cochrane Database of Systematic Reviews*, 1: CD000313. doi:10.1002/14651858.CD000313.pub4.

Sibbald, B., Rogers, A., Lester, H., Harrison, P., Checkland, K., Sutton, M., Campbell, S. and Roland, M. (2010) *National Primary Care Research and Development Centre Final Report: 2005–2010*. Manchester: National Primary Care Research and Development Centre.

Smittenaar, C.R., Petersen, K.A., Stewart, K. and Moitt, N. (2016) 'Cancer incidence and mortality projections in the UK until 2035', *British Journal of Cancer*, 115: 1147–55.

Snell, T., Wittenberg, R., Fernandez, J.L., Malley, J., Comas-Herrera, A. and King, D. (2011) Discussion paper: 'Future demand for social care, 2010 to 2030: projections of demand for social care and disability benefits for younger adults in England', Report to the Commission on Funding of Care and Support, PSSRU 2800/2. Available at: www.pssru.ac.uk/pub/DP2880-3.pdf (last accessed 20 May 2018).

Steel, K., Cox, D. and Garry, H. (2011) 'Therapeutic videoconferencing interventions for the treatment of long-term conditions', *Journal of Telemedicine and Telecare*, 17: 109–17.

Upton, J., Fletcher, M., Madoc-Sutton, H., Sheikh, A., Caress, A.-L. and Walker, S. (2011) 'Shared decision making or paternalism in nursing consultations? A qualitative study of primary care asthma nurses' views on sharing decisions with patients regarding inhaler device selection', *Health Expectations*, 14(4): 374–82.

Whitehead, L.C., Unahi, K., Burrell, B. and Crowe, M.T. (2016) 'The experience of fatigue across long-term conditions: a qualitative meta-synthesis', *Journal of Pain & Symptom Management*, 52: 131e143.

Willis, E. (2013) 'The making of expert patients: the role of online health communities in arthritis self-management', *Journal of Health Psychology*, 0: 1–13. Available at: www.researchgate.net/publication/256289777_The_Making_of_Expert_Patients_The_Role_of_Online_Health_Communities_in_Arthritis_Self-Management (last accessed 20 May 2018).

Wilson, P.M., Kendall, S. and Brooks, F. (2006) 'Nurses' responses to expert patients: the rhetoric and reality of self-management in long-term conditions: a grounded theory study', *International Journal of Nursing Studies*, 43(7): 803–18.

World Health Organization (2011) *Global Status Report on Non-communicable Disease, 2010*. Geneva: WHO.

World Health Organization (2015) *Chronic Obstructive Pulmonary Disease (COPD)*. Geneva: WHO. Available at: www.who.int/respiratory/copd/en (last accessed 22 February 2015).

World Health Organization (2016) *Integrated Care Models: An Overview*. Copenhagen: WHO.

Zanaboni, Z., Hanne Hoaas, H., Aarøen Lien, L.A., 3rd, Hjalmarsen, A. and Wootton, R. (2017) 'Long-term exercise maintenance in COPD via telerehabilitation: a two-year pilot study', *Journal of Telemedicine and Telecare*, 23(1): 74–82.

Zoffmann, V. and Kirkevold, M. (2005) 'Life versus disease in difficult diabetes care: conflicting perspectives disempower patients and professionals in problem solving', *Qualitative Health Research*, 15: 750–65.

Zoffmann, V. and Kirkevold, M. (2007) 'Relationships and their potential for change developed in difficult type 1 diabetes', *Qualitative Health Research*, 17: 625–38.

Zoffmann, V. and Kirkevold, M. (2012) 'Realizing empowerment in difficult diabetes care: a guided self-determination intervention', *Qualitative Health Research*, 22(1): 103–18.

# CARING FOR THE ACUTELY ILL ADULT

## PAUL TIERNEY AND JULIE GREGORY

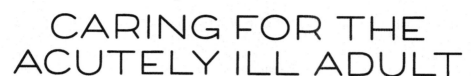

---

### CHAPTER OBJECTIVES

- Define the aims of acute care and identify a variety of settings in which it takes place;
- Identify the knowledge and skills required to work effectively in acute care settings;
- Summarise the components of a comprehensive assessment of an acutely ill adult;
- Explain how to recognise and respond to acutely ill adults using appropriate first aid and evidence-based strategies;
- Define the characteristics of an effective communication strategy when caring for acutely ill adults;
- Highlight the importance of using medical devices safely;
- Explore the use of effective pain assessment and management strategies when caring for patients in pain;
- Consider ways in which a nurse could enhance the patient experience of care within acute settings.

---

## Introduction

All patients, regardless of the setting, have the potential to become acutely unwell. With the general trend of those in hospital being older, sicker and having more complex health issues, the need for skills in recognising and responding to the deteriorating patient are becoming increasingly important. Nurses in all clinical areas, and not just those working in acute care environments, should have the knowledge and skills to recognise and respond competently and confidently to the needs of an acutely ill adult.

Caring for the acutely unwell adult can also be very challenging, not least because it often involves the use of high-tech equipment and monitoring technology which can be a bit worrying to those unfamiliar with such equipment and devices. By exploring the evidence base for the management of acute illness, we will provide you with the underpinning knowledge necessary to be able to provide safe and effective care for such patients. The use of patient scenarios and reflective guidance will also help you consider and acknowledge your own limitations, thereby recognising the need to further develop your skills.

# Related NMC proficiencies for registered nurses

The overarching requirements of the Nursing and Midwifery Council (NMC, 2018) are that all registered nurses should be able to take the lead in providing evidence-based, compassionate and safe nursing interventions. They are required to prioritise the needs of people when assessing and reviewing their mental, physical, cognitive, behavioural, social and spiritual needs. They should use information obtained during assessments to identify the priorities and requirements for person-centred and evidence-based nursing interventions, and are responsible for managing nursing care, being accountable for the appropriate delegation and supervision of care provided by others in the team, including lay carers. They are required to play an active and equal role in the interdisciplinary team, collaborating and communicating effectively with a range of colleagues (NMC, 2018).

 **To achieve entry to the nursing register you must be able to**

- Demonstrate and apply knowledge of all commonly encountered mental, physical, behavioural and cognitive health conditions, medication usage and treatments when undertaking full and accurate assessments of nursing care needs, and when developing, prioritising and reviewing person-centred care plans;
- Demonstrate the ability to manage commonly encountered devices and confidently carry out related nursing procedures to meet people's needs for evidence-based, person-centred care;
- Effectively and responsibly use a range of digital technologies to access, input, share and apply information and data within teams and between agencies;
- Demonstrate the knowledge and skills required to identify and initiate appropriate interventions to support people with commonly encountered symptoms including discomfort and pain;
- Demonstrate the ability to accurately undertake risk assessments in a range of care settings using a range of contemporary assessment and improvement tools;
- Interpret results from routine investigations, taking prompt action when required by implementing appropriate interventions, requesting additional investigations or escalating to others;
- Demonstrate the knowledge and ability to respond proactively and promptly to signs of deterioration or distress in mental, physical, cognitive and behavioural health, and use this knowledge to make sound clinical decisions;
- Demonstrate knowledge of when and how to refer people safely to other professionals or services for clinical intervention or support;
- Demonstrate the ability to coordinate and undertake the processes and procedures involved in routine planning and management of safe discharge home or transfer of people between care settings.

(Adapted from NMC, 2018)

## Background

The term 'acute care' usually refers to care provided when a patient is suffering from an acute episode of a previously undiagnosed problem (e.g. a stroke or appendicitis), an acute exacerbation of a long-term condition (e.g. a diabetic coma or chronic obstructive pulmonary disease [COPD]), or recovering from an accident/trauma or surgery. Acute care environments can be defined as those in which the principal intent is one or more of the following (Organisation for Economic Co-operation and Development [OECD], 2001):

- To cure illness or to provide definitive treatment of injury;
- To perform surgery;
- To relieve symptoms of illness or injury (excluding palliative care);
- To reduce the severity of an illness or injury;
- To protect against the exacerbation and/or complication of an illness and/or injury that could threaten life or normal function;
- To perform diagnostic or therapeutic procedures;
- To manage labour (obstetrics).

The reduction in available hospital beds and an increase in inpatient day-case activity (National Audit Office, 2012) has resulted in greater demands on many acute care services, leading to the introduction of a variety of emergency and urgent care services across the UK, including emergency departments (EDs), minor injury units (MIUs), out-of-hours services, walk-in centres and NHS 111. Accident and Emergency (A&E) departments may now be classified as type 1, 2, 3, 4 or 5 (Table 13.1).

Furthermore, A&E attendances in the UK have continued to rise over the decades. There were approximately 23.4 million A&E attendances in England in 2016–17 (NHS Digital, 2017). This represents a very significant increase of 22% on the figures from 2007 to 2008 (NHS Digital, 2017).

## ACTIVITY 13.1

Access the NHS Digital website (https://digital.nhs.uk) for hospital accident and emergency activity statistics and identify the profile of those who attend A&E (gender and age), and when (most common time of arrival at A&E).

The need to manage acute hospital admissions safely has led to the introduction of medical assessment units (MAUs) and surgical assessment units (SAUs) in some areas, which aim to provide fast-track routes to assessment, diagnosis and subsequent referral to the appropriate specialty.

**Table 13.1**  Accident and emergency department types

| TYPE | DEPARTMENT |
| --- | --- |
| 1 | Emergency departments are a consultant-led 24-hour service with full resuscitation facilities. |
| 2 | Consultant-led mono speciality A&E service (e.g. ophthalmology, dental). |
| 3 | Other type of A&E/minor injury which may be doctor-led or nurse-led treating at least minor injuries and illnesses, and can be routinely accessed without appointment. |
| 4 | NHS walk-in centres. |

*Source:* Health and Social Care Information Centre (2014)

Adult patients are admitted to hospital for a variety of reasons. Admissions can be planned in advance (e.g. for elective surgery or medical investigations/treatment) or may be as a result of an emergency (e.g. accident or injury, acute sudden illness, infectious diseases or an exacerbation of a long-term condition).

Whatever the clinical setting, registered nurses must be able to provide timely, safe and effective care, which includes an ability to recognise the needs of acutely ill patients, the potential for deterioration in their condition and the ability to respond appropriately. It is acknowledged here that you will need to access other specialist literature in order to develop specific knowledge and understanding relating to the care of adults undergoing specific medical treatments and surgical interventions (see 'Further reading' at the end of this chapter). The main focus for this chapter is the systematic assessment and management of an acutely ill patient.

Acute assessment units are often very busy environments and their main aim is to ensure that patients are appropriately assessed to ensure that the right care is provided at the right time by the most appropriate caregiver (e.g. facilitating timely referral to inpatient hospital care within the relevant specialty or on to relevant support teams working in community or primary care settings). As a nurse working in an acute environment you will need to have a good understanding of the altered physiology of illness and the capacity to rapidly observe, assess and monitor patients, interpreting and evaluating your observations and assessments to make sound decisions based on your clinical judgement. Team working and the ability to communicate effectively with patients and their families, as well as other members of the multidisciplinary team, will be crucial in order to help to relieve patient stress and anxiety and to ensure continuity of care.

## Acute medicine

Acute medical emergencies are the most common reason for admission to hospital (Royal College of Physicians, 2007). Acute medicine is now considered a specialism in its own right and many UK hospitals have established acute medical units (AMUs), also known as Medical Assessment Units (MAUs), acute assessment units (AAUs) and early assessment units (EAUs). Scott et al. (2009) suggest that AMUs may reduce inpatient mortality and length of stay, and improve patient and staff satisfaction.

The West Midlands Quality Review Service and the Society for Acute Medicine (2012) recommend that all registered nurses working in such environments should be clinically competent in the following:

Immediate life support (ILS);

Performing an Early Warning Score (EWS) assessment, its interpretation and escalation as appropriate;

Recording an ECG;

Venepuncture;

Intravenous (IV) drug administration;

Urinary catheterisation (male and female);

Aseptic non-touch technique;

Point-of-care testing (e.g. use of small bench analysers for blood glucose, blood gases, coagulation tests);

End of life care;

Handover, transfer and discharge.

However, as outlined in Chapter 2, the NMC (2018) requires adult nurses to be able to demonstrate numerous additional clinical competencies effectively in order to achieve entry to the register.

- Within an acute placement area, what additional skills might you need to the ones outlined above?
- How could you ensure that you are able to develop your clinical skills within an acute area to meet the required NMC (2018) proficiencies?

# Surgery

There have been significant changes in how surgery is performed in a modern healthcare setting. Just like the medical context, patients are older, sicker and have more co-morbidity. There have been considerable modifications to management of wound surgical techniques with advances in the use of technology (robotic surgery), microsurgery and minimally invasive surgical techniques ('keyhole' or laparoscopic surgery). There has also been a significant increase in surgery performed as day cases, after recommendations from the NHS Modernisation Agency (2004) to suggest that day surgery should be considered the norm for elective surgery rather than inpatient surgery. The increased use of day surgery has a number of potential economic benefits, including:

- Shorter hospital stays;
- Release of facilities for more complex and emergency cases;
- Fixed scheduling, reducing cancellations and therefore more efficient theatre use;
- Staff reductions (as overnight staffing is usually not necessary);
- A decrease in both the time taken to perform surgical procedures and their cost, taking advantage of advances in surgical and anaesthetic care;
- Better use of high-cost operating room apparatus and supplies (World Health Organization [WHO], 2007).

The variety of surgical procedures carried out on adults across the UK is vast. However, common surgical procedures include abdominal surgery (e.g. appendicectomy, cholecystectomy, bowel resection), vascular surgery (e.g. varicose vein surgery, aortic repair, insertion of stents), surgical oncology (e.g. resection of tumours), orthopaedic surgery (e.g. joint replacements or fracture repair) and plastic surgery (e.g. skin grafts, surgical repair or reconstruction).

Nursing in a surgical setting involves caring for patients before, during and after surgery, and requires the knowledge and skills outlined above in addition to those in the following list:

- Preoperative, perioperative and postoperative care;
- Anaesthesia;
- Pain management;
- Infection prevention and control (relevant to every setting but particularly important here);
- Wound care, wound healing, dressings and management of wound drains.

Patients undergoing a planned surgical procedure will often be required to present for a 'pre-op' assessment as an outpatient before their admission. Although not all surgery can be planned in

The enhanced recovery pathway

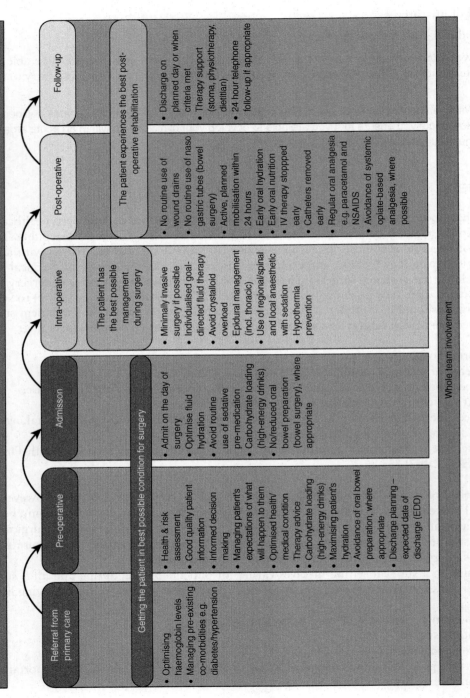

**Figure 13.1** The enhanced recovery pathway (© Crown copyright)

advance in this way, whether a patient is undergoing scheduled or emergency surgery, nurses have a key role in ensuring that patients are not only fully informed about their planned procedure and know what to expect but are also fit enough for surgery (although the time available for preparation will differ). If the opportunity is available, it is also a chance to plan for future discharge arrangements. It has been argued that this approach can help to reduce patient stress, offer an opportunity to provide reassurance and support, and increase the likelihood of an uneventful recovery and a safer, earlier discharge (NHS Institute for Innovation and Improvement, 2008).

'Enhanced recovery' is a relatively new approach that is being promoted in the NHS. It aims to improve the quality of care by helping patients get better sooner after major surgery and reduce the length of stay in hospital (Enhanced Recovery Partnership Programme, 2010). Enhanced recovery addresses issues in preoperative, perioperative and postoperative care. One aim is to ensure that the patient is in the best possible condition for surgery, which encompasses the concept of 'prehabilitation' for surgical patients. Elements of the enhanced recovery pathway can be seen in Figure 13.1 (Enhanced Recovery Partnership Programme, 2010).

Across the NHS, enhanced recovery is being implemented for patients undergoing elective procedures in the four specialties of orthopaedics, colorectal, gynaecological and urological surgery (NHS Improving Quality, 2013). There is a growing body of evidence to support the use of enhanced recovery programmes in patients within these specialties (Aning et al., 2010; Ibrahim et al., 2013; Zhuang et al., 2013; Dwyer et al., 2014).

The Enhanced Recovery Partnership now consider that enhanced recovery should be standard practice for most patients having major surgery, and it has already been implemented in other areas such as emergency surgery and acute medicine (NHS Improving Quality, 2013).

The WHO (2009) advocates the use of the surgical safety checklist in order to promote team work and communication in surgery, with an aim to decrease errors and adverse events.

## Assessing individuals in an acute care setting

Irrespective of the setting where care takes place, it is imperative that as a registered nurse you are able to assess the needs of your patients. This demands an ability to assess and monitor your patient's condition accurately (on admission and continuously thereafter), check vital signs, develop care plans and safely administer oxygen therapy, IV fluids, medications and pain relief as needed.

So far in this book, we have introduced you to some of the systematic frameworks that can assist you in carefully assessing the needs of your patients. Here, we will focus in more depth on the history taking and observation element of assessment.

## Taking a patient history

The assessment of any individual begins by obtaining a clinical history. History taking in the context of the acutely ill individual may need to be briefer and focused. The scope or depth of the history-taking process will need adjusting according to the clinical urgency of the situation. Previously, in Chapter 3 we established that history taking is not just simply a fact-finding mission or compiling a list of questions, but is important in the process of establishing a therapeutic relationship. Recognising the need for patients to feel listened to while also acknowledging the need for focus, there are a number of mnemonics such as 'OLD CARTS', 'PQRST' or 'SOCRATES' that can be used to guide history taking, in order to elicit more specific information from a patient in relation to a complaint such as pain or any other symptom (e.g. dyspnoea, palpitations, nausea).

OLD CARTS (onset, location, duration, character, aggravating/relieving factors, radiation, timing, severity);

PQRST (provoking or relieving factors, quality, radiation, severity, timing);

SOCRATES (site, onset, character, radiation, associations, timing, exacerbating/relieving factors, severity).

Table 13.2 gives an example of some of the questions you may need to consider in taking a history of a patient with chest pain using the 'OLD CARTS' mnemonic.

**Table 13.2** Example of 'OLD CARTS' mnemonic

**Onset**

- What brought this on?
- Did it start suddenly or gradually?

**Location**

- Where exactly is the pain?
- Can you point to where it is?

**Duration**

- How long has it been there?
- Is it constant or intermittent?

**Character**

- What is the pain like? Can you describe it to me?
- Consider offering some examples - sharp, dull, aching, stabbing, burning, heavy. It is important however to avoid 'leading' the patient.

**Aggravating/relieving factors**

- Have you noticed anything that makes it better (e.g. painkillers, other medication such as antacids, positioning)?
- Have you noticed anything that makes it worse (e.g. inspiration, movement, lying down)?

**Radiation**

- Does the pain radiate to any other location? (To the abdomen, arm, jaw etc.?)

**Timing**

- When did it start?
- Is it getting better, worse or staying the same?

**Severity**

- How severe is it?
- Consider using a pain scale (e.g. a 0–10 numeric pain rating).

Other useful questions may ask about associated symptoms, e.g. Do you have any other symptoms with the pain (e.g. dizziness, dyspnoea, nausea)?

Nurses have long been relied on to monitor the condition of patients, thus ensuring the prompt detection of deterioration or delays in recovery. This demands an ability to be able to recognise and interpret subtle and/or significant changes in the normal physiological parameters of the patient by undertaking specific clinical observations (e.g. blood pressure, pulse and respiratory rate, oxygen saturation, temperature and level of consciousness).

1. Do you know how to undertake the following clinical observations correctly?

   - Blood pressure;
   - Pulse rate;
   - Respiratory rate;
   - Oxygen saturation level;
   - Blood glucose level;
   - Temperature;
   - Level of consciousness.

2. Are you aware of the normal parameters for all of the above?

 ACTIVITY 13.2

Many of the clinical observations above can be collated using medical monitoring equipment.
Make a list of all of the medical monitoring equipment available on your placement area.
Are you familiar with the use of all of this equipment?
Can you think of any risks/disadvantages that can be associated with relying on the use of such equipment?
What would you need to do to ensure that this risk was minimised?
Access and read your local trust policy relating to the safe use of medical equipment.
Although we will be exploring some of the frameworks used for detecting patient deterioration later in this chapter, Elliott and Coventry (2012) provide a useful overview of patient monitoring, highlighting the importance of being able to measure and interpret eight vital signs accurately. You may find it useful to access some of the 'Further reading' at the end of this chapter to ensure that you can carry out required clinical observations in the correct manner.

In an emergency setting (e.g. A&E or an ED) the Manchester Triage System (Mackway-Jones et al., 2013) is commonly used across the UK and Europe (Table 13.3). Patients are prioritised into one of five categories (immediate, very urgent, urgent, standard, non-urgent). The assessing nurse uses one of a number of flowcharts based on the patient's symptoms and 'discriminators'. Those patients who fall into the immediate category need instant treatment; very urgent should be treated within 10 minutes, urgent within one hour, standard within two hours and non-urgent within four hours.

**Table 13.3** Manchester triage system

| 1 | Immediate | Red | 0 |
|---|---|---|---|
| 2 | Very urgent | Orange | Within 10 minutes |
| 3 | Urgent | Yellow | Within 1 hour |
| 4 | Standard | Green | Within 2 hours |
| 5 | Non-urgent | Blue | Within 4 hours |

## Recognising patient deterioration

Admission to hospital can be a disruptive and worrying time for patients and their families. Once in hospital patients ought to feel that they are safe and that they will receive optimum care throughout their stay. However, when suffering from acute illness patients may be unstable and at risk of deterioration due to their altered physiological state. They will often manifest abnormal vital signs, indicating cardiovascular, respiratory or neurological deficits. Unfortunately however, there is evidence to suggest that these can go unrecognised by staff, resulting in late treatment, unnecessary admission to critical and intensive care units, and sometimes even death (DH, 2009). Results from the UK National Cardiac Arrest Audit report the incidence of adult cardiac arrest at 1.6 per 1000 hospital admissions (Nolan et al., 2014). Although a significant number of these events occurred in areas such as coronary care units (CCUs) and intensive care units (ICUs), over half of cardiac arrests occurred on general wards (Nolan et al., 2014). It is for this reason that all staff, not just those working in acute areas, need to be able to recognise a patient's deterioration and respond quickly and effectively.

In recognition of growing concerns about suboptimal standards of care within the hospital environment, several clinical guidelines have been published that aim to support healthcare professionals in the assessment and subsequent management of severely ill patients. However, despite regular evidence-based guidelines on resuscitation being produced by the Resuscitation Council UK, and significant amounts of time and money being spent on staff training and equipment, survival rates for cardiac arrest remain low. The National Cardiac Arrest Audit (2017) reported an overall survival rate to discharge of 20.4%. Although undoubtedly there have been significant advances in resuscitation knowledge and practice over the decades, it is not surprising, given the low survival rates, that attention has switched to focusing more on the prevention of cardiac arrest.

Regardless of the setting, nurses need to be aware of the contents of the resuscitation trolley and how to use them:

- How well prepared are you to look after a deteriorating patient?
- Do you know about the contents of the resuscitation trolley?
- Would you know how to safely use each piece of equipment?
- What checks are in place to ensure that this equipment is safe to use?

## Track-and-trigger systems

Most patients who have a serious adverse event, such as an unplanned ICU admission, cardiac arrest or even death, show signs of clinical deterioration in the preceding hours (Schein et al., 1990; Buist et al., 2004). A report from the National Confidential Enquiry into Patient Outcome and Death (NCEPOD) focusing on patients referred to ICUs identified that ward-based recognition of acute illness and its subsequent management was suboptimal (NCEPOD, 2005). The NCEPOD (2005) report considered that 21% of ICU admissions were avoidable and that suboptimal care may have been sufficiently significant to have contributed to 33% of deaths.

Subsequently, the National Institute for Health and Clinical Excellence (NICE) produced the guideline *Acutely Ill Patients in Hospital* (NICE, 2007), addressing the recognition of and response to acute illness in adults in hospital. Similarly, the Scottish Intercollegiate Guidelines Network (SIGN) have also produced the *Care of Deteriorating Patients* guideline (SIGN, 2014). A key priority identified within the NICE (2007: 7) guideline is that 'staff caring for patients in acute hospital settings should have competencies in monitoring, measurement, interpretation and prompt response to the acutely ill patient appropriate to the level of care they are providing'.

NICE (2007) also recommended that physiological track-and-trigger systems should be used to monitor all adult patients in acute hospital settings, suggesting that physiological observations should be monitored at least every 12 hours. Track-and-trigger systems monitor clinical observations ('track') and, if predetermined criteria are met, a clinical response is activated ('trigger'). Track-and-trigger systems allow for monitoring of patients for signs of clinical deterioration, which are frequently similar, regardless of the cause. NICE (2007) identified six physiological parameters to be included in a track-and-trigger system:

1. Respiratory rate;
2. Oxygen saturations;
3. Temperature;
4. Systolic blood pressure;
5. Heart rate;
6. Level of consciousness (AVPU).

A number of track-and-trigger systems exist, but the Royal College of Physicians (2012) proposed a 'National Early Warning Score' (NEWS), which would standardise the assessment of the severity of acute illness in the NHS (Table 13.4). NEWS was not designed to replace some other scoring systems such as the Glasgow Coma Scale (Teasdale and Jennett, 1974), but rather to be used in conjunction with them. This system was updated in late 2017 as NEWS2 (RCP, 2017). The six essential parameters identified by NICE (2007), in addition to an additional score for patients requiring oxygen, are included in NEWS2. Deviations from normal parameters earn a score as outlined in Table 13.4. This provides a total NEWS score.

In addition to the scoring system, the Royal College of Physicians (2017) provide an outline of responses to elevated NEWS2 scores and suggested frequency of monitoring (Table 13.5). The use of NEWS2 can support clinical decision making. It is important to remember that a normal NEWS2 score does not preclude calling for help when you consider that a patient is unwell. NEWS2 does not replace clinical judgement. This graded response strategy provides an escalation in response, with higher NEWS2 scores for those identified as being at risk of clinical deterioration.

**Table 13.4** NEWS2 Score Royal College of Physicians (2017)

| Physiological parameter | Score | | | | | | |
|---|---|---|---|---|---|---|---|
| | 3 | 2 | 1 | 0 | 1 | 2 | 3 |
| Respiration rate (per minute) | ≤8 | | 9–11 | 12–20 | | 21–24 | ≥25 |
| SpO$_2$ Scale 1 (%) | ≤91 | 92–93 | 94–95 | ≥96 | | | |
| SpO$_2$ Scale 2 (%) | ≤83 | 84–85 | 86–87 | 88–92 ≥93 on air | 93–94 on oxygen | 95–96 on oxygen | ≥97 on oxygen |
| Air or oxygen? | | Oxygen | | Air | | | |
| Systolic blood pressure (mmHg) | ≤90 | 91–100 | 101–110 | 111–219 | | | ≥220 |
| Pulse (per minute) | ≤40 | | 41–50 | 51–90 | 91–110 | 111–130 | ≥131 |
| Consciousness | | | | Alert | | | CVPU |
| Temperature (°C) | ≤35.0 | | 35.1–36.0 | 36.1–38.0 | 38.1–39.0 | ≥39.1 | |

(Reproduced from Royal College of Physicians. *National Early Warning Score (NEWS) 2:* Standardising the assessment of acute illness severity in the NHS. Updated report of a working party. London: RCP, 2017. Available at: www.rcplondon.ac.uk/projects/outputs/national-early-warning-score-news-2. Please see the full-colour versions of the NEWS charts before making any clinical use of the information)

**Table 13.5** Clinical response to the NEWS2 trigger thresholds

| NEW score | Frequency of monitoring | Clinical response |
|---|---|---|
| 0 | Minimum 12 hourly | • Continue routine NEWS monitoring |
| Total 1–4 | Minimum 4–6 hourly | • Inform registered nurse, who must assess the patient<br>• Registered nurse decides whether increased frequency of monitoring and/or escalation of care is required |
| 3 in single parameter | Minimum 1 hourly | • Registered nurse to inform medical team caring for the patient, who will review and decide whether escalation of care is necessary |
| Total 5 or more Urgent response threshold | Minimum 1 hourly | • Registered nurse to immediately inform the medical team caring for the patient<br>• Registered nurse to request urgent assessment by a clinician or team with core competencies in the care of acutely ill patients<br>• Provide clinical care in an environment with monitoring facilities |
| Total 7 or more Emergency response threshold | Continuous monitoring of vital signs | • Registered nurse to immediately inform the medical team caring for the patient – this should be at least at specialist registrar level<br>• Emergency assessment by a team with critical care competencies, including practitioner(s) with advanced airway management skills<br>• Consider transfer of care to a level 2 or 3 clinical care facility, i.e. higher-dependency unit or ICU<br>• Clinical care in an environment with monitoring facilities |

## ACTIVITY 13.3

The Royal College of Physicians, together with the Royal College of Nursing and the National Outreach Forum, have developed an online training programme in use of the National Early Warning Score 2 (NEWS2):

- Access and complete the short training course at the following website: https://tfinews.ocbmedia. com.
- Calculate the NEWS scores on the following patients and write down what action you think should be taken.

## MARIANA AND RASHID

Mariana is a 60-year-old woman who is recovering after a minor operation to remove a skin lesion. Her postop observations are:

- (A+B) Respiratory rate: 17 breaths/min;
- (A+B) Oxygen saturation: 97%;
- (C) Blood pressure: 172/84;
- (C) Heart rate: 74 beats/min;
- (D) Level of consciousness: alert ('A' on the ACVPU scale);
- (E) Temperature 36.2°C.

Her dressing is intact and there are no signs of discharge or bleeding from her wound.

Rashid is a 62-year-old man admitted with heart failure. He is complaining of feeling tired and short of breath, and has been commenced on supplementary oxygen 2 litres via nasal cannula, with target saturations of 94–98%. He appears drowsy. His current observations are:

- (A+B) Respiratory rate: 22 breaths/min;
- (A+B) Oxygen saturation: 96% on supplemental oxygen;
- (C) Blood pressure: 96/40;
- (C) Heart rate: 104 beats/min;
- (D) Level of consciousness: responding to voice ('V' on the ACVPU scale);
- (E) Temperature 37.4°C.

Mariana has a NEWS2 total score of 0. The outline clinical response suggested by the Royal College of Physicians (2017) would be to continue routine NEWS monitoring. Although it is worth noting that Mariana has a raised blood pressure, the Royal College of Physicians acknowledges that this is a risk factor for cardiovascular disease, but that a low or falling blood pressure is of more significance in recognising a deteriorating patient.

On the other hand, Rashid has a NEWS2 total score of 10. The urgent or emergency response suggested by the Royal College of Physicians (2017) is outlined in Table 13.5. Although each individual component of Rashid's NEWS2 may not be considered at the extreme, when his condition is considered in its entirety it is evident that he is at considerable risk of clinical deterioration.

- What do you think are the limitations of the track-and-trigger system outlined above?
- What underpinning knowledge and understanding would you need to be able to interpret the above scores effectively?

Although track-and-trigger systems such as NEWS and NEWS2 have been widely introduced across the UK, problems in identifying deteriorating patients still exist. Some studies have found that the application of early warning systems varies between organisations, highlighting issues in incomplete or inaccurate recording of required data, an inability to recognise data trends and the timeliness of communication (Donohue and Endacott, 2010; Massey et al., 2010). Coulter-Smith et al. (2013) also argue that systems such as these tend to focus on the core physiological indicators of severity and that these should be used together with sound clinical judgement based on experience, rather than be seen as a replacement. Therefore, the importance of robust clinical assessment and critical reasoning outlined in Chapter 7 (clinical decision making) should not be overlooked.

## Assessment of the acutely ill or deteriorating patient using the ABCDE approach

Adult nurses need to be able to perform a comprehensive assessment to identify patient deterioration. The Airway, Breathing, Circulation, Disability, Exposure (ABCDE) approach to the assessment of the acutely ill patient is widely advocated (Resuscitation Council UK, 2011; Frost and Wise, 2012).

Thim et al. (2012) suggest that high-quality ABCDE assessment skills among all treating team members can save valuable time and improve team performance. This approach allows for a structured assessment of the patient. The ABCDE approach is beneficial in that it can be used in a variety of settings, for example as a first aid response in non-clinical settings, in the community, pre-hospital and in-hospital when responding to clinical situations (acute medical and surgical emergencies) with adults and children (Thim et al., 2012). The approach therefore forms the basis of current resuscitation guidelines (Brunker, 2010).

### ABCDE principles

The Resuscitation Council UK (2015) details some underlying principles to the ABCDE approach as follows:

1. Use the Airway, Breathing, Circulation, Disability, Exposure approach to assess and treat the patient;
2. Do a complete initial assessment and reassess regularly;
3. Treat life-threatening problems before moving to the next part of the assessment;
4. Assess the effects of treatment;

5. Recognise that you will need extra help. Call for appropriate help early;
6. Use all members of the team. This enables interventions, e.g. assessment, attaching monitors, intravenous access, to be undertaken simultaneously;
7. Communicate effectively. Use an SBAR (Situation, Background, Assessment, Recommendation) or RSVP (Reason, Story, Vital signs, Plan) approach;
8. The aim of initial treatment is to keep the patient alive, and achieve some clinical improvement. This will buy time for further treatment and making a diagnosis;
9. Stay calm. Remember that it can take a few minutes for treatments to work;
10. The ABCDE approach can be used irrespective of your training and experience in clinical assessment or treatment. The detail of your assessment and what treatments you give will depend on your clinical knowledge and skills. If you recognise a problem or are unsure call for help.

## Airway

Walz et al. (2007) recognise that the skill of airway management is important for any healthcare provider caring for acutely and critically ill patients. A patient with a compromised airway will quickly deteriorate (Higginson et al., 2011). Problems with decreased levels of consciousness (assessed as part of Disability) can lead to airway compromise. Sandberg et al. (2013: 20) suggest that 'the awake, alert patient who is able to speak with a normal voice has no immediate threat to the airway'.

Airway obstruction may be partial or complete. With a complete obstruction, a paradoxical respiration pattern may be evident where the chest moves in on inspiration and out on expiration. In the event of airway obstruction Resuscitation Council UK (2015) guidelines for the management of choking may need to be followed:

- Listen for additional noises from the airway such as stridor, snoring or gurgling. Stridor is a high-pitched sound, which usually occurs on inspiration, and is caused by laryngeal or tracheal obstruction (Moore, 2007). Gurgling may indicate fluids in the airway such as blood, vomit or secretions.
- Look in the mouth for any potential cause of obstruction such as food, blood, vomit or loose dentures.
- Foreign objects should be removed where possible. The use of Magill forceps can aid in removing foreign objects from the upper airway, although it is extremely important to ensure that great care is taken to avoid worsening the situation by making the obstruction even more difficult to remove.
- Suctioning can be used to remove any vomit, blood or secretions from the airway. If the patient has vomited or is at risk of vomiting, you should consider putting them into the recovery position (Frost and Wise, 2012).
- Look for any swelling of the lips or tongue, which may be a sign of anaphylaxis. You can assess the ability to cough to clear secretions.

Any significant problems with a patient's airway should be treated before moving on to a Breathing assessment. The management of a compromised airway may include:

- The use of airway manoeuvres such as head tilt/chin lift or jaw thrust;
- The use of airway adjuncts such as oropharyngeal or nasopharyngeal airways;
- Management of choking to appropriate guidelines (back slaps/abdominal thrusts);
- Use of suctioning.

# Breathing

Moore (2007) states that it is essential that nurses can recognise and assess symptoms of respiratory dysfunction to provide early, effective and appropriate interventions. Despite being a sensitive indicator of the deteriorating patient, Ansell et al. (2014) report that nurses admit circumstances in which they miss observing respiratory rate. Taking and recording a patient's respiratory rate is essential for assessing a patient's condition (Ansell et al., 2014), although the respiratory rate should be counted for a full minute rather than trying to estimate. In addition to the respiratory rate, the depth (shallow, normal or deep) and pattern of breathing (e.g. Cheyne–Stokes or Kussmaul's) should be observed:

- Look at the effort of breathing: check for the use of accessory muscles such as the sternocleidomastoid and scalene muscles (which help to raise the sternum and first and second ribs) during inspiration and contraction of abdominal muscles during expiration;
- Look for 'pursed-lip' breathing on expiration and nasal flaring. The patient may be positioned upright to aid chest expansion.
- Normal breathing is usually quiet. Listen for additional breathing noises such as wheeze. Olson (2014) warns that if airflow rates are too low a wheeze may not be audible;
- Assess the patient's ability to speak in complete sentences. Can they answer your questions easily and fully while breathing normally? Observe for signs of cyanosis.

Cyanosis is generally a relatively late finding in the ill patient (McMullen and Patrick, 2013). Moore (2007) notes that central cyanosis usually indicates circulatory or ventilatory problems whereas peripheral cyanosis usually indicates poor circulation. Pulse oximetry is now widely available, and the oxygen saturations should be recorded. '$SpO_2$' refers to the peripheral oxygen saturation (pulse oximetry) whereas '$SaO_2$' refers to the arterial oxygen saturation (obtained from an arterial blood gas [ABG] sample).

Oxygen therapy is a vital element in the care of an acutely ill adult. Oxygen is widely used in the treatment of a variety of conditions and it is vital that nurses are safe, knowledgeable and competent in its use. It is a drug and should be prescribed for an individual patient depending on their condition. It is also important to acknowledge that oxygen is a treatment for hypoxaemia and not breathlessness (British Thoracic Society, 2017). The patient requires a specific dose (concentration). Both an inadequate or excessive oxygen dose may be potentially harmful. However, the amount required varies from patient to patient and indeed within the same patient as their condition changes. The British Thoracic Society (2017) produced guidelines for the emergency use of oxygen in adult patients. One essential element of the guidelines is that oxygen be prescribed according to the target saturation range (e.g. a target saturation range of 94–98% for most acutely ill patients and 88–92% for those at risk of hypercapnic respiratory failure). It is important to remember that in an emergency situation oxygen can be given immediately and documented later (National Patient Safety Agency, 2009; British Thoracic Society, 2017). Those administering oxygen need to monitor the patient and aim to keep saturations within range by adjusting the oxygen delivery devices or flow rates. Monitoring of saturations and respiratory function after the administration of supplemental oxygen is essential.

The nurse administering oxygen needs to consider the following:

- Am I aware of the patient's diagnosis and target saturation?
- Does the flow rate need adjusting to achieve that patient's target saturation?

- Am I familiar with the equipment to do this and have I checked this is in working order (e.g. a facemask/nasal cannulae)?
- Have I recorded the oximetry results (saturation levels)?
- Is the tube connected to the right outlet, i.e. oxygen not air?
- When using cylinders:
  - Have I checked the amount of oxygen in the cylinder before using it?
  - Have I calculated how long the oxygen in the cylinder will last?
  - Do I make sure empty or near-empty cylinders are replaced immediately?

(Adapted from the National Patient Safety Agency, 2009)

There are a number of devices available for the delivery of oxygen including nasal cannula, a simple oxygen mask and a high-concentration reservoir mask (a non-rebreathe mask). It is important to acknowledge that the concentration of oxygen that the patient receives depends not only on the flow rate but also on the type of mask and the patient's breathing pattern.

## Circulation

An assessment of circulation may start with the fundamental pulse and blood pressure check. Although a heart rate may be available from a monitor, a manual pulse check is vital because you can get more information from it such as the character of the pulse and the rhythm:

- Is the pulse fast and weak, which may indicate hypovolaemia?
- Is the pulse regular or irregular?
- Skin temperature can also be assessed while checking the pulse: is the patient cool and clammy or warm to the touch?

Measure the blood pressure. It is advisable to check an abnormal blood pressure reading obtained from a machine with a manual check.

### ACTIVITY 13.4

Access and review the MHRA (2013) top ten tips for measuring blood pressure at www.gov.uk/government/publications/top-10-tips-for-measuring-blood-pressure-poster

The capillary refill time (CRT) should also be assessed. A prolonged CRT may indicate reduced skin perfusion, which may indicate poor circulation. However, Lewin and Maconochie (2008) warn that, although the CRT is a quick and easy bedside test, results cannot be interpreted with any degree of confidence in the adult population and should not be used in isolation.

If a patient has undergone surgical intervention, wound dressings and drains should be checked regularly and observed for sources of blood loss.

IV access is important, particularly if a patient is at risk of hypovolaemia or in need of fluid resuscitation, so it may be necessary to prepare for IV cannulation. The National Institute for Health and Care Excellence (NICE, 2013b) has produced guidelines for IV fluid therapy for adults in hospital. The guidelines suggest that a patient's fluid and electrolyte requirements are identified using the 5Rs: resuscitation, routine maintenance, replacement, redistribution and reassessment. Although many of these guidelines are aimed at prescribers, it is important to acknowledge that managing hydration is a fundamental nursing role (Ugboma and Cowen, 2012). Indicators that a patient may need urgent fluid resuscitation include the following:

- Systolic blood pressure <100 mmHg;
- Heart rate >90 beats/minute;
- CRT >2 seconds or peripheries are cold to the touch;
- Respiratory rate >20 breaths/minute;
- NEWS ≥5;
- Passive leg raising suggests fluid responsiveness (NICE, 2013a).

Urinary output and fluid balance should also be monitored carefully. A decreased urinary output can be a sign of decreased renal perfusion. The NICE (2013a) recognise a urinary output of less than 0.5ml/kg per h as a clinical characteristic of acute kidney injury. IV therapy is a common intervention that does not always get the attention it deserves, and takes place in nearly every healthcare setting (Scales, 2008, 2014). Although very commonplace, it is easy to become complacent, but a NCEPOD (1999) report identified that up to one in five patients receiving IV fluids in hospital could experience complications or morbidity as a result of their inappropriate use.

In an acutely unwell adult, a 12-lead ECG should also be considered. This is not restricted only to those with a suspected cardiac problem, because a 12-lead ECG can help identify other clinical problems such as an electrolyte imbalance (e.g. hypo-/hyperkalaemia).

## Disability

Assess the level of consciousness. This can be done using the AVPU scale or the Glasgow Coma Scale (GCS). Level of consciousness is the earliest and most sensitive indicator of neurological deterioration (Peate, 2013).

### APVU scale

- Alert;
- Responds to verbal stimuli;
- Responds to painful stimuli;
- Unresponsive to all stimuli (Resuscitation Council UK, 2015).

### Glasgow Coma Scale

The GCS should be completed (Table 13.6). The best possible score is 15 out of 15 and the worst 3 out of 15. When documenting the GCS it is important to record not only the total score (i.e. a GCS of 13/15) but also the components of that score (e.g. a GCS of 13/15, i.e. eyes 3, verbal 4, motor 6).

### Stroke

The 'Act FAST' TV campaign in England from Public Health England (PHE, 2014) aims to improve public awareness of the signs of stroke and the need to call emergency services at the onset

**Table 13.6**  The Glasgow Coma Scale

| Score | Eye opening (E) | Best verbal response (V) | Best motor response (M) |
|-------|-----------------|--------------------------|-------------------------|
| 6 |  |  | Obeys commands |
| 5 |  | Orientated to time and place | Localises to pain |
| 4 | Eyes open spontaneously | Confused | Withdrawal from pain |
| 3 | Eyes open to speech | Inappropriate words | Flexion to pain |
| 2 | Eyes open to pain | Incomprehensible sounds | Extension to pain |
| 1 | No eye opening | No verbal response | No motor response |

(*Source:* Teasdale, G. and Jennett, B. (1974) 'Assessment of coma and impaired consciousness: a practical scale', *The Lancet*, 304(7872): 81–4)

of a suspected stroke (Dombrowski et al., 2013). Although the Act FAST campaign seeks to raise public awareness, this simple acronym can be used by a nurse as an aid in recognising some of the common signs of a stroke or transient ischaemic attack (TIA). A stroke is a medical emergency that necessitates immediate attention. It is important to recognise the terrible effects of a stroke and the potential consequences of a delayed response (Kavanagh et al., 2011):

- Facial weakness:

  Can the person smile? Has their face fallen on one side?

- Arm weakness:

  Can the person raise both arms and keep them there?

- Speech problems:

  Can the person speak clearly and understand what you say? Is their speech slurred?

- Time to call 999.

(PHE, 2012)

Examine the pupils. What size are they? Are they equal? Do they react appropriately to light? You should be aware that some drugs can affect pupil size.

- What other conditions might cause a patient to lose consciousness? What other tests or assessment might be useful?

## Check the blood glucose level

The National Diabetes Inpatient Audit for 2016 identified that approximately one in five patients with diabetes reported having one or more hypoglycaemic episodes in the previous seven days (National Diabetes Inpatient Audit, 2017). The audit also identified that early morning (5am–9am) was the most common time for a severe 'hypo' to occur. Diabetes UK advocates the 'make four the floor' rule, signifying a blood glucose reading of 4.0 mmol/L as the lowest acceptable level in people with diabetes. The Joint British Diabetes Societies for Inpatient Care guidelines outlines treatment strategies for the hospital management of hypoglycaemia in adults with diabetes mellitus (Walden et al., 2013).

Review the drug chart to assess for any medications that may have caused an altered level of consciousness. It may be necessary to nurse the patient in the recovery position.

## Exposure

This is a head-to-toe check for anything not already discovered on the ABCD check that may suggest a cause for the patient being unwell:

- Check for any rashes, bruising, bleeding or swelling while ensuring maintenance of the patient's dignity;
- Check temperature;
- Assess if the patient is in any pain.

You should now have some appreciation of how unwell the patient is. Remember, from the principles outlined above that it is important to reassess regularly.

## Evidence-based interventions in acute care

### JIM

Jim is 56-year-old man who has had a bowel resection to remove a tumour. The surgery was uneventful, and the surgeons are confident that the entire tumour has been removed in time, that it has not spread and therefore that this is a curative operation. He has a urinary catheter, one peripheral cannula in his left forearm and a central line. You are the nurse who is looking after him that evening. You have just been given handover. On your initial assessment you find that:

A: he is talking to you.

B: he has a slightly elevated respiratory rate (18) and is receiving 4 L/min of oxygen via nasal specs: his oxygen saturations are 95%.

C: his pulse rate is 92, and manual blood pressure is 135/60; he has no central line monitoring.

D: he is coherent and pain free.

E: there are no obvious rashes, his wound on examination looks clean and dry, and his abdomen looks 'normal'.

An hour later, the patient in the next bed to Jim summons you over, saying that he doesn't think Jim looks well. You re-examine Jim and on examination you find:

A: Jim does answer you.

B: his respiratory rate is now 22, and his oxygen saturations are 92% on 4 L/min nasal specs.

C: his pulse rate is now 125, and his manual blood pressure is 90/40; he appears flushed and his temperature is now 38.4°C.

D: his pain score is 8/10.

E: his wound is looking red, there are obvious signs of bleeding and his abdomen looks more distended.

- What do you think is happening? Write down in detail the physiological responses and consider what is happening and how this has affected his cardiovascular system, e.g. which component (heart, vessels, blood) is compensating for what?
- What would you do next?

---

The changes to Jim's cardiovascular and respiratory function are as a result of his body's responses to infection, which, rather than his presenting symptoms being local (e.g. at the site of infection), they are systemic and affecting the whole body. He is exhibiting three of the physiological symptoms used as criteria for diagnosing sepsis (e.g. a raised temperature, raised respiratory rate and increased heart rate). Sepsis is the body's response to infection. Although the source of this infection appears to be from his wound site, given the information above, Jim has several potential sites of infection that could be the cause of his sepsis: his surgical procedure, his intravenous access and his urinary catheter. Therefore Jim requires early goal-directed treatment to ensure that his sepsis is managed.

Sepsis and severe infection are one of the most common causes of inpatient deterioration (UK Sepsis Trust, 2017). Severe sepsis accounts for approximately a quarter of admissions to general critical care units in the UK (Shahin et al., 2012). Robson and Daniels (2013) consider sepsis a medical emergency and the UK Sepsis Trust (2014) advocate that staff working on all inpatient wards should be aware of the significance of sepsis, and have the skills and knowledge to recognise it early and start treatment.

Sepsis is defined as 'the presence (probable or documented) of infection together with systemic manifestations of infection', whereas severe sepsis is defined as 'sepsis plus sepsis-induced organ dysfunction or tissue hypo-perfusion' (Dellinger et al., 2013: 583). Sepsis arises when the body's response to infection injures its own tissues and organs, and can lead to shock, organ failure and death if not recognised and treated early (UK Sepsis Trust, 2014). The Scottish Intercollegiate Guidelines Network (SIGN, 2014) *Care of Deteriorating Patients'* guideline suggests that any patient whose NEWS2 score triggers action should be screened for sepsis (and delirium). Certainly all patients presenting with abnormal physiological parameters and the signs and symptoms of infection should be screened for sepsis. The UK Sepsis Trust (2014) recommends that sepsis screening be undertaken as a two-part process (e.g. first confirming that sepsis may be present and then screening for severity).

## ACTIVITY 13.5

Access the UK Sepsis Trust website and identify both red and amber flags for sepsis: https://sepsistrust.org/education.

Review the NICE (2016) guideline 'Sepsis: recognition, diagnosis and early management'. Available at: www.nice.org.uk/guidance/ng51.

SIGN (2014) recommend that all patients who screen positively for sepsis should be started on the Sepsis Six care bundle, unless their treatment plan dictates otherwise. The Sepsis Six is a set of interventions to be performed in the first hour of suspected sepsis, which can improve survival. These are as follows:

1.  Give high-flow oxygen;
2.  Take blood cultures;
3.  Give broad-spectrum antibiotics;
4.  Give intravenous fluid challenges;
5.  Take serum lactate and haemoglobin;
6.  Take accurate hourly urine output.

The UK Sepsis Trust (2012) suggests that a useful way to remember the Sepsis Six is to 'give 3 and take 3'. In other words, give oxygen, antibiotics and fluids and take blood cultures, serum lactate and haemoglobin and urine output. It is recommended that you visit the Sepsis Trust UK website to review the latest guidance.

## SBAR communication tool

As we have already outlined the ABCDE assessment aids recognition of the acutely ill patient. An appropriate response together with immediate lifesaving interventions (e.g. oxygen administration) is likely to include a call for help. Clear and effective communication between staff is essential to provide effective care and maintain patient safety and the 'SBAR' communication tool can aid this. The SBAR acronym stands for situation, background, assessment and recommendation. It is a communication tool that can be used to help provide structure to this important conversation on reporting a clinical deterioration in a patient. Originally used by US Navy nuclear submarine personnel, it was adapted for healthcare use by Leonard et al. (2004).

   Beliveau (cited in Buttaro and Barba, 2012) suggests that if SBAR is used consistently, not only will the first responder or nurse understand how to gather, organise and report appropriate information quickly and concisely, but also the recipient can anticipate how the information will be delivered. The use of SBAR helps to deliver critical information effectively to promote patient safety. A study by DeMeester et al. (2013) found that, after the introduction of SBAR across 16 hospital wards, there was an increased perception of effective communication between nurses and doctors and a reduction in unexpected deaths. It is important to remember the listening skills necessary for the receiver.

### ACTIVITY 13.6

Revisit Case Scenario 13.2. How would you report the changes in Jim's condition to the nurse in charge or medical staff? Write down the conversation you would have using the SBAR tool as a guide.

## ACTIVITY 13.7   SBAR ANALYSIS

Your response to Activity 13.6 should have included the following.

### Situation

Identify yourself and where you are calling from. Identify which patient you are calling about and briefly the reason for the call. Leonard et al. (2004) advocate the use of powerful 'critical language' such as 'I'm concerned, this is unsafe', or 'I'm worried' because that will have the effect of gaining the necessary attention of the receiver (e.g. a doctor/senior nurse): 'The reason I am calling is … .'

### Background

You need to relay relevant information, including the reason for admission, relevant past medical/surgical history and current management.

### Assessment

You need to elaborate what you found on your ABCDE assessment of the patient. You should include the NEWS2 score and if it is helpful, bring relevant information such as the observation chart/notes to the phone when making the call to ensure that you have all the relevant information to hand. You can then state what you think is going on: 'I think that they may be ….'

### Recommendation

You should have a clear idea as to what you would like to happen as a result of your call. Are you calling for advice? Do you want an urgent assessment? Or, are you simply providing an update. Do you think that the patient should be transferred to another clinical area such as ICU? You can make suggestions for actions: 'I would like you to ….'

## Acute pain management

The symptom of pain is a common reason for people to seek healthcare.

- Think back to a group of patients you have cared for recently. How many experienced pain?
- Were there any differences in terms of the way your patients expressed their pain? If so, what were the differences? How did you respond to these?

The prevalence of pain in hospitalised patients varies from 37·7% to 84%; surgical patients have a higher prevalence of 48–78% compared with medical patients of between 30% and 55·6% (Gregory and McGowan, 2016). We can therefore see that pain is experienced frequently and it is a significant, distressing and disabling symptom for many hospitalised patients. But what is pain?

Pain is an individual subjective sensation that not only involves a physical sensation, but is also influenced by psychological, environmental and social factors. How an individual interprets the physiological signal depends on numerous factors and includes the type and site of tissue damage, previous experience of pain, age, gender, psychological factors, such as anxiety, and social and environmental influences (Gregory, 2017). The International Association for Pain (IASP, 2017) define acute pain as 'an unpleasant physical and emotional sensation associated with actual or potential tissue damage or described in terms of such damage'. Acute pain is a short-term symptom often described as a warning, for example chest pain, indicating cardiac damage or gastritis. It usually resolves once the cause of pain has been diagnosed and treated; acute pain tends to respond to analgesia and other interventions (Schug et al., 2015). A physiological stress response is stimulated by acute pain, leading to changes in vital signs; increased respiratory rate, heart rate and blood pressure can be indications of pain. These changes should not be relied on when identifying pain. This stress response can be sustained for a certain length of time, which will depend on the general health of the individual patient. The stress response also has a wider effect on bodily systems, which can cause deterioration in patient condition if the pain is not treated effectively (Schug et al., 2015; Swift, 2018) (Table 13.7).

**Table 13.7** The effects of unrelieved pain

| Bodily system | Effects of pain stress response |
|---|---|
| Respiratory | Increased respiratory rate – shallow<br>Avoidance of deep breaths and coughing<br>Increase risk of chest infection |
| Cardiovascular | Increased heart rate and raised BP<br>Increased need for oxygen for cardiac tissue |
| Gastro-intestinal | Slow gastric emptying and peristalsis<br>Nausea and vomiting<br>Constipation<br>Poor nutrition |
| Muscular skeletal | Immobility<br>Loss of muscle tone<br>Joint stiffness<br>Increased risk of pressure ulcers, thrombosis |
| Sleep and rest | Insomnia<br>Poor recovery<br>Reduced ability to cope, irritability |
| Psychological | Increased anxiety and fear<br>Depression<br>Anger<br>Loss of confidence in healthcare professionals' ability |
| Long term | Increased risk of chronic non-malignant pain is associated with poorly controlled acute pain |

## Effects of unrelieved pain

Pain has been advocated as the fifth vital sign since 2000. As such, pain scores are incorporated into patients' monitoring of vital signs, although it is not included in scoring systems used to identify a deteriorating patient. A high pain score and altered vital signs should lead to interventions to reduce pain and lead to a return to an individual's usual physiological measures and prevent potential complications that can occur as a result of the stress response (Schug et al., 2015; Swift, 2018).

Previously in this chapter, enhanced recovery after surgery (ERAS) was described. The protocols and pathways recognise the importance of controlling pain and have incorporated pain management strategies into the preoperative and postoperative pathways to reduce the pain experience, preventing deterioration and ensuring rapid recovery after surgery.

## Assessment of pain

The pain management process begins with the recognition and assessment of pain, followed by analgesia and non-pharmacological interventions which are evaluated with the individual to ensure that they are effective and appropriate (Schug et al., 2015). Lukas et al. (2013) describe the assessment of pain as fundamental to ensuring appropriate and effective pain interventions to improve patient outcomes. This is an important aspect of an adult nurse's role in recognising and assessing an individual patient's pain.

As a consequence of the subjectivity of pain, how it is felt and impacts on an individual need to be communicated to others. Pain scales or tools provide a standard means of assessing pain. They are used to measure or establish the level of pain intensity. Patients use them to communicate their pain experience and they help to evaluate the effect of treatment and indicate when a review of pain therapy is required (Williamson and Hoggart, 2005; Hjermstad et al., 2011). There are many pain assessment scales that ask patients to rate their pain, and these have been found to be easy to use and are described as highly valid and reliable. A small study found that the scales were used in practice and in many cases more than one scale was used in an organisation. If this is the case, it is important that the same scale be used consistently for an individual patient (Gregory and Richardson, 2014). The successful use of these pain scales depends on a patient's ability to use the scales as well as careful interpretation of the scores by healthcare professionals (Williamson and Hoggart, 2005).

- How is pain assessed in your current placement area?
- Have you observed the use of observational pain assessment tools?
- How effective are the tools in identifying and assessing pain?

However, the identification and assessment of pain are more complex than obtaining a pain score by simply asking 'have you any pain today?' According to Hjermstad et al. (2011) pain intensity is the most clinically relevant dimension of the pain experience; hence it is the most commonly assessed element of pain using the one-dimensional scales described in Table 13.8.

**Table 13.8** Self-report pain assessment scales

| The pain assessment tool or scale | Description | Strengths | Limitations |
|---|---|---|---|
| Visual analogue scale (VAS) | Consists of a 10-cm line with anchor words at each end of the line from 'no pain' to 'worst pain imaginable'<br>A mark on the line is made by the patient with a pen or pencil and is measured on the line<br>A plastic or metal slide-ruler may be used as an alternative to paper | Provides an accurate measure of pain<br>Used in research studies<br>Can be written in different languages | It is complicated and requires cognitive skills<br>It is time-consuming, requires special equipment<br>It is difficult to use for people with visual impairment and dexterity problems<br>Is inappropriate for people with cognitive impairment |
| Numerical rating scale (NRS) | Pain is rated as a number (0–10) with 0 indicating no pain and 10 the worse pain imaginable | It is quick and easy to use in patients who can communicate effectively<br>Suitable for all ages<br>Highly valid and reliable<br>The numbers are sensitive to small changes in pain<br>Its use can overcome problems of visual and physical impairment associated with VAS | It is difficult to use with language barriers<br>Some patients have difficulty rating their pain as a number<br>Many older people finding it difficult to use<br>It is inappropriate in the cognitively impaired patient |
| Verbal descriptor scale (VDS) | Patients are asked to indicate which descriptor describes their pain. Examples of descriptors are:<br>No pain<br>Mild pain<br>Moderate pain and severe pain | It is quick and easy to use<br>It is valid and fits with the WHO analgesic ladder<br>Often the preferred scale for use in older people<br>Useful for patients with cognitive impairment | The ratings are subject to the patients' interpretation of the words<br>It lacks the sensitivity of NRS<br>Royal College of Physicians, British Geriatrics Society and British Psychological Society suggested it was useful for older people with mild-to-moderate cognitive impairment |
| Numerical verbal descriptor scale (NVDS) | The patient is asked to indicate which descriptor describes their pain, as above, and this is then given a numerical score.<br>For example:<br>No pain = 0<br>Mild pain = 1<br>Moderate pain = 2<br>Severe pain = 3 | As above for VDS<br>It is quick and easy to use<br>The numerical score enables quick documentation | The ratings are subject to the patients' interpretation of the words<br>It lacks the sensitivity of NRS<br>Some nurses ask the patient to rate their pain between 0 and 3 rather than asking them to describe the pain<br>The numbers can be confused with an NRS |

A more comprehensive assessment would include a number of factors, such as how pain affects the individual's activities of daily living. To explore pain in more depth you could use one of the mnemonics described earlier, such as OLD CARTS or SOCRATES.

When a patient cannot communicate and describe their pain (for example after a stroke or with cognitive impairment, including dementia), pain may be assessed through observing behaviours. Observational behavioural pain assessment tools have been devised, for example the Critical Care Pain Observation Tool (CPOT; Gelinas et al., 2006); in addition to observing facial expression and agitation, the CPOT relies on physiological changes to help identify pain. The Abbey Scale (Abbey et al., 2004) and the Pain Assessment in Advanced Dementia (PAINAD; Warden et al., 2003) have been developed for people living with dementia. The tools devised for people with dementia include verbalisation, facial expression, body movements, changes in interaction, changes in activities of living and mental status changes. The Abbey Tool also includes physiological changes and any physical damage that may be causing pain.

---

## ACTIVITY 13.8

Access and consider the following articles:

- Zwakhalen, S.M.G., Hamers, J.P.H., Abu-Saad, H.H. and Berger, M.P.F. (2006) 'Pain in elderly people with severe dementia: A systematic review of behavioural pain assessment tools', *BMC Geriatrics*, 6: 3. doi:10.1186/1471-2318-6-3.
- Zwakhalen, S.M.G., van't Hof, C.E. and Hamers, J.P. (2012) 'Systematic pain assessment using an observational scale in nursing home residents with dementia: exploring feasibility and applied interventions', *Journal of Clinical Nursing*, 21(21–22): 3009–17.

What could you do to improve your pain assessment skills, particularly for vulnerable groups of patients?

---

## YVONNE

Yvonne is a 65-year-old woman who has fallen down stairs at home and has been admitted into accident and emergency. She has right-sided chest pain and finds it difficult to breathe. (She is suspected of having fractured her ribs as a result of the fall.) On admission her observations are as follows:

A: she can speak to you in full sentences.

B: she has a respiratory rate of 28, her respirations are shallow and her oxygen saturations are 95% on room air.

C: her pulse is 112, strong and regular, and her blood pressure is 185/90.

D: she is coherent but very distressed and her pain score is 9/10.

E: she is very pale and sweaty, has bruising to her right arm and her right ankle is swollen.

*(Continued)*

(Continued)

- What do you think is Yvonne's main problem?
- What might happen if this is not resolved?

The A&E doctor has requested an X-ray of her chest and ankle, and as the nurse responsible for her care:

- Would you be happy to send her straight to radiology?
- What care would be appropriate before transfer?

Yvonne is prescribed the following analgesia:

Morphine IV, 10 mg PRN.

Morphine orally, 10–20 mg 2–4 hourly.

Paracetamol 1 gram, orally or IV, QDS.

What do you feel is the most appropriate analgesia, and by which route would you administer it?

Describe how and what you would monitor for Yvonne: how frequently?

What other possible side effects would you monitor?

Is there any other analgesia that may help?

Once Yvonne's pain is controlled, how would you expect her A–E observations to alter?

## Pain management interventions

Once pain has been identified and assessed it is managed using pharmacological and non-pharmacological interventions, often in combination. It is important that adult nurses understand the pain management options available. We have already established that pain is an individual experience and as such the effectiveness of interventions can vary between individuals, with wide differences in the reaction to interventions – both pharmacological and non-pharmacological pain measures.

## Pharmacological pain management

There is a choice of analgesic drugs available, depending on the nature and severity and the individual patient's reaction to medication. It is important that you advise patients of the benefits of reducing their pain and stress that analgesia needs to be taken regularly to prevent pain rather than waiting for pain and then taking an analgesic. This is because waiting for pain leads to 'chasing the pain' rather than managing or controlling it. The effectiveness of analgesia has been studied and systematic reviews of randomised controlled trials are available for further information at the Oxford Pain Site: www.medicine.ox.ac.uk/bandolier/Extraforbando/APain.pdf.

## The WHO's analgesic ladder

The use of analgesia for all types of pain has been based on the WHO's (1986) analgesic ladder, which was initially introduced for palliative care. It is described as having steps that are used to guide us in the use of analgesia. There are three main classes of analgesia: paracetamol (simple analgesia), non-steroidal anti-inflammatory drugs (NSAIDs) and opioids/opiates. They are well established and are incorporated into the WHO's analgesic ladder. The analgesic ladder relates to the intensity of pain:

Step 1 = mild pain, paracetamol and NSAID;

Step 2 = moderate pain, paracetamol, NSAID and mild opiate;

Step 3 = severe pain, paracetamol, NSAID and strong opiate.

For acute severe pain it is appropriate to start at Step 3, but if the assessment indicates mild pain Step 1 would be appropriate followed by reassessment of the pain to evaluate the effectiveness of the analgesia administered.

### Simple analgesia

Paracetamol can be administered intravenously or taken orally as tablets, capsules, syrup or soluble preparations (although it should be avoided in active liver disease). The daily maximum dose of 4 grams should never be exceeded because it can cause liver damage and/or failure. It is important to stress this aspect and to check that patients are not taking any other medication that may contain paracetamol, such as cough and flu remedies, or combination analgesia, such as co-dydramol.

### Non-steroidal anti-inflammatory drugs

Ibuprofen, diclofenac and naproxen are examples of non-steroidal anti-inflammatory drugs (NSAIDs). They can be taken orally or applied as a gel for mild-to-moderate musculoskeletal pain. They act by blocking the prostaglandins responsible for some of the inflammatory response to tissue damage (Bond and Simpson, 2006). Systematic reviews of randomised controlled trials of NSAIDs have found them to be very effective for the mild-to-moderate pain associated with dysmenorrhoea, joint and muscle pain, post-surgical pain, toothache, etc. They can reduce swelling and pain at site and improve mobility (McQuay and Moore, 1998).

### Opioid analgesia

Opioid analgesia is derived from the opium poppy and is regulated under the Misuse of Drugs Act. Strong opioids are classed as controlled drugs (CDs; see Chapter 5). A prescription is therefore always required for opioid analgesia. Opiates are agonist-type drugs that combine with opiate receptors found mainly in the periphery, spinal cord and brain (Bond and Simpson, 2006). They interfere with the transmission of the pain signal within the spinal cord and change an individual's perception of the pain (Williams and Salerno, 2012). Systematic reviews have found opioids to be more effective when used in combination with paracetamol and NSAIDs (Doherty et al., 2011).

When caring for a patient using opioid analgesia it is important to consider possible side effects and carefully monitor their reaction to the medication. Anticipate constipation and inform the patient of the problem by advising them how to prevent constipation with adequate fluids, etc. Laxatives may be required. Antiemetics may be required initially, and antihistamines can also help with itchiness and any rash, because both symptoms can become less of a problem after a few days. Many healthcare professionals and members of the public fear addiction and will avoid using opioid analgesia as a result. However, addiction is rare when analgesia is required, and the importance of good pain control should always be emphasised (Gregory, 2014).

Morphine is considered the cornerstone of pain relief for severe pain. It is relatively cheap and available in many forms, orally and parentally. The dose of morphine required for individuals varies in its ability to provide similar pain relief. Therefore, this needs to be adjusted according to a patient reaction (Bond and Simpson, 2006). Patient-controlled analgesia (PCA) is a system, commonly used after surgery, which aims to overcome some of this individual variation. PCA is a device (usually electronic) that enables the patient to deliver a small predetermined dose of morphine IV (usually 1–2 mg) via a demand button or handset. There is a 'lockout' safety feature which means that the patient does not receive morphine more than every five minutes.

Nitrous Oxide 50% and Oxygen 50% (Entonox) is a medical gas indicated for procedural pain. It has been traditionally used in maternity and emergency departments, and increasingly in hospital wards and departments for painful procedures such as wound care. It is quickly effective, within a few deep breaths, easy to use and provides the patient with an element of control and distraction from the procedure. It has few side effects (mainly nausea), can be used with other analgesics, and is considered safe for all age groups (Gregory, 2008).

## Non-pharmacological pain interventions

Pain is not just a physical event. It responds to a variety of treatments and often a combination of strategies to give pain relief. This section examines some of the non-pharmacological and less invasive interventions that can be used alongside analgesia to help pain.

 Relating back to Case Scenario 13.3, can you think of any non-pharmacological interventions you might use to help Yvonne deal with her pain?

Psychological interventions help people to cope with pain. Also known as cognitive-behavioural therapies, they can be relatively simple or complex interventions. The aim of these interventions is to decrease or change the individual's perception of pain. It is important to remember that an ability to distract an individual from the pain does not indicate that the pain is not real; believing the patient during the assessment and encouraging the use of distraction are therapeutic. Some of the strategies include the use of distraction, music therapy, meditation, guided imagery and relaxation. If the individual focuses their attention on the painful stimulus it becomes more intense. Distraction is easily applied and basically takes the patient's mind off the pain. It is a useful strategy that is frequently used during procedures such as a dressing change. Focusing the mind on other stimuli reduces the pain intensity. Mental distraction involves carrying out a mental activity, such as counting, reciting a poem or prayer, and behavioural task distraction, like reading a book, or listening to the radio, watching TV or playing a computer game. Music has also been found to be effective in reducing pain by distraction and relaxation, reducing anxiety and allowing increased feelings of control. The choice of music is important and should be suitable to ensure that it helps the patient relax. Pain, muscle tension and anxiety are closely linked and helping an individual reduces muscle tension, anxiety and therefore the pain intensity. A simple technique is deep breathing exercises, because they are a form of distraction and help patients to relax (Hawthorn and Redmond, 1998).

Physical therapy can be used to help reduce pain. Exercise helps to maintain joints and muscles, and it stimulates the body's natural pain relief, endorphins. The use of hot or cold can help alleviate pain. Heat in the form of a heat pad or a warm bath can help a patient to relax. Heat increases vasodilatation and increases the blood supply to the affected area. Cold packs have the opposite effect and cause constriction of the blood vessels; in acute inflammation this can reduce swelling and pain. Seek advice before using either heat or cold therapy, especially in patients with vascular impairment. A transelectrical nerve stimulation (TENS) machine stimulates touch sensations, which can override some of the pain stimulus, it also acts as a distraction. TENS machines have been found to be effective for musculoskeletal pain, such as back pain, and are used for many patients with chronic, ongoing pain conditions. Complementary therapies can also be helpful for some patients and include acupuncture, aromatherapy and reflexology; these therapies can be provided only by therapists who have undergone approved training programmes.

Evaluation or reassessment of pain to establish the effectiveness of interventions is as important as the initial assessment. Has the pain score reduced? Is the patient able to complete their normal activities of daily living (ADLs)? It is important to include monitoring side effects, such as gastric irritation and constipation, as part of the evaluation to ensure patients continue with their medication. Experience has found that, if nausea and vomiting are severe, patients refuse to continue with analgesia because they can tolerate the pain better than the vomiting. Alternative medications may be required, and/or if the analgesia is not effective then a gradual increase or titration of the dose may be necessary to provide adequate pain relief with less severe side effects. The use of non-pharmacological interventions can be suggested and encouraged once the pain has become tolerable. For many patients an increase or improvement in activity may be as important as the reduction of pain intensity and should be included in the evaluation of pain management interventions.

## Caring for a group of patients

A survey of nine European countries by Aiken et al. (2014) assessed the link across nurse staffing, training and patient mortality. Although the main finding of the survey was that higher levels of nurse staffing and training were associated with lower patient mortality, it also revealed significant variations in nurse-to-patient staffing levels across Europe. The survey reported an average patient:nurse ratio of 8.8:1 (a 5.5–11.5 range). The National Institute for Health and Clinical Excellence (2014) has produced guidance for safe nurse staffing levels for adult inpatient wards in acute hospitals. Although much of the guidance provides information relevant from an organisational perspective, there are recommendations for nurses in charge of shifts to assess if the nursing staff available on the day can meet patients' nursing needs. Aston et al. (2010: 108) identify a series of items that the nurse needs to consider when caring for a group of patients:

- How you utilise information that has been handed over to you by previous staff;
- Deciding if you need more information;
- Assessing or reassessing patients;
- Prioritising care;
- Planning care;
- Deciding what to delegate and to whom you can delegate;
- How to manage time efficiently;
- How to respond to changes/incidents/issues that arise;
- Adapting your initial plans.

There are a number of factors to consider in prioritising care for a group of patients or indeed one patient. Time management and prioritising care are interlinked. Although you should have a patient-centred approach to care and avoid considering patient care as simply 'tasks to be done', a 'to-do list' can help you focus. Making a list can also make it easier to prioritise and delegate. This prioritisation can lead to a plan of care. As you are no doubt aware, it is important to acknowledge that this plan of care is devised in collaboration with the patient, because what the patient considers most important may vary from your perspective on what is important. It is the individual and not the tasks that are the priority. It is important that this plan of care is not considered a fixed or permanent schedule, because patient priorities can and do change.

In thinking about how to manage time effectively you should consider if there is the potential for multi-tasking. It is important that you use the best evidence available to support your decision making. Priority setting is based on assessment. As a nurse you will need to be flexible and able to adapt to changing priorities and demands. You should remember that you are providing care as part of a team and consider decision making as part of a team. Effective team work can impact on patient outcomes. A nurse needs to be able to work in a collaborative manner as part of a team to ensure patient safety.

## Acute hospital care of the older person

Although the UK population is ageing, it is those aged over 85 who are showing the fastest population increase (Office for National Statistics [ONS], 2017a). Indeed, although only representing 1%, the population in the UK of those aged 90 and over has been seen to grow at a quicker rate than younger age groups (ONS, 2017b). Conroy and Cooper (2010) recognise that the acute clinical problems and needs of older patients are often substantially different from those of younger patients. The King's Fund (2014: 27) report, *Making Our Health and Care Systems Fit for an Ageing Population*, emphasises that 'acute hospital care must meet the needs of older patients with complex co-morbidities, frailty and dementia'. The older adult may be considered at higher risk of issues concerning patient safety while in the acute setting. Although the National Patient Safety Agency (2010) reports an average of 5.6 falls per 1000 bed days in acute hospitals, over 80% of reported falls happened in those aged over 65 years, with those aged over 85 at highest risk.

The Alzheimer's Society (2009) report provides some interesting statistics:

- 97% of nursing staff and nurse managers reported that they always or sometimes care for someone with dementia;
- 47% of carer respondents said that being in hospital had a significant negative effect on the general physical health of the person with dementia which wasn't a direct result of the medical condition;
- Over a third of people with dementia who go into hospital from living in their own homes are discharged to a care home setting;
- 77% of carer respondents were dissatisfied with the overall quality of dementia care provided;
- 89% of nursing staff respondents identified working with people with dementia as very or quite challenging.

The report above identified key areas of dissatisfaction identified by carer respondents: nurses not recognising or understanding dementia; a lack of person-centred care; not being helped to eat and drink; a lack of opportunity for social interaction; not as much involvement in decision making as wished for (for both the person with dementia and the carer); and the person with dementia being treated with a lack of dignity and respect. Key areas of concern as identified by nursing staff respondents were managing difficult/unpredictable behaviour; communicating; not having enough time to spend with patients and provide one-to-one care; wandering/keeping people on the ward; and ensuring patient safety. Bridges et al. (2010: 89) warn that 'older patients in hospital may feel worthless, fearful or not in control of what happens, especially if they have impaired cognition or communication difficulties'. The Royal College of Nursing (2011) provides five principles to supporting good dementia care in the hospital setting:

1. Staff who are skilled and have time to care;
2. Partnership working with carers;
3. Assessment and early identification;
4. Care that is individualised;
5. Environments that are dementia friendly.

# Enhancing the patient experience

Within the NHS there has been a progression in the way that the 'quality' of the care being provided is assessed. Although traditional measures looking at clinical effectiveness (e.g. standardised mortality ratios) and safety have unquestionable significance, the importance of the patient experience is now recognised. The National Institute for Health and Care Excellence (2012a, 2012b) has produced clinical guidance and a set of quality standards on improving the experience of care for people using adult NHS services. These documents contain some key themes, including providing an individualised service, family and carer involvement, getting the basics right and clear communication.

Access some of the friends and family test data from the website below:
www.england.nhs.uk/publication/friends-and-family-test-data-december-2017
As an adult nurse working in an acute care setting, what could you do to try to enhance the experience of the patients for whom you care?

## Chapter summary

Nurses have a central role in ensuring safe patient care. This chapter has discussed the knowledge, skills and attributes needed by adult nurses working in an acute care setting. We have also focused on the knowledge and skills needed in the assessment and recognition of the acutely ill adult. The signs of clinical deterioration can happen many hours before a cardiac arrest. Early detection of patient deterioration gives an opportunity to improve patient outcomes by providing timely and appropriate care. NEWS2 is a valuable tool in achieving this, but it is important to remember that, if you are concerned about a patient's safety and are not sure what to do, you should call for help. A comprehensive assessment using the ABCDE approach and use of the SBAR communication tool can help you in these situations.

Medical technology is part of the modern healthcare environment and is not limited to critical care areas. Although the 'technical' aspects of nursing may be appealing to nurses working in acute care, these cannot and must not be promoted at the expense of providing compassionate nursing care. A nurse should use appropriate technology for the benefit of patients but also be aware of the potential of over-reliance. For example, a nurse should not have to rely on pulse oximetry to be able to identify that a patient with an increased respiratory rate, who is cyanotic, using accessory muscles and unable to talk in complete sentences with an audible wheeze, is unwell.

Pain assessment and management are a fundamental aspect of the registered nurse's role. Sometimes this can be difficult particularly when dealing with acutely ill and vulnerable patients. However, there are tools and strategies available to help us to manage pain effectively, thereby improving the overall patient experience of acute care.

The profile of patients in the acute care setting and the way that care is provided are changing. Patients who have a greater level of acuity tend to be older and have more co-morbidity. Acute care environments need to adapt to these changes. It is important to remember that the acute care environment can be a scary place for patients and their families.

## Further reading

Bickley, L.S. (2017) *Bates' Guide to Physical Examination and History Taking*, 12th edn. Philadelphia, PA: Lippincott, Williams & Wilkins.
British Geriatric Society (2012) *Quality Care for Older People with Urgent Care Needs (The 'Silver Book')*. Available at: www.bgs.org.uk/campaigns/silverb/silver_book_complete.pdf (last accessed 20 May 2018).
Brooker, C. and Nichol, M. (2011) *Alexander's Nursing Practice*, 4th edn. London: Churchill Livingstone.
O'Driscoll, B.R., Howard, L.S., Earis, J. and Mak, V., on behalf of the British Thoracic Society (2017) 'BTS guideline for oxygen use in adults in healthcare and emergency settings', *Thorax*, 72(Suppl 1).
Page, K. and McKinney, A. (2012) *Nursing the Acutely Ill Adult*. London: Sage.
Resuscitation Council UK (2016) *Immediate Life Support Manual*, 4th edn. London: Resuscitation Council UK.

# References

Abbey, J.A., Piller, N., DeBellis, A., Esterman, A., Parker, D., Giles, L. and Lowcay, B. (2004) 'The Abbey Pain Scale: a 1-minute numerical indicator for people with late-stage dementia', *International Journal of Palliative Nursing*, 10(1): 6–13.

Aiken, L., Sloane, D., Bruyneel, L., Van de Heede, K. et al. for the RN4CAST Consortium (2014) 'Nurse staffing and education and hospital mortality in nine European countries: a retrospective observational study', *The Lancet*, 383(9931): 1824–30.

Alzheimer's Society (2009) *Counting the Cost: Caring for People with Dementia on Hospital Wards*. London: Alzheimer's Society.

Aning, J., Neal, D., Driver, A. and McGrath, J. (2010) 'Enhanced recovery: from principles to practice in urology', *BJU International*, 105(9): 1199–201.

Ansell, H., Meyer, A. and Thompson, S. (2014) 'Why don't nurses consistently take patient respiratory rates?', *British Journal of Nursing*, 23(8): 414–18.

Aston, L., Wakefield, J. and McGown, R. (eds) (2010) *The Student Nurse Guide to Decision Making in Practice*. Maidenhead: Open University Press.

Bond, M.R. and Simpson, K.H. (2006) *Pain: Its Nature and Treatment*. Edinburgh: Churchill Livingstone.

Bridges, J., Flatley, M. and Meyer, J. (2010) 'Older people's and relatives' experiences in acute care settings: systematic review and synthesis of qualitative studies', *International Journal of Nursing Studies*, 47: 89–107.

British Thoracic Society (2017) 'BTS Guideline for oxygen use in adults in healthcare and emergency settings', *Thorax*, 72(Suppl 1).

Brunker, C. (2010) 'A brief history of resuscitation and beyond: as easy as ABCDE', *British Journal of Neuroscience Nursing*, 6(5): 232–5.

Buist, M., Bernard, S., Nguyen, T., Moore, G. and Anderson, J. (2004) 'Association between clinically abnormal observations and subsequent in-hospital mortality: a prospective study', *Resuscitation*, 62: 137–41.

Buttaro, T.M. and Barba, K.M. (eds) (2012) *Nursing Care of the Hospitalized Older Patient*. Oxford: Wiley-Blackwell.

Conroy, S. and Cooper, N. (2010) *Acute Medical Care of Elderly People*. London: British Geriatric Society.

Coulter-Smith, M.A., Smith, P. and Crow, R. (2013) 'Critical review: a combined conceptual framework of severity of illness and clinical judgement for analysing diagnostic judgement in critical illness', *Journal of Clinical Nursing*, 23: 784–98.

Dellinger, R., Levy, M., Rhodes, A., Djillali, A., Gerlach, H., Opal, S.M., Sevransky, J.E., Sprung, C.L. et al., and the Surviving Sepsis Campaign Committee including the Pediatric Subgroup (2013) 'Surviving Sepsis Campaign: international guidelines for the management of severe sepsis and septic shock: 2012', *Critical Care Medicine*, 41(2): 580–637.

DeMeester, K., Verspuy, M., Monsieurs, K.G. and Van Bogaert, P. (2013) 'SBAR improves nurse–physician communication and reduces unexpected death: a pre and post intervention study', *Resuscitation*, 84: 1192–6.

Department of Health (2009) *Competencies for Recognising and Responding to Acutely Ill Patients in Hospital*. Leeds: DH.

Doherty, M., Hawkey, C., Goulder, M., Gibb, I., Hill, N., Aspley, S. and Reader, S. (2011) 'A randomised controlled trial of ibuprofen, paracetamol or a combination tablet of ibuprofen/paracetamol in community-derived people with knee pain', *Annals of Rheumatic Disease*, 70: 1534–41.

Dombrowski, S.U., Mackintosh, J., Sniehotta, F., Arajo-Soares, V., Rodgers, H., Thomson, R., Murtagh, M., Ford, G., Eccles, M. and White, M. (2013) 'The impact of the UK Act FAST stroke awareness campaign: content analysis of patients, witness and primary care clinicians' perceptions', *BMC Public Health*, 13: 915.

Donohue, L.A. and Endacott, R. (2010) 'Track, trigger and teamwork: communication of deterioration in acute medical and surgical wards', *Intensive Critical Care Nursing*, 26(1): 10–17.

Dwyer, A.J., Thomas, W., Humphry, S. and Porter, P. (2014) 'Enhanced recovery programme for total knee replacement to reduce the length of hospital stay', *Journal of Orthopedic Surgery (Hong Kong)*, 22(2): 150–4.

Elliott, M. and Coventry, A. (2012) 'Critical Care: The eight vital signs of patient monitoring', *British Journal of Nursing*, 21(10): 621–5.

Enhanced Recovery Partnership Programme (2010) *Delivering Enhanced Recovery: Helping Patients to Get Better Sooner After Surgery*. Available at: https://assets.publishing.service.gov.uk/government/uploads/system/uploads/attachment_data/file/215511/dh_128707.pdf (last accessed 20 May 2018).

Frost, P. and Wise, M. (2012) 'Early management of acutely ill ward patients', *British Medical Journal*, 345: e5677.

Gelinas, C., Fillion, L., Puntillo, K., Viens, C. and Fortier, M. (2006) 'Validation of a critical care pain observational tool in adults', *American Journal of Critical Care*, 15(4): 420–7.

Gregory, J. (2008) 'Using nitrous oxide and oxygen to control pain in primary care', *Nursing Times*, 104(37): 24–6.

Gregory, J. (2014) 'Dealing with acute and chronic pain: part one – assessment', *Journal of Community Nursing*, 28(5): 83–6.

Gregory, J. (2017) 'Assessing pain for cognitive impaired patients in acute care', *Nursing Times*, 113(10): 18–21.

Gregory, J. and McGowan, L. (2016) 'An examination of the prevalence of acute pain for hospitalised adult patients: a systematic review', *Journal of Clinical Nursing*, 25(5–6): 583–98.

Gregory, J. and Richardson, C. (2014) 'The use of pain assessment tools in clinical practice: a pilot survey', *Journal of Pain Relief*, 3(2): 140–6.

Hawthorn, J. and Redmond, K. (1998) *Pain: Causes and Management*. Oxford: Blackwell Sciences Ltd.

Health and Social Care Information Centre (2014) *Accident and Emergency Department Types*. Available at: www.datadictionary.nhs.uk/data_dictionary/attributes/a/acc/accident_and_emergency_department_type_de.asp?shownav=1 (last accessed 17 October 2014).

Higginson, R., Jones, B. and Davies, K. (2011) 'Emergency and Intensive care: assessing and managing the airway', *British Journal of Nursing*, 20(16): 973–7.

Hjermstad, M.J., Fayers, P.M., Haugen, D.T., Caraceni, A., Hanks, G.W., Loge, J.H. et al. (2011) 'Studies comparing numerical rating scales, verbal rating scales and visual analogue scales for assessment of pain in adults: a systematic literature review', *Journal of Pain and Symptom Management*, 41: 1073–93.

Ibrahim, M.S., Alazzawi, S., Nizam, I. and Haddad, F.S. (2013) 'An evidence-based review of enhanced recovery interventions in knee replacement surgery', *Annals of the Royal College of Surgeons England*, 95(6): 386–9.

International Association for Pain (2017) *IASP Terminology*. Updated from 'Part III: Pain terms, a current list with definitions and notes on usage'. In H. Merskey and N. Bogduk (eds), *Classification of Chronic Pain*, 2nd edn. Seattle, WA: IASP Press, pp. 209–14. Available at: www.iasp-pain.org/Education/Content.aspx?ItemNumber=1698#Pain (last accessed 20 August 2018).

Kavanagh, S., Cambell, J. and Rudd, A. (2011) 'Impact of the FAST campaign', *British Journal of Neuroscience Nursing*, 7(5): 626.

King's Fund (2014) *Making Our Health and Care Systems Fit for an Ageing Population*. London: The King's Fund.

Leonard, M., Graham, S. and Bonacum, S. (2004) 'The human factor: the critical importance of effective teamwork and communication in providing safe care', *Quality Safety Healthcare*, 13(Suppl).

Lewin, J. and Maconochie, I. (2008) 'Capillary refill time in adults', *Emergency Medicine Journal*, 25: 325–6.

Lukas, A., Niederecker, T., Günther, I., Mayer, B. and Nikolaus, T. (2013) 'Self- and proxy report for the assessment of pain in patients with and without cognitive impairment: experiences gained in a geriatric hospital', *Zeitschrift für Gerontologie und Geriatrie*, 46(3): 214–21.

Mackway-Jones, K., Marsden, J. and Windle, J. (2013) *Emergency Triage: Manchester Triage Group*, 3rd edn. Chichester: Wiley.

Massey, D., Aitken, L.M. and Chaboyer, W. (2010) 'Literature review: do rapid response systems reduce the incidence of major adverse events in the deteriorating ward patient?', *Journal of Clinical Nursing*, 19: 3260–73.

McMullen, S.M. and Patrick, W. (2013) 'Cyanosis', *American Journal of Medicine*, 126(3): 210–12.

McQuay, H. and Moore, A. (1998) *An Evidence-based Resource for Pain Relief*. Oxford: Oxford University Press.

Moore, T. (2007) 'Respiratory assessment in adults', *Nursing Standard*, 21(49): 48–56.

National Audit Office (2012) *Healthcare Across the UK: A Comparison of the NHS in England, Scotland, Wales and Northern Ireland*. Available at: www.nao.org.uk/wp-content/uploads/2012/06/1213192.pdf (last accessed 20 May 2018).

National Cardiac Arrest Audit (2017) *Key Statistics from the National Cardiac Arrest Audit 2016–17*. Available at: www.icnarc.org/Our-Audit/Audits/Ncaa/Reports/Key-Statistics (last accessed 16 February 2018).

National Confidential Enquiry into Patient Outcome and Death (NCEPOD) (2005) *An Acute Problem?* Available at: www.ncepod.org.uk/2005report/summary.pdf (last accessed 20 May 2018).

National Confidential Enquiry into Perioperative Deaths (NCEPOD) *Extremes of Age: The 1999 Report of the National Confidential Enquiry into Perioperative Deaths*. Available at: www.ncepod.org.uk/pdf/1999/99full.pdf

National Diabetes Audit (2017) *National Diabetes Inpatient Audit (NaDIA) 2016*. Available at: https://digital.nhs.uk/data-and-information/clinical-audits-and-registries/our-clinical-audits-and-registries/national-diabetes-inpatient-audit (last accessed 20 May 2018).

National Institute for Health and Care Excellence (2007) *Acutely Ill Patients in Hospital: Recognition of and Response to Acute Illness in Adults in Hospital*, NICE Clinical Guideline 50. London: NICE.

National Institute for Health and Care Excellence (2012a) *Patient Experience in Adult NHS Services: Improving the Experience of Care for People using Adult NHS Services*, NICE Clinical Guidance 138. London: NICE.

National Institute for Health and Care Excellence (2012b) *Quality Standard for Patient Experience in Adult NHS Services*, NICE Quality Standards (QS15). London: NICE.

National Institute for Health and Care Excellence (2013a) *Acute Kidney Injury: Prevention, Detection and Management of Acute Kidney Injury up to the Point of Renal Replacement*, NICE Clinical Guideline 169. London: NICE.

National Institute for Health and Care Excellence (2013b) *Intravenous Fluid Therapy in Adults in Hospital*, Clinical Guideline 174. Available at: www.nice.org.uk/guidance/cg174 (last accessed 20 August 2018).

National Institute for Health and Care Excellence (2014) *Safe Staffing for Nursing in Adult Inpatient Wards in Acute Hospitals*, NICE Safe staffing guideline [SG1]. London: NICE.

National Patient Safety Agency (2009) *Rapid Response Report: Oxygen Safety in Hospitals*. Available at: www.nrls.npsa.nhs.uk/resources/type/alerts/?entryid45=62811&p=2 (last accessed 20 May 2018).

National Patient Safety Agency (2010) *Slips, Trips and Falls Data Update June 2010*. Available at: www.nrls.npsa.nhs.uk/resources/patient-safety-topics/patient-accidents-falls (last accessed 20 May 2018).

NHS Digital (2017) *Hospital Admitted Patient Care Activity 2016–17*. Available at: https://digital.nhs.uk/data-and-information/publications/statistical/hospital-admitted-patient-care-activity/2016-17 (last accessed 20 May 2018).

NHS Improving Quality (2013) *Enhanced Recovery Care Pathway: A Better Journey for Patients Seven Days a Week and a Better Deal for the NHS*. Progress review (2012/2013) and level of ambition (2014/2015). London: NHS.

NHS Institute for Innovation and Improvement (2008) *Enhanced Recovery Programme*. Available at: www.institute.nhs.uk/quality_and_service_improvement_tools/quality_and_service_improvement_ tools/enhanced_recovery_programme.html (last accessed 2 December 2014).

NHS Modernisation Agency (2004) *10 High Impact Changes for Service Improvement and Delivery: A Guide for NHS Leaders*. Available at: www.nursingleadership.org.uk/publications/ HIC.pdf (last accessed 17 October 2014).

Nolan, J., Soar, J., Smith, G., Gwinnutt, C., Parrott, F., Power, S., Harrison, D., Nixon, E. and Rowan, K., on behalf of the National Cardiac Arrest Audit (2014) 'Incidence and outcome of in-hospital cardiac arrest in the United Kingdom National Cardiac Arrest', *Resuscitation*, 85: 987–92.

Nursing and Midwifery Council (2018) *Future Nurse: Standards of Proficiency for Registered Nurses*. London: NMC.

Office for National Statistics (2017a) *Overview of the UK Population: July 2017*. Available at: https://www.ons.gov.uk/peoplepopulationandcommunity/populationandmigration/populationestimates/articles/overviewoftheukpopulation/july2017 (last accessed 26 February 2018).

Office for National Statistics (2017b) *Estimates of the Very Old (including Centenarians): 2002 to 2016*. Available at: www.ons.gov.uk/peoplepopulationandcommunity/birthsdeathsandmarriages/ageing/bulletins/estimatesoftheveryoldincludingcentenarians/2002to2016 (last accessed 26 February 2018).

Olson, K. (2014) *Oxford Handbook of Cardiac Nursing*, 2nd edn. Oxford: Oxford University Press.

Organisation for Economic Co-operation and Development (2001) 'Acute care'. In *Glossary of Statistical Terms*. France: OECD. Available at: https://stats.oecd.org/glossary/search.asp (acute care) (last accessed 20 August 2018).

Peate, I. (2013) *The Student Nurse Toolkit: An Essential Guide for Surviving Your Course*. Chichester: Wiley-Blackwell.

Public Health England (2012) Act FAST. Available at: https://campaigns.dh.gov.uk/category/act-fast (last accessed 20 May 2018).

Public Health England (2014) Act FAST TV Campaign. Available at: www.gov.uk/government/ news/act-fast-campaign (last accessed 20 May 2018).

Resuscitation Council UK (2011) *Immediate Life Support Manual*, 3rd edn. London: Resuscitation Council UK.

Resuscitation Council UK (2015) *The ABCDE Approach*. Available at: www.resus.org.uk/resuscitation-guidelines/abcde-approach (last accessed 24 February 2018).

Robson, W. and Daniels, R. (2013) 'Diagnosis and management of sepsis in adults', *Nurse Prescribing*, 11(2): 76–82.

Royal College of Nursing (2011) *Dementia: Commitment to the Care of People with Dementia in Hospital Settings*. Available at: www.rcn.org.uk/development/practice/dementia/commitment_ to_the_care_of_people_with_dementia_in_general_hospitals (last accessed 2 December 2014).

Royal College of Physicians (2007) *Acute Medical Care: The Right Person, in the Right Setting, First Time*. Available at: www.acutemedicine.org.uk/wp-content/uploads/2014/04/RCP-Acute-Medicine-Task-Force-Report.pdf (last accessed 20 May 2018).

Royal College of Physicians (2012) *National Early Warning Score (NEWS): Standardising the Assessment of Acute-illness Severity in the NHS*. Available at: www.england.nhs.uk/nationalearlywarningscore/#links-to-relevant-documents (last accessed 20 May 2018).

Royal College of Physicians (2017) *National Early Warning Score (NEWS) 2. Standardising the Assessment of Acute-illness Severity in the NHS*. Available at: www.rcplondon.ac.uk/projects/outputs/national-early-warning-score-news-2 (last accessed 15 February 2018).

Sandberg, M., Nakstad, A., Berlac, P., Hyldmo, P.K. and Boylan, M. (2013) 'Airway assessment and management'. In T. Nutbeam and M. Boylan (eds), *ABC of Prehospital Emergency Medicine*. London: BMJ Books, pp. 20–6.

Scales, K. (2008) 'Intravenous therapy: a guide to good practice', *British Journal of Nursing*, 17(19, Suppl): S4–12.

Scales, K. (2014) 'IV fluid therapy', *Nursing Standard*, 28(23): 19.

Schein, R.M., Hazday, N., Pena, M., Ruben, B.H. and Sprung, C.L. (1990) 'Clinical antecedents to in-hospital cardiopulmonary arrest', *Chest*, 98(6): 1388–92.

Scott, I., Vaughan, L. and Bell, D. (2009) 'Effectiveness of acute medical units in hospitals: a systematic review', *International Journal for Quality in Healthcare*, 21(6): 397–407.

Scottish Intercollegiate Guidelines Network (SIGN) (2014) *Care of Deteriorating Patients*. Available at: www.sign.ac.uk/assets/sign139.pdf (last accessed 20 May 2018).

Schug, S.A., Palmer, G.M., Scott, D.A., Halliwell, R. and Trinea, J. (2015) *Acute Pain Management: Scientific Evidence*, 4th edn. Melbourne: Australian and New Zealand College of Anaesthetists.

Shahin, J., Harrison, D. and Rowan, K. (2012) 'Relation between volume and outcome for patients with severe sepsis in United Kingdom: retrospective cohort study', *British Medical Journal*, 344: e3394.

Swift, A. (2018) 'Understanding the effect of pain and how the human body responds', *Nursing Times*, 114(3): 22–6.

Teasdale, G. and Jennett, B. (1974) 'Assessment of coma and impaired consciousness: a practical guide', *The Lancet*, 304(7872): 81–4.

Thim, T., Krarup, T., Grove, E., Rohde, C. and Lofgren, B. (2012) 'Initial assessment and treatment with the Airway, Breathing, Circulation, Disability, Exposure (ABCDE) approach', *International Journal of General Medicine*, 5: 117–21.

Ugboma, D. and Cowen, M. (2012) 'Managing hydration'. In I. Bullock, J. Clark and J. Rycroft-Malone (eds), *Adult Nursing Practice: Using Evidence in Care*. Oxford: Oxford University Press, pp. 328–42.

UK Sepsis Trust (2012) *The Sepsis Six*. Available at: https://sepsistrust.org/education/ (last accessed 20 May 2018).

UK Sepsis Trust (2014) *General Ward Toolkit*. Available at: https://sepsistrust.org/wp-content/uploads/2018/02/ED-toolkit-2016-Final-2.pdf (last accessed 20 May 2018).

UK Sepsis Trust (2017) *The Sepsis Manual*, 4th edn. Available at: https://sepsistrust.org/education/educational-tools/ (last accessed 26 February 2018).

Walden, E., Stanisstreet, D., Jones, C. and Graveling, A., on behalf of the Joint British Diabetes Societies for Inpatient Care (2013) *The Hospital Management of Hypoglycaemia in Adults with Diabetes Mellitus*. Available at: https://abcd.care/joint-british-diabetes-societies-jbds-inpatient-care-group (last accessed 20 May 2018).

Walz, J.M., Zayaruuzny, M. and Heard, S.O. (2007) 'Airway management in critical illness', *Chest*, 131(2): 608–20.

Warden, V., Hurley, A.C. and Volicer, L. (2003) 'Development and psychometric evaluation of the Pain Assessment in Advanced Dementia (PAINAD) Scale', *Journal of the American Medical Directors*, Jan/Feb: 9–15.

West Midlands Quality Review Service and the Society for Acute Medicine (SAM) (2012) *Quality Standards for Acute Medical Units (AMUs)*. Available at: www.acutemedicine.org.uk/ resources/quality-standards (last accessed 20 May 2018).

Williams, C. and Salerno, S. (2012) 'The patient in pain'. In D. Tait, D. Barton, J. James and C. Williams (eds), *Acute and Critical Care in Adult Nursing*. London: Sage, pp. 88–101.

Williamson, A. and Hoggart, B. (2005) 'Pain: a review of three commonly used pain rating scales', *Journal of Clinical Nursing*, 14: 798–804.

World Health Organization (1986) *Cancer Pain Relief*. Geneva: WHO.

World Health Organization (2007) *Policy Brief. Day Surgery: Making it Happen*. Available at: www.euro.who.int/__data/assets/pdf_file/0011/108965/E90295.pdf (last accessed 20 May 2018).

World Health Organization (2009) *WHO Guidelines for Safe Surgery: Safe Surgery Saves Lives*. Geneva: WHO. Available at: http://whqlibdoc.who.int/publications/2009/9789241598552_eng.pdf?ua=1 (last accessed 20 May 2018).

Zhuang, C.L., Ye, X.Z., Zhang, X.D., Chen, B.C. and Yu, Z. (2013) 'Enhanced recovery after surgery programs versus traditional care for colorectal surgery: a meta-analysis of randomised controlled trials', *Diseases of the Colon and Rectum*, 56(5): 667–78.

# CARING FOR THE CRITICALLY ILL ADULT

## SAMANTHA FREEMAN, COLIN STEEN AND GREG BLEAKLEY

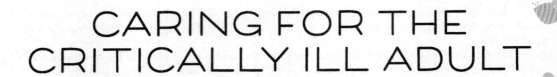

---

**CHAPTER OBJECTIVES**

- Critically discuss the comprehensive assessment of a critically ill adult;
- Recognise and respond to critically ill adults using appropriate evidence-based strategies;
- Appreciate the importance of using medical devices safely;
- Demonstrate a critical understanding of legal and ethical issues relating to the individual in acute care settings, including consent, confidentiality and best interest principles.

---

## Introduction

Chapter 13 focused on the care of the 'acutely ill' adult. This chapter will now explore the care of those who require specialist treatment within a critical care environment. The critical care environment is a constantly changing field with emerging technologies and therapies to aid patient recovery through a potentially life-threatening illness. As an adult nurse you will be required to understand and recognise the need to respond to those requiring critical care, ensuring that you assess the patient thoroughly, identify their problems and devise a plan of care based on their needs. The requirements to support a critically ill patient mean that a multidisciplinary team approach to care is needed. The coordination of the different disciplines is often the responsibility of the nurse who is able to constantly observe and interact with the patient. By exploring the evidence base for the management of critical illness we will provide you with the underpinning knowledge necessary to be able to assist in the safe and effective care for such patients. The use of patient scenarios and reflective guidance will help you consider and acknowledge your own limitations, thereby recognising the need to develop your skills.

# Related NMC proficiencies for registered nurses

The overarching requirements of the Nursing and Midwifery Council (NMC) are that all nurses must use information obtained during assessments to identify the priorities and requirements for person-centred and evidence-based nursing interventions, prioritising the needs of people when assessing and reviewing their mental, physical, cognitive, behavioural, social and spiritual needs. They ensure that the care they provide and delegate is person centred and of a consistently high standard. Working in partnership with people, families and carers, they must be able to evaluate whether care is effective and the goals of care have been met in line with patient wishes, preferences and desired outcomes (NMC, 2018).

 **To achieve entry to the nursing register you must be able to**

- Demonstrate the ability to accurately process all information gathered during the assessment process to identify needs for individualised nursing care and develop person-centred, evidence-based plans for nursing interventions with agreed goals;
- Demonstrate an understanding of co-morbidities and the demands of meeting people's complex nursing and social care needs when prioritising care plans;
- Interpret results from routine investigations, taking prompt action when required by implementing appropriate interventions, requesting additional investigations or escalating to others;
- Demonstrate the knowledge and ability to respond proactively and promptly to signs of deterioration or distress in mental, physical, cognitive and behavioural health, and use this knowledge to make sound clinical decisions;
- Demonstrate knowledge of when and how to refer people safely to other professionals or services for clinical intervention or support;
- Effectively assess a person's capacity to make decisions about their own care and to give or withhold consent, and understand and apply the principles and processes for making reasonable adjustments and best interest decisions where people do not have capacity;
- Demonstrate the knowledge, communication and relationship management skills required to provide people, families and carers with accurate information that meets their needs before, during and after a range of interventions;
- Effectively and responsibly use a range of digital technologies to access, input, share and apply information and data within teams and between agencies;
- Understand and recognise the need to respond to the challenges of providing safe, effective and person-centred nursing care for people who have co-morbidities and complex care needs;
- Demonstrate the ability to coordinate and undertake the processes and procedures involved in routine planning and management of safe discharge home or transfer of people between care settings;
- Understand how to monitor and evaluate the quality of people's experience of complex care.

(Adapted from NMC, 2018)

## Background

An admission to an adult critical care unit (ACCU) is a traumatic and potentially life-altering event. The underlying causes for admission are vast in range. The commonality is that the individual is

**Table 14.1**   Classification of critical care

| Level | Standard |
|---|---|
| 0 | Patients whose needs can be met through normal ward care in an acute hospital |
| 1 | Patients at risk of their condition deteriorating, or those recently relocated from higher levels of care, whose needs can be met on an acute ward with additional advice and support from the critical care team |
| 2 | Patients requiring more detailed observation or intervention, including support for a single failing organ system or postoperative care and those 'stepping down' from higher levels of care |
| 3 | Patients requiring advanced respiratory support alone or basic respiratory support, together with support of at least two organ systems. This level includes all complex patients requiring support for multi-organ failure |

From Intensive Care Society (2015)

experiencing illness so severe that they cannot be managed elsewhere and require drastic intervention. The system of critical care classification outlined in Table 14.1 is not universally employed or nationally validated, yet it is referred to by national authorities as a useful means of defining the varying needs of the critically ill patient. 'Normally', intensive care unit (ICU) Level 3 care or high dependency unit (HDU) level 2 collective is referred to as critical care.

The guideline for the provision of critical care services describes the environment as a, 'specially staffed and equipped, separate and self-contained area of a hospital dedicated to the management and monitoring of patients with life-threatening conditions' (Intensive Care Society, 2015). Level 3 patients require a minimum registered nurse:patient ratio of 1:1 to deliver direct care, with level 2 patients requiring a 1:2 ratio (Intensive Care Society, 2015). In the UK there is a National Competency Framework for Registered Nurses in Adult Critical Care. The competences are in three steps: step 1 starts when the nurse starts in critical care with no experience of the speciality and works up to step 3 working independently within critical care (Critical Care 3 Network, 2015). In addition to the nursing requirement, a complex multiprofessional team works together to provide care to patients within a critical care setting, including doctors, advanced critical care practitioners, physiotherapists, dieticians, infection control and microbiology specialists, and pharmacists, with further input from other specialisms such as renal or burns, as well as occupational therapy, speech and language therapy, and clinical psychology.

## Outreach services

Critical care needs to be viewed as more than a dedicated unit but a resource that supports patients within the wider hospital environment (Department of Health [DH]/Emergency Care, 2005). The introduction of critical care outreach services developed from the 'critical care without walls' (DH, 2000) concept of care. It focused on patients' needs rather than location. As a result of this document two key developments occurred: first the early warning scoring systems (discussed in Chapter 13) were developed.; second, critical care outreach services were introduced. The National Institute for Health and Care Excellence (NICE, 2015) guideline on the effectiveness of outreach services suggests critical care outreach teams may provide a benefit in increased numbers of 'Do Not

Attempt Resuscitation' (DNAR) orders issued, but there was no clear evidence that the service improved in-hospital mortality, avoidable adverse events such as cardiac arrest, unplanned intensive care unit (ICU) admission or ICU admissions. The current research exploring the effectiveness of outreach services is of low or medium quality, which may be why there can be significant variations in the composition of critical care outreach teams (Pattison and Eastham, 2011).

## ACTIVITY 14.1

Research the outreach service within your placement area.

- Who is on the team?
- What is their aim and how do they provide the service?

## Medical technology

Inevitably critical care areas will have a higher degree of medical technology for you to contend with. Adult nurses are responsible for ensuring that all the medical devices/equipment they are likely to use are checked regularly to ensure that everything is in working order. You will need to be aware of the potential pitfalls of using medical devices and the impact that these can have on patient safety.

- How many medical devices have you already used in clinical practice?
- Do you know how to use them safely?
- What should you do if things went wrong?
- Where would you go to access training in the use of medical devices?

## ACTIVITY 14.2

Before reading the next section you may want to revisit an anatomy and physiology textbook to refresh your memory of the respiratory system. It is important to understand normal respiratory function before we care for those who need respiratory support.

It would also be worth accessing the NMC (2018) *Standards of Proficiency* document and identifying all of the clinical competencies (Annexes A and B) required of registered nurses.

Within a critical care environment how could you ensure that you are able to develop your clinical skills to meet the required competencies outlined?

## Airway

When an airway problem is identified, as outlined in Chapter 13, there are a range of interventions. If these interventions and basic manoeuvres are not successful, then the patient will require more advanced airway care through the use of artificial airways such as an endotracheal tube (ETT) or a tracheostomy tube. Mechanical ventilation is one of the various interventions the patient may encounter during their admission (Chen et al., 2014). Nursing a patient with an artificial airway in place presents many challenges. These challenges are mainly related to maintaining patient safety through ensuring the patency of the artificial airway, preventing aspiration of any secretions and decreasing potential trauma to the trachea.

## Endotracheal intubation

Intubation involves inserting a tube directly into the trachea with the aid of a laryngoscope. The tube is secured by the use of cotton tape, or similar, tying the tube in position, and the use of a balloon situated, and integral to, the distal end of the ETT, which is inflated. This balloon is called the cuff. It is important to measure the pressure in the cuff to detect over-inflation, which may cause tracheal damage. Once inserted and secured the nurse's role is to monitor and maintain the position and patency of the ETT.

The length of the tube visible should be noted at either the lips or the teeth. This gives you a baseline position and there is then a need to check frequently to see whether it has moved, particularly after patient movement or re-positioning. This will help identify whether the tube has moved or dislodged. Diligent mouth care and suction of oral secretions are vital to maintain patient comfort and hygiene. It may also reduce the risk of ventilator-associated pneumonia (Hellyer et al., 2016).

Endotracheal suctioning is one of the most common procedures performed in patients with artificial airways. There are many things you need to consider before, during and after endotracheal suctioning.

### ACTIVITY 14.3

For further information on suctioning take a look at this guidance: www.evidence.nhs.uk/search?q=endotracheal+suctioning.

There may be post-intubation complications you need to be aware of such as:

- Hypoxia;
- Trauma to lips, teeth and vocal folds;
- Transient cardiac arrhythmias due to vagal nerve stimulation;
- Hypertension, tachycardia or raised intracranial pressure;
- Aspiration;
- Missed placement: potential oesophageal intubation;
- Infection;
- Reduced cough reflex;
- Bronchial and tracheal ulceration or stenosis;
- Laryngeal oedema;
- Bronchospasm;
- Discomfort and patient anxiety;
- ETT kinked or damaged;
- Measurement of cuff pressure.

# Tracheostomy

This is a tube that is inserted through the anterior wall of the trachea, just below the larynx and cricoid cartilage.

The indications for a temporary tracheostomy to be sited are (Intensive Care Society, 2008):

- To protect the airway;
- To aid the removal of excessive secretions;
- To aid weaning from mechanical ventilation.

For further information you are advised to visit the following website: www.tracheostomy.org.uk.

Many patients in need of critical care will have a temporary tracheostomy sited. They may require this to remain *in situ* when discharged from the ICU to the ward. In fact, some patients with a tracheostomy are nursed in other clinical environments such as community settings (Freeman, 2011). As an adult nurse you will need to be aware of the additional equipment required, the potential risk and how to manage these.

## JAN

Jan is 42 years old. She was admitted to the ICU for management of respiratory failure. She had a prolonged recovery, which required a temporary tracheostomy to be inserted. She is no longer requiring ventilation and is breathing unsupported via her tracheostomy with 35% humidified oxygen. She is due to be transferred to your ward.

- What additional equipment do you think you will need at this patient's bedside to ensure the safety of the patient?
- In relation to caring for someone with a temporary tracheostomy, what are the nursing implications?
- What are the potential complications of a tracheostomy?
- What symptoms of complications would you look for when caring for this patient?

According to the Intensive Care Society (2008), when caring for a patient with a temporary tracheostomy it is important that nursing staff are familiar with and able to use the following additional equipment, which should be immediately available:

- An operational suction unit, which should be checked at least daily, with suction tubing attached;
- Appropriately sized suction catheters;
- Non-powdered, latex-free gloves, aprons and eye protection;
- Spare tracheostomy tubes of the same type as inserted: one the same size and one a size smaller;
- Tracheal dilators;
- Re-breathing bag with tubing and a connection to an oxygen supply;
- Catheter mount or connection;

- Tracheostomy disconnection wedge;
- Tracheostomy tube holder and dressing;
- 10-ml syringe (if tube cuffed);
- Artery forceps;
- Resuscitation equipment;
- Manometer to measure cuff pressure.

The potential complications of a temporary tracheostomy are (Intensive Care Society, 2008):

- Airway occlusion;
- Displaced tubes;
- Blocked tubes;
- Air leaks;
- Impaired cough;
- Impaired swallow reflex which increases the risk of aspiration;
- Surgical emphysema;
- Infection wound/chest;
- Haemorrhage;
- Tracheal stenosis;
- Ulcerated tissue damage;
- Altered body image.

You should note that there are some differences in resuscitation approaches for individuals who have a temporary tracheostomy. If effective ventilation can be provided with a bag/valve, then continual chest compressions should be carried out and the patient ventilated with approximately 10 breaths/minute (Resuscitation Council (UK), 2015).
   If not then ask the following:

- Is the tube patent?
- Can a suction catheter be passed down?
- Can you change the inner cannula? (Some tracheostomies have an inner cannula);
- If the tracheostomy is occluded or displaced, remove and cover stoma and ventilate via the patient's mouth.

## Breathing

Normal respiration is quiet, effortless and rhythmical. It happens automatically without any conscious effort and any changes indicate abnormal breathing. In order for gas exchange to occur there needs to be a neurological stimulus from the respiratory centre in the brain. This stimulus triggers contraction of the diaphragm downwards and contraction of the intercostal muscles drawing the rib cage upwards and outwards. The overall effect is an increase in intrathoracic space, resulting in a decrease in intrathoracic pressure. The pressure in the thoracic cavity is now less than atmospheric pressure and this results in air being drawn into the lungs. In order for air to reach the alveoli, air sacks of the lungs where gas exchange takes place, a patent airway is needed, along with a patent respiratory tree. This means that, as both lungs expand, there is no obstruction to gas flowing into the lungs.

When caring for patients, consider what you can do to improve chest expansion to aid air entry into all areas of the lungs.

What could be the possible reason for an obstruction in airflow?

Are there any possible reasons that may cause an obstruction to the airflow to the alveoli?

You can access this e-portfolio of professional learning resources, which will enhance your learning in related areas: http://chss-elearning.info/

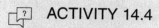 **ACTIVITY 14.4**

Mary is 68 and has been admitted to your ward with shortness of breath. Her oxygen saturation is low. Mary was being treated by her GP for a chest infection. She has no other medical history. Mary is diagnosed with type 1 respiratory failure.

- Why is Mary's oxygen saturation low?
- What is the likely barrier to the gas exchange in the lungs?
- What can you do about this to improve her breathing?

## Respiratory assessment

A patient experiencing critical illness may have a multitude of symptoms, some specific to the respiratory system. It is important to ascertain a good history to diagnosis respiratory problems or disease correctly. In addition to the physical examination, a detailed respiratory assessment can help focus the correct plan of care. Some patients on mechanical ventilation have a prescribed number of breaths that the ventilator delivers; however, patients can breathe independently while being supported by the ventilator, so it is important to conduct frequent breathing assessment. An important element of the respiratory assessment is to inspect the chest for symmetry of movement. The nurse closely observes the chest wall for symmetrical movement during each respiration. Abnormal chest wall expansion during respiration, for example only one side of the chest wall inflating, could indicate underlying pathology, including previous surgical removal of lung or pneumothorax (collapsed lung) (Arshad et al., 2016).

Enhanced respiratory assessment includes chest auscultation but this skill is often challenging in a busy and noisy critical care environment. Normally, chest auscultation occurs with the patient in a sitting position but this may not be possible during critical illness. With use of a stethoscope, chest auscultation allows the nurse to detect normal airflow sounds, which change if airways are blocked, narrowed or filled with fluid (Singh, 2016).

## Arterial blood gas interpretation

An arterial blood gas (ABG) contains lots of information about the patient, we are just focusing on respiratory function which includes four elements:

1. The pH;
2. Partial pressure of oxygen ($PaO_2$);
3. Partial pressure of carbon dioxide ($PaCO_2$);
4. Bicarbonate ($HCO_3^-$).

The pH is the measure of acidity or alkalinity of a substance; the normal range for blood is 7.35–7.45. During normal cellular metabolism, $CO_2$ carried in the blood to the lungs combines with $H_2O$ to give carbonic acid $H_2CO_3$. Therefore the blood pH changes according to the level of carbonic acid present and this allows the person to compensate for any changes. Compensation can either be quick by increasing or decreasing respiratory function or slowly as the kidney either retains or excretes bicarbonate ($HCO_3^-$) to maintain pH in a normal range. It's worth remembering that when a patient is unwell the body will respond by trying to maintain normal homoeostasis through compensating for the changes. Detecting these compensatory mechanisms provides vital information that illness is present and its severity.

The reading of the partial pressure of oxygen ($PaO_2$) dissolved in arterial blood should be >10 kPa (kilopascals) and the partial pressure of carbon dioxide ($PaCO_2$) dissolved in arterial blood should be between 4.5 kPa and 6.1 kPa. The bicarbonate ($HCO_3^-$) reading should be between 22 mmol/L and 26 mmol/L.

There are some basic steps to interpreting a simple ABG result. But before we start to answer these questions it is important to understand the context of the patient's results, i.e. what oxygen therapy, if any, the patient is receiving. There is a difference between the levels of oxygen we breathe in and the partial pressure ($PaO_2$) of oxygen dissolved in arterial blood. The difference is normally around 10 kPa. In a person with damage to their lungs, by either infection or illness, this difference will be bigger. The larger the gap between what concentration of oxygen the person inhales and their $PaO_2$ the more the degree of damage. This difference is referred to as the alveolar–arterial (A–a) gradient. For example, we would expect a person with a healthy lungs receiving 60% oxygen to have a $PaO_2$ of approximately 50 kPa (60 – 50 = 10). Once we have all the information we need, we can then start to interpret the ABG using five questions:

1. Is the patient hypoxic?
2. How does this relate to the inspired $O_2$?
3. Do they have an acidosis or alkalosis (the pH level)?
4. Is the cause respiratory or metabolic (determined by $PaCO_2$ and $HCO_3^-$)?
5. Is there any attempt at compensation (determined by $PaCO_2$ and $HCO_3^-$)?

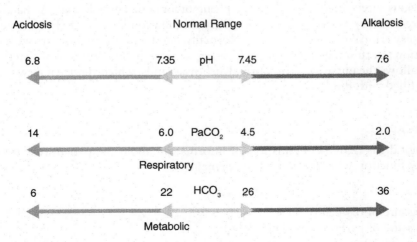

**Figure 14.1**    Plot the results

These last two questions can sometimes be more challenging. Read the scenario below and mark the results on Figure 14.1. If the result is marked on the same side as the pH then it's the cause of the deterioration; if the result is on the opposite side it's the compensatory mechanism trying to correct the pH.

---

### ☐ ACTIVITY 14.5

A 65-year-old man presents in the emergency department complaining of increased breathlessness. The paramedics have put him on an oxygen mask to give 40% oxygen due to his breathlessness and initial low saturations.

Significant findings on your examination are a drowsy patient with a:

- Respiratory rate of 28;
- $O_2$ saturation of 85%;
- Widespread coarse crackles on auscultation.

Arterial blood gas analysis reveals:

- $PaO_2$: 7.0;
- pH: 7.25;
- $PaCO_2$: 8.9;
- $HCO_3^-$: 35.

Work though the five steps and plot the result on Figure 14.1.

---

## Invasive ventilation

Invasive or mechanical ventilation aims to assist with the movement of gases into and out of a patient's lungs, while minimising the effort of breathing (Scholz et al., 2011). Most mechanical ventilators used in the UK today are positive-pressure ventilators, where lung volumes and gas exchange are achieved by applying oxygen/air in a positive pressure through the trachea, via an artificial airway (Higginson et al., 2011), effectively blowing gas into the lungs inflating them.

There are many different types of positive-pressure ventilation strategies and ventilator modes. It is important that the nurse understands the different modes of ventilation and why the patient is receiving a particular mode. Different modes affect the pattern of breathing to optimise gas exchange while reducing the risk of lung injury. Some modes also permit patients to breathe spontaneously through the ventilator.

Nurses need to be aware of the complications of mechanical ventilation and the nursing interventions that can minimise the risk. Common complications associated with mechanical ventilation include ventilator-induced lung injury, ventilator-associated pneumonia (VAP), blocked artificial airways and unplanned extubations.

VAP is a life-threatening nosocomial infection and a major complication of mechanical ventilation. There is a VAP care bundle that nursing staff should deliver to reduce the risk of patients developing VAP. Care bundles are evidenced-based practices that are grouped together to encourage the consistent delivery of these practices.

Recommended bundle of interventions for the prevention of VAP (Hellyer et al., 2016; Neuville et al., 2017):

- Elevation of head of bed (30–45°);
- Daily sedation interruption and assessment of readiness to extubate;
- Use of subglottic secretion drainage;
- Avoidance of scheduled ventilator circuit changes;
- Oral hygiene;
- Stress ulcer prophylaxis;
- Thromboembolism prophylaxis.

## Positioning

Patients experiencing critical illness are often immobile due to therapeutic interventions and sedation. Body positioning is one of the most important nursing considerations to prevent complications of immobility (Alcan et al., 2016). Unless cervical spine injury or lesion is suspected, critically ill patients are nursed with 30–45° head of bed elevation to prevent aspiration of gastric contents (Hellyer et al., 2016). Moreover, aspiration of gastric contents is linked to the pathogenesis of VAP. In addition, prolonged periods of immobility are known to cause thromboembolic occlusion, muscle weakness, pressure ulcer development and pulmonary insufficiency (Makic, 2015). Critically ill patients are at increased risk of developing chest infection because endotracheal intubation and mechanical ventilation bypass normal anatomical defences (Benson et al., 2013). Therefore acute respiratory failure (ARF) is a common phenomenon within the critical care setting, and prolonged connection to mechanical ventilation increases the risk of VAP (Scaravilli et al., 2015).

To prevent further cellular hypoxia, prone positioning during mechanical ventilation has been demonstrated to enhance arterial oxygenation in the most severe cases of acute respiratory distress syndrome (ARDS). Prone positioning, the opposite of supine, results in the patient lying face downward (Drahnak and Custer, 2015). In addition, prone positioning can be used to aid surgical procedures, and improve lymphatic drainage and secretion removal. However, prone positioning introduces the risk of dislodging an ETT and specialised airway securement devices should be considered (Drahnak and Custer, 2015).

## Non-invasive ventilation

Non-invasive ventilation refers to the administration of ventilatory support without using an invasive artificial airway.

- CPAP: continuous positive airway pressure;
- BiPAP: bilevel positive airway pressure.

These are types of non-invasive modes of ventilation requiring the patient to wear a very tightly fitting mask. Patients can find this very difficult to cope with, because the oxygen is humidified, and therefore warm, and patients find the mask uncomfortable and claustrophobic. Both of these treatments are for spontaneously breathing patients.

CPAP delivers oxygen via a continuous one pressure setting with the aim to:

- Increase oxygen levels;
- Recruit redundant alveoli.

Throughout the whole respiratory cycle, CPAP maintains a positive pressure within the respiratory circuit as a pressure higher than atmospheric pressure. It increases intrathoracic pressure, which reduces venous return to the heart. This can lower blood pressure, increasing the workload of the heart. The improved blood oxygen levels should compensate for this increase in workload. However, it may be a treatment of choice to manage patients with left ventricular failure because CPAP can reduce the workload of the left ventricle by reducing the resistance against which the left ventricle has to pump, known as the afterload.

BiPAP uses CPAP but also provides extra support to reduce the work of breathing. As the patient breathes in, the machine supports this effort by blowing gas under positive pressure to improve the volume of air inspired and oxygen levels, and reduce the $PaCO_2$ and respiratory workload.

Before reading the next section you may want to revisit an anatomy and physiology textbook to refresh your memory of the circulatory system. It is important to understand normal circulatory function before we care for those with abnormal circulatory function. Chapter 12 in Boore et al. (2016) is a useful resource.

# Circulation

In order for the heart to function normally, it has to have three main systems functioning in unison. It requires an electrical system, a mechanical pump and a valve system.

## The electrical system

The electrical system is recorded using an electrocardiograph or ECG. This shows the route the electricity flows through the cells that make up the muscle of the heart. Where there is any damage to these cells, the route the electricity has to take is either delayed or deviates and these changes can be seen in the ECG. The electricity is generated by the movement of positively and negatively charged electrolytes passing into and out of the cell. This shift in charged electrolytes creates an electrical impulse that results in contraction of the muscle. If there is an imbalance in the electrolytes in the body then the electrical system may become unstable and disrupted, causing either minor symptoms or a risk to life.

## MARY

Mary is 72 and is complaining of palpitations in her chest. She says that sometimes it feels as though her heart is racing or she feels extra strong, pounding beats. She also complains of tiredness and occasional dizziness.

- What could be causing Mary's symptoms?
- What investigations could be done to determine whether there's an electrical problem with her heart?
- What simple observations could you make to detect an abnormal heart rhythm?
- How could an imbalance in electrolytes be diagnosed?

There are various different electrical disorders of the heart, some of which are simple and some imminently life threatening. One major electrical disorder of the heart that is linked to a variety of co-morbidities, with incidence that increases with age, is atrial fibrillation. This occurs when there is erratic electrical flow through the upper chambers, the atria of the heart. The consequence of this is that these chambers do not contract or pump properly, and this creates turbulent blood flow through the heart. The result of turbulent blood flow is blood clots, which leave the heart and affect other parts of the body, especially the brain, causing stroke. Untreated, atrial fibrillation is a major contributing factor to the cause of stroke in the UK (NICE, 2014).

- Have you cared for a patient with an arrhythmia? Reflect on what could have been the cause of this arrhythmia, and how it was diagnosed and monitored. What observations did you perform to help with the diagnosis and monitoring?

## ECG monitoring

There are six basic steps to assist you in interpreting a basic ECG:

1. Is there a pulse?
2  Is there any electrical activity?
3. What is the ventricular (QRS) rate?

When recording speed and calculating the rate, check that the ECG is recorded at the standard UK paper speed of 25 mm/s for 1 minute of recording = 300 large squares. Each large square (5 mm) = 0.2 s, each small square (1 mm) = 0.04 s.

Regular rhythm: count number of large squares between two consecutive R waves then divide 300 by the number, e.g. if there are 5 large square intervals between R waves, heart rate = 300/5 = 60 beats/min or b[m.

Irregular rhythm: count the number of QRS in 30 large squares (QRS in 6 s) × 10 = rate/min (bpm).

4. Is the QRS rhythm regular or irregular?
5. Is the QRS width normal or broad?
6. Is atrial activity present?

If so:

- Is it regular?
- Is there more than one P wave?
- Is there any other atrial activity?
- How is atrial activity related to ventricular activity?
- Does it appear in front of every QRS complex?
- Is there any delay between the P wave and the QRS complex?

### ACTIVITY 14.6

Look at the following website for further information: https://bjcardio.co.uk/2014/03/my-top-10-tips-for-ecg-interpretation.

# The heart as a mechanical pump

The heart is a muscle and therefore requires a blood supply to the muscle itself so that it can contract and relax. The efficiency in the contraction of the heart is dependent on the muscle of the heart being undamaged, the amount of blood that is flowing into the heart and the resistance against which the heart has to pump the blood out. It is reliant on the valves that separate the four chambers of the heart working efficiently.

The amount of blood that flows into the heart is an indication of the patient's hydration. If a patient is dehydrated there is insufficient blood entering the heart, the efficiency of the contraction of the heart is reduced, and consequently the volume and pressure of blood leaving the heart are reduced, resulting in poor oxygen and nutrient delivery to the cells of the body.

In order to determine whether the patient is dehydrated or not there are a number of measurements that nurses can make:

1. Measure the fluid intake and urine output, i.e. the fluid balance;
2. Measure the pulse rate (heart rate): as the blood volume declines the heart rate increases to compensate in an attempt to maintain a normal oxygen and nutrient supply to the cells;
3. Feel the patient's skin to determine whether they are cold and peripherally shut down. This is an autonomic compensation system the body uses in an attempt to maintain oxygen and nutrient supply to the cells of the vital organs;
4. Measure the patient's blood pressure. Please note that a low blood pressure is a late indication of the patient being short of blood or fluid;
5. The patient may state that they are thirsty;
6. The patient's eyes may appear sunken;
7. The patient's skin loses its elasticity;
8. The patient's mucous membranes, i.e. their tongue and mouth, will appear dry and coated;
9. In some more severe cases the patient may become confused.

All of the above are simple observations that nurses can make to determine whether their patient is dehydrated.

## AHMED

Ahmed is 72 years old and has been admitted to your ward feeling unwell. He is a little confused and lives alone. He's been feeling unwell for a few days and has struggled to look after himself at home.

- How would you assess Ahmed's hydration status?
- Which of your observations would tell you that Ahmed may be dehydrated?
- How would you help to rehydrate Ahmed?
- What records would you need to make to continue the management of Ahmed's hydration?

Where patients are unable to take sufficient fluids orally or through an alternative enteral feeding system, then an intravenous drip can be used to administer fluids and electrolytes where necessary. In these circumstances a clear and accurate record of the patient's fluid balance is vitally important. A detailed record of all fluids and diet taken orally and through an intravenous drip should be documented, along with all the patient's outputs such as urine, vomit, the nature and consistency of faeces, and whether the patient is excessively diaphoretic. The difference between intake and output should be calculated every 24 hours and the result used to inform the next 24-hour fluid management. Regular testing of the patient's blood electrolyte levels will determine whether specific electrolytes need to be added to the intravenous fluid.

In critical care, the assessment of circulation is invasive and detailed. It uses both central venous lines and arterial lines to assess the hydration status of the patient, the function of the heart and the vascular tone, i.e. vasoconstriction, vasodilatation.

What are the factors that influence the flow of blood around the body and the diseases or conditions that may affect this?

In critical care, patients may suffer acute renal failure as a result of poor fluid management before admission. These patients will receive a gentle form of dialysis called haemofiltration. This form of dialysis is less likely to cause major shifts in blood volume adversely affecting the blood pressure.

In addition to IV fluid critically ill patients can also receive blood products. Blood and blood product transfusions are frequently administered to critically ill patients. Transfusions can help increase oxygen delivery to the tissues and improve the oxygen demand/supply balance, but may also have some harmful effects (Vincent et al., 2018). The various blood products that you may see administered are:

- Packed red blood cells;
- Platelets;
- Fresh frozen plasma;
- Albumin;
- Cryoprecipitate.

Globally there are clear differences in transfusion practice (Vincent et al., 2018).

- What is your placement's policy on blood and blood product transfusion?
- What are the risk factors and what safety measures are taken to manage these risks during transfusion?

Consider patients who do not wish to receive blood or blood products. How have you seen this managed? Look at the NICE guidelines on alternatives to blood products:
www.nice.org.uk/guidance/ng24/chapter/Key-priorities-for-implementation#alternatives-to-blood-transfusion-for-patients-having-surgery.

## Nutrition

During an episode of critical illness most patients are unable to eat due to the presence of an artificial airway and the need to be sedated. The nutritional needs in critically ill individuals are poorly understood and can vary at different stages of illness. During critical illness profound metabolic changes occur and malnutrition is associated with impaired immune function and muscle weakness, and results in increased ventilator-dependent days and length of stay in intensive care (McDonald et al., 2012). Nutrition support refers to enteral or parenteral provision of calories, protein, electrolytes, vitamins, minerals, trace elements and fluids. Enteral feeding, either through an oral or a nasal tube, or directly into the gastrointestinal tract via a gastrostomy or jejunostomy is the preferred method in critical care (McDonald et al., 2012).

What are the differences between enteral nutrition and parenteral nutrition? What are the advantages and disadvantages of each method and what are the nursing implications?
During your time on placement discuss your findings with a dietician.

# Sedation

The care and treatments provided in critical care can often be painful and invasive. To ensure that the level of intervention is tolerated, sedation is administered to the patient and is deemed an essential component of care (Whitehouse et al., 2014). In some cases a paralysing agent is also required. This ensures comfort, assists recovery and enables treatment to be carried out in a humane manner (Mehta et al., 2012). As the patient recovers, the level of sedation is reduced, enabling the patient to breathe, allowing a decrease in the dependency on mechanical ventilation (Intensive Care Society, 2008). The level and type of sedation will vary from patient to patient, with the most common sedative agents being opioids, benzodiazepines, and intravenous and, occasionally, inhaled general anaesthetic agents, neuroleptic drugs, phencyclidine derivatives, phenothiazines, α agonists and barbiturates (Whitehouse et al., 2014). The main aim of the sedation strategy is to use the minimal dose to ensure treatment compliance. The Intensive Care Society (2014) stated that the following were indications for the use of sedation:

- To alleviate pain;
- To facilitate the use of an otherwise distressing treatment and minimise discomfort, e.g. tolerance of ETTs and ventilation;
- To augment the effectiveness of a treatment, e.g. inverse ratio ventilation;
- As a treatment in its own right, e.g. seizure control or management of intracranial pressure;
- To reduce anxiety;
- To control agitation;
- For amnesia during neuromuscular block.

## Assessment of sedation

There are many sedation scoring tools available, but the most commonly used are the Ramsay Sedation Scale (RSS) and the Richmond Agitation Sedation Score (RASS). Using a sedation scoring tool, the nursing team can titrate the doses of sedation to achieve a pre-prescribed sedation score. Table 14.2 illustrates the RASS scoring system.

There are many complications with continuous sedation and the clinical team will often give the patients a break from sedation.

**Table 14.2**   The Richmond Agitation Sedation Score (RASS)

| Score | |
|---|---|
| +4 | Combative, violent, danger to staff |
| +3 | Pulls or removes tube(s) or catheters; aggressive |
| +2 | Frequent non-purposeful movement, fights ventilator |
| +1 | Anxious, apprehensive, but not aggressive |
| 0 | Alert and calm |
| −1 | Awakens to voice (eye opening/contact) >10 s |
| −2 | Light sedation, briefly awakens to voice (eye opening/contact) <10 s |
| −3 | Moderate sedation, movement or eye opening. No eye contact |
| −4 | Deep sedation, no response to voice, but movement or eye opening to physical stimulation |
| −5 | Unrousable, no response to voice or physical stimulation |

(Adapted from Barr et al., 2013)

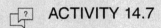 **ACTIVITY 14.7**

If you want to read the evidence around the effectiveness of sedation break, then take a look at the Standards and Guideline issued by the Intensive Care Society at: www.ics.ac.uk.

# Legal and ethical considerations in critical care

Nurses in critical care environments may be faced with a number of situations or decisions that have ethical or legal considerations. The nurse must approach these situations with due care and deliberation.

## Consent

Although we briefly covered the concepts of consent and mental capacity in Chapter 3, it is worthwhile revisiting these concepts here within the context of critical care provision. Consent should be obtained by any healthcare professional before any examination, treatment or care is provided to a patient. 'Consent' is the patient's agreement or permission for the examination, treatment or care to occur. It is based on the fundamental principle of autonomy, whereby the patient has the right to choose what happens to his or her own body. The Department of Health (DH, 2009: 9) guidance on consent considers that,

> For consent to be valid, it must be given voluntarily by an appropriately informed person who has capacity to consent to the intervention in question (this will be the patient or someone with parental responsibility for a patient under the age of 18, someone authorised to do so under a Lasting Power of Attorney (LPA) or someone who has the authority to make treatment decisions as a court appointed deputy).

Considering this statement, three key questions need to be considered:

1. Does the person have capacity?
2. Has the consent been given voluntarily?
3. Has the person received sufficient information?

## Does the person have capacity?

The assessment of the patient's capacity to give or withhold consent is considered in relation to a specific decision. Although the patient may not have capacity to make some decisions they may still retain capacity for other decisions. For example, a patient may not have capacity to make a decision about a surgical procedure but could retain capacity to consent (or not) to having their clinical observations (e.g. blood pressure) checked.

The Mental Capacity Act 2005 (see www.legislation.gov.uk/ukpga/2005/9/contents) provides guidance on the issue of capacity and has five key principles (Office of the Public Guardian: www. legislation.gov.uk/ukpga/2005/9/section/1):

1. Every adult has the right to make his or her own decisions and must be assumed to have capacity to make them unless it is proved otherwise;
2. A person must be given all practicable help before anyone treats them as not being able to make their own decisions;
3. Just because an individual makes what might be seen as an unwise decision, they should not be treated as lacking capacity to make that decision;
4. Anything done or any decisions made on behalf of a person who lack capacity must be done in their best interest;
5. Anything done for or on behalf of a person who lacks capacity should be the least restrictive of their basic rights and freedoms.

If the patient lacks capacity a decision may be made in the patient's best interests. The Code of Practice (The Stationery Office, 2007) of the Mental Capacity Act 2005 provides guidance on how best to establish a patient's best interests. This will include trying to establish the patient's previous wishes and feelings, and may involve consulting carers, family or friends.

## Is the consent given voluntarily?

Consent should be obtained voluntarily without coercion. Healthcare providers can be considered to be in a position of power, whereas patients may be in a vulnerable or stressed state. Likewise, family members can place undue pressure on a patient about decision making and this needs to be considered. Ideally, patients should not feel pressurised into making a decision quickly, without having had adequate time to consider their options. The patient has the right to withdraw consent at any time.

## Has the person received sufficient information?

Information should be provided to a patient in a way that they can readily understand. The use of highly technical or medical jargon should be avoided. Information should be balanced, outlining potential benefits and the risks along with potential alternatives (if any). The use of interpreting services should be considered when appropriate.

In the emergency situation consent should still be sought from competent patients, but if this is not possible (e.g. unconscious patient) care can be provided that is in the patient's *best interests*, i.e. that which is lifesaving or aimed at preventing serious deterioration.

## JACK

Jack is 65; he is in type II respiratory failure and his condition is deteriorating. He has had a previous admission to the ICU and is refusing artificial ventilation. Some colleagues believe Jack is delirious which is affecting his decision making.

Jot down your thoughts about this case in relation to the following:

- Complexity in care delivery;
- Complexity in care management;
- Complexity in ethical decision making.

Do you know the difference between type I and type II respiratory failure?

Jack has type II respiratory failure, which refers to poor carbon dioxide excretion from the lungs. Type I respiratory failure relates to low oxygen levels passing through the lungs into the blood-stream. Type I is referred to as hypoxaemia and type II as hypercapnia, but patients can have both. Jack will require increased observation and as noted earlier, due to the potential for the need for advanced respiratory support, may need to be moved to a higher level of care. His wish not to be artificially ventilated may be due to impaired decision making as a result of his deteriorating respiratory function or to his past ICU experience. This will need to be assessed carefully to establish if Jack does have the capacity to make an informed decision. The team will need to support and advocate for a patient in situations such as this, and the involvement of family members is also key to ensuring that treatment and care are in the best interests of the patient.

## Pain, agitation and delirium

Delirium is a very common problem in the acute setting, with Ryan et al. (2013) estimating that it may affect one in five of general hospital inpatients. It is defined by Maldonado (2008) as an acute change in cognition, inattention and a disturbance of consciousness. Delirium can develop over a short period of hours or days and fluctuate over time (Griffiths and Jones, 2007). The NICE (2010) guidelines for delirium identify those at risk as:

- Aged 65 years or older;
- Having cognitive impairment (past or present) and/or dementia;
- Having a current hip fracture;
- Having a severe illness.

In addition, Ely et al. (2001) noted that patients receiving care within an intensive care setting have a high probability of developing delirium due to multi-system illness, their co-morbidities, the use of psychoactive medications and age. Delirium is the most common neurological diagnosis among adult patients within the ICU (Guenther et al., 2012) and yet is often missed by staff. This is possibly due to each patient with delirium displaying different clinical symptoms. Patients can be restless, agitated and aggressive, possibly trying to remove a line and catheters, often referred to as hyperactive delirium (NICE, 2010). These patients are easily identified; however, a group who are often missed are those patients experiencing hypoactive delirium. These patients become quiet, withdrawn and sleepy (NICE, 2010). It is vital that this patient group be adequately assessed, diagnosed and treated. The CAM-ICU tool is one of the most common tools for identifying delirium in the ICU, which can be used by nursing staff, and has been found to be a valid and reliable measure (Krahne et al., 2006).

## Promotion of a natural sleep

Poor sleep is a frequent occurrence in the ICU; patients are known to have disrupted sleep and circadian rhythms (Ding et al., 2017). Reasons for sleep disruption may include the underlying illness, uncomfortable therapy, psychological stress or the environment (Hu et al., 2015).

One of the challenges is to restore the patient's normal sleep–wake cycle. The promotion of sleep can include pharmacological and non-pharmacological interventions. Non-pharmacological interventions may include noise reduction strategies such as the use of an eyemask and earplugs, grouping of care activity to minimise disruption, music therapy, complementary therapy, and using social and family support. Pharmacological approaches may include the use of melatonin and regular review of medication, which may have a negative impact on the patient's ability to sleep.

- How can you reduce the noise levels in the clinical environment?
- How do you plan your nursing interventions to reduce the number of interactions?
- How can you reduce the light levels in an ICU?

## Decisions about CPR

Although most people would prefer to die in their 'own home' currently most people who die in the UK die in hospital (Public Health England, 2015). In acknowledging this, there are issues about decision making at the end of life including those encompassing cardiopulmonary resuscitation (CPR). The British Medical Association (BMA), the Resuscitation Council (UK) and the Royal College of Nursing's (2014) decisions relating to CPR provide some guidance. Some of the main points identified in the document are as follows:

1. 'Where no explicit decision about CPR has been considered and recorded in advance, there should be an initial presumption in favour of CPR';
2. 'Every decision about CPR must be made on the basis of a careful assessment of each individual's situation';
3. 'Clear and full documentation of decisions about CPR, the reasons for them, and the discussions that informed those decisions are an essential part of high-quality care';
4. 'Each decision about CPR should be subject to review based on the person's individual circumstances';

5. 'Any decision about CPR should be communicated clearly to all those involved in the patient's care';
6. 'A DNACPR (Do Not Attempt CPR) decision does not override clinical judgement in the unlikely event of a reversible cause of the person's respiratory or cardiac arrest that does not match the circumstances envisaged when that decision was made and recorded. Examples of such reversible causes include but are not restricted to: choking, a displaced tracheal tube or a blocked tracheostomy tube';
7. 'Making a decision not to attempt CPR that has no realistic prospect of success does not require the consent of the patient or of those close to the patient. However, there is a presumption in favour of informing a patient of such a decision'.

---

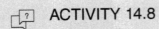 ACTIVITY 14.8

Access the following websites and read the above documents related to CPR:

Decisions relating to cardiopulmonary resuscitation – guidance from the British Medical Association, the Resuscitation Council and the Royal College of Nursing:

file://nask.man.ac.uk/home$/20160123%20Decisions%20Relating%20to%20CPR%20-%20 2016.pdf;

www.resus.org.uk/pages/dnar.pdf.

Access and read the following British Psychological Society document: Joyce, T. (2007) *Best Interests Guidance on Determining the Best Interests of Adults who Lack the Capacity to Make a Decision (or Decisions) for Themselves (England and Wales)*. Leicester: The British Psychological Society.

---

• How could you use the guidance above to inform the decision-making process when considering Jack's 'best interests'?

## Organ and tissue donation

The UK has approximately 600,000 deaths annually, 290,000 occurring within the hospital environment (Office for National Statistics [ONS], 2017; NHS Blood and Transplant, 2017a). A small group of patients being cared for in critical care environments have the potential to become organ donors after death. During the financial year 2016–17, 1413 patients donated their organs to help other people with lifesaving and life-enhancing transplant operations (NHS Blood and Transplant, 2017b). The number of patients waiting for an organ transplant far outstrips the number of donated organs. As at 31 March 2017, 6388 patients were on the active transplant waiting list. Many of these patients have to wait months, even years, for their transplant and, sadly, some patients die while waiting. On average, three people on the transplant waiting list die every day because no suitable donor organ had been identified (NHS Blood and Transplant, 2017b).

The three categories of organ donation include donation following brainstem death (DBD), donation following circulatory death (DCD) and living donation. Deceased organ donation is only possible from the DBD and DCD route, usually within the critical care areas. Clinically, the patient is often on mechanical ventilation and vasoactive drugs. DBD arises when brainstem death testing confirms the absence of brainstem reflexes (Academy of Medical Royal Colleges, 2008; Bleakley, 2017). DCD occurs following the withdrawal of life-sustaining treatment (WLST). Living donation occurs when a healthy person donates an organ to an identified recipient, as either a directed donation (the donor may have genetic or pre-existing emotional relationship) or a directed altruistic donation, whereby the donor and recipient have no qualifying genetic or pre-existing emotional relationship (Human Tissue Authority, 2017).

---

### ACTIVITY 14.9

The Organ Donation and Transplantation (ODT) clinical website provides online learning resources that are useful and informative. Access the website below and search for the different types of organs and tissue that can be donated: www.odt.nhs.uk.

---

A clinical plan to perform brainstem death testing or planned withdrawal of life-sustaining treatment on a critically ill patient should trigger an urgent referral to the on-call specialist nurse–organ donation (SNOD). The SNOD is specifically trained to facilitate all aspects of the donation process, including initiating donation conversations with distressed relatives/carers. The refusal rate for organ donation in the UK is significantly higher than other European countries, fixed at 42%. Refusal of family consent for organ and tissue donation is the single greatest barrier to lifesaving and life-enhancing transplants (Hulme et al., 2016). Consent rates for donation are significantly higher if the approach is made by the SNOD, working collaboratively with the clinical team.

NHS Blood and Transplant have produced guidance on how best to approach a relative/carer with an organ donation request. As identified by Kübler-Ross (1969), normal grief response observes the relative/carer enter a primary state of denial after the delivery of bad news. Nurses need to be mindful of the inner turmoil experienced by relatives/carers before making an approach. Best practice encourages nurses to make a referral to the on-call SNOD and gain expert advice (NICE, 2011; Bleakley, 2010). Critical care areas often have extensive resources regarding organ and tissue donation, including the pager/telephone number for the on-call specialist. Figure 14.2 provides a suitable structure to plan for difficult donation discussions.

Organ donation occurs with a specific and small number of deaths in critical care areas, but nearly every other death in a hospital or community setting has the potential for tissue donation. It is helpful to establish known wishes before initiating donation discussion. This requires nurses to routinely check the organ donor register (ODR) after the death of a patient. The ODR is a confidential NHS database that can be accessed 24 hours a day, 7 days a week, allowing clinical staff to assess whether a patient has already made their donation wishes known. Even if the patient has a known absolute contraindication to donation, it is helpful to inform the relative/carer that donation was not possible due to a specific clinical reason. This approach ensures that donation is embraced as a normal part of end of life care within the clinical setting and, more importantly, does not leave the relative/carer wondering whether or not donation was possible (DH, 2008). Many clinical settings are specialised, with intricate disease processes contributing to the death of a

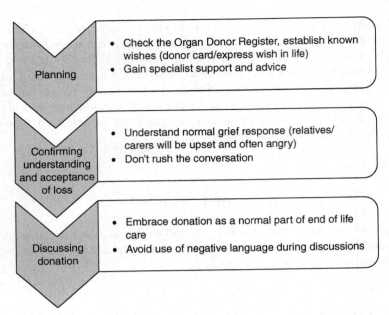

**Planning**
- Check the Organ Donor Register, establish known wishes (donor card/express wish in life)
- Gain specialist support and advice

**Confirming understanding and acceptance of loss**
- Understand normal grief response (relatives/carers will be upset and often angry)
- Don't rush the conversation

**Discussing donation**
- Embrace donation as a normal part of end of life care
- Avoid use of negative language during discussions

**Figure 14.2** Consent: the family approach. (Adapted from NHS Blood and Transplant, 2017b). More details available at: www.odt.nhs.uk/deceased-donation/best-practice-guidance/consent-and-authorisation

patient. It is important that nurses do not to make any judgement on whether the patient is a suitable candidate for organ and tissue donation. Remember to gain specialist advice from the SNOD or specialist nurse in the National Referral Centre (NRC) for tissue donation and allow these professionals to make the clinical judgement on suitability.

 **ACTIVITY 14.10**

Access the following link and identify the process for contacting the NHS Blood and Transplant Duty Office to check the Organ Donor Register (ODR): http://odt.nhs.uk/donation/deceased-donation/organ-donation-services/odt-duty-office-functions.

If you are working within an acute NHS hospital care setting, find out the contact details for the SNOD who can be contacted for professional advice, training and further support.

## GEORGE

You are a student nurse working on the acute medical unit (AMU). Working with your mentor, you admit 59-year-old George who has increasing shortness of breath (dyspnoea) with underlying ischaemic heart disease (IHD). His clinical condition rapidly deteriorates and he experiences a cardiorespiratory arrest. Despite advanced life support (ALS) from the resuscitation team, the decision is taken to stop CPR and death is confirmed. Following your involvement with the cardiac arrest, you discuss care after the death process with your practice supervisor. You have a thought that tissue donation might be an option. It appears no one has considered donation as an end of life option and notice that George's partner is tearful and distressed at the bedside. You mention donation to your mentor who agrees to support you with a donation request.

- How would you check the Organ Donor Register to establish if George has made his donation wishes clear?
- What are your immediate plans to initiate the donation discussion with George's partner?
- What words are you going to use during the donation request?

## Supporting the families of critically ill patients

When a person is acutely unwell the psychological distress within family members is an inherent factor that a nurse needs to be mindful of and they should do their utmost to provide appropriate support. Informing an individual that their loved one has become acutely unwell and is possibly moving to a department such as an ICU can illicit the same response outlined elsewhere in the book when breaking bad news. The ability to calm feelings of panic and distress felt by patients, family and friends is an important aspect of care that cannot be overlooked, and will place significant demands on your communication skills and ability to demonstrate empathy, compassion and understanding. For example, the society we currently live in is diverse and as a nurse you will encounter very different types of 'family'. In fact, due to this the term 'significant other' is often used. A lot of high care areas such as ICUs have very strict visiting rules related to family only, and yet as adults we have more than family who may want to visit and support the acutely unwell person. These restrictions can put increased strain on an already stressed individual trying to visit. In addition, families may be left waiting while interventions are carried out, such as a line insertion or X-rays. Nursing staff must remain vigilant in updating families and visitors about the reasons why they have been asked to wait.

The families of those admitted to an ICU are often in a highly anxious state and are confronted with a highly technical environment with their loved one at the centre, so it is vital they are adequately supported. Families can provide a crucial contribution to the person's care. Many patients, after an ICU stay, have problems recalling elements of their illness and care and families can provide this insight into the experience. More importantly families can be provided with reassurance and support. A study conducted by Kean (2014), which explored how ICU nurses perceived families, found that patients' families made a notable contribution to patient care; however, the nursing staff felt they needed to remain in control of that involvement.

If the patient or the patient's 'significant other' is happy with a visitor then do you think we should be able to gate keep in this way?

What factors would influence your decision to limit visiting?

How do you feel about families witnessing resuscitation? Find out what the policy is in your placement area in relation to families witnessing resuscitation.

You may want to read the guidance from the Resuscitation Council (UK) at www.resus.org.uk.

Reflect on the placements you have already experienced:

What sort of reception do families and visitors get?

Access and read the Intensive Care Society's (1998) *Guidelines for Bereavement Care in Intensive Care Units*.

## After critical care

Patients and their families can often feel anxious and apprehensive about the move from critical care to a ward environment. The patient and the family will need lots of reassurance and may have many questions about their care. The patient may be experiencing significant changes in their body image or mobility, appetite and sleep, as well as the physiological impact of surviving a critical illness. Many ICU patients have difficulty remembering their time during their critical illness, and some departments use patient diaries compiled by family and staff to support and address these gaps in memories. To ensure continuity of care, the patient's rehabilitation care pathway should be coordinated and communicated to the new nursing team.

### The NICE (2017) document on rehabilitation after critical illness in adults states that

*Quality statement 1: Rehabilitation goals*: adults in critical care at risk of morbidity have their rehabilitation goals agreed within 4 days of admission to critical care or before discharge from critical care, whichever is sooner;

*Quality statement 2*: Transfer from critical care to a general ward: adults at risk of morbidity have a formal handover of care, including their agreed individualised structured rehabilitation programme, when they transfer from critical care to a general ward;

*Quality statement 3*: Information on discharge from hospital: adults who were in critical care and at risk of morbidity are given information based on their rehabilitation goals before they are discharged from hospital;

*Quality statement 4*: Follow-up after critical care discharge: adults who stayed in critical care for more than 4 days and were at risk of morbidity have a review 2–3 months after discharge from critical care.
(Reproduced with permission under the NICE UK Open Content Licence)

Although the guidelines are clear and useful for healthcare staff, they address the care and rehabilitation of the patient only within the hospital setting. Stepping down from critical care is challenging for the patient, family and ward-based staff. The needs of a patient post-critical illness are complex and the patient is often vulnerable. It is well documented that patients experience intense anxiety when being discharged from the critical care unit (Kauppi et al., 2018). Readmission to critical care is associated with increased mortality. Discharging the patient too quickly, without appropriate resources and poor communication, contributes towards poor patient outcomes. Stepping down from critical care has to be planned, controlled and appropriate (Kauppi et al., 2018).

## NASAR

Nasar is a 58-year-old man who had a 3-month stay in ICU admission due to sepsis. He required the insertion of a temporary tracheostomy and was sedated and ventilated for a number of weeks. He had a long period of time being weaned from his ventilator. He was transferred to the ward where he stayed for a further two weeks. During this time his tracheostomy was removed; however, he remained weak with a significant loss of muscle mass and experiences nightmares and flashbacks from ICU admission. He also has residual renal impairment following his illness.

He is now fit for discharge.

Consider the implications of this patient being discharged home. What do the community nursing team need to be aware of?

How effective do you think our current strategies of communicating patient history across services are?

## Chapter summary

Nurses have a central role in ensuring safe patient care. This chapter has discussed some of the knowledge, skills and attributes needed by adult nurses working in a critical care setting. Medical technology is part of the modern healthcare environment and is not limited to critical care areas. A nurse should use appropriate technology for the benefit of patients but also be aware of the potential of over-reliance. It is important to remember that the critical care environment can be a scary place for patients and their families, so the importance of compassion in nursing cannot be over-emphasised. An admission to a critical care environment can be the result of a vast range of reasons that we are unable to cover in this chapter, but we hope this will provide a springboard for your interest in critical care nursing.

Remember the ABG question? The patient was hypoxic, with respiratory acidosis and chronic renal compensation – did you get the same answer?

## Useful websites

For information on different types of arrhythmias, their causes and treatments, see the following websites:

www.nhs.uk/conditions/arrhythmia/Pages/arrhythmia.aspx.

www.bhf.org.uk/heart-health/conditions/abnormal-heart-rhythms.aspx.

www.bhf.org.uk/publications/heart-conditions/m111a-inherited-heart-conditions---sudden-arrythmic-death-syndrome.

www.bhf.org.uk/publications/heart-conditions/heart-rhythms.

www.heartrhythmalliance.org/aa/uk.

## Further reading

Bickley, L.S. (2013) *Bates' Guide to Physical Examination and History Taking*, 11th edn. Philadelphia, PA: Lippincott, Williams & Wilkins.

Brooker, C. and Nichol, M. (2011) *Alexander's Nursing Practice*, 4th edn. London: Churchill Livingstone.

National Institute for Health and Care Excellence (2012) *Patient Experience in Adult NHS Services: Improving the Experience of Care for People Using Adult NHS Services*. NICE Clinical Guidance 138. London: NICE.

O'Driscoll, B.R., Howard, L.S. and Davison, A.G., on behalf of the British Thoracic Society (2008) 'Guideline for the emergency oxygen use in adult patients', *Thorax*, 63(Suppl VI).
Resuscitation Council (UK) (2011) *Immediate Life Support Manual*, 3rd edn. London: Resuscitation Council.
Tait, D., James, J., Williams, C. and Bartion, D. (2016) *Acute and Critical Care in Adult Nursing*, 2nd edn. London: Sage.

# References

Academy of Medical Royal Colleges (2008) *A Code of Practice for the Diagnosis of Death*. Portsmouth: PPG Design and Print Ltd.
Alcan, A., Giersbergen, M.Y., Dinscarslan, G., Hepcivici, Z., Kaya, E. and Uyar, M. (2016) 'Effect of patient position on endotracheal cuff pressure in mechanically ventilated critically ill patients', *Australian Critical Care*, 30(5): 267–72.
Arshad, H., Young, M., Adurty, R. and Singh, A.C. (2016) 'Acute pneumothorax', *Critical Care Nursing*, 39(2): 176–89.
Barr, J., Fraser, G.L., Puntillo, K., Ely, E.W., Gélinas, C., Dasta, J.F., Davidson, J.E., Devlin, J.W., Kress, J.P., Joffe, A.M. et al. (2013) 'Clinical practice guidelines for the management of pain, agitation, and delirium in adult patients in the intensive care unit', *Critical Care Medicine*, 41(1): 263–306.
Benson, S., Johnson, A. and Petera, C. (2013) 'VAP Free for 1000 days, it can be done', *Critical Care Nursing*, 36(4): 421–4.
Bleakley, G. (2010) 'Implementing minimum notification criteria for organ donation in an acute hospital's critical care units', *Nursing in Critical Care*, 15(4): 185–91.
Bleakley, G. (2017) 'Understanding brainstem death testing', *British Journal of Neuroscience Nursing*, 13(4): 172–7.
Boore, J., Cook, N. and Shepard, A. (2016) *Essentials of Anatomy and Physiology for Nursing Practice*. London: Sage.
British Medical Association, the Resuscitation Council (UK) and the Royal College of Nursing (2014) *Decisions Relating to Cardiopulmonary Resuscitation*, 3rd edn. (Guidance from the British Medical Association, the Resuscitation Council (UK) and the Royal College of Nursing [previously known as the 'Joint Statement']). Available at: http://resus.org.uk/pages/dnacpr.htm.
Chen, H.-B., Liu, J., Chen, L.-Q. and Wang, G.-C. (2014) 'Effectiveness of daily interruption of sedation in sedated patients with mechanical ventilation in ICU: a systematic review', *International Journal of Nursing Sciences*, 1(4): 346–51.
Critical Care 3 Network (2015) *National Competency Framework (steps 1–4)*. Available at: http://cc3n.org.uk/competency-framework/4577977310 (last accessed 21 August 2018).
Department of Health (2000) *Comprehensive Critical Care. A Review of Adult Critical Care Services*. London: DH.
Department of Health (2008) *Organs for Transplant: A Report from the Organ Donation Taskforce*. London: DH.
Department of Health (2009) *Consent for Examination, Treatment or Care*. London: DH. Available at: https://www.health-ni.gov.uk/articles/consent-examination-treatment-or-care (last accessed 20 May 2018).
Department of Health/Emergency Care (2005) *Quality Critical Care – Beyond 'Comprehensive Critical Care'*. London: DH/Emergency Care. Available at: http://webarchive.nationalarchives.gov.uk/20130124071030/http://www.dh.gov.uk/prod_consum_dh/groups/dh_digitalassets/@dh/@en/documents/digitalasset/dh_4121050.pdf (last accessed 21 August 2018).
Ding, Q., Redeker, N.S., Pisani, M.A., Yaggi, H.K. and Knauert, M.P. (2017) 'Factors influencing patients' sleep in the intensive care unit: perceptions of patients and clinical staff', *America Journal of Critical Care*, 26(4): 278–86.
Drahnak, D.M. and Custer, N. (2015) 'Prone positioning of patients with acute respiratory distress syndrome', *Critical Care Nurse*, 35(6): 29–37.

Ely, E.W., Inouye, S.K., Bernard, G.R., Francis, J., May, L., Truman, B., Speroff, T., Gautam, S., Margolin, R., Hart, R.P. and Dittus, R. (2001) 'Delirium in mechanically ventilated patients: validity and reliability of the Confusion Assessment Method for the Intensive Care Unit (CAM-ICU)', *Journal of the American Medical Association*, 286: 2703–10.

Freeman, S. (2011) 'Care of adult patients with a temporary tracheostomy', *Nursing Standard*, 26(2): 49–56.

Griffiths, R.D. and Jones, C. (2007) 'Deliriums, cognitive dysfunction and posttraumatic stress disorder', *Current Opinion in Anaesthesiology*, 20(2): 124–9.

Guenther, U., Weykam, J., Andorfer, U., Theuerkauf, N., Poop, J., Ely, W. and Putensen, C. (2012) 'Implications of objective vs subjective delirium assessment in surgical intensive care patients', *American Journal of Critical Care*, 21(1): 12–20.

Hellyer, T.P., Ewan, V. and Wilson, P. (2016) 'The Intensive Care Society recommended bundle of interventions for the prevention of ventilator-associated pneumonia', *Journal of the Intensive Care Society*, 17(3): 238–43.

Higginson, R., Jones, B. and Davies, K. (2011) 'Emergency and intensive care: assessing and managing the airway', *British Journal of Nursing*, 20(16): 973–7.

Hu, R.-F., Jiang, H.R.F., Chen, J., Zeng, Z., Chen, X.Y., Li, Y., Huining, X. and Evans, D.J. (2015) 'Non pharmacological interventions for sleep promotion in the intensive care unit', *Cochrane Database of Systematic Reviews*, doi:10.1002/14651858.CD008808.pub2.

Hulme, W., Allen, J., Manara, A.R., Murphy, P., Gardiner, D. and Poppitt, E. (2016) 'Factors influencing the family consent rate for organ donation in the UK', *Anaesthesia*, 17(9): 1053–63.

Human Tissue Authority (2017) *Types of Living Donation*. Available at: www.hta.gov.uk/guidance-public/living-organ-donation/types-living-organ-donation (last accessed 18 July 2017).

Intensive Care Society (1998) *Guidelines for Bereavement Care in Intensive Care Units*. London: The Intensive Care Society.

Intensive Care Society (2008) *Standards for the Care of Adult Patients with a Temporary Tracheostomy*. London: The Intensive Care Society.

Intensive Care Society (2014) *Review of Best Practice for Analgesia and Sedation in Critical Care*. London: Intensive Care Society.

Intensive Care Society (2015) *Guidelines for the Provision of Intensive Care Services*. London: Intensive Care Society.

Kauppi, W., Proos, M. and Olausson, S. (2018) 'Ward nurses' experiences of the discharge process between intensive care unit and general ward', *Nursing in Critical Care*, 23(3): 127–33.

Kean, S. (2014) 'How do intensive care nurses perceive families in intensive care? Insights from the United Kingdom and Australia', *Journal of Clinical Nursing*, 23(5–6): 663–72.

Krahne, D., Heymann, A. and Spies, C. (2006) 'How to monitor delirium in the ICU and why it is important', *Clinical Effectiveness in Nursing*, 269–79.

Kübler-Ross, E. (1969) *On Death and Dying*. London: Tavistock Publications.

McDonald, K., Page, K., Brown, L. and Bryden, D. (2012) 'Parenteral nutrition in critical care', *Continuing Education in Anaesthesia Critical Care & Pain*, 13(1): 1–5.

Makic, M.B.F. (2015) 'Rethinking mobility and intensive care patients', *Journal of Perianesthesia Nursing*, 30(2): 151–2.

Maldonado, J.R. (2008) 'Delirium in the acute care setting: characteristics, diagnosis and treatment', *Critical Care Clinics*, 24: 657–722.

Mehta, S., Bury, L. and Cook, D. (2012) 'Daily sedation interruption in mechanically ventilated critically ill patients cared for with a sedation protocol: a randomized controlled trial', *Journal of the American Medical Association*, 308(19): 1985–92.

National Institute for Health and Care Excellence (2010) *Delirium: Diagnosis, Prevention and Management*. London: NICE.

National Institute for Health and Care Excellence (2011) *Organ Donation for Transplantation: Improving Donor Identification and Consent Rates for Deceased Organ Donation*, Clinical Guidance 135. London: NICE. Available at: www.nice.org.uk/guidance/cg135.

National Institute for Health and Care Excellence (2014) *Atrial Fibrillation: Management*, Clinical Guidance CG180. London: NICE. Available at: www.nice.org.uk/guidance/cg180.

National Institute for Health and Care Excellence (2015) *Critical Care Outreach Teams Emergency and Acute Medical Care in Over 16s: Service Delivery and Organisation*. London: NICE. Available at: www.nice.org.uk/guidance/ng94/evidence/27.critical-care-outreach-teams-pdf-172397464640 (last accessed 21 August 2018).

National Institute for Health and Care Excellence (2017) *Rehabilitation after Critical Illness*, Clinical Guidance QS158. London: NICE. Available at: www.nice.org.uk/guidance/qs158.

Neuville, M., Mourvillier, B., Bouadma, L. and Timsit, J.-F. (2017) 'Bundle of care decreased ventilator-associated events: implications for ventilator-associated pneumonia prevention', *Journal of Thoracic Disease*, 9(3): 430–3.

NHS Blood and Transplant (2017a) *Transplant Activity Report*. Available at: https://nhsbtdbe.blob.core. windows.net/umbraco-assets-corp/4657/activity_report_2016_17.pdf (last accessed 15 March 2018).

NHS Blood and Transplant (2017b) *Consent: The Family Approach*. Available at: www.odt.nhs.uk/deceased-donation/best-practice-guidance/consent-the-family-approach (last accessed 16 June 2017).

Nursing and Midwifery Council (2018) *Future Nurse: Standards of Proficiency for Registered Nurses*. London: NMC.

Office for National Statistics (2017) *Deaths Registered in England and Wales: 2015*. Available at: www.ons. gov.uk/peoplepopulationandcommunity/birthsdeathsandmarriages/deaths/bulletins/deathsregistrationsum marytables/2015 (last accessed 18 July 2017).

Pattison, N. and Eastham, E. (2011) 'Critical care outreach referrals: a mixed-method investigative study of outcomes and experiences', *Nursing in Critical Care*, 17(2): 71–82.

Public Health England (2015) *National End of Life Care Intelligence Network. What we know now 2014*. London: PHE.

Resuscitation Council (UK) (2015) *Immediate Life Support Manual*, 3rd edn. London: Resuscitation Council (UK).

Ryan, D.J., O'Regan, N.A., Caoimh, R.Ó., Clare, J., O'Connor, M., Leonard, M., McFarland, J., Tighe, S., O'Sullivan, K., Trzepaczk, P.T. et al. (2013) 'Delirium in an adult acute hospital population: predictors, prevalence and detection', *BMJ Open*, 3: e001772. doi:10.1136/bmjopen-2012-001772.

Scaravilli, V., Grasselli, G., Castagna, L., Zanella, A., Isgro, S., Lucchini, A., Patroniti, N., Bellani, G. and Pesenti, A. (2015) 'Prone positioning improves oxygenation in spontaneously breathing nonintubated patients with hypoxemic acute respiratory failure: a retrospective study', *Journal of Critical Care*, 30(6): 1390–4.

Scholz, A.W., Weiler, N., David, M. and Markstaller, K. (2011) 'Respiratory mechanics measured by forced oscillations during mechanical ventilation through a tracheal tube', *Physiological Measures*, 32(5): 571–83.

Singh, S. (2016) 'Respiratory symptoms and signs', *Medicine*, 44(4): 205–12.

Stationery Office, The (2007) *Mental Capacity Act Code of Practice*. London: TSO. Available at: www.gov. uk/government/publications/mental-capacity-act-code-of-practice (last accessed 21 August 2018).

Vincent, J.-L., Jaschinski, U., Wittebole, X., Lefrant, J.-Y., Jakob, S.M., Almekhlafi, G.A. et al., on behalf of the ICON Investigators (2018) 'Worldwide audit of blood transfusion practice in critically ill patients', *Critical Care*, 22: 102.

Whitehouse, T., Snelson, C., Grounds, M., Willson, J., Tulloch, L., Linhartova, L., Shah, A., Pierson, R. and England, K. (2014) *Review of Best Practice for Analgesia and Sedation in Critical Care*. Available at: www.ics.ac.uk/ICS/Guidelines___Standards/ICS/guidelines-and-standards.aspx?hkey=4ed20a1c-1ff8-46e0-b48e-732f1f4a90e2.

# THE PROVISION OF EFFECTIVE PALLIATIVE CARE FOR ADULTS

## JOHN COSTELLO

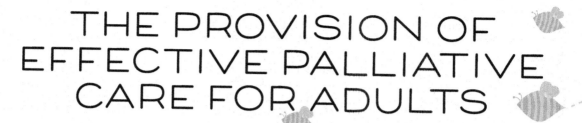

---

**CHAPTER OBJECTIVES**

- Demonstrate a clear understanding of the way in which palliative care for adults has been developed in the UK;
- Explain the principles of palliative care and identify key policies and standards that underpin an evidence-based approach;
- Discuss the importance of effective communication and therapeutic relationships in exploring patient choice and preferences in end of life care;
- Discuss the legal and ethical issues associated with end of life care and advanced planning decisions;
- Describe and discuss what constitutes a good death for the patient, the family and health practitioners;
- Describe the role of the nurse in meeting the needs of informal caregivers;
- Describe effective end of life care for the patient and the family, including how to initiate, implement and carry out culturally competent care effectively and sensitively.

---

Most people in the UK die in hospital (National End of Life Care Intelligence Network, see www.endoflifecare-intelligence.org.uk/home [accessed 8 October 2013]), with around 58% of people dying in acute hospital settings (Gardiner et al., 2013). An essential part of adult nursing involves you having the competence and confidence to care for patients with a life-limiting illness, providing them with high-quality palliative care. The challenges associated with this lie in your ability not only to give high-quality care to the patient but also to offer psychosocial support to the family. In many respects palliative care constitutes the essence of what is referred to as holistic care, in the real sense of enabling both the patient and the family to experience what is referred to as a good death (Costello, 2006).

This chapter introduces some of the key issues relating to palliative care for adults, providing explanations about terms such as 'a good death' and how these can be applied in the context of adult nursing. End of life care should reflect contemporary developments in policy and practice, as well as considering the challenges of caring for patients who live with a life-limiting illness and are cared for in hospitals, community and hospice settings.

The main focus of the chapter will be based on the acute hospital context because this is where most patients in the UK die. The essence of much of end of life care for adults has been to transfer the gold standards of care often seen in hospices into the acute hospital care context. Strategies and contemporary developments that have formed part of contemporary palliative care (e.g. Integrated Care Pathways, the Gold Standard Framework and Preferred Priorities of Care; Department of Health [DH], 2004) will be explained and discussed. There is an assumption here that you are aware that end of life care (in the past referred to as terminal care) is an integral and important part of the palliative care approach. One of the central features of end of life care is the ability of a registered nurse to demonstrate effective communication skills with the patient, family and other multiprofessional team colleagues. The development of a therapeutic relationship with the patient forms a significant part of the final section of the chapter and constitutes a key element of its take-home message.

## Related NMC proficiencies for registered nurses

The overarching requirements of the Nursing and Midwifery Council (NMC) are that all registered nurses must act in the best interests of people, putting them first and providing nursing care that is person centred, safe and compassionate. They must take the lead in providing evidence-based, compassionate and safe nursing interventions, managing the complex nursing and integrated care needs of people at any stage of their lives, across a range of organisations and settings. They must work in partnership with people, families and carers to evaluate whether the goals of care have been met in line with their wishes, preferences and desired outcomes (NMC, 2018a).

 **To achieve entry to the nursing register you must be able to**

- Take appropriate action to ensure privacy and dignity at all times;
- Understand and apply DNACPR (Do Not Attempt Cardiopulmonary Resuscitation) decisions and verification of expected death;
- Engage in difficult conversations, including breaking bad news, and support people who are feeling emotionally or physically vulnerable or in distress, conveying compassion and sensitivity;
- Identify and assess the needs of people and families for care at the end of life, including requirements for palliative care and decision making related to their treatment and care preferences;
- Understand and apply advanced planning decisions, living wills and health, and lasting powers of attorney;
- Assess and review preferences and care priorities of the dying person and their family and carers;
- Demonstrate the knowledge and skills required to prioritise what is important to people and their families when providing evidence-based, person-centred nursing care at the end of life, including the care of people who are dying, families, the deceased and the bereaved;
- Provide care for the deceased person and the bereaved, respecting cultural requirements and protocols.

(Adapted from NMC, 2018a)

# Background

The term 'palliative' in its Latin translation means 'to cloak' and can cause confusion among health professionals and lay caregivers. It is often used by medical staff when other active methods of intervention are ineffective, or when it is clear that the patient's condition is no longer susceptible to curative methods of treatment. The confusion about when and what constitutes palliative care is part of the problem that many nurses have in explaining to families what is happening to patients. Palliative care is focused on patients with a life-limiting illness (not necessarily cancer) when the chances of curative treatment are diminished.

Historically, palliative care emerged from the hospice movement during the 1960s when one of the first hospices (St Christopher's) was built in 1967 based on the pioneering work of Dame Cecily Saunders. Saunders trained as a nurse in 1948, became a medical social worker and finally a physician. Not only did she care for dying patients, but she was also a prolific writer, publishing her work internationally. She is regarded as the founder of St Christopher's Hospice, the first research and teaching hospice linked with clinical care and focused on palliative medicine. Saunders was dismayed when, as a nurse, she cared for dying patients experiencing distress at the end of life. Her motivation to improve standards partly stemmed from the poor prescribing habits of medical staff who, at the time, were reluctant to prescribe morphine to patients in pain. Saunders wanted patients to receive what is referred to as tender loving care (TLC) and for both patients and family members to experience a good death (Saunders et al., 2003). Her famous quote – 'You matter because you are you, and you matter to the end of your life. We will do all we can not only to help you die peacefully, but also to live until you die' – epitomises her concept of total pain and the notion that patients are more than a set of symptoms. Her philosophy was based on the provision of physical, psychological, social and spiritual care from the time of diagnosis until death.

Before reading and working with this chapter, it is appropriate to point out that some of the content and interactive text could potentially cause some readers to become emotional because the case studies reflect authentic situations. The text may cause you to recall sad and painful experiences or you may feel empathy with what is being discussed. It is entirely natural that you may feel this way. As a way of helping you consider your feelings in relation to thinking about loss, try to reflect on your past loss experiences and consider undertaking Activity 15.1 below. The completion of this should help you focus on the loss and its impact. It is not uncommon for nurses to feel emotional and upset when managing patients with a life-limiting illness, it is an indication that we feel for others. It is perhaps more worrying when we do not feel slightly emotional when working with patients and families at the end of life.

## ACTIVITY 15.1

We are all affected by loss, be it the death of a family pet or the death of a relative, grandparent, friend or a patient to whom we felt emotionally close. The impact of loss can influence our thoughts, feelings and ideas and how we approach palliative provision. It is useful to reflect on your own losses. This activity requires you to make a short list of three or four significant losses that have occurred in your life. 'Loss lines' (Figure 15.1) asks you to draw a line for every loss that you have experienced in your life. The length of each horizontal line denotes its emotional intensity. Some lines may be shorter than others. The aim of the activity is to get you to reflect on loss and its impact on how you felt. It's also worth considering what sources of support were available and how you used these.

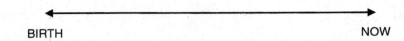

**Figure 15.1**  Loss line

Loss lines are a useful exercise to do with family members who may be feeling confused or uncertain about what their feelings are. It can help put their thoughts and ideas into perspective. It is therefore helpful if you do the exercise yourself and consider what helped you manage the loss and how you feel as a result of it (Figure 15.2). Do you still feel that there are issues that you could and should have resolved, or do you, as the proverb states, feel stronger as a result of the experience on the basis of that which does not kill you makes you stronger?

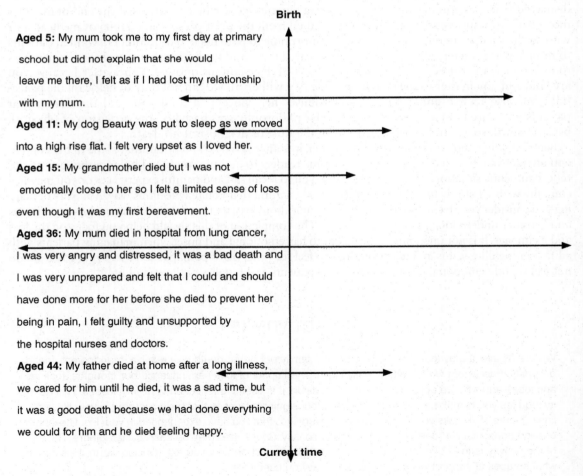

**Figure 15.2**  Author's loss line

# Diagnosing dying

A major challenge for palliative care practitioners is knowing when a patient is approaching death. The need for preparation and planning is important if the patient's death is to be well managed. Effective palliative care involves closely monitoring patients whose medical condition has become life threatening. Moreover, one of the major challenges facing many healthcare practitioners, and particularly nurses, has always been to identify when a patient has reached the point where active treatment is no longer an option (Broeckaert, 2008).

Ellershaw et al. (2010) point out that, when it is suspected that a patient is dying because of a significant deterioration in their condition, a number of considerations need to be made. In the early days of the Liverpool Care Pathway, ideas around when a patient was dying were based on key criteria. These consisted of a series of questions such as: 'Is the patient bed bound?' 'What is the patient's level of consciousness, are they semi-comatose?' 'Are they able to swallow and take sips of water?' Finally, 'can they take oral medication?' Should the patient fulfil two of these criteria then it may be considered that they are likely to be in the advanced stages of dying or near to death. Elliott and Nicholson (2017) suggest that practitioners considering patients' proximity to death ask the 'surprise' question: 'Would you be surprised if the patient were to die in the next few months, weeks or days?' If the answer is 'no' then the patient may be considered to be entering the dying phase.

Successful assessment of a patient's illness trajectory involves a thorough multidisciplinary team (MDT) assessment. Initially this is carried out when the patient is showing signs of deterioration. It is important to eliminate potentially reversible causes for the deterioration (such as an infection or opioid toxicity).

- Identify the role of each member of the multidisciplinary team in the assessment highlighted above. Which professionals might contribute to the assessment process and what might their individual roles involve?

The nurse would probably be the first person to recognise deterioration in a patient's condition. Assessment may involve the speech and language therapist assessing swallowing ability, or the physiotherapist assessing respiratory function. A patient who is very dehydrated, especially an older person who has stopped eating and drinking for whatever reason, may show signs consistent with an acute deterioration and be temporarily confused and unable or unwilling to drink. All reversible causes should be acted upon where possible to improve the patient's condition. Second, should the patient not respond positively to such steps, the next step is the clinical decision-making stage. This is where the MDT decide if the patient is to receive palliative care. Third, and most importantly, it is at this stage that this decision involves the patient if appropriate, and/or the family, relatives and significant others. For many healthcare practitioners this can be the most difficult situation which requires tact, sensitivity and a good relationship with the family.

Once a patient is considered to be no longer eligible for active treatment, it is important to communicate this effectively with them and/or their relatives, family or significant others. This can be one of the most challenging situations a healthcare practitioner can face.

# The importance of communication

Developing effective communication with patients and families about the diagnosis and prognosis of a life-limiting illness, not just cancer, is an essential part of quality care (Wilkinson, 2002; Skilbeck and Payne, 2003; Davies et al., 2003; Fallowfield, 2005; Kurtz et al., 2005; Seymour and Horne, 2013). Hospitals in particular have been criticised for not providing effective communication to patients and examples of poor communication such as 'blocking behaviour', where nurses avoid discussing perceived sensitive areas of care or answer questions such as 'What is wrong with me?' or 'Do I have cancer?' by changing the subject and blocking attempts at communication. Failure to develop more open communication with patients has resulted in the UK health ombudsman receiving complaints from the public about poor end of life communication (Department of Health [DH], 2008). The study by Rogers et al. (2000), nearly two decades ago, highlighted the issues of poor communication, still evident today, that influenced the development of advanced communication courses throughout the UK. These courses use up-to-date, humanistic communication methods to train healthcare staff, emphasise the need for hospital staff to develop compassion and for nurses and doctors to demonstrate empathy. and develop what O'Connell (2008) and others call therapeutic relationships with patients. We will revisit this concept again later in the chapter.

## Disclosing sensitive information

Often referred to as breaking bad news, this term has been used for many years to identify the point at which the diagnosis of a life-threatening illness is disclosed (Arnautska, 2010). However, as many patients and family members may have become aware of the condition, the disclosure will not be news but a confirmation. Moreover, in terms of the extent to which sensitive information can be disclosed, there are many other things that practitioners can tell a patient/family that are just as sensitive, such as the withdrawal/withholding of treatment, or a decision not to resuscitate in the event of a cardiac/respiratory arrest, which can have a devastating impact on their wellbeing. It seems logical, therefore, to consider some guidance based on published work around breaking bad news. Numerous authors have identified ways of disclosing sensitive information: including Buckman (1992), Baile et al. (2000) and Fallowfield (2005). Notable among these is the SPIKES model (Baile et al., 2000), which offers a clear and concise series of steps to follow that are both understandable and sensitive.

Step 1: S – SETTING UP the interview;

Step 2: P – Assessing the patient's PERCEPTION;

Step 3: I – Obtaining the patient's INVITATION;

Step 4: K – Giving KNOWLEDGE and information to the patient;

Step 5: E – Addressing the patient's EMOTIONS with empathic responses;

Step 6: S – STRATEGY and SUMMARY.

However, taking an eclectic approach by utilising the key components of a number of models, various principles emerge that can be seen as guidance for best practice. These principles are summarised in the following illustration.

## ———— PRINCIPLES OF BREAKING BAD NEWS ————

Preparation of the setting, including the availability of documents, such as medical notes: this can include giving the patient the opportunity to invite a friend.

Warning shot: this is an important principle that helps prepare the patient psychologically: 'I am afraid the news is rather bad; I am sorry but the results are not good'.

Pause: allow the patient time to consider the news.

Provide a clear/concise account: 'I am afraid you have cancer' or 'The results indicate cancer.'

Clarify: 'The cancer is malignant, meaning that it is possible that it will spread.'

Elicit the patient's concerns: 'You may be feeling shocked by this result.'

Express treatment aspirations: 'We can and will provide treatment and care.'

## BRENDA

In the following situation consider what you, as a nurse, could do to help a patient in relation to trying to provide comfort and improve their wellbeing without being patronising.

Brenda was in bed and was just having a wash. While undertaking his usual ward round, Brenda's consultant decided to give her the result of her recent bronchoscopy. As the consultant was reading Brenda's medical notes, he gestured to the staff nurse to close the curtains. Then, without looking up from the notes, he initially told Brenda in a very matter of fact manner that the result of the bronchoscopy showed that she had a large mass in her windpipe that was causing the problem with breathing, but (then looked up and said) 'We have no way of removing a cancer this large as it has progressed rather rapidly'.

Brenda went pale and sagged in the bed 'What does that mean?' she said. The consultant replied that in his opinion she had a few weeks or months left and she should consider being admitted to a hospice for further care. The consultant pointed out that he appreciated that it was a difficult time but suggested she discuss things with the nurse and the hospital social worker. He then went on to continue with his rounds, leaving you alone with Brenda.

This sad and insensitive situation was obviously badly managed but could and should have been carried out in a more sensitive way. What could have been done to improve the situation in light of your reading and understanding of the SPIKES model?

Nurses will rarely disclose a diagnosis to a patient but many will deal with the aftermath of the encounter with another healthcare professional, something Costello (2004) refers to as the emotional rescue. Evidence suggests that, despite many years of education and training to improve communication about a life-threatening illness, many healthcare practitioners get it wrong (Smith et al., 2012). The role of the nurse in relation to receiving bad news is to provide comfort, sometimes in the form of reassurance arising not from platitudes that things will be all right but from clear reassurance and knowledge based on sound evidence. Moreover, nurses are in a position to provide information about the diagnosis and the likely reactions people make when they are given bad news.

Responding to a patient's emotions is one of the most difficult challenges of breaking bad news because their emotional response may vary from silence to disbelief, crying, denial or anger. When told bad news, a patient's emotional reaction can be expressed in many ways such as anger, shock, isolation and grief. The role of the nurse is to try to accurately identify the patient's reaction and make an empathic response. An empathic response consists of observing the patient's emotions, identifying their emotions (be they sad, angry or very distressed), and by expressing this in an understanding way (e.g. 'You sound very angry'). It is important to make an empathic response such as 'I can understand your anger' or 'You have every right to feel angry'. It is also important to connect the feeling with the response, e.g. 'I can see you are angry and this is justified'. Throughout the period after the bad news is broken the patient should be allowed time to express their feelings. Use open questions if you are unsure of what emotions are being expressed.

## Breaking bad news: where things go wrong

Sadly, breaking bad news is very difficult to get right because what may work for one patient will not always work every time. Having a set of principles such as the SPIKES model is useful to enable a consistent approach to be made, based on sound evidence. In relation to the previous case scenario, it is easy to pick out what went wrong here. However, it is more difficult to work out why the consultant chose to disclose the bad news then and there. For example, why did he not choose a more private place, with the patient's family there to provide support? Why did he not provide a sense of hope and discuss the possibility of palliative radiotherapy to arrest the growth and enable the patient to have some hope?

You will already be aware after reading Chapter 2 that the development of therapeutic relationships involves the promotion of trust and understanding between the patient and the nurse. Central to the development of such relationships is mutual respect for the patient and their situation. Considering the patient's situation and expressing empathy are very important, although difficult to achieve in some cases. A therapeutic relationship is often focused on enabling the patient's needs to be met in their current situation (O'Connell, 2008). By finding out what the patient's needs are (e.g. for dignity, privacy and respect) nurses can tangibly help to improve their situation.

In practical terms, developing and maintaining a therapeutic relationship with a patient requires the nurse to consciously spend time actively listening to that patient, allowing time to develop trust and respect for each other, and for the nurse to elicit the patient's needs and concerns about care and treatment. The development of empathy is a very difficult thing to do because often there may be many barriers to understanding a patient's situation, such as age, gender, culture, beliefs, religion, and a lack of understanding of the attitude and relationship between the patient and others. Many nurses find this hard to understand and have little empathy for patients who attempt suicide, take drugs and self-harm (McAllister et al., 2002).

The development of empathy is central to the provision of effective palliative care. Nyatanga (2013) points out that empathy for others is an ability to identify the emotional experience of others. In doing so we need to try to see things from the other person's viewpoint or to stand in their shoes and see the world as they see it. Sharing the suffering and grief of others and considering what it may be like to have a limited time left to live are a very challenging prospect for any individual, but are especially difficult if you are young. Noddings (2002) states that care providers must step out of their frame of reference and into the patient's situation and worldview. Although very noble and idealistic, this is by no means an easy task.

However, one way of helping to develop empathy is through education and training. The 'SAGE & THYME' model of communication (Connolly et al., 2010) was designed to assist healthcare professionals to learn to recognise and respond effectively to psychological distress, avoiding causing psychological harm, communicating honestly and compassionately, and knowing when they have reached the boundary of their competence. 'SAGE & THYME' is a mnemonic that guides healthcare professional/care workers into and out of a conversation with someone who is distressed or concerned. It provides a structure for psychological support by encouraging the health worker to hold back with advice and prompting the concerned person to consider their own solutions (Connolly et al., 2010).

## Contemporary end of life policy and standards

Contemporary end of life care has received a lot of attention through the government's strategy to develop, maintain and improve end of life care, encapsulated in the *End of Life Care Programme* (DH, 2008) which sets out to improve end of life care through effective communication, education and the development of high-quality, evidence-based care. The evidence is encapsulated in the quality standards from the National Institute for Health and Care Excellence (NICE, 2018), where quality end of life care for adults indicates the best practice to adopt for patients at the end of life. This covers all settings and services, providing end of life care to adults in the UK, including adults who die suddenly or after a very brief illness. The quality standard gives specific guidance on patients with advanced cancer, with special reference to the following areas:

- Patient and carer involvement;
- Psychological, social and spiritual support services;
- General and specialist palliative care services;
- Rehabilitation services;
- Complementary therapy services;
- Services for families and carers;
- Workforce development.

The guidance makes it clear that many patients in the past have unfortunately experienced suboptimal care because of poor interprofessional communication and lack of coordination. For these reasons, communication between MDTs as well as among patients, staff and caregivers needs to focus on involving patients and caregivers in decisions about their current and future care. The guidance also highlights a need for psychological, social and spiritual support services to be made available.

In the hospital context, this involves access to psychologists who can offer a range of services including psychosexual counselling. Hospital services should also offer access to a social work team who can provide help about issues from practical financial support up to and including bereavement after-care. For example, providing information and help to ensure access to Fast Track Continuing Healthcare ensures that a package of care can be agreed, arranged and funded to cover the cost of additional support for patients who have ongoing significant health needs, including those requiring palliative care (Age UK, 2017). Spiritual care services are provided in hospitals by spiritual care teams (traditionally referred to as the chaplains department). Hospitals and community services provide general and specialist palliative care services. These include nurses with no specialist palliative care experience up to and including Macmillan and Marie Curie nurse services, the latter being provided by hospital specialist palliative care services (HSPCS).

Often hospitals can transfer or offer beds for patients receiving palliative care, referred to as continuing care, which may be situated outside the hospital site, or in specialist units that offer rehabilitation. These may be disease specific, such as cancer care centres in regions throughout the UK that offer outpatient services to patients and their families. The availability of complementary therapy services is becoming widespread in the UK, especially in specialist oncology centres but also in many hospitals and all hospices. The latter services focus on care and emotional support for families and patients.

Furthermore, the NICE (2018) guidance stipulates a need for workforce development in order to provide training and education for hospital staff in palliative care. In many hospitals staff training takes place on a range of issues and palliative care is often among a range of topics offered. The role of education in palliative care is often the remit of the hospital specialist palliative care team, who often make a contribution to workforce development.

## Principles of palliative care

Palliative care is focused on a number of key principles that are largely associated with quality of life. Becker (2009) discusses the importance of ensuring that the patient is considered to be the central feature of care management, with the needs of the family a close second.

Many of the key principles of palliative care are encapsulated in Box 15.1. These principles suggest that, like other nursing specialisms, holistic care is required in order to ensure that the philosophy described by Saunders et al. (2003) is adhered to. In order to do this, nurses providing palliative care need to consider the needs of the family/significant others as very important.

There may come a point in the patient's illness trajectory when they are not conscious or in a persistent vegetative state (PVS). In such circumstances, the nurse provides all the care to the patient, but should also pay attention to the emotional needs of the family who may require as much emotional support as possible (Main, 2002). In circumstances whereby the patient does not have any meaningful social contact with those around them, it is important to enhance communication with family members. Sweeting and Gilhooly (1992) refer to patients unable to have any significant social contact with others as being 'socially dead'. This could include patients receiving artificial ventilation and/or those with advanced dementia. It is in such cases that the nurse and the rest of the team need to focus closely on family needs. Working as a team and collaborating together is one of the ideals of palliative care, although as McIlfatrick (2013) points out embracing this ideal is easier said than done. Despite this, working together as a team (including social workers, physiotherapists and the spiritual care team) is vital to the provision of high standards of care. The last is often more successful in hospice contexts than in hospitals where a curative ideology prevails (Costello, 2004).

## BOX 15.1   PRINCIPLES OF PALLIATIVE CARE

- Neither hastens nor postpones death
- Views death as a natural healthy process
- Emphasise the importance of quality of life

- Embraces the notion of team working
- Control of symptoms is a priority
- Focuses on the patient and the family
- Considers spiritual and psychosocial needs

(Adapted from Becker, 2010)

## Patient choices and preferences for end of life care

In 2015, the government commissioned a group of UK palliative care experts to advise them on what choices were important to patients and families at the end of life and after death. The group known as the Choice in End of Life Care Programme Board (2015) produced a report based on engagement with the public about their choices for end of life care. The report addresses the following issues:

- Patients wanted to die and be cared for in a place of their choice;
- They wanted involvement in and control over decisions relating to end of life care;
- Patients wanted access to high-quality care provided by well-trained staff and access to the right services when they were needed;
- Support for physical, emotional, social and spiritual needs;
- Support for those important to the patient and their involvement in care;
- Information about the patient to be shared with the right people at the right time.

Choice at the end of care is encapsulated in the notion of experiencing a good death (Costello, 2006). The Choice in End of Life Care Programme Board came up with a national choice offer. This is essentially what should be offered to all patients approaching end of life, and should be based on honest conversations with health- and social care staff, which could form part of advance care planning. Moreover, the board advises that the choices made should be consistently reviewed and documented through conversations with end of life care staff.

## Policy context: advance care planning

Advance care planning (ACP) is a key part of end of life care. Improving the pre-planning of care is one of the most important ways that nurses can ensure reliable patient-focused care. ACP is an integral part of the NHS End of Life Care Strategy (DH, 2008). Effective palliative care includes open discussion and ACP in order to enable the patient to experience a good death. This includes the use of a number of relatively recent innovations such as integrated care pathways (ICPs), the Gold Standard Framework (GSF) and the use of the Preferred Priorities of Care (PPC) document (DH, 2004). Such organisation can be very difficult to initiate if, for example, the patient is not aware that they are dying (Skilbeck and Payne, 2003). In such situations, the notion of ACP becomes problematic. Once it is established that curative treatment is no longer an option and this has been discussed with the patient and/or family, it is recommended that ACP can become a feature of the patient's end of life care (Ellershaw et al., 2010). However, when a patient dies suddenly or when the patient's death is unexpected, ACP is not possible. The three innovations are important aspects of ACP in end of life care and provide a broad structure of how effective care can be organised.

## Advance care planning 1: integrated care pathways

Up until 2013, one of the most significant elements of ACP was the Liverpool Care Pathway or LCP. For many years, the LCP was considered the epitome of good care at the end of life. The pathway provided a documentary framework that helped to guide and facilitate practitioners to ensure completeness of care. It did this through devising procedures to enable patients with life-limiting illness, near the time of death, to be provided with the highest standard of care resources allowed. However, due to a series of media portrayals of the pathway not doing what it was supposed to, its use was discontinued in the UK towards the end of 2013. In an independent review of the LCP, Neuberger et al. (2013: 3) commented that: 'what we have heard at relatives' and carers' events ... that there have been repeated instances of patients dying on the LCP being treated with less than the respect that they deserve'. The academic response was the withdrawal of the LCP, which questioned the lack of research underpinning the pathway (Hughes et al., 2013), together with the lack of communication and multidisciplinary collaboration by clinical practitioners (Seymour and Horne, 2013).

Much of the media publicity focused around the latest changes to the document (version 12), and centred on hydration. The LCP guidance advocated that clinicians should not over-hydrate patients towards the end of life, but correct dehydration wherever possible. In clinical practice many hospital wards adopted an approach based on non-hydration. As a result, a small number of patients were portrayed in the media as being left to die without adequate food and hydration. The LCP came under sustained criticism, with some authors citing that it was a back door to euthanasia (Granger, 2012). After a number of highly publicised cases where family members were not made aware that the patient was dying (*Newsweek*, 2013), the use of the LCP was discontinued. On reflection, it may be argued that the pathway was an excellent tool for monitoring the patient's progress, although issues such as the diagnosis of dying remained problematic, and the communication of the purpose of the pathway across health professionals, the patient and the family was not all that it could have been.

We will now shift our emphasis from hospital-based care to focus on community care where approximately 20% of patients are cared for at the end of life.

## Advance care planning 2: the Gold Standards Framework

The Gold Standards Framework is a community-based model of best practice originally designed by Kerri Thomas (2003), a GP concerned about the need to develop and coordinate care for those at the end of life in the community. The GSF has been adopted by almost a third of GP practices in the UK, and the model consists of seven components (known as the 7Cs: communication, coordination, control (of symptoms), continuity, continued learning, carer support and care in the dying phase – Box 15.2). Each is interlinked to ensure that community resources and support for those at the end of life, who choose to be cared for at home, can be optimised by community care staff using available resources. It begins with communication and is summarised in Box 15.2.

## BOX 15.2  COMPONENTS OF THE GOLD STANDARDS FRAMEWORK

1. Communication: a supportive care register is compiled to record, plan and monitor patient care. This is used as a tool for discussion at healthcare team meetings, which are held regularly to improve the flow of information
2. Coordination: a nominated coordinator (e.g. a district nurse, practice manager or GP) is appointed to maintain a register of concerns and problems. The coordinator also organises team meetings for discussion, planning, case analysis and education
3. Control of symptoms: patient symptoms are assessed, discussed and treated. Anticipatory prescribing is practised
4. Continuity: palliative care patient details are passed on to local palliative care specialists with transfer of information to the local out-of-hours service. Patients and carers are given information about the contacts needed for out-of-hours advice
5. Continued learning: meetings are organised to discuss patients' care and to share ideas and problems. Significant event analysis takes place to consider good examples of care and possible improvements for future work
6. Carer support: carers are supported, listened to, encouraged and educated to play as full a role in the patient's care as they wish. A link with social services is made to ensure that practical support is available. Healthcare professionals plan support for the carer when bereavement occurs
7. Care in the dying phase: the period when the patient is approaching the terminal phase (death is likely in the next two weeks) is recognised and this information communicated to the family and carers. Medicines for symptom control of all terminal symptoms are made available in the home

(Adapted with permission Amass, 2006)

## Advance care planning 3: Preferred Priorities of Care document

Palliative care practice upholds the right of the individual to express their autonomy and places high regard for the wishes of the patient and the family. The Preferred Priority of Care document (PPC) originated in the Lancashire and South Cumbria Cancer Network in June 2004 and was endorsed by the NHS End of Life Care Programme (DH, 2008), which supported the view that patient choice was important and encapsulated this in the End of Life Care Strategy published in 2008 (DH, 2008).

The PPC is a patient-held document designed to facilitate individual choice at end of life care. Documenting and responding to individual preferences and wishes can enable both the person and their carers to express their desires, beliefs and wishes to be cared for in the place of their choice. The PPC document is part of the wider assessment made of a patient at the end of life. Moreover, it is part of a process of care and assessment designed to empower patients at the end of life and to enable and encourage nurses to ensure that the patient's wishes are included in advance care planning.

The document encourages patients to state their individual preferences. Moreover, its importance lies more in the fact that it demonstrates that the practitioner and patient had had a discussion about the wishes of the patient, so it represents that the patient has been involved in the decision-making process when it becomes clear that the patient is nearing the end of life. Once documented, it is necessary (with the individual's permission) that these wishes be shared with key care facilitators such as community nurses. The PPC document provides the opportunity to discuss concerns that may not otherwise be addressed. As such, it is a very useful tool to enable nurses to initiate and record the patient's wishes. The explicit recording of individual wishes can form the basis of care planning in multidisciplinary teams and other services, therefore reducing unplanned admissions and avoiding inappropriate and/or unwanted interventions. The PPC document is used more widely in the community as a means of enabling patients to exercise choice over where they receive care at the end of life (Reynolds and Croft, 2011).

## Legal and ethical issues

The PPC document provides patients with the freedom to express their preferences, but it does not constitute a legal document binding nurses to carry out all the patient's wishes. For example, it is not the appropriate place to record decisions concerning a refusal of treatment. Furthermore, should the person lose capacity to make a decision about issues, the previously completed PPC acts as an advanced statement. An Advance Decision (Living Will) allows you to write down any treatments that you don't want to have in the future, in case you later become unable to make or communicate decisions for yourself. Advance Decisions are legally binding in England and Wales, as long as they meet certain requirements. Information included within the PPC can be used as part of an assessment of a person's best interests when making decisions about their care. However, from a legal and ethical perspective, the PPC document is not the place to state the patient's refusal to have, for example, a nasogastric tube or to comment on DNAR (Do Not Resuscitate) orders. The latter are medical directives and form part of the overall treatment medically determined by competent medical practitioners. This does not mean that the patient is excluded from such discussions. They are, however, separate issues. Evidence suggests that the PPC is having a significant impact and enabling individuals to receive care in their preferred place at the end of life.

# Enabling patients to experience a good death in hospital

The concept of the so-called good death is ambiguous and the attributes numerous. Good death concepts have received a lot of attention since the hospice movement and the development of palliative care focused on the quality of care for dying patients (Conway, 2007). What constitutes a good death includes various attributes that have been described by numerous authors, such as open and honest communication about end of life care (McNamara, 2004), effective pain and other symptom control (Tadman and Roberts, 2007), and enabling the patient and family to be involved in decision making about end of life care (Morrison and Garland, 2004; Smith et al., 2012). Further attributes of the good death include upholding the patient's dignity and self-respect (Stringer, 2007), as well as focusing on spiritual wellbeing (Mootoo, 2005; Murray, 2010; Milligan, 2011).

• **What does the term 'a good death' mean to you?**

The literature has drawn attention to the differing perceptions of good death and some authors have asked for whom is the death good (Gazelle, 2003; Schwartz et al., 2003)? Specifically, what the patient may regard as a good death in terms of a quick and sudden departure from life may leave the family and hospital staff shocked, unprepared and grief stricken. The literature relating to the good death concept has grown rapidly in the last decade, with writers highlighting the difficulties of being able to achieve a good death for all (Ellershaw et al., 2010), and the importance of context in shaping the experience of good death (Costello, 2004; Paddy, 2011). What in fact many describe as a good death is often a term meaning the process of dying and not the actual death event itself (Costello, 2006).

One of the key features of enabling patients and families to experience good death is recognising advanced disease and the inevitability of death (Gadoud and Johnson, 2011). The sooner ACP can take place, for example in an ideal situation from the time of diagnosis, the more likely it will be that steps can be taken to ensure that the patient's wishes become an integral part of end of life care and treatment. Evidence suggests that it is often too late to include the patient in care planning when their illness becomes more advanced (Skilbeck and Payne, 2003). Dying well should involve the patient and the family.

Others have focused on the influence of context in shaping the experience of good death, with hospitals being the most challenging areas for good deaths to occur (Costello, 2006). The time spent once the life-limiting illness has been diagnosed (also known as the dying trajectory) may help to prepare both the patient and the family for death. If the wishes of the patient and family in relation to dying are considered and implemented, despite the sadness that this involves, death may be seen as appropriate or good. In some cases, the death of some patients who have suffered and experienced pain and other adverse symptoms may be seen as a blessing and a relief to families.

Enabling patients to experience a good death often means finding out what their wishes are and what they consider to be in their best interests. This could mean discharging them to die at home or a place of their choice, utilising the PPC documentation (DH, 2004), if home is not appropriate due to a lack of care facilities or vulnerability of family care. Patient and family perceptions of a good death experience can also involve a range of scenarios, for example not attempting to resuscitate, providing the patient with adequate symptom relief, and considering and responding to requests for assisted dying.

As a way of clarifying how nurses and others can help patients to experience a good death, the following case study of an authentic patient experience illustrates some of the difficulties associated with experiencing a good death in an acute hospital context.

## JESSIE

Jessie was a 58-year-old woman admitted to the surgical ward, with a suspected acute abdomen, in pain and acute distress resulting from a prolonged period at home where her symptoms became out of control. Her husband John was her primary carer and they received help from friends, neighbours and their daughter who lived 60 miles away. Jessie did not want to be in hospital and was hoping to be cared for at home. On admission, she was found to be in pain, distressed and tearful. After being settled into the ward and medically examined, it was confirmed that Jessie was dehydrated and constipated, and had been experiencing nausea and vomiting for two weeks. As a consequence of her

*(Continued)*

(Continued)

symptoms, she was not eating well, had lost weight, and her heels, sacrum and hips were red from prolonged periods in bed. She also had a urinary tract infection. Psychologically she was depressed and felt frustrated at having to be admitted when she wanted to be at home. On examination it was found that she had an acute abdomen and a hard mass suggestive of an obstruction or tumour. Ultrasound investigations indicated a need for an explorative laparotomy, which was performed as an emergency procedure and revealed an inoperable tumour and widespread metastases.

The case study highlights a reasonably typical situation of a patient being cared for at home under the medical treatment of the GP and being cared for by a relative. Having diagnosed a life-limiting illness, the priority was to manage her symptoms, specifically pain and nausea and vomiting, and to prevent further problems. Clearly Jessie required palliative care.

---

Nurses and others in the team can help patients like Jessie experience a good death by actively listening to them and enabling the patient and relatives to express their needs, wishes and fears. If in doubt about what to do about situations like Jessie's, the medical staff could refer her to the hospital's palliative care support team for advice on further treatment. All hospitals in the UK have such teams. Patients like Jessie need to have each symptom (physical and psychosocial) responded to and treated.

Once her physical symptoms had been well managed, a discussion with her and her family would need to take place about future care. This would involve the multidisciplinary care team and involve the husband and the patient. John, as the primary caregiver, may feel upset at not being able to meet her needs. Jessie needed to have the news broken sensitively with her husband and possibly other family members present. Explanations and information about her care and treatment needed to be provided in a careful and sensitive way.

Future care depended on what her wishes were for palliation. A stay in a hospice could be in her best interests. Jessie may wish to stay in hospital and possibly be transferred to a ward more appropriate to her needs. Moreover, Jessie needed to have her psychosocial needs assessed and responded to in a professional and sensitive way. At this stage she and her husband needed a compassionate approach based on her need for comfort, symptom management, and an acknowledgement that her and her husband were experiencing a crisis. Her situation required the highest quality of communication.

## The role of the nurse providing palliative care

The contemporary development of therapeutic relationships with patients represents a response to the objectification of patients in hospital (May, 1992). In particular, palliative care is the area of nursing in which using a relatively new vocabulary focuses on holistic and personal care. Palliative care nurses advocate the use of therapeutic relationships because they represent the essence of holistic care. Central to such care is the ability of the nurse to develop emotional intelligence, and to elicit and consider the patient's feelings and how they influence the dynamics of the relationship (Goleman, 1995). In relation to nursing patients at the end of life and supporting their families, emotional intelligence can be utilised to help nurses consider the situation and distress of the family, how they may be feeling and how the nurses can help them.

As we have already established elsewhere in the book, a therapeutic relationship between the patient and the healthcare practitioner involves the practitioner focusing their attention on the needs of the patient at the expense of the needs and demands of the organisation. A key element of interpersonal relationships between healthcare practitioners and patients in contemporary times has been the development of a more meaningful level of emotional engagement between nurses and patients, especially at the end of life. In palliative care, this is seen as especially poignant and resonates with others writing about nursing care for vulnerable patients (Dexter and Walsh, 2001; O'Connell, 2008). O'Connell argues that the development of therapeutic nurse–patient relationships in certain contexts can expose nurses to emotional pain. However, by reflecting on their situation through, for example, clinical supervision, nurses have an opportunity to learn about the emotional intelligence required to develop and maintain this important relationship.

As the social group with the most contact with the patient, nurses who form therapeutic relationships can become what Peplau (1996) and others call a professional friend.

## ACTIVITY 15.2

Drawing on your knowledge and understanding from reading this and previous chapters, consider what attributes are required to fulfil the important role of a professional friend. Make a list of the things you consider to be important in order to develop a therapeutic relationship.

Becoming a 'professional friend' requires the nurse consciously to spend time actively listening to the patient, with the patient and nurse developing trust and respect for each other, and for the nurse to elicit the patient's needs and concerns about care and treatment. By undergoing training such as the SAGE & THYME model of communication we referred to earlier in the chapter (Connolly et al., 2010), nurses can learn to recognise and respond effectively to psychological distress, avoiding causing psychological harm, communicating honestly and compassionately, and knowing when they have reached the boundary of their competence.

In the recommendations to improve the safety and wellbeing of patients, the Berwick report (DH, 2013) pointed out the need for nurses to treat patients with respect and enable respect to develop from the basis of compassion for and understanding of vulnerable patients (DH, 2013). It may be argued, therefore, that nurses have a professional duty to develop therapeutic relationships with patients and their families, not only at the end of life but also at the beginning of their illness trajectory. Moreover, at the end of life, there is only one chance to get it right and therefore it is essential that patients and their informal caregivers receive high-quality competent care, from committed practitioners who demonstrate a desire to ensure that the patient, the family and lay caregivers are given emotional support that becomes the professional aim of all practitioners.

## The role of informal caregivers at the end of life

There are approximately 6·5 million known individuals in the UK providing the role of family caregiver (Costello, 2017). Hulme et al. (2016) estimate that informal and family caregivers save the UK £119 billion per year. These figures identify how informal and family caregivers make a major contribution to palliative care. Professional caregivers need to acknowledge this contribution, and deal sensitively and professionally with lay caregivers, many of whom are family members, when a patient has to be admitted for end of life care in hospital.

The challenge of managing healthcare for people who have long-term medical conditions (LTMCs), many of whom have no chance of cure, is very significant worldwide. There are estimated to be over 36 million deaths each year, many of which may be premature and occurring before the age of 60 (Nicol, 2015). The Department of Health (2012) estimates that the number of cases of LTMCs will rise from 1.9 million in 2008 to 2.9 million in 2018. These disease include cancer, diabetes, chronic kidney disease and dementia (Nicol, 2015). These statistics inform us of the need for nursing care and extra resources. Many patients with LTMCs are cared for at home by family members and friends, often referred to as lay or informal caregivers. Lay caregivers take on the caregiver role either as a family member or on behalf of the family (Leow et al., 2015). Evidence suggests that the role of the informal caregiver was one of the key determinants in the provision of effective end of life care (Gagyor et al., 2015).

## Caregiver concerns

As professional practitioners, we exercise our duty of care to patients, although we have a duty of care to lay caregivers as well. These informal caregivers make a significant contribution to patient care, and nurses should also consider their concerns and needs when caring for people in the palliative phase of their illness experience (Sampson et al., 2014). Lay caregivers may have a range of concerns and needs that vary according to the patient's quality of life (Simon et al., 2015). These may include the caregivers' personal circumstances (Horne et al., 2012) and their physical and psychosocial needs (Van Beek et al., 2016). A significant concern for many lay caregivers, particularly those caring for patients with advanced cancer, is their need for information and knowledge about impending end of life (Wright et al., 2016).

Caregiver concerns often focus around their ability to carry out activities of daily living (Lee et al., 2015), as well as worries about pain and symptom control (Nissen et al., 2016) and lack of resources or funding/facilities (Kent et al., 2016). A concern often shared by many caregivers is around caring for people at home, because most patients when asked state a preference to stay at home when their prognosis is made clear to them (Morris et al., 2015). Caregivers point out that information giving and being kept up to date about prognosis are helpful when considering future planning (Parker et al., 2007). Evidence suggests that many caregivers requested information about what to expect in the future (Clayton et al., 2005; Enzinger et al., 2015).

## Meeting caregiver concerns: the role of the professional

In the palliative phase of a patient's illness, caregivers need guidance from professionals in terms of information and emotional support (Luker et al., 2000; Georges et al., 2002; Mok and Chiu, 2004; Law, 2009; De Haes and Teunissen, 2005; Bridges et al., 2013; Griffiths, 2013). Professionals can and do make a significant contribution to supporting caregivers by establishing therapeutic relationships (as previously discussed) with the family and patient from their initial contact. These need to be sustained during the palliative phase and after death to include bereavement support. The establishment and maintenance of such relationships require effective interpersonal interactions, with nurses engaging emotionally with the caregivers to form partnerships based on trust and mutual respect (McQueen, 2000). During the palliative journey, the patient and their family or lay caregiver will experience times of distress, such as when decisions are made to stop or with-draw treatment. Moreover, the evidence suggests that patients and families experience distress when the patient is managing the coping transition between the end of active treatment and the start of palliative care (Hardy and Brown, 2016). This is often a time when it becomes clear that cure is no longer a viable option, and concerns and needs about the future focus on end of life care.

## Nursing competence in end of life pathophysiology

For most nurses, their knowledge base of pathophysiology is limited to understanding how the body functions in health and how to return the patient's homoeostasis to normal. However, at the end of life when caring for a dying patient and supporting the family, knowledge of how the patient's dying body undergoes changes is central to providing effective end of life palliative care. Two key issues stand out in relation to palliative care at the end of life and after death. Towards the end of life patients may experience a number of bodily changes that can be expressed mentally in the form of agitation, also referred to as terminal restlessness/delirium. This is explained in Case Scenario 15.3. Second, nurses also need to understand what happens to the body *post mortem* in order to provide a broader evidence base, as well as to enable them to educate the family about changes that will have occurred when they view the body after death. Approximately 2 hours after death, rigor mortis (the process of muscle stiffness caused by a lack of bodily ATP) begins throughout the body. For this reason, in most cases it is necessary to conduct last offices before rigor mortis has set in in order to move the body and enable any dentures to be placed in the mouth. The patient's skin will become mottled as blood begins to be withdrawn from peripheral organs – a process known as lividity.

## THOMAS

Thomas was 92 and had suffered from chronic obstructive pulmonary disease (COPD) for most of his life. He was admitted to hospital after an exacerbation of his condition brought on by pneumonia. His son Joe and daughter Rachel were told their father had end-stage pulmonary disease (ESPD). They wanted to stay with him because it was felt that he was near the end of life and likely to die soon. Thomas was unconscious, receiving oxygen (24%) via a nasal cannula, and seemed a little agitated. Joe and Rachel understood that the oxygen was having a minimal effect. They were aware that their father was not having intravenous fluid due to his chronic chest condition and the need not to overload his pulmonary circulation with fluid. It had already been discussed a few weeks ago that he should not be given artificial fluids but receive regular mouth and skin care. After an hour at his bedside, Thomas's breathing had become erratic and noisy. He had also begun to show signs of agitation and his movements became jerky. Rachel and Joe were distressed by their father's mental and physical state and called the nurse.

As the qualified nurse, what would you have done?

## Nursing response

As the nurse on duty, it is necessary to provide the family with information to help them cope with the distress while at the same time calling for medical help to alleviate the patient's condition.

Thomas was experiencing a situation called terminal delirium or terminal restlessness. The symptoms include physical ones such as myoclonic movements in his limbs, agitation expressed physically and psychologically, emotional or spiritual distress, and anxiety. You would need to explain that, because Thomas was nearing death, his bodily responses were deteriorating. End of life often produces physical changes that result partly from the patient's deteriorating condition, which, coupled with their dehydrated state, creates challenges for effective symptom control. You should point out that, to help provide comfort and reduce the symptoms, palliative sedation can be prescribed to aid breathing, reduce agitation and make Thomas more comfortable. In the UK, it is common to find that patients in such situations are given low doses of drugs such as morphine 5 mg subcutaneously, to help manage breathing and/or a sedative such as midazolam to control terminal restlessness or terminal agitation (Rietjens et al., 2018). Terminal restlessness in a dying person is a distressing situation to observe, especially if you are a loved one. It can have a negative impact on the family and professional caregivers (Hall et al., 2014). Of course, you would need to base your practice and patient/family education on a sound knowledge of bodily changes at the end of life and an awareness of the body's homeostatic status. You would need to be able to explain how the body is affected by the dying process, both before and after death, in order to educate family members appropriately about the changes in the bodily symptoms the patient is experiencing.

## Respecting cultural requirements at the end of life

In relation to the NMC proficiencies (NMC, 2018a) associated with end of life care for the deceased and the bereaved, three key issues should be focused on in relation to respecting the cultural requirements and protocols of quality palliative care. The first is to respect the patient's dignity at all times. The NMC (2018b: 6) remind us that, as a registered nurse, it is important to respect a patient's human rights at all times and treat them (and their families) with kindness and compassion (NICE, 2011: 13). The need for dignity is fundamental to all aspects of nursing care, although at the end of life empathy and compassion should be expressed and made explicit.

The second issue associated with expressing respectful cultural need for the deceased and bereaved is the discussion of their preferences and choices for end of life care. This can be included in advance care planning (previously discussed with the patient and family). If, for example, a Muslim family wish to say prayers for the dead by reading from the Koran while the patient is dying, it is important to discuss with the Imam how this can be done. Practically, this may require the patient to be in a side room and involve the use of audio equipment, to ensure privacy for the patients. In a similar way the need to wash before prayers can involve the patient being given a jug and bowl and assisted sensitively to carry out this important ritual.

The third issue in providing quality of care at the end of life is meeting patients' expectations. What patients may expect as good end of life care may not always be provided. An example is the need for an orthodox Muslim's need to face Mecca when dying (Neuberger, 2004). In hospital this can be managed by discussing this with the religious leader (the Imam), and turning the bed to face south-west. In a similar way, meeting cultural needs and expectations can be met by ensuring that a patient's request sacrament of the sick is met in advance of their death. When a patient dies, it is also important to maintain the same standard of dignity in relation to their cultural beliefs. An example is a patient of the Jewish faith who wishes not to be touched by those outside their faith. Again this is something very likely to be facilitated by the attending rabbi. Should nurses need to move the patient for safety reasons, then the use of gloves shows respect for the person's culture. In a similar way many eastern faiths and Asian ethnic groups prefer nurses of the same sex as the deceased to carry out last offices. Families of patients who follow orthodox Buddhist culture may also have specific cultural rituals that should be adhered to. The corpse of a Buddhist should not be touched for 3–8 hours after breathing ceases because the belief is that the spirit lingers on for some time. Orthodox followers of Hinduism believe the body of the dead must be bathed, massaged in oils, dressed in new clothes and then cremated before the next sunrise. Cremation would be acceptable in a faith where the soul will be released to find another body to inhabit. In practical terms, it is appropriate where possible to either keep the body in a side room or transfer untouched on a trolley to the mortuary. Nurses can and should offer the bereaved family member the opportunity to assist them in washing the patient after death, inviting them to take part if they prefer. This may involve same-sex involvement. It is also a respectful way of ensuring that the families' wishes are recognised. However, nurses should be sensitive in the way the invitation is expressed and avoid making the family feel obliged to take part in the last offices.

In a similar way, dealing with the deceased's personal belongings should be conducted with sensitivity and respect. Special circumstances, for example requests for organ donation, should be managed by specialist practitioners with nurses facilitating discussion before any intervention (Neuberger, 2004). In all instances, it is necessary for nurses to respect the wishes of the patient (made in advance of their death) and the bereaved family.

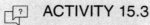

## ACTIVITY 15.3

Access the NMC (2018a) *Standards of Proficiency for Registered Nurses* document and identify all of the clinical skills required of registered nurses.

Within a palliative care environment, how could you ensure that you are able to develop skills to meet the clinical competencies required (i.e. annexes A and B)?

Now make a list of things you can do to develop your overall competence in palliative care nursing.

No doubt you will have identified a number of things that you can do to help you achieve and maintain your competence in this area of nursing. Your list may include the following:

- Maximising opportunities for improving services by improving your knowledge and experience, such as volunteering to work in a hospice, through selective spoke placements;
- Shadowing those who have a specialist role in palliative care;
- Keeping up to date can be achieved by reading journals, books and short research reports;
- Attending seminars and study days;
- Enrolling on a palliative care course at your school of nursing;
- Attending additional education and training in the form of study days, short courses and conferences. These are helpful to ensure that your practice not only is based on up-to-date evidence but will also help you to develop the confidence required to provide effective palliative care.

## Chapter summary

This chapter has focused on the importance of palliative care for ensuring that experiences at the end of life are positive, involve the patient's choices, wishes and preferences, and are fulfilling for the patient and the family as well as the healthcare professional. Nurses are often the group who have the most intimate contact with and spend a lot of time with patients and families. It is worth considering the famous quote from Cecily Saunders: 'You matter because you are you, and you matter to the end of your life. We will do all we can not only to help you die peacefully, but also to live until you die.' The chapter has highlighted the importance of enabling all those involved in end of life care, including lay and family caregivers, to experience a good death. In particular, advance care planning, effective symptom control from the time of diagnosis, respect for patient autonomy and engaging in frank discussion is important, and made easier when the nurse is enabled to develop a therapeutic relationship with the patient and family. The six Cs (Cummings, 2012), often discussed and publicised, particularly in the wake of the Francis report (Francis, 2010), are central features of effective palliative care. We have only one chance to get it right for patients with a life-limiting illness, and we can get it right by enabling the patient and the family to play an active part in the planning and implementation of care by respecting their wishes and putting their needs at the forefront of planning.

## Further reading

Albarran, A.J.W. and Hills, M. (2012) 'Managing end of life care'. In I. Bullock, J. Macleod-Clark and J. Rycroft-Malone (eds), *Adult Nursing Practice*. Oxford: Oxford University Press, pp. 302–7.

Baldwin, M.A. and Woodhouse, J. (2011) *Key Concepts in Palliative Care*. London: Sage.

Department of Health, Social Services and Public Safety (DHSSPS) (2010) *Living Matters, Dying Matters: A Palliative and End of Life Care Strategy for Adults in Northern Ireland*. Belfast: DHSSPS.

NHS Wales (2013) *Together for Health: Delivering End of Life Care*. Cardiff: Welsh Assembly Government.

Payne, S., Seymour, J. and Ingelton, C. (2008) *Palliative Care Nursing*, 2nd edn. Milton Keynes: McGraw-Hill Open University Press.

Scottish Government (2008) *Living and Dying Well: A National Action Plan for Palliative and End of Life Care in Scotland*. Edinburgh: The Scottish Government.

Wiienberg-Lyles, E., Goldsmith, J., Ferrell, B. and Ragan, S.L. (2013) *Communication in Palliative Nursing*. Oxford: Oxford University Press.

## References

Age UK (2017) *NHS Continuing Healthcare and NHS-funded Nursing Care*. Factsheet 20 (amended April 2018). London: Age UK.

Amass, J. (2006) 'The Gold Standard Framework', *Pharmacological Journal*, 276: 353–4. Available at: www.pharmaceutical-journal.com/libres/pdf/articles/pj_20060325_goldstandards.pdf (last accessed 22 August 2018).

Arnautska, E. (2010) 'Breaking bad news', *Trakia Journal of Sciences*, 8(Suppl 2): 491–2.

Baile, W., Buckman, B., Renato, L., Globera, G., Bealea, E.A. and Kudelka, B. (2000) 'SPIKES: a six step protocol for delivering bad news: application to the patient with cancer', *Clinical Journal of Oncology Nursing*, 14(4): 302–11.

Becker, R. (2009) 'Palliative care 1: principles of palliative care nursing and end-of-life care', *Nursing Times*, 105(13): 14–16.

Becker, R. (2010) *Fundamental Aspects of Palliative Care Nursing*, 2nd edn. London: Quay Books.

Bridges, J., Nicholson, C., Maben, J., Pope, C., Flatley, M., Wilkinson, C., Meyer, J. and Tziggili, M. (2013) 'Capacity for care: meta-ethnography of acute care nurses' experiences of the nurse–patient relationship', *Journal of Advanced Nursing*, 69(4): 760–72.

Broeckaert, B. (2008) 'Treatment decisions at the end of life: a conceptual framework'. In S. Payne, J. Seymore and C. Ingleton (eds), *Palliative Care Nursing*, 2nd edn. Maidenhead: McGraw-Hill/Open University Press, pp. 402–22.

Buckman, R. (1992) *Breaking Bad News: A Guide for Healthcare Professionals*. Baltimore, MA: Johns Hopkins University Press.

Choice in End of Life Programme Board (2015) *What's Important to Me. A Review of Choice in End of Life Care*. Available at: www.gov.uk/government/uploads/system/uploads/attachment_data/file/407244/CHOICE_REVIEW_FINAL_for_web.pdf (last accessed 28 April 2018).

Clayton, J.M., Butow, P.N., Arnold, R.M. and Tattersall, M.H.N. (2005) 'Discussing end-of-life issues with terminally ill cancer patients and their carers: a qualitative study', *Support Care Cancer*, 13: 589–99.

Connolly, M., Perryman, J., McKenna, Y., Orford, J., Thomson, L., Shuttleworth, J. and Cocksedge, S. (2010) 'SAGE & THYME: a model for training health and social care professionals in patient-focussed support', *Patient Education and Counseling*, 79: 87–93.

Conway, S. (2007) 'The changing face of death: implications for public health', *Critical Public Health*, 17(3): 195–202.

Costello, J. (2004) *Nursing the Dying Patient: Caring in Different Contexts*. London: Palgrave.

Costello, J. (2006) '"Dying well": nurses' experiences of good and bad deaths in hospital', *Journal of Advanced Nursing*, 54(5): 1–8.

Costello, J. (2017) 'The role of informal caregivers at the end of life: providing support through Advance Care Planning', *International Journal of Palliative Nursing*, 23(2): 60–5.

Cummings, J. (2012) 'I want to achieve pride in the profession. The 6 Cs of nursing'. Available at: www.nursingtimes.net/nursing-practice/leadership/jane-cummings-i-want-to-achieve-pride-in-the-profession/5048241.article# (last accessed 20 May 2018).

Davies, J., Kristjanson, L.J. and Blight, J. (2003) 'Communication with families of patients in an acute hospital with advanced cancer: problems and strategies identified by nurses', *Cancer Nursing*, 26: 337–45.

De Haes, H. and Teunissen, S. (2005) 'Communication in palliative care: a review of recent literature', *Current Opinion in Oncology*, 17(4): 345–50.

Department of Health (2004) *Preferred Place of Care*. London: DH. (Revised December 2007 by the National PPC Review Team.)

Department of Health (2008) *Promoting High Quality Care for Adults at the End of their Lives*. London: DH.

Department of Health (2012) *Long Term Conditions: Compendium of Information*, 3rd edn. London: DH.

Department of Health (2013) *The Berwick Report into Patient Safety*. London: DH.

Dexter, G. and Walsh, M. (2001) *Psychiatric Nursing: A Patient Centred Approach*. Bath: Nelson Thornes.

Ellershaw, J.E., Dewar, S. and Murphy, D. (2010) 'Achieving a good death for all', *British Medical Journal*, 341: c4861.

Elliott, M. and Nicholson, C. (2017) 'A qualitative study exploring use of the surprise question in the care of older people: perceptions of general practitioners and challenges for practice', *British Medical Journal Support Palliative Care*, 7(1): 32–8.

Enzinger, A.C., Baohui Zhang, B., Schrag, D. and Prigerson, H.G. (2015) 'Outcomes of prognostic disclosure: associations with prognostic understanding, distress, and relationship with physician among patients with advanced cancer', *Journal of Clinical Oncology*, 33(32): 3809–17.

Fallowfield, L. (2005) 'Learning how to communicate in cancer settings', *Support Cancer Care*, 13: 349–50.

Francis, R. (2010) *Mid Staffordshire NHS Foundation Trust Enquiry*. London: HMSO.

Gadoud, A. and Johnson, M. (2011) 'Recognising advancing disease', *British Journal of Hospital Medicine*, 78(2): 432–6.

Gagyor, I., Himmela, W., Pieraua, A. and Chenotb, J.F. (2015) 'Dying at home or in the hospital? An observational study in German general practice', *European Journal of General Practice*, 22(1): 9–15.

Gardiner, C., Gott, M., Ingelton, C., Seymour, C. and Cobb, M. (2013) 'Extent of palliative care need in the acute hospital setting: a survey of two hospitals in the UK', *Palliative Medicine*, 27(1): 76–83.

Gazelle, G. (2003) 'A good death: not just an abstract concept', *Journal of Clinical Oncology*, 2(9): 95–6.

Georges, J., Grypdonck, M. and Casterle, B.D.D. (2002) 'Being a palliative care nurse in an academic hospital: a qualitative study about nurses' perceptions of palliative care nursing', *Journal of Clinical Nursing*, 11: 785–93.

Goleman, D. (1995) *Emotional Intelligence*. London: Bloomsbury.

Granger, K. (2012) 'The Liverpool Care Pathway for the dying patient improves the end of life', *The Guardian*, 13 November.

Griffiths, R. (2013) 'Professional boundaries in the nurse–patient relationship', *British Journal of Nursing*, 22(18): 1087–8.

Hall, S.H., Leonard, M.M., Agar, M., Spiller, J.A., Hosie, A., Wright, D.K., Meagher, D.J., Currow, D.C., Bruera, E. and Lawler, P.G. (2014) 'End-of-life delirium: issues regarding recognition, optimal management, and the role of sedation in the dying phase', *Journal of Pain and Symptom Management*, 48(2): 215–30.

Hardy, K. and Brown, M. (2016) 'Care planning and changing care needs'. In M. Brown (ed.), *Palliative Care in Nursing and Health Care*. London: Sage, pp. 44–60.

Horne, G., Seymour, J. and Payne, S. (2012) 'Maintaining integrity in the face of death: a grounded theory to explain the perspectives of people affected by lung cancer about the expression of wishes for end of life care', *International Journal of Nursing Studies*, 49(6): 718–26.

Hughes, S., Preston, N. and Payne, S. (2013) 'What went wrong with the Liverpool Care Pathway and how can we avoid making the same mistakes again?', *International Journal of Palliative Nursing*, 19(8): 372–3.

Hulme, C., Carmichael, F. and Meads, D. (2016) 'What about informal carers and families?'. In J. Round (ed.), *Care at the End of Life*. Heidelberg: Springer, pp. 167–76.

Kent, E.E., Rowland, J.H., Northouse, L., Litzelman, K., Chou, W.Y.S., Shelburne, N., Timura, C., O'Mara, A. and Huss, K. (2016) 'Caring for caregivers and patients: research and clinical priorities for informal cancer caregiving', *Cancer*, 122(13): 1987–95.

Kurtz, S., Silverman, J. and Draper, J. (2005) *Teaching and Learning Communications Skills in Medicine*. Oxford: Radcliffe Publishing.

Law, R. (2009) '"Bridging worlds": meeting the emotional needs of dying patients', *Journal of Advanced Nursing*, 65(12): 2630–41.

Lee, K.C., Yin, J.J., Lin, P.C. and Lu, S.H. (2015) 'Sleep disturbances and related factors among family caregivers of patients with advanced cancer', *Psycho-oncology*, 24(12): 1632–8.

Leow, M., Chan, S. and Moon, F.C. (2015) 'A pilot randomized, controlled trial of the effectiveness of a psychoeducational intervention on family caregivers of patients with advanced cancer', *Oncology Nursing Forum*, 42: E63–72 (supplement online exclusive).

Luker, K.A., Austin, L., Caress, A. and Hallett, C.E. (2000) 'The importance of "knowing the patient": community nurses' constructions of quality in providing palliative care', *Journal of Advanced Nursing*, 31(4): 775–82.

Main, J. (2002) 'Management of relatives of patients who are dying', *Journal of Clinical Nursing*, 11(6): 794–801.

May, C. (1992) 'Individual care? Power and subjectivity in therapeutic relationships', *Sociology*, 26(4): 589–602.

McAllister, M., Creedy, D., Moyle, W. and Farrugia, C. (2002) 'Nurses' attitudes towards clients who self-harm', *Journal of Advanced Nursing*, 40(5): 578–86.

McIlfatrick, S. (2013) 'Interprofessional collaboration in palliative care: rhetoric or reality? (Editorial)', *International Journal of Palliative Nursing*, 19(9): 419.

McNamara, B. (2004) 'Good enough death: autonomy and choice in Australian palliative care', *Social Science and Medicine*, 58(5): 929–38.

McQueen, A. (2000) 'Nurse–patient relationships and partnership in hospital care', *Journal of Clinical Nursing*, 9(5): 723–31.

Milligan, S. (2011) 'Addressing the spiritual needs of people near the end of life', *Nursing Standard*, 26(4): 12–15.

Mok, E. and Chiu, P.C. (2004) 'Nurse–patient relationships in palliative care', *Journal of Advanced Nursing*, 48(5): 475–83.

Mootoo, J.S. (2005) 'A guide to cultural and spiritual awareness', *Nursing Standard*, 19: 17.

Morris, S.M., King, C., Turner, M. and Payne, S. (2015) 'Family carers providing support to a person dying in the home setting: a narrative literature review', *Palliative Medicine*, 1–9. doi:10.1177/0269216314565706.

Morrison, J. and Garland, E. (2004) 'Developing palliative care services in partnership', *Cancer Nursing Practice*, 3(31): 22–5.

Murray, R.P. (2010) 'Spiritual care, beliefs and practices of special care and oncology RNs at patients end of life', *Journal of Hospice and Palliative Nursing*, 12(1): 12–14.

National Institute for Health and Care Excellence (2011) *Quality Standard for End of Life Care in Adults*. London: NICE. Available at: http://guidance.nice.org.uk/QS13 (last accessed 20 January 2016).

National Institute for Health and Care Excellence (2018) *End of Life Care for Adults*. London: NICE. Available at: https://pathways.nice.org.uk/pathways/end-of-life-care-for-people-with-life-limiting-conditions#path=view%3A/pathways/end-of-life-care-for-people-with-life-limiting-conditions/caring-for-an-adult-at-the-end-of-life.xml&content=view-index.

Neuberger, J. (2004) *Caring for People of Different Faiths*. Washington: DC: CRC Press, Taylor & Francis.

Neuberger, J., Guthrie, C., Aaronovitch, D., Hameed, K., Bonser, T., Harris, R., Jackson, E. and Waller, S. (2013) *More Care, Less Pathway A Review of the Liverpool Care Pathway*. Independent review of the Liverpool Care Pathway. Available at: www.gov.uk/government/publications/review-of-liverpool-care-pathway-for-dying-patients (last accessed 22 August 2018).

*Newsweek* (2013) 'BBC Death in hospital'. BBC Television programme, May 2013.

Nicol, J. (2015) *Nursing Adults with Long Term Conditions*, 2nd edn. London: Sage.

Nissen, K.G., Trevino, K. and Prigerson, H.G. (2016) 'Family relationships and psychosocial dysfunction among family caregivers of patients with advanced cancer', *Journal of Pain and Symptom Management*, 52(5): 841–9.

Noddings, N. (2002) *Starting at Home: Caring and Social Policy*. Berkeley, CA: University of California Press.

Nursing and Midwifery Council (2018a) *Future Nurse: Standards of Proficiency for Registered Nurses*. London: NMC.

Nursing and Midwifery Council (2018b) *The Code*. London: NMC.

Nyatanga, B. (2013) 'Empathy in palliative acre: is it possible to understand another person (editorial)', *International Journal of Palliative Nursing*, 19(10): 471.

O'Connell, E. (2008) 'Therapeutic relationships: a reflection on practice', *Critical Care Nursing*, 13(3): 138–43.

Office of National Statistics (2013) *2012-based National Population Projections* (Released 6 November 2013). London: ONS.

Paddy, M. (2011) 'Influence of location on a good death', *Nursing Standard*, 26(3): 12–13.

Parker, S.M., Clayton, J.M., Hancock, K. et al. (2007) 'A systematic review of prognostic/end-of-life communication with adults in the advanced stages of a life-limiting illness: patient/caregiver preferences for the content, style, and timing of information', *Journal of Pain and Symptom Management*, 34: 81–93.

Peplau, H. (1996) *Interpersonal Relations in Nursing*. New York: Springer.

Reynolds, J. and Croft, S. (2011) 'Applying the preferred priorities for care document in practice', *Nursing Standard*, 25: 36.

Rietjens, J.A.C., van Delden, J.J.M. and van der Heide, A. (2018) 'Palliative sedation: the end of heated debate? (editorial)', *Palliative Medicine*, March: 1–2.

Rogers, A., Karlsen, S. and Addington-Hall, J. (2000) 'All the services were excellent. It is when the human element comes in that things go wrong: dissatisfaction with hospital care at the end of life', *Journal of Advanced Nursing*, 31(4): 768–74.

Sampson, C., Finlay, I., Byrne, A., Snow, V. and Nelson, A. (2014) 'The practice of palliative care from the perspective of patients and carers', *BMJ Supportive and Palliative Care*, 4: 291–8.

Saunders, Y., Ross, J.R. and Riley, J. (2003) 'Planning for a good death: responding to unexpected events', *British Medical Journal*, 327(7408): 204–6.

Schwartz, C.E., Mazor, K., Rogers, J., Ma, Y. and Reed, G. (2003) 'Validation of a new measure of concept of good death', *Journal of Palliative Medicine*, 6(4): 575–84.

Seymour, J. and Horne, G. (2013) 'The withdrawal of the Liverpool Care Pathway in England: implications for clinical practice and policy', *International Journal of Palliative Nursing*, 19(8): 369–71.

Simon, J.E., Ghosh, S., Heyland, D., Cooke, T., Davison, S., Holroyd-Leduc, J., Wasylenko, E., Howlett, J. and Fassbender, K. (2015) 'Evidence of increasing public participation in advance care planning: a comparison of polls in Alberta between 2007 and 2013', *BMJ Supportive and Palliative Care*, 0: 1–8.

Skilbeck, J. and Payne, S. (2003) 'Emotional support and the role of clinical nurse specialist in palliative care', *Journal of Advanced Nursing*, 43: 521–30.

Smith, S., Pugh, E. and McEvoy, M. (2012) 'Involving families in end of life care', *Nursing Management*, 19(4): 72–7.

Stringer, S. (2007) 'Quality of death: humanisation v medicalisation', *Cancer Nursing Practice*, 6(3): 12–19.

Sweeting, H. and Gilhooly, M. (1992) 'Doctor, am I dead? A review of social death in modern societies', *Omega: Journal of Death and Dying*, 24(4): 251–69.

Tadman, M. and Roberts, D. (2007) *Oxford Handbook of Cancer Nursing*. Oxford: Oxford University Press.

Thomas, K. (2003) *Caring for the Dying at Home. Companions on the Journey*. Oxford: Radcliffe Medical Press.

Van Beek, K., Siouta, N., Preston, N., Hasselaar, J., Hughes, S., Payne, S., Radbruch, L., Centeno, C., Csikos, A., Garralda, E. et al. (2016) 'To what degree is palliative care integrated in guidelines and pathways for adult cancer patients in Europe: a systematic literature review', *BMC Palliative Care*, 15: 26. doi:10.1186/s12904-016-0100-0.

Wilkinson, S. (2002) 'The essence of cancer care: the impact of training on nurses' ability to communicate effectively', *Journal of Advanced Nursing*, 40(6): 731–38.

Wright, A.A., Keating, N.L., Ayanian, J.Z., Chrischilles, E.A., Kahn, K.L., Ritchie, C.S., Weeks, J.C., Earle, C.C. and Landrum, M.B. (2016) 'Family perspectives on aggressive cancer care near the end of life', *Journal of the American Medical Association*, 315(3): 284–92.

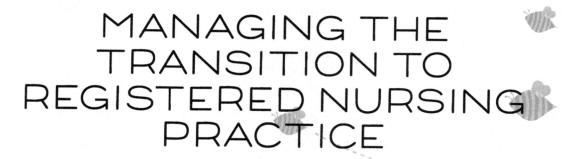

# MANAGING THE TRANSITION TO REGISTERED NURSING PRACTICE

## KAREN HEGGS AND SAMANTHA FREEMAN

---

### CHAPTER OBJECTIVES

- Consider how best to approach your final placement;
- Describe the process of application for employment and explain how best to promote yourself to prospective employers;
- Begin to develop and enhance your personal statement;
- Consider strategies for self-care and personal development;
- Outline the process of revalidation;
- Explain how preceptorship can support you in your transition from student nurse to registrant;
- Explore the role of a registered nurse when responding to a major incident.

---

The transition from nursing student to registered nurse is a busy and exciting time. However, this transition period can sometimes feel challenging and stressful and you may start to feel apprehensive about your pending change in role. This chapter will explore the challenge of managing role transition and help you to prepare for the start of your professional career. We will explore the theory and evidence base around role transition as well as practical aspects of:

- Your final placement;
- Applying for employment;
- Self-care;
- Becoming a registered nurse;
- Preceptorship;
- Nursing and Midwifery Council (NMC) revalidation.

The primary shift is that you will have developed skills of leadership, management and decision making and yet conducted them only in the supervised student role. Most of your concerns may stem from feelings of needing to know everything. Within this chapter, you should find useful guidance to support you during this time and the reassurance that none of us know everything!

 **To achieve entry to the nursing register you must be able to**

- Act as an ambassador, upholding the reputation of your profession and promoting public confidence in nursing, and health- and care services;
- Understand the demands of professional practice, acknowledge the need to accept and manage uncertainty, and demonstrate an understanding of strategies that develop resilience in self and others;
- Understand and maintain the level of health, fitness and wellbeing required to meet people's needs for mental and physical care;
- Demonstrate how to recognise signs of vulnerability in yourself or your colleagues and the action required to minimise risks to health;
- Take responsibility for continuous self-reflection, seeking and responding to support and feedback to develop their professional knowledge and skills;
- Support and supervise students in the delivery of nursing care, promoting reflection and providing constructive feedback, and evaluating and documenting their performance;
- Contribute to supervision and team reflection activities to promote improvements in practice and services;
- Demonstrate effective supervision, teaching and performance appraisal through the use of:

  - clear instructions and explanations when supervising, teaching or appraising others;
  - unambiguous, constructive feedback about strengths and weaknesses and potential for improvement;
  - encouragement to colleagues that helps them to reflect on their practice;
  - active listening when dealing with team members' concerns and anxieties;
  - understand the role of registered nurses and other health and care professionals at different levels of experience and seniority when managing and prioritising actions and care in the event of a major incident.

(Adapted from NMC, 2018a)

## Approaching the end of your nurse education

It may seem at the start of your nursing degree programme that the point of registration is a long way off. But time on a nurse degree programme will pass quickly and, before you know it, you are approaching the end of your programme and the point of registration.

This can be an exciting time with the opportunity to begin to develop your own practice and move forward in your career, with a wealth of opportunities available to you. It can also be a time of apprehension, uncertainty and worry as the responsibility of becoming a registrant becomes a reality. Often, student nurses worry that they are not ready to become registrants; they do not feel prepared and are concerned that they may not have the skills that they need in order to begin their role as a newly registered staff nurse.

## Expectations of yourself and others

Do these expectations that students have of themselves reflect the reality of what is expected of them as a newly registered nurse?

- Competent in skills specific to new role;
- Knowledge base specific to new role;
- Confidence in abilities;
- Highly skilled;
- Able to 'hit the ground running'.

In reality it is important to remember to be kind to yourself as you approach the end of your nursing degree programme, acknowledging the skills and knowledge that you have acquired throughout your programme and the value that this has to employers.

What do employers expect from newly registered nurses? What skills and knowledge do they seek:

- Critical thinking;
- Adaptable;
- Open to development and change;
- Collegiate;
- Professional.

In your role, you will be supported in your development as a newly qualified practitioner when you undertake your preceptorship. We will discuss this in more detail later on in this chapter.

## This is the beginning of your journey of lifelong learning

An important factor to consider as you approach the end of your nurse education is that lifelong learning is a key part of your role as a professional. In line with *The Code* (NMC, 2018b), it is essential that you continue to engage in learning and development throughout your career. It is helpful to view your nurse degree programme as a foundation for your lifelong learning.

Consider your nursing degree programme and your nurse education as the roots and trunk of your nursing career (Figure 16.1). They are vital to provide you with deep-rooted knowledge and skills, and the stability to begin to grow and develop as a registered nurse. Nursing requires you to be a lifelong learner. Look back on learning throughout your programme and identifying gaps in knowledge. Consider how you can address these gaps and develop a personal development plan.

Can the gaps you have identified be addressed on your final placement?

It is good to ask questions and to not be frightened to admit if you don't know something. Developing skills in clinical judgement and decision making are guided by our experiences and by seeking information on which to base these decisions.

Earlier in this book (Chapter 7), we identified the role of the theory developed by Benner (1984) in the development of the experiential learner and the skills of clinical judgement and decision making.

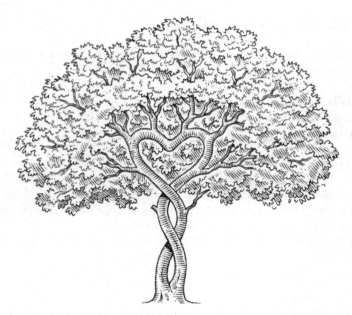

**Figure 16.1**    What do you consider to be the roots and trunk of your nursing career?

*Source:* iStock

It would be appropriate to consider the work of Benner here again, but in the context of your identity as a student and as a newly qualified nurse.

In her intuitive–humanistic theory, Benner (1984) identifies stages of development from novice through to expert via the development of knowledge base and experience. It is useful to consider this model in the context of your current identity as a student and your upcoming new identity as a newly qualified registered nurse. There is no expectation that you will complete your nursing degree programme and be an expert in your identified field of nursing; this takes time and experience. But you may have knowledge and experience that you bring with you from before the commencement of your programme, through study and exposure to the role of the nurse; you will also have skills, knowledge and experience that you gain from the programme itself and the range of exposure to practice experience and theoretical experiences offered to you. Finally, you may have supplementary knowledge, skills and experience that you gain through your life: hobbies, personal life, interests, voluntary work. All of these add to the rich and unique map that is your own identity as a registered nurse.

Consider Benner's model (Figure 16.2) and your perception of yourself.

Think about your skills, knowledge and experiences that you bring to your role as a student nurse and think about your future identity as a registered nurse. Where do you see yourself within the context of Benner's model? Take time to identify the value that you bring to the nursing role. Does this match your previous expectations of where you feel you should be?

You will find it incredibly helpful to look back and consider your learning and experiences on your nursing programme to help you in identifying gaps in your knowledge. Looking back through reflections that you have developed would be an interesting and insightful exercise, and offer the

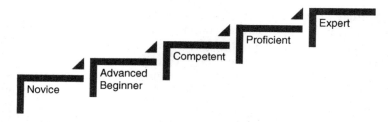

**Figure 16.2**   Novice to expert stages 1–5 (Adapted from Benner, 1984)

opportunity to consider how far you have come and where you want to go. This may support you to consider your learning needs for your final placement. One tool that can facilitate you in this process is the use of a SWOT analysis (Figure 16.3); originally developed in the 1960s by Humphrey, the SWOT analysis has been developed further over time and is utilised in a wide range of different contexts such as decision making, evaluation and change management.

By taking the time to consider your own strengths and opportunities, alongside areas for development and threats to this, you will find it a supportive and facilitative process that may support you to consider how best to utilise the learning opportunities available to you.

It may also be helpful to link your SWOT analysis to the development of a personal development plan (PDP) to support you in identifying any specific personal learning needs for your final practice learning experiences on your nurse degree programme. Your PDP will require you to develop SMART objectives in your plan so that your action plan objectives are:

Specific

Measurable

Achievable

Relevant

Time-based

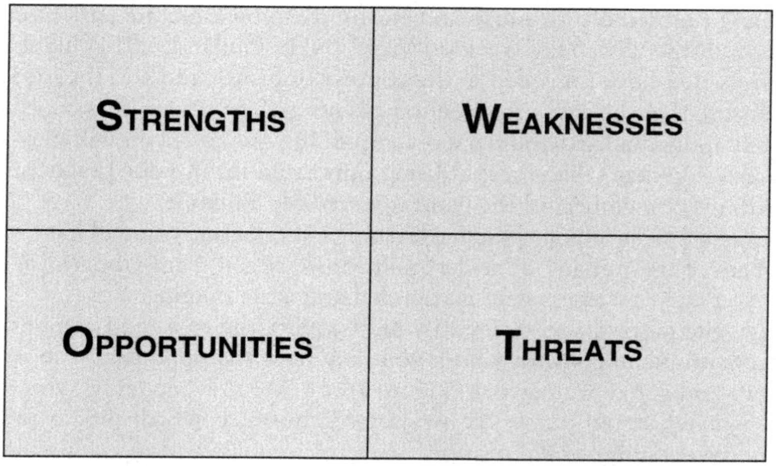

| **Strengths** | **Weaknesses** |
|---|---|
| **Opportunities** | **Threats** |

**Figure 16.3**   SWOT analysis tool

You may remember that we introduced the idea of SMART objectives in previous chapters and it is worth recognising again that these have been applied in a wide range of contexts. For example, you may find that your employer encourages you to use SMART objectives in your annual personal performance reviews, or you may have considered using SMART objectives when implementing a change in practice or a service improvement. Using this same approach here helps you to identify your own personal objectives, and can help ensure that you maintain motivation and focus in your development.

The completion of SWOT and PDP may also support you in identifying your career plans and moving forward into your preceptorship, which we will consider later on in this chapter.

---

### 🗩 ACTIVITY 16.1

Using the SWOT analysis framework highlighted in Figure 16.3, complete your own SWOT analysis of the nursing knowledge and skills you have developed so far, and then reflect on how you may address the areas for development and threats to this.

Now use your completed SWOT analysis to support you in developing a short-term PDP for the next 12 months. What do you feel you need to achieve? What do you want to achieve? How will you do this?

---

## Opportunities for multiprofessional learning and development

One key factor to consider as you approach the end of your nursing programme is your future role as a core member of the multiprofessional team. As a registered nurse, you will be pivotal in leading and supporting the multiprofessional team and their collaborative work in managing the provision of care for the patient and service users whom you meet. It is vital that you understand roles and respect colleagues in the delivery of effective and safe patient care. Having a good understanding of the role of the various team members is vital to ensure that you can move forward in your role as a newly registered staff nurse and ensure that you facilitate patient-centred care.

The introduction of the 'Five Year Forward View' (NHS England, 2014) highlights the need to break down barriers that have prevailed in the context of health and social care across a range of care settings, to ensure that the care provided to patients and service users is coordinated, effective, safe, and ultimately individualised and person-centred. In your role, you will play a pivotal role in this vital service development; therefore, utilising opportunities in your practice, learning experiences to work with other members of the team is incredibly valuable.

As part of your assessment in your practice learning experiences, you will have no doubt worked with other members of the nursing or wider multi-professional team who will feed back to your practice assessor so that your assessment is rounded and wide ranging.

In Chapter 4 we encouraged you to identify and explore the roles and responsibilities of other multiprofessional team members with whom you may have the opportunity to work as a student nurse within a hub-and-spoke framework (Figure 16.4). We now encourage you to consider these again, this time as a registered nurse. As a registered nurse, you will play a pivotal role in the facilitation of interprofessional collaboration, assessing, managing and evaluating care provision,

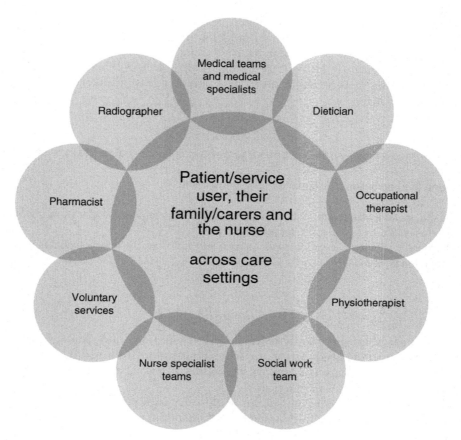

**Figure 16.4** Hub-and-spoke placement framework

and collaborating with colleagues to successfully and significantly impact on the safe delivery of care and positive outcomes for patients (Martin et al., 2010).

Your own exposure to the expertise and valuable input of the wider team will vary dependent on your individual practice learning experience, and your role and where you choose to work, nevertheless, by now you will no doubt have recognised that it is essential that you take the time to work and learn alongside each member of the team in order that you respect the value of the input that they offer in the delivery of individualised, person-centred care. Learning from each other in practice is a valuable part of learning and development as a nurse. Later in this chapter we will consider the importance of self-care and reflective practice, but it is important here also to highlight the value of engaging the wider team in group reflection; this is particularly valuable after involvement in a stressful or difficult situation such as a major trauma. There is a growing body of evidence to support this as a very valuable learning opportunity for all. One example from practice is that of 'Schwartz rounds' which are supported by the Point of Care Foundation in the UK and are being utilised across many organisations nationally. They are an excellent example of the value of supported group reflection, where teams come together to discuss a situation and share their experiences, learning about the input and role of each team member and the value of their involvement. A greater appreciation of roles and experiences can lead to more effective team working, improved staff health and wellbeing; this, in turn, can have a significant impact on the quality of care provision and patient experience (Point of Care Foundation, 2015: 13). Goodrich (2012: 120) also identified that by sharing experiences team members have a greater understanding, appreciation and respect for each other.

- By now you should have had the opportunity to work with members of the multiprofessional team?

List them and then consider your understanding of their role.

- Try to place yourself as a leader of this team. How would you apply what you know about their role and responsibilities to assist you in leading the team?
- Can you identify any gaps in your knowledge here and if so consider how you plan to find out more about each team member?

## What to expect from your final placement

Your final placement is an opportunity to enhance and build on your prior learning and also to identify your future learning needs as you approach registration. Your practice assessor may have completed specific postgraduate education programmes to ensure that they are adequately prepared to support student nurses in practice.

It is important to be aware that you will not work solely with your practice assessor but as part of the wider team with nurses and other members of the multiprofessional team (practice supervisors), who will feed back to your assessor to provide a holistic approach and breadth to your final assessment.

## Embracing learning opportunities in your final placement

It may be the case that your final student placement is not your identified area of employment on registration. However, it is perhaps important to consider that this is your final placement as a student and to take every learning opportunity offered to you, embracing this final student experience. The skills, knowledge and experience from this practice learning experience are transferable into any area of nursing practice, alongside those achieved and gained throughout your nurse education.

When you begin your new post as a registered nurse, your employer and team should support you in developing the skills, knowledge and experience that will be specific to your role; you may not have encountered these during your nurse education depending on your practice learning journey, but you will have a solid grounding of core skills, knowledge and experience (Figure 16.5) that will be a solid foundation on which to build, adapt and develop as you progress through your career.

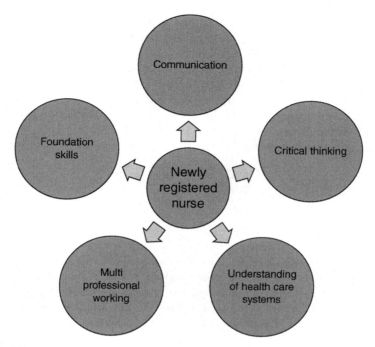

**Figure 16.5** Core skills, knowledge and experience of a newly registered nurse (NMC, 2018a)

---

## ⬚? ACTIVITY 16.2

It would be worth revisiting the NMC (2018a) proficiencies required for entry to the nursing register and considering what evidence you have that demonstrates your achievements of these here.

- Are there any areas that you consider need further development on your final placement?
- How might you address this in your final sign-off placement?

---

## Application for employment

You may have already started to think about your career plans for the future. This may have been influenced by your experiences in practice throughout your nurse degree programme, or you may have had a very clear idea of your career direction from the very start of the programme. Whatever your thoughts on your career plans, it is necessary to consider applying for employment as you approach the end of the programme. It is worth remembering here when considering your career path: your first job might not be your forever job! Be mindful that there is an incredible amount of flexibility and career routes within nursing as a profession, and you may make the decision to change your specialty as you progress through your career. Many skills in nursing are transferable and can be utilised and developed in a wide range of specialities.

You may wish to take some time at the end of the programme to have a break after years of study, to travel or to consider further your career plans (see 'Further reading' at the end of this chapter about working internationally). If this is the case, you will need to check to ensure that you register to practise with the NMC within the required timescales (usually within five years of completion of your nursing programme). Currently, if you apply to join the register after six months, you will be required to complete a new application because the application sent on your behalf from your higher education institute will no longer be valid. The NMC provides very clear and up-to-date guidance about the process of registration on its website:

www.nmc.org.uk/registration/joining-the-register/trained-in-the-uk.

## Developing your curriculum vitae and personal supporting statement

Your curriculum vitae (CV) is a fluid tool that will develop with you throughout your career. You may already have a developed CV from your employment before commencing your degree programme, or you may have never developed a CV. Whatever your situation, it is useful to begin to structure and develop your CV before beginning to look for employment. It can take time to pull together all of the relevant information, and you are advised to consider allowing time to complete your CV in the first instance. Once you have the basic outline structure of your CV, this will then grow and develop with you as you progress through your nursing career journey, wherever that may take you.

The basic outline structure for a CV has not changed over many years. The key is to keep it clean and simple and to keep to a minimum length. Writing in a succinct manner is a skill and this will reflect well to prospective employers. Ideally your initial CV should be no longer than two sides of A4 paper. Ensure that you check for spelling and grammatical errors – prospective employers will notice this!

---

### BOX 16.1   CV TEMPLATE

But what should be included and how should this be set out? This list will help you to begin to develop your outline CV structure:

1. Title and name
2. Address
3. Date of birth and age
4. A brief statement about yourself, including key drivers and positive statements (really sell yourself here)
5. Education:

    a. Institution attended (school/college/further education/higher education)
    b. Qualifications gained
    c. Grades/outcome

6. Details of relevant courses attended

7. Details of employment (starting with the most recent)

   a. Organisation
   b. Job title
   c. Dates of employment
   d. Brief outline of key roles and responsibilities

8. A brief overview of activities that you enjoy out of work
9. Contact details of two referees

The initial information will remain the same as you progress through your career, with additions to qualifications and details of employment that can be added and amended as you progress and move along. Investment in your CV now is an investment in your future.

Have you started to develop your CV?

Think about the information that you will need to begin to populate your CV.

Do you have access to certificates and contact details for any previous employment?

Begin to develop your CV by asking your personal tutor or your support person in practice to review this for you.

Do you need to make any changes or amendments?

Your personal statement is a key aspect of the job application process; it is your opportunity to sell yourself to your prospective employer, to stand out from the crowd and to highlight the reasons why they should consider you for employment. It is important that you take time to develop your personal statement and that this links clearly to both the person specification and the role description that are linked to the job itself. You will find both attached to the advertisement for the job and it is vital that you read these thoroughly. Depending on the role, employer and environment, there may be some variation in the person specification and the job description, but there are common factors that employers identify as key in their search for an employee. Bright et al. (2014: 70) have identified what they feel are the eight key qualities that are identified in person specifications:

1. Effective communication skills: both verbal and written;
2. The ability to work in a team and be a team player;
3. Attention to detail;
4. Enthusiasm and passion;
5. The ability to use initiative;
6. The ability to work under pressure;
7. Energy and drive;
8. Evidence of leadership skills.

When you have reviewed the job description and person specification, begin to make notes and ensure that you take time to consider how you can demonstrate your suitability for the job, and what skills and attributes you can bring to the role through reflection on your experiences in practice, theory and extracurricular activities in which you engage.

The use of a simple spider diagram is a helpful tool (Figure 16.6) to begin the development of your personal statement.

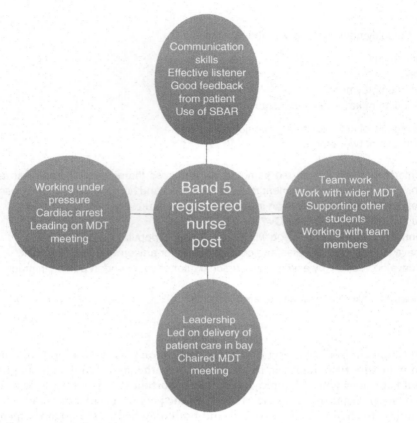

**Figure 16.6**   Spider diagram example

You will also find that reviewing and revisiting any reflections on your experiences will be a huge help to you in the development of your personal statement. For example, you may have recorded reflections in your practice assessment document, ongoing achievement record or portfolio.

 What do your reflections tell you about your experiences? Have you had feedback that could be incorporated to strengthen your personal statement?

Take time to read through your reflections on practice and feedback in your practice assessment documents.

Look through the job specification of a job in an area of practice you are interested in. You can source these on organisational web pages and/or recruitment sites.

Are there key reflections that you feel will contribute towards your personal statement?

## Applying for your first post

Many organisations now utilise online websites to facilitate the process of application, seeking references and offering posts. For example, if applying for a post within the NHS in England,

Scotland and Wales, websites such as NHS Jobs (www.jobs.nhs.uk) or Health & Social Care jobs in Northern Ireland (www.hscrecruit.com) offer a great opportunity to search for posts that may be of interest to you. Some also offer the option to receive notifications when posts are advertised on the site, which is a useful tool to support you in your search for posts.

Ensure that you have your outline CV to hand and that you have an outline personal statement available. If you see a post that interests you, it is best to apply sooner; you may miss the opportunity to apply if the advert is closed before the deadline due to a high number of applicants.

You will find that online systems offer the opportunity to save relevant information that you may need again for future applications. Although it may take time to collate information on the system in the first instance, you will save time in the future when completing applications because much of the information can be taken from the information you have previously submitted.

Not all employers use online systems for application for employment and some may use paper-based application processes. In these situations, it is important that you use black ink to complete your form (unless otherwise indicated) and that you do not complete the form when you may be rushed and with little time. Nothing looks worse to prospective employers than a poorly completed application form. If you do have to complete a handwritten form, ensure that you have the time and space to undertake the task in hand and all the relevant information to hand. Use clear writing and ensure that you read the form thoroughly; do you need to use block capitals?

## Attending open days

There have been some changes in recent years in the methods of application for employment for nurses, with many organisations now offering open days, with the opportunity to interview 'on the spot' for posts within the organisation.

If you have attended a practice placement during your degree programme and enjoyed your experience, you may be interested to attend an open day at the organisation to find out more about employment and development opportunities. This is also a great opportunity to meet with senior nursing staff from the organisation and to make a good impression that would be beneficial for your future employment opportunities. Open days offer the chance to ascertain what benefits and opportunities the organisation can offer you as a member of their team.

It is important to remember when attending an open day that you have a good understanding of the organisation and their values before the day. Access the organisation's website and take time to read about the organisation so you are prepared for the open day; this may prompt questions and further information on your part.

Attend the open day in smart clothing and take along relevant information (e.g. a copy of your current CV) so that prospective employers can view this if you are happy for them to do so, should the opportunity for interview arise on the day. It is valuable to make a good first impression to prospective employers.

## Interview skills

You have submitted a successful application and have been invited to attend for an interview. What do you do now? At this stage it would be useful to ask practice colleagues, other students and your practice supervisors and assessors, and academic staff what questions they think you might be asked at interview. You may want to start collating a bank of questions with a small group of peers. As you go to interviews write down the questions. Then try out answering these again, asking peers, clinicians in practice and family to ask you questions and test out the way you answer. Most universities will have career support service so seek this out and see what general interview support is available.

---

### BOX 16.2   INTERVIEW TIPS

Some general interviewing tips:

- Make eye contact with all members of the interview panel. Try not to just focus on the person who has asked the question you are answering;
- Smile!;
- Be clear and concise in your responses;
- If your mishear, don't understand the question or lose your train of thought don't panic, just say so. Ask for the question to be repeated;
- Link the question back to your own experience (and your portfolio!);
- Sell yourself and be reflective; give real examples of 'how' you have achieved a positive outcome and how this impacted on your practice;
- Read around and demonstrate that you understand the organisation's mission or goal. Link this to your own practice;
- Be aware of your body language. You want to convey that you're enthusiastic, positive and energetic. Try to keep fidgety hands still.

Try to prepare a question you want to ask at the end; it helps demonstrate that you are keen and want the job, for example 'What preceptorship programme does the organisation provide?'.

---

## Accepting a post

Following the process of application and interview, you may find that you are in the position where you have more than one offer of employment. At this point, you will have a choice to make about which role you want to accept and which you do not wish to accept. It is important to be considerate of your potential employers in this situation and to inform them as soon as possible of your decision, so they can offer the position to an alternative suitable candidate or re-advertise the position in a timely manner in order that the vacancy can be filled and the service not affected.

Be mindful of your professional responsibility in this situation and the need to consider the needs of the wider service. Although it can sometimes be difficult to make a final decision for your first post as a registered nurse, as we have identified, this may not be your 'forever' role and there are a wide range of opportunities available to you in your career. The decision to accept a role and then to decline this at the last minute could lead to a missed opportunity for the organisation to fill a post and may impact on the service that they provide.

## Starting your role as a registered nurse

Once you have successfully competed your programme of study, your university will inform the NMC. You need to be mindful that there may be a slight delay in you completing your studies and receiving your personal identification number (PIN). Once you receive your PIN number, you will need to alert your employer and you can then practise as a registered nurse.

# Preceptorship

There is a growing body of evidence to support the need to ensure that healthcare practitioners have a clear plan of support in the transition period, to facilitate their growth and development as a practitioner and to help them identify their ongoing learning needs as a developing practitioner.

'Preceptorship' is the term used to outline the structured period of time in which you are supported in your new employment as a newly registered nurse. The NMC (2006) suggest that this period of time will allow for the development of confidence in practice and allows the newly qualified nurse to be supported to practise in line with *The Code* (NMC, 2018b). However, you need to be aware that the term and provision of the preceptorship period applies only to NHS employment. Currently, there is no requirement for a similar provision in the private sector. This does not mean a private sector employer will not support you during this transition period, but it may be a point of discussion to have if this is your first role. Within the NHS provision the period and method of preceptorship will vary, so it is useful that you enquire about the model of preceptorship at interview in order that you are aware of the support that the organisation will offer you as you begin your role as a newly qualified nurse.

There have been many developments in the drive for preceptorship over recent years. In 2009, the Department of Health (DH) published the *Preceptorship Framework for Nursing*. This provided guidance and potential structure to support those developing and facilitating preceptorship programmes for nurses within NHS organisations. The definition of preceptorship presented within the framework provided greater clarity, and also identified what is meant by an effective preceptorship and the benefits that it can offer to newly registered nurses in support of their transition from student to registrant. Here preceptorship is defined as:

> A period of transition for the newly registered nurse during which time he or she will be supported by a preceptor, to develop their confidence as an autonomous professional, refine skills, values and behaviours and to continue on their journey of life-long learning.
>
> (DH, 2009: 11)

This framework was superseded in 2010 by the introduction of a framework that also included midwifery and other allied health professions, acknowledging the value of preceptorship for nursing and beyond. The Department of Health (2010) also took the opportunity to highlight that preceptorship requires clarity in its boundaries, and that its introduction is to enhance the confidence and competence of the newly qualified and accountable practitioner through support.

Across the UK, there are a range of new initiatives being developed to facilitate preceptorship; in some areas this is within individual organisations and in some regions there are collaborative approaches that are being developed to embrace a standardised approach.

- What do you know about preceptorship? Does your current knowledge and understanding of preceptorship meet with the definition highlighted here?
- How might preceptorship assist you in your transition into registered practice?
- What elements of preceptorship would be particularly important to you?

## Utilising preceptorship to support your development

Through the completion of your degree programme, you will be required to meet the *Standards of Proficiency for Registered Nurses* (NMC, 2018a). Throughout this book, so far you have been introduced to a range of these standards in the openings to each chapter.

Embracing the opportunity for preceptorship will allow you the opportunity to build on your developing knowledge and skill base, through the support of your preceptor and your employing organisation.

The Department of Health (2010) highlight a wide range of ways in which preceptorship can support your development as a newly registered practitioner:

- Confidence in applying evidence-based practice;
- Develop confidence and self-awareness;
- Implement the code of professional values;
- Increase knowledge and clinical skills;
- Integrate prior learning into practice;
- Understand policies and procedures;
- Reflection and receiving feedback;
- Develop an outcome-based approach to continuing professional development;
- Advocacy;
- Interpersonal skills;
- Managing risk and not being risk adverse;
- Equality and diversity;
- Negotiation and conflict resolution;
- Leadership and management development;
- Team working;
- Decision making.

Throughout your time on your nursing programme you will have experience and exposure to many of these aspects, both theoretically and through exposure to clinical practice. Preceptorship allows to you build on your prior learning, acknowledging that you will continue to develop all of these aspects of your professional practice as you move through your nursing career.

The utilisation of a period of preceptorship will also feed forward into your first revalidation with the NMC and will encourage you to maintain supporting evidence of your achievements.

## Nursing and Midwifery Council: revalidation

Revalidation as a requirement of the NMC was introduced in 2016 (NMC, 2016). It is the way in which nurses demonstrate to the NMC that they have continued to practise safely and effectively via a process of gathering feedback on their ability. Nurses are also required to apply critical reflective skills to continually develop as a practitioner, with clear links to *The Code* (NMC, 2018b) and its application to professional practice. This is evidenced via a professional portfolio and is required to be formally reviewed every three years.

The NMC have developed a useful microsite that contains all the information you will need to undertake revalidation, and provides templates that will support you in the building and development of your professional portfolio from the point of registration. During your preceptorship, your new employer should also be able to give you guidance on how the process of revalidation is managed within the organisation.

---

### ☐? ACTIVITY 16.3

Take some time to visit the NMC's Revalidation webpage and read through the guidance provided on revalidation. Look through and familiarise yourself with the documentation/templates provided and consider how you would start to create and further develop and enhance your professional portfolio to support you in your revalidation.

http://revalidation.nmc.org.uk/welcome-to-revalidation

http://revalidation.nmc.org.uk/download-resources/forms-and-templates

---

## Self-care and the demands of professional practice

After reading the previous chapters in this book, you will no doubt have recognised that adult nursing is a demanding role, both physically and emotionally. This is acknowledged by the NMC (2018a: 8) when they require that as a registered nurse you must be able to:

Understand the demands of professional practice and demonstrate how to recognise signs of vulnerability in themselves or their colleagues and the action required to minimise risks to health.

In addition, *The Code* (NMC, 2018b: 19) also identifies that, as a nurse, you:

maintain the level of health you need to carry out your professional role.

The Royal College of Nursing (RCN, 2018) booklet *Rest, Rehydrate and Refuel* provides some useful tips on what you can do to help yourself stay well at work. In addition, although we have explored the need for emotional resilience in previous chapters, it is worth revisiting the important aspects again as you begin your role as a registered nurse.

Resilience is considered to be an important attribute in healthcare professionals (McGowan and Murray, 2016). However, there is little agreement on what being resilient entails, and how we develop into resilient practitioners. What it isn't is absorbing all that you witnessed or experienced and just 'getting on with it'. It is important that you share your experiences with your colleagues, have open dialogue and seek support from your peers and senior colleagues. Remember that you should not have to feel that you have to manage everything on your own. Looking after yourself allows you to remain healthy and well, so that you can practise safely and effectively. If you do feel that you are finding things difficult and recognise vulnerability in yourself, there is value in sharing this with your peers and to know that you will be supported. In turn, too, it is important that you also look out for your colleagues and encourage them to seek support and help if you feel that they are finding things difficult.

- Can you remember some of the things you might be able to do to increase your resilience?

As a newly registered nurse you will possibly be working in a new environment, faced with change and reorganisation, and you will have to be able to deal with this, in addition to the role and responsibility of providing care to patients and their families. A multifaceted approach will help you cope with this potentially challenging time. Jackson et al. (2007) identified key strategies in the development of resilience:

- Positive relationships;
- A sense of humour;
- Self-awareness;
- A sense of balance;
- Developing as a reflective practitioner.

The benefits of working in a team and developing effective working relationships with your peers are a valuable approach to ensuring support and a sense of belonging throughout your nursing career.

## Reflection and self-care

Earlier in this chapter, the use of Schwartz rounds (Point of Care Foundation, 2015) was identified as a positive model to facilitate effective team working and to enhance respect and communication through reflective discussion. In addition to this there are other ways in which you can engage in supportive reflection.

At the very start of this book, we introduced you to the concept of reflection as a process to facilitate understanding, knowledge and development, and the varying models that may support this process. In addition to this, it is also appropriate to consider here how the process of reflection can be utilised in the facilitation of self-care and also, in some cases, the engagement of others, so this is a shared process where learning and support are encouraged within the wider team.

Through the process of revalidation, the NMC (2016) encourages nurses to engage in written reflection to demonstrate learning and development through experiences in practice. There are a number of ways in which you can engage in written reflection and you may have undertaken this as part of your nurse degree programme. Some nurses enjoy the process of written reflection, taking the time to focus on their learning through experiences. Some find written reflection a challenge and acknowledge that the skill of written reflection takes time to develop and hone over many years.

It is important to acknowledge that, through the process of reflective writing, it is not simply a case of recording an event, but that the writing itself is the process of reflection (Bolton and Delderfield, 2018: 135). There are a range of ways that reflective writing can be developed: the use of a journal or diary is often the most common method. Some find the structure of a model for example Gibbs (1988) can help in the development of reflection. In their recently updated book on reflective practice, Bolton and Delderfield (2018) discuss in detail the practice of reflective writing; in this they identify the process of developing your reflective writing and the value of time and space to develop this practice. This would be a valuable activity to begin to develop as a student and as a registered nurse.

## ACTIVITY 16.4    SIX-MINUTE WRITING TASK

1. Write whatever is in your head – do not edit this;
2. Write for 6 minutes – don't stop writing during this time, let the words flow;
3. Don't stop, re-read or be critical during this 6 minutes;
4. Don't worry about spelling, grammar, punctuation;
5. Allow yourself the permission to write anything;
6. Importantly, whatever you write is right: it belongs to you and you don't have to share it with anyone.

(Bolton and Delderfield, 2018: 160)

## Clinical supervision

Clinical supervision is the process of reflection through discussion with an identified colleague or an independent professional. In 2013, the Care Quality Commission (CQC) acknowledged the value of clinical supervision in the delivery of safe and effective patient care, identifying the purpose of clinical supervision to be:

a safe and confidential environment for staff to reflect on and discuss their work… The focus is on supporting staff in their personal and professional development and in reflecting on their practice.

(CQC, 2013: 4)

Clinical supervision can be on a one-to-one basis or as part of a group, and is a valuable aspect of support for nurses. Bifarin and Stonehouse (2017) acknowledge the incredible value that effective clinical supervision can offer to each nurse who engages with the activity, but, ultimately, it can have a significantly positive impact on working relationships and patient care through stress reduction, and a feeling of value and satisfaction in the role of the nurse.

## Your future career

Consider how you felt about becoming a nurse at the beginning of your nurse degree programme. Do you feel that your professional identity has changed?

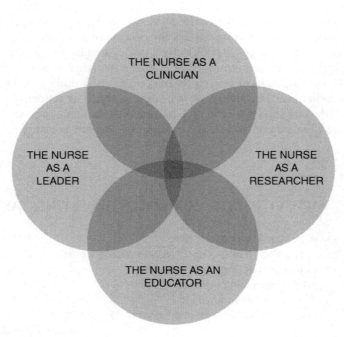

**Figure 16.7**   The nurse's role

Through the reading of this book, you will have been introduced to the many potential roles and pathways of your future nursing career. You will also have had exposure to the vast array of options open to you from your own experiences in your practice placements, and through the theoretical context of your nursing degree programme.

Figure 16.7 depicts the overlapping spheres of the four key aspects of the registered nurse's role. As you can see, none are in isolation and there is overlap between the varying aspects of the role.

## ACTIVITY 16.5

Consider your reading from the book so far and also your experiences from your degree programme, and apply this to the four key aspects of the nurse's role identified as:

1. Clinician;
2. Educator;
3. Researcher;
4. Leader.

Identify examples of nurses whom you have met through your experience and reading, and how they fit within the different aspects of the role identified above.
   Think about which aspects are of interest to you?

## Continuing your professional development

Nursing requires lifelong commitment to personal learning and development to ensure that the best patient care is provided. As a registered nurse, you will develop skills and experience new professional responsibilities, developing relationships and becoming part of a team. There will be opportunity to access a range of continuing professional development opportunities:

- Organisational education and training;
- Education relating to your specific role;
- Individual postgraduate study at university.

This can further enhance and extend your clinical and leadership skills to maintain and develop the delivery of high-quality care across a range of settings. You should be guided by your continuing professional development needs through your annual performance development review, the process of revalidation and the identification of areas of specific interest for you as a nurse.

# Supporting and supervising others in practice

As a qualified nurse and a registrant you will be involved and engaged in the process of supporting learners in practice. *The Code* (NMC, 2018b) stipulates the professional responsibility of nurses to engage in the education and support of learners and colleagues. As a nurse, you should support students' and colleagues' learning to help them develop their professional competence and confidence. You will know from your current experiences as a student that engagement with learners provides an excellent opportunity to share knowledge; engagement in the process of supporting learners as a registered nurse will serve to support your own continuing professional development.

You may find, as you move through your own degree programme, that you become engaged in the support of learners in your practice experiences; these may be students who are new to the area, who have not had a similar experience and who may be at an earlier point in their own degree programme. You may also meet learners from other professions whom you can support in your role.

Peer support is incredibly valuable in your learning and can allow the opportunity to share knowledge and experiences from your learning in both practice and theory. It could be argued that the utilisation of peer support lends itself well to the concept of coaching; that being so, it promotes problem solving and learning through experience. In some situations, clinical supervision can be peer led, and can allow registered nurses and teams to work through and learn from challenging situations in practice.

Coaching is defined as 'unlocking a person's potential to maximise their own performance' (Whitmore, 2009: 10). Rather than teaching, showing and telling; the coach supports the learner to identify their learning needs and to achieve those through empowerment and with the use of a nurturing approach. This approach to supporting learners not only serves to enhance and develop the autonomous practitioner, but also lends itself to the development of self-esteem and self-belief.

- Have you ever been coached?
- If so in what context were you coached? Was this during your nurse education, in a sport activity, at school?
- What skills do you think you need to have to be an effective coach?

There are a range of ways in which you can engage in the support and development of students in the placement area, which have been clearly identified by the NMC (2018c). They clearly identify two practice-based roles in the support and assessment of student nurses in the practice setting. As a registered nurse, you will engage in the support and supervision of students as a practice supervisor, and may undertake the role of practice assessor as you progress in your career and after suitable preparation for the role (Box 16.3). It is important to remember that students are valuable team members, working and learning alongside the team. There is also significant opportunity to learn from students who bring with them a developing knowledge and understanding. Through reciprocity in the relationship between student and supervisor and assessor, there is great value in acknowledging that we can all learn from each other.

---

### BOX 16.3   ROLES OF PRACTICE SUPERVISOR AND ASSESSOR

**Practice supervisor**

- A role model
- Supporting learning
- Working within own scope of practice
- Current knowledge and experience
- Contributing to assessment via feedback to assessor and recording experience of observing student in practice

**Practice assessor**

- Assessing achievement and providing feedback
- Working in partnership with the academic assessor and practice supervisors
- Gathering and coordinating feedback from the wider team
- Understanding the students' learning needs and outcomes
- Current knowledge and experience
- Undertaking preparation or evidence of prior experience that would facilitate the role.

NMC (2018c)

---

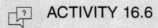 ACTIVITY 16.6

Visit NMC (2018c) and read *Part 2: Standards for Student Supervision and Assessment*
  How could you develop an effective practice learning environment for students?
  Consider how you could be involved in the supervision of students in practice as a newly qualified nurse.
  What requirements would you need in the future to become an assessor?

---

## Major incident response: your responsibilities as a registrant

A major incident is defined by the Joint Emergency Service Interoperability Programme (JESIP) as 'beyond the scope of business-as-usual operations, and is likely to involve serious harm, damage, disruption or risk to human life or welfare, essential services, the environment or national security' (JESIP, 2016). It is widely accepted that major incidents such as terrorist attacks, natural disasters, traumatic events or industrial accidents with multiple casualties cannot be managed within routine service arrangements. Most organisations have contingency plans in place so that they can respond appropriately in the event of a major incident. As a registered nurse you have a professional responsibility to be aware of such plans and the expectations placed upon you in the overall response to a major incident (NMC, 2018a). However, it is important to remember that, even in such situations, you must act only within the limits of your knowledge and competence (NMC, 2018b) and always follow the local major incident policies. If an incident happens away from your normal place of work, you are advised to follow current NMC guidance (NMC, 2017). In addition, witnessing or being involved in a major incident can be a highly traumatic experience. Talking about your experiences within a supportive environment is one of the strongest predictors of recovery after psychological trauma (Brewin et al., 2000) and the NMC (2017) advocate seeking support and help from your employer or GP if needed.

## ACTIVITY 16.7

Access and read the major incident policy or plan for your employer organisation. How well prepared are you? How might you be called upon to contribute to a major incident response? Find out what support services might be available for staff affected.

## Chapter summary

The transition from student nurse to registered nurse is supported through the process of preceptorship. It is acknowledged that this period of transition can be a period of challenge and uncertainty, but, with the support of peers and the wider team, the period of transition can be facilitated in a nurturing and safe environment. It is important that newly qualified nurses continue to engage in personal development, through the process of preceptorship and moving into revalidation. It is also important to engage in reflective activities and you will encounter a range of ways to facilitate this. As a registered nurse, you will also be expected to support and eventually assess learners in the practice environment; you are best placed to consider your own experiences as a student nurse and the influence of this on your own enactment of this aspect of your role. As a student nurse approaching the end of your degree programme, you are encouraged to consider the many options available to you, but importantly acknowledging your own self-care and supporting those around you in what is a challenging but incredibly rewarding career. As you begin your journey as a registered nurse, you will have a wide range of career options available to you and your career journey will be unique to you, taking on board the four aspects of the role of the nurse within this.

## Further reading

Bolton, G. and Delderfield, R. (2018) *Reflective Practice: Writing and Professional Development*, 5th edn. London: Sage.

Boychuck Duchscher, J.E. (2008) 'Transition shock: the initial stage of role adaptation for newly graduated registered nurses', *Journal of Advanced Nursing*, 65(5): 1103–13.

Clark, T. and Holmes, S. (2007) 'Fit for practice? An exploration of the development of newly qualified nurses using focus groups', *International Journal of Nursing Studies*, 44: 1210–20.

Mooney, M. (2006) 'Facing registration: the expectations and the unexpected', *Nurse Education Today*, 27: 840–7.

Royal College of Nursing (2016) *Students: Thinking about Your Career*. London: RCN.

Royal College of Nursing (2017) *Working Internationally. A Guide to Humanitarian and Development Work for Nurses and Midwives*. London: RCN.

# References

Benner, P. (1984) *From Novice to Expert: Excellence and Power in Clinical Nursing Practice*. Melno Park, CA: Addison-Wesley.

Bifarin, O. and Stonehouse, D. (2017) 'Clinical supervision: an important part of every nurse's practice', *British Journal of Nursing*, 26(6): 331–5.

Bolton, G.E.J. and Delderfield, R. (2018) *Reflective Practice: Writing and Professional Development*, 5th edn. London: Sage.

Brewin, C.R., Andrew, B. and Valentine, J.D. (2000) 'Meta-analysis of risk factors for posttraumatic stress disorder in trauma-exposed adults', *Journal of Consulting Clinical Psychologists*, 68(5): 748–66.

Bright, J., Earl, J. and Winter, D. (2014) *Brilliant Graduate CV: How to Get Your First CV to the Top of the Pile*. Harlow: Pearson Education.

Care Quality Commission (2013) *Supporting Information and Guidance: Supporting Effective Clinical Supervision* [online]. Available at: www.cqc.org.uk/sites/default/files/documents/20130625_800734_v1_00_supporting_information-effective_clinical_supervision_for_publication.pdf (last accessed 20 May 2018).

Department of Health (2009) *Preceptorship Framework for Nursing*. Available at: webarchive.nationalarchives.gov.uk/+/www.dh.gov.uk/prod_consum_dh/groups/dh_digitalassets/@dh/@en/@abous/documents/digitalasset/dh_109794.pdf (last accessed 19 April 2018).

Department of Health (2010) *Preceptorship Framework for Newly Registered Nurses, Midwives and Allied Health Professionals*. Available at: https://matrix.rcn.org.uk/__data/assets/pdf_file/0010/307756/Preceptorship_framework.pdf (last accessed 20 January 2018).

Gibbs, G. (1988) *Learning by Doing, A Guide to Teaching and Learning Methods*. Oxford: Further Education Unit, Oxford Brookes University.

Goodrich, J. (2012) 'Supporting hospital staff to provide compassionate care: do Schwartz rounds work in English hospitals?', *Journal of the Royal Society of Medicine*, 105: 117–22.

Jackson, D., Firtko, A. and Edenborough, M. (2007) 'Personal resilience as a strategy for surviving and thriving in the face of workplace adversity: a literature review', *Journal of Advanced Nursing*, 60(1): 1–9.

Joint Emergency Service Interoperability Programme (JESIP) (2016) *Definitions of Terms Used: Glossary*. Available at: www.jesip.org.uk/ (last accessed 8 May 2018).

Martin, J.S., Ummenhofer, W., Manser, T. and Spirig, R. (2010) 'Interprofessional collaboration among nurses and physicians: making a difference in patient outcome', *Swiss Medical Weekly*, 140: w13062. https://doi.org/10.4414/smw.2010.13062.

McGowan, J.E. and Murray, K. (2016) 'Exploring resilience in nursing and midwifery students: a literature review', *Journal of Advanced Nursing*, 72(10): 2253–68.

NHS England (2014) *Five Year Forward View* [online]. Available at: www.england.nhs.uk/wp-content/uploads/2014/10/5yfv-web.pdf (last accessed 1 January 2018).

Nursing and Midwifery Council (2006) *Preceptorship Guidelines*. NMC Circular 21/2006, published 4 October 2006. Available at: www.nmc.org.uk/globalassets/sitedocuments/circulars/2006circulars/nmc-circular-21_2006.pdf (last accessed 19 April 2018).

Nursing and Midwifery Council (2016) *Revalidation.* Available at: http://revalidation.nmc.org.uk/welcome-to-revalidation (last accessed January 2018).

Nursing and Midwifery Council (2017) *Information for Nurses and Midwives on Responding to Unexpected Incidents or Emergencies.* Available at: www.nmc.org.uk/news/news-and-updates/information-for-nurses-and-midwives-on-responding-to-unexpected-incidents-or-emergencies (last accessed 18 April 2018).

Nursing and Midwifery Council (2018a) *Future Nurse: Standards of Proficiency for Registered Nurses.* London: NMC. Available at: www.nmc.org.uk/globalassets/sitedocuments/education-standards/future-nurse-proficiencies.pdf (last accessed 18 May 2018).

Nursing and Midwifery Council (2018b) *The Code: Professional Standards for Practice and Behaviour for Nurses and Midwives.* London: NMC. Available at: www.nmc.org.uk/globalassets/sitedocuments/nmc-publications/nmc-code.pdf (last accessed 18 April 2018).

Nursing and Midwifery Council (2018c) *Realising Professionalism: Standards for Education and Training. Part 2: Standards for Student Supervision and Assessment.* Available at: www.nmc.org.uk/globalassets/sitedocuments/education-standards/student-supervision-assessment.pdf (last accessed 18 May 2108).

Point of Care Foundation (2015) *Staff Care: How to Engage Staff in the NHS and Why it Matters.* Available at: https://s16682.pcdn.co/wp-content/uploads/2014/01/POCF_FINAL-inc-references.pdf. (last accessed 22 April 2018).

Royal College of Nursing (2018) *Rest, Rehydrate, Refuel.* London: RCN.

Whitmore, J. (2009) *Coaching for Performance: GROWing People, Performance and Purpose*, 4th edn. London: Nicholas Breale.

# INDEX